Cardio-Nephrology

Janani Rangaswami · Edgar V. Lerma
Claudio Ronco
Editors

Cardio-Nephrology

Confluence of the Heart and Kidney in Clinical Practice

Springer

Editors
Janani Rangaswami
Department of Internal Medicine, Einstein Medical Center
Sidney Kimmel College of Thomas Jefferson University
Philadelphia, PA
USA

Claudio Ronco
Department of Nephrology Dialysis and Transplantation
International Renal Research Institute, San Bortolo Hospital
Vicenza
Italy

Edgar V. Lerma
Department of Medicine, Section of Nephrology
University of Illinois at Chicago
Chicago, IL
USA

ISBN 978-3-319-56040-3 ISBN 978-3-319-56042-7 (eBook)
DOI 10.1007/978-3-319-56042-7

Library of Congress Control Number: 2017938627

Printed on acid-free paper

This Springer imprint is published by Springer Nature
The registered company is Springer International Publishing AG
The registered company address is: Gewerbestrasse 11, 6330 Cham, Switzerland

I would like to thank Appa and Amma for their innumerable sacrifices and love that have allowed me to be the physician I am today. Without them, none of the contributions I have directly or indirectly made to my profession or patients would be possible. I thank my teachers and mentors for emphasizing to me that asking the right questions in clinical practice and academic medicine are the only way to achieve meaningful outcomes. The monumental task of editing this textbook would not be possible without the support and understanding of my husband Ram, and the patience and love of little Aniruddh who gives me new strength everyday. My co-editors Profs. Ronco and Lerma have been an inspiration to work alongside this project, and I value their guidance and support immensely. Most importantly, I thank my patients who are open textbooks of medicine in everyday life, from whom I continue to learn each day.

Janani Rangaswami

To all my mentors, and friends, at the University of Santo Tomas College of Science, University of Santo Tomas Faculty of Medicine and Surgery in Manila, Philippines, and Northwestern University Feinberg School of Medicine in Chicago, IL, who have in one way or another, influenced and guided me to become the physician that I am ...

To all the medical students, interns, and residents at Advocate Christ Medical Center whom I have taught or learned from, especially those who eventually decided to pursue Nephrology as a career...

To my parents and my brothers, without whose unwavering love and support through the good and bad times, I would not have persevered and reached my goals in life ...

Most especially, to my two lovely and precious daughters Anastasia Zofia and Isabella Ann, whose smiles and laughter constantly provide me unparalleled joy and happiness; and my very loving and understanding wife Michelle, who has always been supportive of my endeavors both personally and professionally, and who sacrificed a lot of time and exhibited unwavering patience as I devoted a significant amount of time and effort to this project. Truly, they provide me with motivation and inspiration.

Edgar V. Lerma

To Federico, my son and my preferred cardiologist

Claudio Ronco

Foreword

It is becoming ever more apparent with the aging of adult populations and the increasing overlay of illnesses such as diabetes, hypertension, atherosclerosis, heart failure, and chronic kidney disease that the heart and the kidneys are at the center of most case discussions involving critically ill patients. The heart and the kidneys have vital, lifelong relationships in both health and disease. In this edition of *Cardio-Nephrology*, Drs. Ronco, Lerma, and Rangaswami have assembled the world's most preeminent experts on the full spectrum of topics that cover cardiorenal interactions. Importantly, the epidemiology, pathophysiology, prognosis, and implications for management are woven into a comprehensive and tractable text that will be essential for students, residents, and attending physicians as they further their knowledge and expertise in this complicated area of medicine. The reader is encouraged to find the time to unpack the key conceptual frameworks upon which to build understanding, conduct future investigation, and translate progress to the bedside. Greater interest in this field with a lead to an ever-increasing critical mass of intellectual effort that will bring great advances to patients and their families impacted by cardiorenal syndromes. On behalf of all the beneficiaries of this work, I offer my thanks to the venerable and iconic leaders in this field—Claudio Ronco, MD, Edgar Lerma, MD, and Janani Rangaswami, MD, for the conception and creation of this wonderful text for libraries and offices across the globe.

Peter A. McCullough, MD, MPH, FACC, FACP, FCCP, FAHA, FNKF, FNLA
Baylor University Medical Center, Baylor Heart
and Vascular Institute, Baylor Jack and Jane Hamilton Heart
and Vascular Hospital, Dallas, TX, USA
The Heart Hospital Baylor Plano, Plano, TX, USA

Preface

The increasing prevalence of vascular risk factors such as diabetes, obesity, and hypertension coupled with increased longevity has resulted in a worldwide epidemic of cardiovascular and kidney disease. Never has the implication of one organ system on the other been so profound, as in the current context of the cardio-nephrology symbiosis: complex interventional strategies for vascular disease, identification of novel biomarkers of renal and cardiac injury, the ever-increasing transplantation potential of patients with complex cardiac and renal disease, and the mutually significant prognostic implications between these organ systems. Despite the expanded understanding of the nuances of both these organ systems, there still remains a "vacuum" in the interface between cardiology and nephrology in key overlap areas. Ironically, these decisions involve day to day management in patients with complex disease burden involving both systems.

This textbook brings together a diverse group of extraordinary clinicians and scientists in cardiology, nephrology, hypertension, and lipidology and summarizes their collective experience and contributions in this field. The scope of this textbook extends from the outpatient management of cardiovascular and kidney disease, to hospital-based decision-making in patients with cardio-renal disease and complex interfaces such as hemodialysis in patients with ventricular assist device support. This book is intended to serve as a "one stop shop" for cardiology and nephrology clinicians and researchers dealing with the significant overlap areas between these two specialties. It should also be relevant to medical students, trainee physicians, and general internists. More importantly, the emphasis on the confluence of these specialties should translate into increased cardio-nephrology clinical and research cross-communication, which is the ultimate goal of such an endeavor.

We wish to acknowledge the invaluable contributions of each author and group that has contributed their time and writing effort to embellish this textbook. Springer International has supported the concept of cardio-nephrology immensely by bringing out this textbook, and we thank their leadership, specifically Gregory Sutorius, for all their support through this process. This textbook would not be possible without the diligence and hard work of the developmental editorial team headed by Sarah Simeziane and Barbara Lopez-Lucio, and we appreciate all their efforts in giving this textbook its current form. We truly hope this textbook will foster increased awareness, interest, and applicability of key concepts in cardio-nephrology to patient care in everyday practice.

The editors would like to acknowledge the following for their specialty editorial input in cardiology, for select sections of this textbook:

- Igor Palacios, MD (Massachusetts General Hospital)
- Christian Witzke, MD (Einstein Medical Center)

Philadelphia, USA — Janani Rangaswami, MD
Chicago, USA — Edgar V. Lerma, MD
Vicenza, Italy — Claudio Ronco, MD

Contents

Part I Cardiovascular Disease Spectrum in Chronic Kidney Disease

1 **Endothelial Dysfunction and Nitric Oxide: Albuminuria as a Central Marker** 3
Jolanta Malyszko, Hanna Bachorzewska-Gajewska, and Jacek Malyszko

2 **Vascular and Valvular Calcification in Chronic Kidney Disease: Pathogenesis and Clinical Outcomes** 11
Hope Caughron, Jose F. Condado, and Vasilis Babaliaros

3 **Sudden Cardiac Death in CKD and ESKD: Risk Factors, Mechanisms, and Therapeutic Strategies** 21
Darren Green, Diana Y.Y. Chiu, and Philip A. Kalra

4 **Coronary Artery Disease in CKD: Traditional and Nontraditional Risk Factors, Diagnosis and Management** 35
Christian Witzke, Igor Palacios, and Andre Macedo Dias

5 **CKD Associated Cardiomyopathy: Molecular Mechanisms, Imaging Modalities, Disease Evolution and Interventions** 45
Nicola C. Edwards, Manvir Kaur Hayer, Charles J. Ferro, Jonathan N. Townend, and Richard P. Steeds

Part II Chronic Kidney Disease and CAD: Two Sides of the Same Coin

6 **CKD as CAD Equivalent: Inflammatory Milieu and Vascular Oxidative Stress** 61
Shien Wen Sheryl Gan and Christopher T. Chan

7 **Phosphorus and Mortality: Do We Have the Panacea?** 71
Tatsuo Shimosawa and Rika Jimbo

8 **Inhibition of the Renin–Angiotensin System: How Far Have We Come?** . . . 77
Jay Ian Lakkis and Matthew R. Weir

9 **Vitamin D and Its Role in CKD and CAD: A Novel Therapeutic Target** . . . 97
Kenneth Lim, Thomas F Hiemstra, and Ravi Thadhani

10 **Association of Catalytic (Labile) Iron with Cardiovascular Morbidity and Mortality** 109
Mohan Rajapurkar, Suhas S. Lele, Nasim Khan, and Sudhir V. Shah

11 **Erythropoietin and Its Cardiovascular Effects** 119
Nupur Gupta and Jay B. Wish

Part III Cardio-Renal Syndrome

12 **Pathophysiology of the Cardiorenal Syndromes Types 1–5: Updates from the Eleventh Consensus Conference of the Acute Dialysis Quality Initiative (ADQI)** 131
Luca Di Lullo, Antonio Bellasi, and Mario Cozzolino

13 **Hemodynamic Cross-Talk in Cardiorenal Syndrome: Era of Biomarkers** . . . 145
Faeq Husain-Syed, Salvador Lopez-Giacoman, and Horst-Walter Birk

14 **Kidney Attack: Is NGAL Set to Take the Stage with Troponins?** 155
Prasad Devarajan

15 **Ultrafiltration Therapy in Decompensated Heart Failure** 163
Dan Negoianu

16 **Bioimpedance Vectorial Analyses in Cardiorenal Syndrome** 171
Nadia Aspromonte, Francesco Monitillo, Roberto Valle, and Massimo Iacoviello

17 **Novel Therapies for Acute Decompensated Heart Failure** 177
Bryan A. Smith and John E.A. Blair

18 **Kidney Injury in Patients with Ventricular Assist Devices** 191
Ami M. Patel, Karan Kapoor, and Michael R. Rudnick

19 **Palliation with Dual Burden of Heart and Kidney Failure: An Underutilized Strategy** 205
Robin Turner and Hesham Shaban

Part IV Cardiac Evaluation of the Renal Transplant Candidate

20 **Screening Strategies for Coronary Artery Disease (CAD) in Candidates for Kidney Transplants** 219
Guilherme Vianna Silva, John D. Allison, and Francisco Yuri Bulcao Macedo

21 **Cardiac Pre-operative Evaluation as an Opportunity to Optimize Risk Factors in Kidney Transplant Candidates** 229
Amer Kasim Ardati

22 **Revascularization in Patients on the Renal Transplant List: When and What Is Appropriate?** 235
Pablo Rengifo-Moreno, Alexandre C. Ferreira, and Eduardo de Marchena

23 **Pulmonary Hypertension in the Potential Kidney Transplant Recipient** 243
Sourin Banerji and Anjali Vaidya

24 **Cardiac Surveillance Whilst Listed for Renal Transplantation** 251
Karen L. Keung, Madhav C. Menon, and Barbara Murphy

25 Post-Kidney Transplant Modification of Cardiovascular Risk 259
Mythili Ghanta, Swati Rao, Iris Lee, and Serban Constantinescu

26 Cardiomyopathy in the Potential Kidney Transplant Candidate 271
Burhan Mohamedali

Part V Anticoagulation and Antiplatelet Therapy in CKD

27 Anticoagulation in Patients with Atrial Fibrillation and Chronic Kidney Disease 283
Michelle D. Carlson and Gautam R. Shroff

28 Anticoagulation-Related Nephropathy: Tip of the Iceberg 295
David S. Wheeler

29 Impact of Antiplatelet Therapy and Platelet Reactivity Testing on Cardiovascular Outcomes in Patients with Chronic Kidney Disease 301
Sandeep Nathan and Brian Conway

Part VI Interventional Strategies in Cardiovascular Disease in CKD

30 Revascularization Strategies in Chronic Kidney Disease: Percutaneous Coronary Intervention Versus Coronary Artery Bypass Graft Surgery 317
Amit V. Patel and Sripal Bangalore

31 Revascularization Strategies in CKD: Antiplatelet Therapy, Stent Type, Timing, and Complications of PCI 329
Marwan Y. Qattan and Somjot S. Brar

32 Peripheral Arterial Disease in CKD: Disease Burden, Outcomes and Interventional Strategies 337
Bhalaghuru Chokkalingam Mani and Nicholas J. Ruggiero II

33 Contrast Induced Nephropathy 347
Jatinder Kohli, Akash N. Sethi, and Michael R. Rudnick

34 Acute Kidney Injury After Cardiac Surgery 355
Andrea Perrotti, Benoit Barrucand, and Sidney Chocron

Part VII The Cardiorenometabolic Spectrum

35 Dyslipidemias in CKD and ESKD: Outcomes and Management 369
David Carruthers and Anand Rohatgi

36 The Cardiac Impact of Atherosclerotic Renovascular Disease (ARVD) 377
Diana Vassallo, Darren Green, and Philip A. Kalra

37 Preeclampsia: A Mirror into Future Cardiovascular and Renal Health 385
Scott Blumhof and Janani Rangaswami

38 Obstructive Sleep Apnea: A Unifying Link Between Cardiovascular and Renal Disease 395
Parasuram Melarcode Krishnamoorthy, Virend K. Somers, and Abel Romero-Corral

Part VIII Dilemmas in Hypertension

39 Chronic Kidney Disease and BP Goals 403
Debbie L. Cohen and Raymond R. Townsend

40 Renal Artery Stenosis: Diagnosis and Management 411
Harold M. Szerlip and Bhupinder Singh

41 Renal Denervation: Current Opinions and Practice 419
Markus P. Schlaich

Index 427

Contributors

John D. Allison Department of Medicine - Cardiology, Baylor College of Medicine, Houston, TX, USA

Amer Kasim Ardati Department of Medicine, Jesse Brown Veterans Affairs Medical Center, University of Illinois- Chicago, Chicago, IL, USA

Nadia Aspromonte Division of Cardiology, San Filippo Neri Hospital, Rome, Italy

Vasilis Babaliaros Department of Cardiology, Emory University Hospital F606, Atlanta, GA, USA

Hanna Bachorzewska-Gajewska Department of Invasive Cardiology, Medical University, Białystok, Poland

Sourin Banerji Division of Cardiology, Department of Medicine, Christiana Care Medical Center, Newark, DE, USA

Sripal Bangalore Department of Medicine, Division of Cardiology, New York University School of Medicine, New York, NY, USA

Benoit Barrucand Department of Anesthesiology and Surgical Critical Care Medicine, University Hospital Jean Minjoz, Besançon, France

Antonio Bellasi Nephrology and Dialysis, S. Anna Hospital, Cantù, Como, Italy

Horst-Walter Birk Division of Nephrology, Pulmonology and Critical Care Medicine, Department of Internal Medicine II, University Clinic Giessen and Marburg (UKGM) – Campus Giessen, Giessen, Hessen, Germany

John E.A. Blair Department of Medicine, Section of Cardiology, University of Chicago Pritzker School of Medicine, Chicago, IL, USA

Scott Blumhof Department of Pulmonary, Allergy, and Critical Care Medicine, UAB, Birmingham, AL, USA

Somjot S. Brar Department of Cardiology and Regional Cardiac Cath Lab, Kaiser Permanente, Los Angeles Medical Center, Los Angeles, CA, USA

Michelle D. Carlson Cardiology Division, Hennepin County Medical Center, Minneapolis, MN, USA

David Carruthers Department of Cardiology, University of Texas Southwestern, Dallas, TX, USA

Hope Caughron Structural Heart and Valve Center, Emory University Hospital F606, Atlanta, GA, USA

Christopher T. Chan University Health Network, University of Toronto, Toronto, ON, Canada

Diana Y. Y. Chiu Department of Renal Medicine, Salford Royal NHS Foundation Trust, Salford, UK

Sidney Chocron Department of Thoracic and Cardio-Vascular Surgery, University Hospital Jean Minjoz, EA3920, University of Franche-Comté, Besançon, France

Debbie L. Cohen Renal Division, Perelman School of Medicine at The University of Pennsylvania, Philadelphia, PA, USA

Jose F. Condado Cardiovascular Disease Fellowship Program, Emory University School of Medicine, Emory University, Atlanta, GA, USA

Serban Constantinescu Department of Medicine, Section of Nephrology, Hypertension and Kidney Transplantation, Lewis Katz School of Medicine, Temple University, Philadelphia, PA, USA

Brian Conway Department of Medicine/Section of Cardiology, University of Chicago Medicine, Chicago, IL, USA

Mario Cozzolino Department of Health Sciences, Hospital of San Paolo, University of Milan, Milan, Italy

Prasad Devarajan Department of Nephrology and Hypertension, Cincinnati Children's Hospital Medical Center, University of Cincinnati School of Medicine, Cincinnati, OH, USA

Luca Di Lullo Department of Nephrology and Dialysis, L. Parodi-Delfino Hospital, Colleferro, Rome, Italy

Andre Macedo Dias Einstein Medical Center, Philadelphia, PA, USA

Eduardo de Marchena University of Miami Hospital, Miami, USA

Nicola C. Edwards Department of Cardiology, Queen Elizabeth Hospital Birmingham, Birmingham, UK

Alexandre C. Ferreira Jackson Memorial Hospital, Miami, USA

Charles J. Ferro Department of Nephrology, Queen Elizabeth Hospital Birmingham, Birmingham, UK

Shien Wen Sheryl Gan Department of Renal Medicine, Singapore General Hospital, Singapore, Singapore

Mythili Ghanta Department of Internal Medicine, UT Southwestern Medical Center, Dallas, TX, USA

Darren Green Department of Renal Medicine, Salford Royal NHS Foundation Trust, Salford, UK

Nupur Gupta Division of Nephrology, Indiana University School of Medicine, Indianapolis, IN, USA

Manvir Kaur Hayer Department of Nephrology, Queen Elizabeth Hospital Birmingham, Birmingham, UK

Thomas F. Hiemstra Cambridge Clinical Trials Unit, University of Cambridge, Cambridge, UK

Faeq Husain-Syed Division of Nephrology, Pulmonology and Critical Care Medicine, Department of Internal Medicine II, University Clinic Giessen and Marburg (UKGM) – Campus Giessen, Giessen, Hessen, Germany

Massimo Iacoviello Cardiothoracic Department, Policlinic Hospital of Bari, Bari, Italy

Rika Jimbo Department of Internal Medicine, Tohto Bunkyo Hospital, Bunkyo-ku, Tokyo, Japan

Philip A. Kalra Department of Renal Medicine, Salford Royal NHS Foundation Trust, Salford, UK

Karan Kapoor Department of Internal Medicine, University of Maryland Medical Center, Baltimore, MD, USA

Karen L. Keung Centre for Transplant and Renal Research, The Westmead Institute for Medical Research, University of Sydney at Westmead Hospital, Sydney, NSW, Australia

Nasim Khan Department of Internal Medicine Division of Nephrology, University of Arkansas for Medical Sciences and Central Arkansas Veterans Healthcare System, Little Rock, AR, USA

Jatinder Kohli Renal, Electrolyte and Hypertension Division, Department of Medicine, Hospital of University of Pennsylvania, Philadelphia, PA, USA

Parasuram Melarcode Krishnamoorthy Department of Cardiology, Einstein Medical Center, Philadelphia, PA, USA

Jay Ian Lakkis Department of Medicine, John A. Burns School of Medicine, University of Hawaii at Manoa, Maui Memorial Medical Center, Kahului, HI, USA

Iris Lee Department of Medicine, Section of Nephrology, Hypertension and Kidney Transplantation, Lewis Katz School of Medicine, Temple University, Philadelphia, PA, USA

Suhas S. Lele Department of Internal Medicine Division of Nephrology, University of Arkansas for Medical Sciences and Central Arkansas Veterans Healthcare System, Little Rock, AR, USA

Kenneth Lim Massachusetts General Hospital, Harvard Medical School, Boston, MA, USA

Salvador Lopez-Giacoman Hospital General Issste Zacatecas, Zacatecas, Zacatecas, Mexico

Francisco Yuri Bulcao Macedo Department of Medicine - Cardiology, Baylor College of Medicine, Houston, TX, USA

Jacek Malyszko First Department of Nephrology, Medical University, Białystok, Poland

Jolanta Malyszko Second Department of Nephrology, Medical University, Białystok, Poland

Bhalaghuru Chokkalingam Mani Jefferson Heart and Vascular Institute, Thomas Jefferson University Hospital, Sidney Kimmel College of Medicine, Philadelphia, PA, USA

Madhav C. Menon Division of Nephrology and Recanati-Miller Transplantation Institute, Mount Sinai Hospital, New York, NY, USA

Burhan Mohamedali Department of Internal Medicine, Rush University Medical Center, Chicago, IL, USA

Francesco Monitillo Cardiology Unit, Veris Delli Ponti Hospital, Scorrano, LE, Italy

Barbara Murphy Icahn School of Medicine, Mount Sinai, New York, NY, USA

Sandeep Nathan Department of Medicine/Section of Cardiology, University of Chicago Medicine, Chicago, IL, USA

Dan Negoianu Renal Electrolyte and Hypertension Division, Hospital of the University of Pennsylvania, Philadelphia, PA, USA

Igor Palacios Massachusetts General Hospital, Boston, MA, USA

Ami M. Patel Division of Nephrology, Department of Medicine, University of Maryland Medical Center, Baltimore, MD, USA

Amit V. Patel Department of Medicine, Division of Cardiology, NYU Langone Medical Center, New York, NY, USA

Andrea Perrotti Department of Thoracic and Cardio-Vascular Surgery, University Hospital Jean Minjoz, EA3920, University of Franche-Comté, Besançon, France

Marwan Y. Qattan Department of Cardiology, Kaiser Permanente, Los Angeles Medical Center, Los Angeles, CA, USA

Mohan Rajapurkar Department of Internal Medicine Division of Nephrology, University of Arkansas for Medical Sciences and Central Arkansas Veterans Healthcare System, Little Rock, AR, USA; Department of Nephrology, Muljibhai Patel Urological Hospital, Nadiad, Gujarat, India

Swati Rao Department of Medicine, Section of Nephrology, Hypertension and Kidney Transplantation, Lewis Katz School of Medicine, Temple University, Philadelphia, PA, USA

Janani Rangaswami Department of Medicine, Einstein Medical Center, Philadelphia, PA, USA; Sidney Kimmel College, Thomas Jefferson University, Philadelphia, PA, USA

Pablo Rengifo-Moreno Department of Medicine Phoebe Memorial Hospital, Medical College of Georgia, Augusta University, Albany, GA, USA

Anand Rohatgi Department of Cardiology, University of Texas Southwestern, Dallas, TX, USA

Abel Romero-Corral Department of Cardiology, Einstein Medical Center, Philadelphia, PA, USA

Michael R. Rudnick Department of Medicine, Penn Presbyterian Medical Center, Perelman School of Medicine of the University of Pennsylvania, Philadelphia, PA, USA

Nicholas J. Ruggiero II Jefferson Angioplasty Center, Thomas Jefferson University Hospital, Philadelphia, PA, USA

Markus P. Schlaich Dobney Hypertension Centre, School of Medicine and Pharmacology – Royal Hospital Unit, University of Western Australia, Perth, WA, Australia

Akash N. Sethi Renal, Electrolytes and Hypertension, Hospital of University of Pennsylvania, Philadelphia, PA, USA

Hesham Shaban Palliative Care, Duke University Hospital, Durham, NC, USA

Sudhir V. Shah Department of Internal Medicine Division of Nephrology, University of Arkansas for Medical Sciences and Central Arkansas Veterans Healthcare System, Little Rock, AR, USA

Tatsuo Shimosawa Department of Clinical Laboratory, Faculty of Medicine, International University of Health and Welfare, Narita, Chiba, Japan; Department of Clinical Laboratory, Mita Hospital, IUHW, Minatoku, Tokyo, Japan

Gautam R. Shroff Cardiology Division, Hennepin County Medical Center, Minneapolis, MN, USA

Guilherme Vianna Silva Department of Medicine - Cardiology, Baylor College of Medicine, Houston, TX, USA

Bhupinder Singh Cardio Renal Society of America, Phoenix, AZ, USA

Bryan A. Smith Department of Medicine, Section of Cardiology, University of Chicago Pritzker School of Medicine, Chicago, IL, USA

Virend K. Somers Department of Cardiovascular Diseases, Mayo Clinic, Rochester, MN, USA

Richard P. Steeds Department of Cardiology, Queen Elizabeth Hospital Birmingham, Birmingham, UK

Harold M. Szerlip Department of Nephrology, Baylor University Medical Center, Dallas, TX, USA

Ravi Thadhani Massachusetts General Hospital, Harvard Medical School, Boston, MA, USA

Jonathan N. Townend Department of Cardiology, Queen Elizabeth Hospital Birmingham, Birmingham, UK

Raymond R. Townsend Renal Division, Perelman School of Medicine at The University of Pennsylvania, Philadelphia, PA, USA

Robin Turner Internal Medicine/Palliative Medicine, Duke University Health System, Durham, NC, USA

Anjali Vaidya Advanced Heart Failure and Cardiac Transplant, Division of Cardiology, Department of Medicine, Temple University Lewis Katz School of Medicine, Philadelphia, PA, USA

Roberto Valle Department of Cardiology, Ospedale Civile, Chioggia, VE, Italy

Diana Vassallo Department of Renal Medicine, Salford Royal NHS Foundation Trust, Salford, UK

Matthew R. Weir Division of Nephrology, Department of Medicine, University of Maryland School of Medicine, Baltimore, MD, USA

David S. Wheeler Department of Internal Medicine, Einstein Medical Center Philadelphia, Philadelphia, PA, USA

Jay B. Wish Division of Nephrology, Indiana University School of Medicine, Indianapolis, IN, USA

Christian Witzke Einstein Medical Center, Philadelphia, PA, USA

Part I

Cardiovascular Disease Spectrum in Chronic Kidney Disease

1 Endothelial Dysfunction and Nitric Oxide: Albuminuria as a Central Marker

Jolanta Malyszko, Hanna Bachorzewska-Gajewska, and Jacek Malyszko

Endothelial Function

Human endothelial cells were first propagated in culture in the early 1970s [1]. To date, there have been major subsequent advances in our understanding of endothelial cell (EC) biology based upon this critically important technology. However, it is still apparent that ECs tend to dedifferentiate and lose their specialized characteristics in culture. Endothelial cells (ECs) form the lining of all blood and lymphatic vessels within the vascular tree. In the last two decades, one of the major achievements in medicine has been defining the biology of vascular endothelium. The endothelium is not a simple, inert semipermeable structure, which merely served to line blood vessels. Strategically located between the wall of blood vessels and the blood stream, it forms an active organ with endocrine and paracrine functions. The human body contains approximately 10^{13} endothelial cells weighing approximately 1 kg, covering a surface area of 4000–7000 m^2 equivalent to a football playground. The endothelial cell monolayer forming the inner lining of all blood vessels within the vascular tree, covering glycocalyx, and underlying basement membrane constitutes the endothelium. Due to the complex nature of the endothelium, studies on its function transcend all existing organ-specific disciplines (Fig. 1.1). The endothelium first functions as a physical barrier, defining the components of the vessel wall and the contents of the vessel lumen. Second, this barrier affords movement of small solutes in preference to large molecules, therefore it is involved in regulating cellular and nutrient trafficking. The endothelium also mediates vasoactivity, maintains blood fluidity, and contributes to the local balance between pro- and anti-inflammatory mediators as well as pro- and anticoagulant activity (Fig. 1.1). Finally, the endothelium takes part in angiogenesis, and mediates adherence of platelets and leukocytes to the vessel wall during injury and inflammation. Each of these activities is differentially regulated both in location and time, a phenomenon that has been variably termed endothelial cell heterogeneity or vascular diversity. Phenotypic heterogeneity is a central feature of the endothelium, and includes variations in morphology, biosynthetic repertoire, and behavior. Specialized functions of the endothelium can be anatomically specific, i.e., in the glomeruli. In cardiovascular medicine, endothelial biology is critical in the pathophysiology of coronary artery disease (CAD) as well as fundamental to the mechanisms of thrombolysis.

Over 30 years ago, Furchgott and Zawadzki [1] found that acetylcholine requires the presence of endothelial cells to elicit vasodilatation. Since then, there have been enormous advances in our understanding of endothelial cell biology in different settings. It appears that vasodilation is largely a function of vasodilatory endothelium-derived nitric oxide (EDNO) and to a lesser extent, prostacyclin, C-type natriuretic peptide, and several endothelium-derived hyperpolarizing factors. Vasoconstriction is mediated by several peptides including thromboxane A_2, endothelins, and angiotensin II. Inflammatory modulators elaborated by the endothelium include adhesion molecules like ICAM-1 (intercellular adhesion molecule-1), VCAM-1 (vascular adhesion molecule-1), E-selectin, nitric oxide (NO) and nuclear factor κ[kappa]B (NF-κ[kappa]B) Plasminogen activator (t-PA), its inhibitor (PAI-1). Von Willebrand factor (vWF), prostacyclin, thromboxane A_2, tissue factor pathway inhibitor (TFPI), and fibrinogen are some of the factors through which the endothelium regulates hemostasis [2].

J. Malyszko (✉)
Second Department of Nephrology, Medical University, Sklodowskiej-Curie 24a, 15-276 Białystok, Poland
e-mail: jolmal@poczta.onet.pl

H. Bachorzewska-Gajewska
Department of Invasive Cardiology, Medical University, Sklodowskiej-Curie 24a, 15-276 Białystok, Poland
e-mail: hgajewska@op.pl

J. Malyszko
First Department of Nephrology, Medical University, Zurawia 14, 15-276 Białystok, Poland
e-mail: jackmaly@pczta.onet.pl

J. Rangaswami et al. (eds.), *Cardio-Nephrology*,
DOI 10.1007/978-3-319-56042-7_1

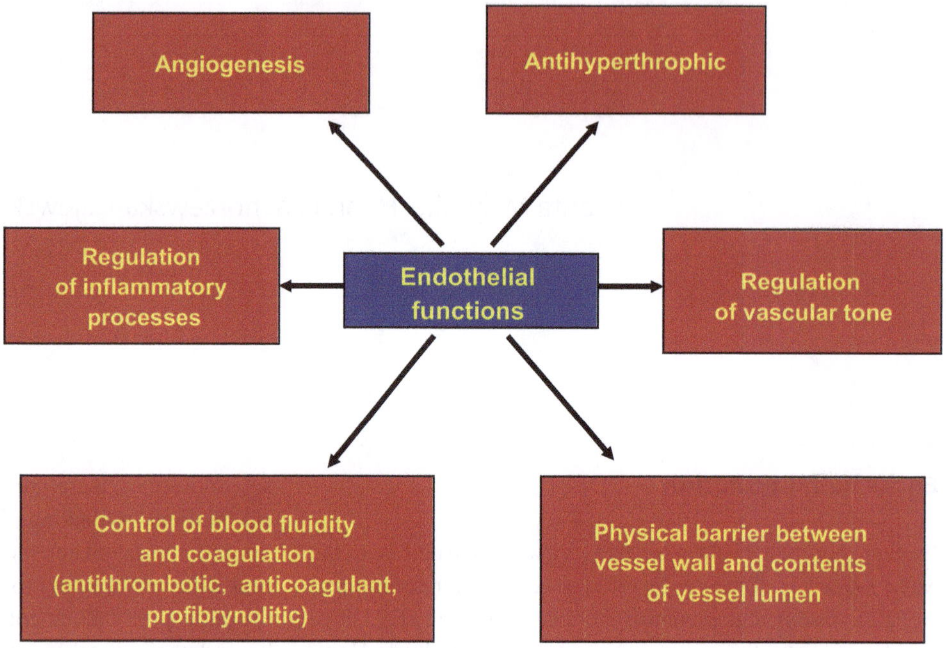

Fig. 1.1 Biological spectrum of endothelial function

The principal physiologic stimulus for endothelial nitric oxide (NO) synthesis is blood-flow-induced shear stress, a process termed "flow-mediated vasodilation". In the quiescent state, nitric oxide and prostacyclin directly inhibit platelet aggregation, and thrombomodulin inactivates thrombin. Nitric oxide also reduces endotoxin- and cytokine-induced expression of tissue factor, thus reducing the prothrombotic potential of the endothelial cell. While the endothelium maintains the vessel in a relatively dilated state in the basal conditions, it also possesses the capacity to respond to various physiological stimuli such as shear stress. In the response to the latter stimulus and other stressors, on one hand the endothelium becomes prothrombotic, secreting platelet-activating factor and expressing thromboplastin on cell membranes, but on the other hand, blood vessels dilate, in the process called flow-mediated dilation (FMD) [3]. In the clinical practice, assessment of FMD is a measure of endothelial function. However, despite its important role in a wide range of homeostatic processes and its potential as a therapeutic target, the assessment of endothelial function continues to be underutilized in clinical practice. This bench to bedside gap is mainly due to the fact that endothelial function is difficult to assess optimally due to several clinical confounders such as food, temperature, drugs, sympathetic stimuli and intra- and interobserver variance. In addition, endothelial dysfunction occurs in the absence of reliable circulating markers, while with concurrent target organ damage, endothelial dysfunction is generally associated with changes in either blood chemistry and/or imaging.

Endothelial Activation and Endothelial Dysfunction

"Endothelial cell activation" was described on the basis of increased leukocyte adhesion following exposure to inflammatory mediators in cultured endothelial cells (ECs). Later, a wider spectrum of phenotypic changes, including decreased thromboresistance, altered vasomotor tone, and loss of barrier function were demonstrated. According to this paradigm, quiescent ECs display a thromboresistant, anti-adhesive and vasodilatory phenotype, whereas activated ECs have procoagulant, pro-adhesive, and vasoconstricting properties. Activation of endothelial cells may occur both in pathological and in physiological conditions, and neither is an all-or-none response. Endothelial cell dysfunction was observed early in the course of structural vascular changes, particularly in atherosclerosis. Later, it was indicated that the intact endothelium might actively contribute to disease initiation and/or progression [4].

EC dysfunction referred to structural changes, loss of integrity, or hyper-adhesiveness of the vascular lining toward platelets, as might be seen in atherosclerosis. It was also initially defined also as an impaired vasodilation to specific stimuli such as acetylcholine or bradykinin. Paradoxical vasoconstriction of coronary arteries induced by acetylcholine was described in early and advanced human atherosclerosis, suggesting that an abnormal vascular response to acetylcholine may represent a defect in endothelium vasodilatory function, due to, at least in part, a reduced endothelial cell production of nitric oxide.

Besides shear stress, a variety of agonists such as acetylcholine, histamine, thrombin, serotonin, adenosine diphosphate (ADP), bradykinin, and norepinephrine could stimulate endothelial nitric oxide synthesis. These stimuli lead to vasorelaxation when the endothelium is intact, and vasoconstriction if the endothelium is injured or dysfunctional [5]. The endothelium responds to stress in ways that differ according to the nature of the pathogen in a case of sepsis/infection, host genetics (in the case of sepsis/inflammation), underlying comorbidity, age, gender, and the location of the vascular bed. These responses may include structural changes, such as nuclear vacuolization, cytoplasmic swelling, cytoplasmic fragmentation, denudation, and/or detachment. However, functional changes in the endothelium are even more common and include shifts in hemostatic balance, increased leukocyte adhesion and trafficking, altered vasomotor tone, loss of barrier function, and programmed cell death.

Inducible endothelial–leukocyte adhesion molecules in atherosclerosis (so-called athero-ELAMs) are identified by inducible endothelial cell-specific antigens that binds predominantly to monocytes. Human vascular cell adhesion molecule (VCAM)-1, previously cloned as a cytokine-inducible protein in endothelial cells, is one of the ELAMs. Moreover, other substances such as VCAM-1, ICAM-1, P-selectin, E-selectin, are expressed on the endothelial cell surface in specific vascular beds in response to inflammatory mediators. VCAM-1 was localized to the endothelium overlying atherosclerotic lesions in a hyperlipidemic rabbit model and was shown to be a risk factor for venous thrombosis in a kindred with protein C deficiency, highlighting the role of endothelial dysfunction as a primary determinant of atherosclerosis, and stresses the inflammatory nature of the atherosclerotic process [5].

Vascular endothelial growth factor (VEGF), produced by a number of different cell types, acts selectively on vascular endothelial cells. VEGF is a well-known promoter of angiogenesis and an endogenous regulator of endothelial integrity. Moreover, VEGF acts on the endothelium by stimulation of endothelial mitogenesis, promotion of endothelial survival, and control of vascular permeability. VEGF is 50,000 times more potent in inducing vascular leakage in comparison with histamine. VEGF receptor 1, also known as soluble Flt-1 (sFlt-1), is a potent antagonist of VEGF. The major sources of sFlt-1 are endothelial cells, monocytes, and the placenta. Soluble Flt-1 has been found to cause endothelial dysfunction, decrease angiogenesis, impair capillary repair, and increase proteinuria, and correlate with the severity of the clinical pre-eclampsia phenotype (see Chap. 37). Moreover, it has been suggested that increased VEGF might be evidence of the early stages of atherosclerosis [6].

Endothelial cells express a range of complement receptors and complement regulatory proteins, and are subject to injury by the complement cascade. The C5b-9 membrane attack complex (MAC) can induce endothelial cell lysis, while sub-lytic amounts of MAC activate these cells to release pro-inflammatory P-selectin and procoagulant von Willebrand factor, and disturb the normal endothelial cell barrier function [7]. Complement-mediated thrombotic microangiopathy (TMA), also called complement-mediated hemolytic uremic syndrome (HUS), is associated with mutations or autoantibodies that lead to excessive complement activation. Renal endothelial cells appear to be especially sensitive to complement-mediated injury, thus providing a possible rationale for the efficacy of complement inhibition in this setting. Additionally, in antibody-mediated transplant rejection, antibodies directed against endothelial cell antigens, most often HLA-A, B, C and DR, may kill or disable endothelial cells by excessive activation of complement.

In the past, the main focus of endothelial biology research was on the measurement of endothelium-derived vasoactive substances, inflammatory markers, or adhesion molecules. Biomarkers represent only the net result of activity from multiple vascular beds, wherein localized "hot spots" in specific sites of the vasculature could be overlooked. The current focus is now on bone-marrow-derived progenitor cells (EPCs) participating in repairing the endothelium, circulating endothelial cells and endothelial microparticles as markers of endothelial cell activation/injury [8]. However, we should bear in mind that endothelial dysfunction usually results from maladaptive responses, which became excessive, sustained, or misplaced (temporally or spatially). Accordingly, the transition between endothelial cell function and dysfunction is not always clear.

Evaluation of Endothelial Dysfunction

The assessment of endothelial cell function/injury in vivo is complex due to multifunctional nature of these cells. Studies in vivo on endothelial cell function/dysfunction involve the use of strategically placed catheters that allow the examiner to sample blood from a specific vascular bed. In clinical practice, coronary endothelial function in humans can be assessed by selective infusion of acetylcholine into the epicardial coronary arteries, followed by measurement of vessel diameter and doppler-derived velocities to calculate coronary blood flow. Based on this approach, coronary endothelial dysfunction was demonstrated to be common in patients with coronary artery disease [9]. Many imaging techniques, such as doppler measurements of blood flow, magnetic resonance angiography, and CT scanning are likely to be employed in the study of endothelial cell (dys)function. It appears that molecular imaging and linking the power of proteomics with advanced labeling techniques are likely to revolutionize the diagnosis of endothelial-based disorders [10].

Circulating endothelial cells (CEC) and their progenitors may yield insight into their function or their bed of origin [11]. It has been suggested that imbalance between circulating endothelial cells (indicative of endothelial injury) and bone-marrow-derived progenitor cells (which can potentially repair injured endothelium) might be more indicative of overall vascular endothelial health. Bone-marrow-derived endothelial progenitor cells (EPC) constitute an endogenous vascular repair system protecting against atherosclerosis. In 1997, Asahara et al. [8] in their landmark study demonstrated for the first time, the existence of cells in the circulation that could differentiate into endothelial cells. They expressed endothelial cell surface markers, VEGF receptor and, endothelial nitric oxide synthase mRNA, and produced nitric oxide upon stimulation [8]. A prior history of cardiovascular disease and increased endothelial dysfunction markers were related to lower EPC levels in patients with hypertension or diabetes.

Nitric Oxide and Endothelium

Nitric oxide (NO) produced by endothelial cells through the endothelial nitric oxide synthase (eNOS) pathway plays a major role in maintenance of endothelial function, and that decreased NO production and bioavailability largely contribute to endothelial dysfunction in diabetes [12]. Experimental studies have suggested that development and/or progression of diabetic kidney disease is associated with alterations in eNOS expression and activity. eNOS was shown to be the major NOS enzyme in the renal vasculature, and eNOS expression was shown to be upregulated in early (1–6 weeks) diabetic kidneys, especially in the afferent arteriolar and glomerular endothelium. Studies assessing NO production or responses in renal vasculature and glomerulus demonstrated decreased eNOS and NO activity in DN, even when eNOS expression is upregulated. The eNOS uncoupling caused by reactive oxygen species has been suggested to be a mechanism underlying this paradox. In humans, upregulated eNOS expression in glomerular endothelium was demonstrated in nephropathy patients with type 2 diabetes. In their elegant study, Taahashi and Harris [12] showed that eNOS-deficient diabetic mice exhibited advanced nephropathic changes with distinct features of progressive diabetic kidney disease, including pronounced albuminuria, nodular glomerulosclerosis, mesangiolysis, and arteriolar hyalinosis. These studies clearly defined a critical role of eNOS in diabetic kidney disease.

Albuminuria and Endothelium

Albuminuria is measured using a specific assay for albumin, as the urine dipstick is a relatively insensitive marker for albuminuria, not reflecting albumin excretion $\leq$s 300 mg/day. The normal rate of albumin excretion is <30 mg/day); persistent albumin excretion between 30 and 300 mg/day is called microalbuminuria) [13]. Albumin excretion above 300 mg/day is considered to represent overt albuminuria. Chronic kidney disease is considered by many to be a coronary artery disease (CAD) equivalent that should be managed according to secondary prevention goals [13, 14].

Albuminuria in kidney disease is thought to be mediated by complex and manifold pathophysiological mechanisms [15]. It is also thought to be a reflection of generalized increase in endothelial permeability or dysfunction [16]. Microalbuminuria and a fall in eGFR are independently associated with cardiovascular disease [17]. Decrease in albuminuria by renin–angiotensin system blockade results in a diminished cardiovascular mortality.

The gold standard for the detecting albuminuria is a 24-h hour urine collection [18]. For simplicity and to avoid the confounding effect of variations in urine volume on the urine, albumin concentrations of the albumin-to-creatinine ratio in an untimed spot urine specimen are used. A value 30–300 mg/g of the albumin/creatinine ratio suggests that albumin excretion is between 30 and 300 mg/day and therefore is diagnostic of microalbuminuria. Values above 300 mg/g are indicative of overt albuminuria.

Confounders that may affect the reliability of a spot microalbumin-to-creatinine ratio must be kept in mind when interpreting this data: (1) vigorous exercise causes a transient increase in albuminuria. Thus urine albumin excretion should be performed at least 24 h after strenuous exercise. (2) The optimal time to measure the urine albumin-to-creatinine ratio is not established yet. Both first morning void and before bedtime as well as first morning void and collections at other times [19] correlated with a 24-h urine collection. (3) In a case when creatinine excretion is substantially different from the expected value, the accuracy of the urine albumin-to-creatinine ratio will be diminished. This is in particular in patients with borderline values. In addition, muscle mass should also be taken into account as albumin excretion will be underestimated in a muscular man with a high rate of creatinine excretion and overestimated in a cachectic female in whom muscle mass and creatinine excretion are markedly reduced. Despite these limitations, urine albumin-to-creatinine ratio in an untimed urinary sample is the preferred approach to screen for albuminuria as it does not require early morning or timed collections, it gives a quantitative result that correlates with the 24-h urine values over a wide range of protein excretion, it is simple to perform and reproducible [20].

Albuminuria and Cardiovascular Disease

Albuminuria is an important risk factor for cardiovascular disease and early cardiovascular mortality in patients with and without diabetes and/or hypertension [21–23]. Albuminuria reflects the generalized increase in endothelial permeability or dysfunction, which drives progression of kidney disease and cardiovascular disease. A key mechanism that contributes to this process is the loss of the glycocalyx—a polysaccharide gel that lines the luminal endothelial surface and that normally acts as a barrier against albumin filtration. Degradation of the glycocalyx in response to endothelial activation can lead to albuminuria, and subsequent renal and vascular inflammation, thus providing a pathophysiological framework for the clinical association of albuminuria with renal and cardiovascular disease progression [24].

There is increasing evidence that glomerular endothelial cell injury plays a major role in the development and progression of diabetic kidney disease [25]. Alteration of the glomerular endothelial cell surface layer, including its major component, glycocalyx, is a leading cause of albuminuria observed in early diabetic kidney disease. The glomerular endothelium is also likely to indirectly influence glomerular albumin handling by modifying podocyte behavior. The importance of the glomerular endothelium and endothelial surface layer in albumin handling also sheds light on the relationship between albuminuria and vascular disease [26]. Many studies suggest a presence of cross talk between glomerular cells, such as between glomerular endothelial cell and mesangial cells or glomerular endothelial cell and podocytes. These superficially discordant paradigms can be assimilated by the emerging concept of endothelial–podocyte cross talk across the glomerular filtration barrier, whereby the actions of one type of cell may profoundly influence the function of the other. Platelet-derived growth factor B-(PDGF-B), and its receptor PDGFR-β[beta] are major mediators in glomerular endothelial cell and mesangial cell cross talk, while vascular endothelial growth factor (VEGF), angiopoietins, and endothelin-1 are the major mediators for glomerular endothelial cell and podocyte communication. The bidirectional nature of this paracrine network is illustrated by the actions of the vascular endothelial growth factor-A (VEGF-A)/VEGF receptor-2 and activated protein C systems, among others [27] (Fig. 1.2). On the other hand, in diabetic kidney disease, glomerular endothelial cell injury may lead to podocyte damage, while podocyte loss further exacerbates glomerular endothelial cell injury, forming a vicious cycle [25]. Therefore, glomerular endothelial cell injury may predispose to albuminuria in diabetes either directly or indirectly by communication with neighboring podocytes and mesangial cells via secreted mediators [25].

In essential, hypertension abnormalities in kidney include the development of a medium- and small-size arteriolopathy characterized by intimal hyperplasia, hyalinosis, and smooth muscle cell hypertrophy (nephroangiosclerosis). The latter one could be an expression of a systemic dysfunction of vascular endothelium. It seems to be the basic anatomic disturbance that may eventually lead to disastrous vascular events in the heart, brain, and the kidney. Moreover, the small and medium size vessels respond inappropriately to vasodilatory stimuli such as acetylcholine mediated by nitric oxide. Similarly, in clinically healthy subjects with moderately increased albuminuria, vasodilation in response to certain stimuli is relatively reduced relative to those with lower levels of albumin excretion. In addition, nondiabetic hypertensive patients with increased albuminuria had higher plasma levels of von Willebrand factor (vWF) antigen, a marker of endothelial dysfunction, than patients with normal albumin excretion [28]. Endothelial dysfunction is frequently found in diabetic patients, and the degree of coronary endothelial dysfunction appears to be correlate with albuminuria [29]. In diabetes, endothelial function can be modulated by several factors including the degree of hyperglycemia, duration of disease, accumulation of advance glycation end products, and albuminuria [29]. In addition, hyperglycemia stimulates increased VEGF expression, known to be a mediator of endothelial injury in human diabetes. VEGF blockade improved albuminuria in an experimental model of diabetic nephropathy supporting a potentially pathogenic role for VEGF in diabetic nephropathy.

The Heart and Soul Study evaluated circulating soluble endothelial cell-selective adhesion molecule (sESAM), a marker of endothelial dysfunction, as a risk factor for kidney function decline and albuminuria. Park et al. [30] reported that elevated levels of sESAM were strongly and independently associated with baseline reduced eGFR <60 mL/min per 1.73 m^2 and urine albumin to creatinine ratio ≥ 30 mg/g ($P < 0.0001$). They concluded that as sESAM was associated with albuminuria and reduced kidney function in both cross-sectional and longitudinal analyses, implicating endothelial dysfunction as a potential contributor to the elevated kidney disease risk in persons with cardiovascular disease. The HOPE trial demonstrated that moderately increased albuminuria was associated with an increased relative risk of the primary aggregate end point (myocardial infarction (MI), stroke, or cardiovascular death) independently of presence of diabetes. Similarly in the LIFE trial, the albumin-to-creatinine ratio was associated with the risk of the composite end point of cardiovascular death, myocardial infarction, or stroke in both nondiabetics and diabetics. In PREVEND, a population-based study on 40,548 participants followed for a median of 2.6 years [20],

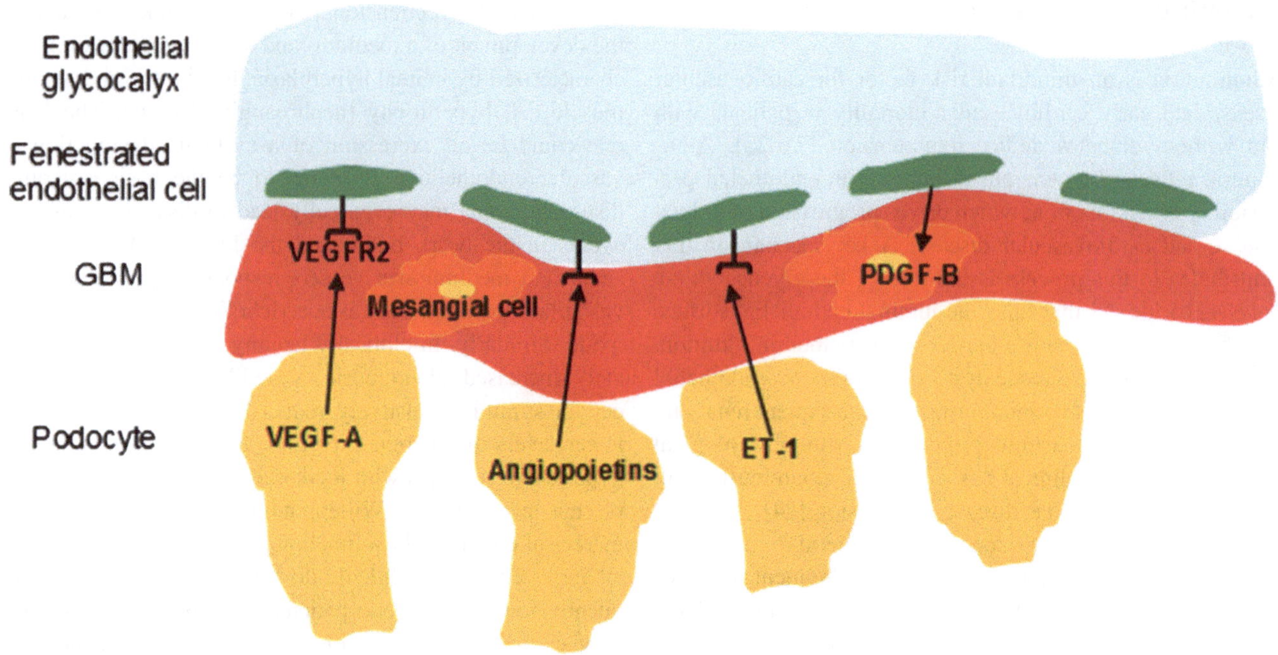

Fig. 1.2 Glomerular filtration barrier cross talk (endothelium–mesangium, endothelium–podocyte)

there was a graded increase in the relative risk of cardiovascular mortality of 1.35 for each doubling of urinary albumin excretion, when adjusted for age and sex. Roest et al. [23] in a cohort of 12,239 postmenopausal women observed a higher cardiovascular mortality in those in the highest quintile of urinary albumin excretion [>21 mg/g creatinine (>2.41 mg/mmol)], independently of presence of diabetes and hypertension.

Summary

Albuminuria of any degree is associated with cardiovascular disease that is additive to conventional risk factors in both nondiabetic and diabetic patients. The mechanism by which albuminuria is associated with cardiovascular disease is not fully explained. Endothelial dysfunction together with abnormalities in endothelial–podocyte cross talk across the glomerular filtration barrier may play an important role in pathogenesis of albuminuria. Regardless of whether albuminuria is present in isolation or co-exists with a decline in GFR, it is clearly associated with an increase in cardiovascular risk. Albuminuria should be treated aggressively with renin–angiotension–aldosterone axis blocking agents and adjunct therapy, and pursued as an independent modifiable risk factor to favorably alter cardiovascular risk profiles. This is critical to improving cardiovascular outcomes and optimizing endothelial function, as a whole.

References

1. Furchgott RF, Zawadzki JV. The obligatory role of endothelial cells in the relaxation of arterial smooth muscle by acetylcholine. Nature. 1980;288:373–6.
2. Verma S, Anderson TJ. Fundamentals of endothelial function for the clinical cardiologist. Circulation. 2002;105:546–9.
3. Panza JA, Quyyumi AA, Brush JE Jr, Epstein SE. Abnormal endothelium-dependent vascular relaxation in patients with essential hypertension. N Engl J Med. 1990;323:22–7.
4. Schwartz SM, Gajdusek CM, Reidy MA, Selden SC 3rd, Haudenschild CC. Maintenance of integrity in aortic endothelium. Fed Proc. 1980;39:2618–25.
5. Bombeli T, Mueller M, Haeberli A. Anticoagulant properties of the vascular endothelium. Thromb Haemost. 1997;77:408–23.
6. Jarray R, Pavoni S, Borriello L, Allain B, Lopez N, Bianco S, Liu WQ, Biard D, Demange L, Hermine O, Garbay C, Raynaud F, Lepelletier Y. Disruption of phactr-1 pathway triggers pro-inflammatory and pro-atherogenic factors: new insights in atherosclerosis development. Biochimie. 2015;118:151–61.
7. Kerr H, Richards A. Complement-mediated injury and protection of endothelium: lessons from atypical haemolytic uraemic syndrome. Immunobiology. 2012;217:195–203.
8. Asahara T, Murohara T, Sullivan A, Silver M, van der Zee R, Li T, Witzenbichler B, Schatteman G, Isner JM. Isolation of putative progenitor endothelial cells for angiogenesis. Science. 1997;275:964–7.
9. Ludmer PL, Selwyn AP, Shook TL, Wayne RR, Mudge GH, Alexander RW, Ganz P. Paradoxical vasoconstriction induced by acetylcholine in atherosclerotic coronary arteries. N Engl J Med. 1986;315:1046–51.
10. Zoccali C, Bode-Böger S, Mallamaci F, Benedetto F, Tripepi G, Malatino L, Cataliotti A, Bellanuova I, Fermo I, Frölich J, Böger R. Plasma concentration of asymmetrical dimethylarginine and

mortality in patients with end-stage renal disease: a prospective study. Lancet. 2001;358:2113–7.
11. Shantsila E, Blann AD, Lip GY. Circulating endothelial cells: from bench to clinical practice. J Thromb Haemost. 2008;6:865–8.
12. Takahashi T, Harris RC. Role of endothelial nitric oxide synthase in diabetic nephropathy: lessons from diabetic eNOS knockout mice. J Diabetes Res. 2014;2014:590541.
13. KDIGO. Chapter 1: definition and classification of CKD. Kidney Int Suppl 2013;3:19. http://www.kdigo.org/clinical_practice_guidelines/pdf/CKD/KDIGO_2012_CKD_GL.pdf. Accessed 29 Jan 2016.
14. Glassock RJ. Debate: CON position. Should microalbuminuria ever be considered as a renal endpoint in any clinical trial? Am J Nephrol. 2010;31:462–5.
15. Comper WD, Hilliard LM, Nikolic-Paterson DJ, Russo LM. Disease-dependent mechanisms of albuminuria. Am J Physiol Renal Physiol. 2008;295:1589–600.
16. Stehouwer CD, Henry RM, Dekker JM, Nijpels G, Heine RJ, Bouter LM. Microalbuminuria is associated with impaired brachial artery, flow-mediated vasodilation in elderly individuals without and with diabetes: further evidence for a link between microalbuminuria and endothelial dysfunction—the Hoorn Study. Kidney Int. 2004;92(Suppl):S42–44.
17. Stenvinkel P, Carrero JJ, Axelsson J, Lindholm B, Heimburger O, Massy Z. Emerging biomarkers for evaluating cardiovascular risk in the chronic kidney disease patient: how do new pieces fit into the uremic puzzle? Clin J Am Soc Nephrol. 2008;3:505–21.
18. Mogensen CE, Vestbo E, Poulsen PL, Christiansen C, Damsgaard EM, Eiskjaer H, Frøland A, Hansen KW, Nielsen S, Pedersen MM. Microalbuminuria and potential confounders. A review and some observations on variability of urinary albumin excretion. Diabetes Care. 1995;18:572–81.
19. Tani Y, Nakayama M, Terawaki H, Iseki K, Watanabe T. Comparison of albuminuria test and urine test strip in Japanese hypertensive patients: AVA-E study. Clin Nephrol. 2015;84:270–3.
20. Witte EC, Lambers Heerspink HJ, de Zeeuw D, Bakker SJ, de Jong PE, Gansevoort R. First morning voids are more reliable than spot urine samples to assess microalbuminuria. J Am Soc Nephrol. 2009;20:436–43.
21. Bartz SK, Caldas MC, Tomsa A, Krishnamurthy R, Bacha F. Urine albumin-to-creatinine ratio: a marker of early endothelial dysfunction in youth. J Clin Endocrinol Metab. 2015;100:3393–9.
22. Hillege HL, Fidler V, Diercks GF, van Gilst WH, de Zeeuw D, van Veldhuisen DJ, Gans RO, Janssen WM, Grobbee DE, de Jong PE, Prevention of Renal and Vascular End Stage Disease (PREVEND) Study Group. Urinary albumin excretion predicts cardiovascular and noncardiovascular mortality in general population. Circulation. 2002;106:1777–82.
23. Roest M, Banga JD, Janssen WM, Grobbee DE, Sixma JJ, de Jong PE, de Zeeuw D, van Der Schouw YT. Excessive urinary albumin levels are associated with future cardiovascular mortality in postmenopausal women. Circulation. 2001;103:3057–61.
24. Rabelink TJ, de Zeeuw D. The glycocalyx-linking albuminuria with renal and cardiovascular disease. Nat Rev Nephrol. 2015;11:667–76.
25. Fu J, Lee K, Chuang PY, Liu Z, He JC. Glomerular endothelial cell injury and cross talk in diabetic kidney disease. Am J Physiol Renal Physiol. 2015;308(4):F287–97.
26. Satchell S. The role of the glomerular endothelium in albumin handling. Nat Rev Nephrol. 2013;9:717–25.
27. Siddiqi FS, Advani A. Endothelial–podocyte crosstalk: the missing link between endothelial dysfunction and albuminuria in diabetes. Diabetes. 2013;62:3647–55.
28. Khaleghi M, Singletary LA, Kondragunta V, Bailey KR, Turner ST, Mosley TH Jr, Kullo IJ. Haemostatic markers are associated with measures of vascular disease in adults with hypertension. J Hum Hypertens. 2009;23:530–7.
29. Petrica L, Vlad A, Gluhovschi G, Gadalean F, Dumitrascu V, Vlad D, Popescu R, Velciov S, Gluhovschi C, Bob F, Ursoniu S, Petrica M, Jianu DC. Glycated peptides are associated with the variability of endothelial dysfunction in the cerebral vessels and the kidney in type 2 diabetes mellitus patients: a cross-sectional study. J Diabetes Compl. 2015;29:230–7.
30. Park M, Vittinghoff E, Ganz P, Peralta CA, Whooley M, Shlipak MG. Role of soluble endothelial cell-selective adhesion molecule biomarker in albuminuria and kidney function changes in patients with coronary artery disease: the Heart and Soul Study. Arterioscler Thromb Vasc Biol. 2014;34:231–6.

2 Vascular and Valvular Calcification in Chronic Kidney Disease: Pathogenesis and Clinical Outcomes

Hope Caughron, Jose F. Condado, and Vasilis Babaliaros

Introduction

Patients with chronic kidney disease (CKD) are two to four times as likely to have cardiovascular disease (CVD) compared to the general population, when adjusted for traditional CVD risk factors [1]. CVD is the leading cause of death in these patients, with vascular and valvular calcification being an integral part of its pathophysiology. Calcium phosphate crystals are deposited through a multifactorial dynamic process that leads to the development of atherosclerosis, arteriosclerosis, and valvular calcification. This chapter will discuss the pathogenesis of vascular and valvular calcification, focusing on the unique risk factors associated with the milieu of chronic kidney disease. Utilizing this knowledge, this chapter will delve into the clinical manifestations, complications, treatments, and outcomes associated with vascular and valvular calcification in CKD and end-stage kidney disease (ESKD).

Vascular Calcification

Vascular calcification can be classified into intimal calcification and medial calcification according to the location of calcium deposition within the arterial wall. Intimal calcification is commonly associated with atherosclerotic plaques that partially occlude the arterial lumen, reducing blood flow and resulting in peripheral ischemia, myocardial infarction, stroke, and sudden death [2, 3]. Alternatively, medial calcification is deposited circumferentially along the elastic lamellae, which damages the elastic collagen resulting in an increase in wall stiffness and a decrease in vascular compliance [4, 5]. Clinically, medial calcification is more commonly seen in patients who are older, diabetic, and those with CKD [6].

Valvular Calcification

Valvular calcification is an independent predictor of CVD, heart failure, and death [7, 8], and is often responsible for leaflet and annular thickening with resulting valve dysfunction (i.e., stenosis). Calcification is more common in the aortic and mitral valves due to the higher pressures, turbulence, and mechanical stress seen on the left side of the heart compared to the right side. In the aortic valve, the increased calcium deposition often causes aortic stenosis (AS). Though symptoms of AS (angina, syncope, and dyspnea) are identical in patients regardless of baseline kidney function, the natural course of the disease is accelerated in patients with CKD and as a result these rapid progressors have severe, symptomatic AS at a younger age than the non-CKD population [9, 10].

In the mitral valve, mitral annular calcification (MAC) arises early in the course of renal insufficiency and often has clinical consequences prior to the onset of ESKD [11]. In most patients, MAC is initially isolated to the ventricular base under the posterior mitral leaflet, and can spread to involve the entire posterior annulus [12, 13]. Advanced posterior MAC can cause mitral regurgitation (MR) due to restriction of the posterior leaflet movement, while the anterior leaflet remains mobile (Fig. 2.1). In patients with ESKD, MAC can progress further to involve the anterior annular ring. This circumferential calcific ring restricts the

H. Caughron
Structural Heart and Valve Center, Emory University Hospital F606, 1364 Clifton Road, Atlanta, GA 30322, USA
e-mail: hope.caughron@emory.edu

J.F. Condado
Cardiovascular Disease Fellowship Program, Emory University School of Medicine, Emory University, 101 Woodruff Circle, WMB 308. MS:190-001-1AJ, Atlanta, GA 30322, USA
e-mail: jfcondado@emory.edu

V. Babaliaros (✉)
Department of Cardiology, Emory University Hospital F606, 1364 Clifton Road, Atlanta, GA 30322, USA
e-mail: vbabali@emory.edu

J. Rangaswami et al. (eds.), *Cardio-Nephrology*,
DOI 10.1007/978-3-319-56042-7_2

movement of both the anterior and posterior leaflets resulting in mitral stenosis [12, 13] (Fig. 2.1).

Pathogenesis of Vascular Calcification

Extraskeletal calcification was previously believed to be an inert process that resulted from an increase in serum levels of calcium and phosphate. It is now understood that both intimal and medial calcification share a common downstream pathway involving the de-differentiation of vascular smooth muscle cells (VSMCs) into cells with osteogenic capability [14, 15]. Despite similar risk factors, medial and intimal calcification are likely initiated through different primary mechanisms.

Intimal calcification, seen in atherosclerosis, has a patchy morphology composed of calcium crystal aggregates within atherosclerotic plaques [16]. The primary event in atherosclerosis is endothelial dysfunction due to physical or chemical stressors. The breakdown of the endothelial barrier allows lipids to become trapped and oxidized within the sub-endothelial space, inducing an inflammatory response that results in the production of a fatty streak. A fatty streak is composed of foam cells or fat-laden macrophages, lipids, and necrotic tissue surrounded by leukocytes. Necrotic tissue and the formation of matrix vesicles likely serve as nucleation sites for intimal calcification [16].

In contrast, medial calcification consists of a focal, circumferential sheet of calcium crystals surrounded by VSMCs in the absence of lipid aggregation or inflammatory mediators [16]. Evidence suggests that elastin degradation by matrix metalloproteinases (MMP) may be the initial step facilitating medial calcification [17]. Elevated MMP is correlated with increased arterial stiffness and severity of medial calcification [18].

Once the aforementioned initial stimulus has occurred, the mechanism of calcium deposition downstream is the same regardless of the location (intimal vs. medial). In normal human development, mesenchymal stem cells differentiate into osteoblasts, chondrocytes, adipocytes, and VSMCs. Chemical stressors such as diabetes, dyslipidemia, inflammation, and other cytotoxins promote de-differentiation of VSMCs into cells with an osteochondrogenic phenotype. Bone associated-proteins such as osteocalcin, osteopontin, matrix γ-carboxyglutamic acid protein, bone morphogenic protein, and osteoprotegerin have been found in atherosclerotic plaques and mineralized heart valves [15, 19–21]. Transcription factors essential to osteoblastic differentiation such as runt related transcription factor (Cbfa1/RUNX2) and muscle segment homeobox (MSX-2) are upregulated in cells surrounding calcified arterial walls and are indicative of phenotypic de-differentiation [14, 19, 21]. VSMCs expressing these osteogenic indicators deposit collagen and non-collagenous proteins in a mechanism similar to osteoblastic bone formation. VSMCs then form matrix vesicles similar to exosomes that contain calcium, phosphate, alkaline phosphatase, and annexin to initiate calcification [2, 5, 19]. Calcium and phosphorus are further mineralized into hydroxyapatite in the vesicles.

Pathogenesis of Valvular Calcification

Valvular calcification results from the deposition of calcium-phosphate crystals on the annulus and the leaflets of the valves, at sites of inflammation or mechanical stress [22]. Similar to vascular calcification, valvular calcification is also an active process that involves de-differentiation of matrix cells into cells with osteoblastic potential. Although the pathogenesis of valvular calcification is not fully understood, it is believed to be similar to that of atherosclerosis, explaining the shared risk factors between these two conditions [23]. Cardiac valves, particularly on the left side of the heart, are subject to cyclic mechanical stress from high pressure gradients and turbulent flow related to high peak velocities and rapid acceleration [10]. The mechanical stress on the valve with each cardiac cycle leads to endothelial microfractures that cause rearrangement of elastin and breakdown of the collagen structure [10, 22]. Over time, the repetitive damage to the valve will result in fibrosis and calcification via mechanisms similar to those described in vascular calcification.

Pathogenesis of Vascular and Valvular Calcification in CKD and ESKD

In CKD, the contributions of traditional risk factors such as hypertension, dyslipidemia, smoking, diabetes, gender, and older age do not fully account for the high incidence of calcification associated CVD, suggesting that there is a unique set of calcification promoting risk factors in the CKD milieu [6, 24]. In the early stages of renal impairment, the complex balance between promoters and inhibitors of osteogenesis begins to breakdown, resulting in the deposition of calcium in extraskeletal organs. In CKD, calcium deposition is partially attributed to a disturbance in mineral metabolism, an alteration in inhibitory regulation, an increase in MMP concentration, the presence of chronic inflammation, and the effect of mechanical stress (Fig. 2.2).

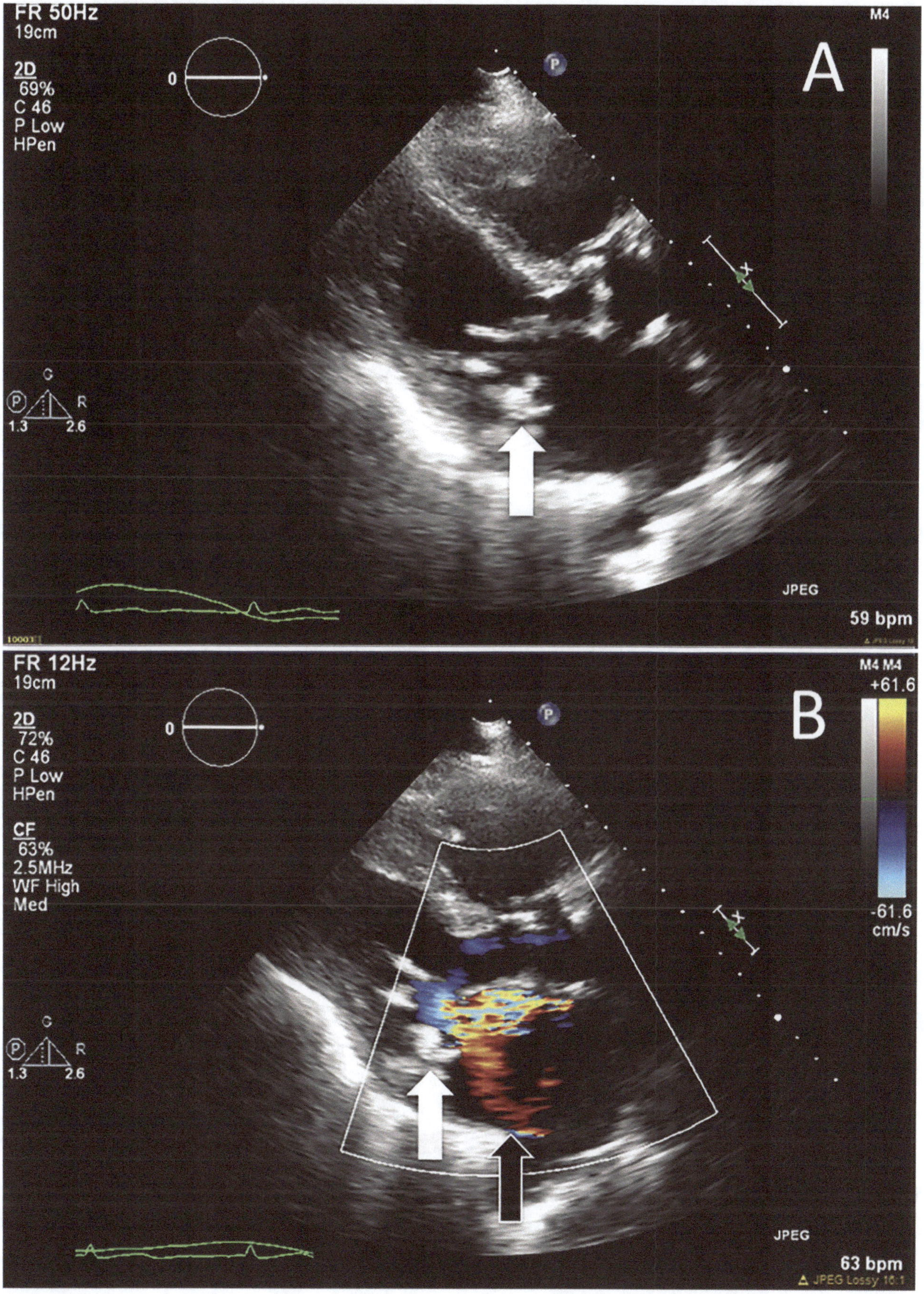

Fig. 2.1 Transthoracic echocardiogram (TTE) revealing posterior mitral annular calcification (MAC, *white arrows* **a**, **b**) causing restriction of the posterior mitral leaflet with the resulting severe mitral regurgitation on Doppler (b, *black arrow*)

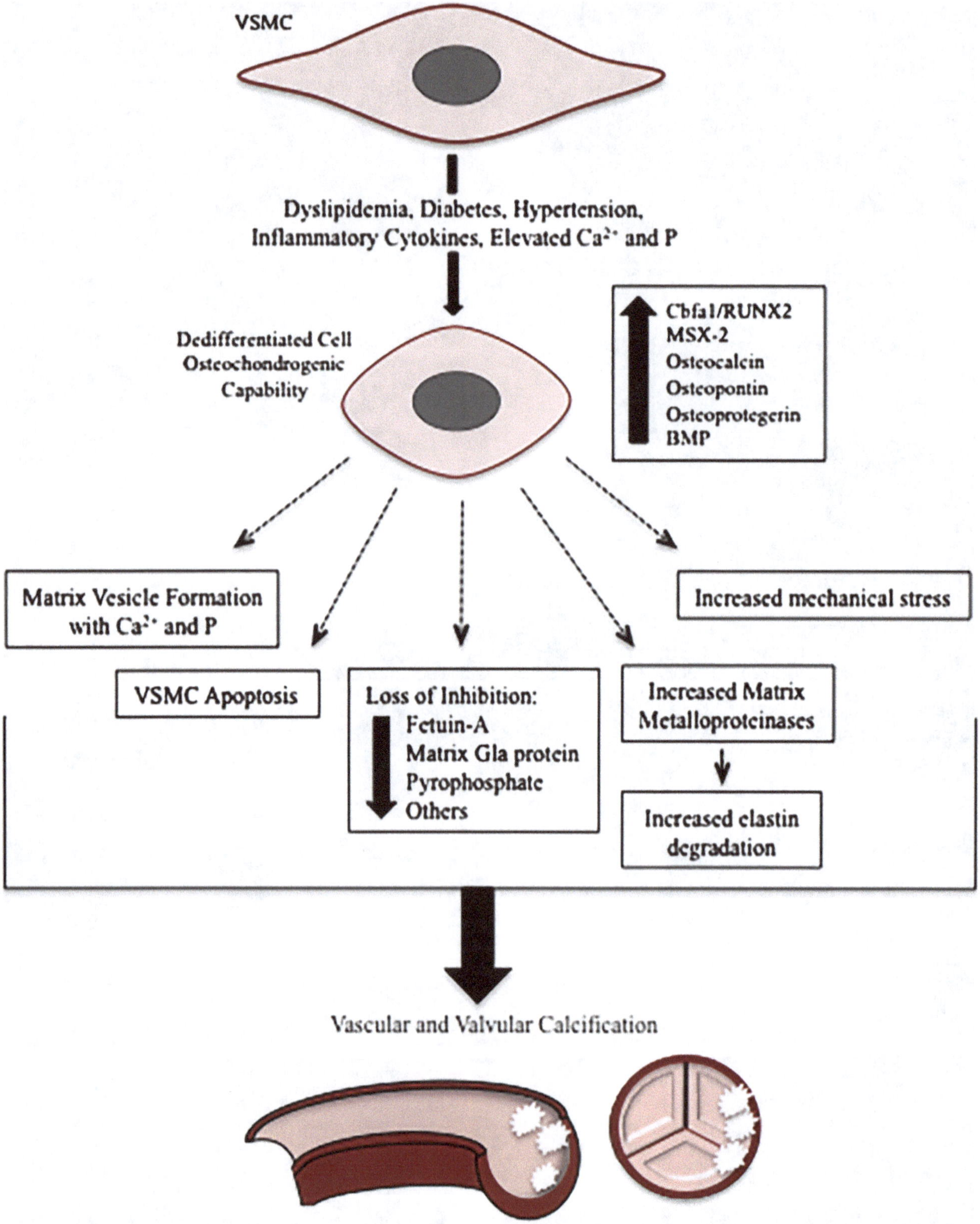

Fig. 2.2 Pathophysiology of vascular/valvular calcification in patients with chronic kidney disease

Disturbance in Mineral Metabolism

Early in CKD, disturbances in mineral metabolism result in a positive calcium and phosphate balance. Increases in fibroblast growth factor-23 (FGF-23) cause inhibition of 1-α hydroxylase, decreasing 1,25-dihydroxyvitamin D_3 (calcitriol) synthesis. Calcitriol, which is produced by the proximal tubular cells of the nephron, normally inhibits the renin–angiotensin system (RAS) and has anti-inflammatory effects. The decrease in calcitrol also decreases calcium absorption in the stomach resulting in a decrease in total body calcium. This triggers secondary hyperparathyroidism caused by hyperplasia of the parathyroid gland, which promotes osteoclast resorption of bone to release calcium and phosphate. PTH directly stimulates the renin–angiotensin system causing a hypertensive state that may further promote endothelial damage and calcification [25]. Increases in PTH and FGF-23 also promote increased phosphate excretion from the kidney; therefore, hyperphosphotemia is only a clinical finding in late CKD when GFR is significantly reduced. Elevated levels of calcium, phosphate, FGF-23, and PTH are all associated with increased vascular and valvular calcification in patients with CKD and are almost ubiquitous in advanced CKD [3, 26]. Some patients with CKD may develop a relative resistance to PTH and resultant adynamic bone disease. Despite elevated levels of PTH compared to the normal population, these patients have decreased osteoblast and osteoclast activity, which can cause skeletal abnormalities and increased CVD [27, 28].

The presence of hyperphosphotemia in ESKD is associated with increased mortality rates, particularly when the serum phosphorous levels are higher than 6.5 mg/dl [26, 29]. Elevated phosphate promotes VSMC de-differentiation to osteogenic cells and induces mineralization of VSMC.

The increase in total body calcium and phosphate in patients with CKD have independent and additive effects promoting extraskeletal calcification. Serum calcium concentrations however, can be misleading because patients on dialysis can have an increase in total calcium balance despite a normal serum calcium [3]. Calcium is deposited within and on the surface of matrix vesicles, which enables calcium-phosphate nucleation via matrix proteins. The increase in cytoplasmic calcium induces VSMC apoptosis, releasing the hydroxyapatite matrix vesicles and forming a nidus for vascular calcification [30].

Alteration in Inhibitory Regulation

Proteins that are responsible for inhibiting calcification such as *Fetuin-A*, *matrix Gla protein* (MGP), and *inorganic pyrophosphate* are often reduced in patients with CKD. Fetuin-A is a circulatory defense mechanism, working to prevent systemic inflammation and vascular calcification without affecting bone mineralization. Fetuin-A binds to both calcium and phosphorus in the serum to promote removal through the reticuloendothelial system. This prevents matrix vesicle formation and increases phagocytosis of matrix vesicles by VSMCs [31]. In ESKD patients, serum Fetuin-A levels are inversely associated with carotid artery plaques, coronary artery calcification, valvular calcification, and death [19].

MGP is a vitamin K dependent regulator of vascular calcification that is normally expressed in arteries and bone. The role of MGP is not well understood, but it is generally accepted that MGP inhibits arterial calcification [15]. High calcium levels are associated with CKD overwhelm endogenous MGP activity, thereby reducing inhibition of calcification in matrix vesicles. Warfarin, a vitamin K antagonist, is believed to promote calcification in the aorta and in the arterial elastic lamina due to its effect on MGP [15, 32]. This hypothesis has been further corroborated by studies showing that supplementation with vitamin K in patients on hemodialysis can increase carboxylated MGP levels and to reduce vascular calcification [33].

Pyrophosphate is another calcification inhibitor, which prevents VSMC formation of hydroxyapatite. Increased levels of alkaline phosphatase, which hydrolyzes pyrophosphate, may be responsible for the decrease in pyrophosphate in patients with renal insufficiency and are negatively associated with arterial calcification in these patients [34].

Increase in Matrix Metalloproteinases (MMP)

Elevated MMP may cause an increase in medial elastic fiber fragmentation, which promotes medial calcification by preventing excess elastin degradation. In patients on hemodialysis, there is an increase in MMP-2 and an associated increase in elastin fragmentation [35]. MMP-2 is also elevated in patients with advanced CKD and is correlated with increased arterial stiffness and increased calcification [18, 35]. The role of MMP in elastin degradation may explain why medial calcification is more prevalent in patients with renal insufficiency and may be a target for future therapy [6, 24].

Chronic Inflammation

In ESKD, protein–energy malnutrition (PEM) and inflammation often occur concomitantly as malnutrition–inflammation complex syndrome (MICS) or malnutrition atherosclerosis. Chronic inflammation is thought to contribute to the decrease in total body protein and reduced functional capacity seen in PEM [36]. The chronic inflammatory state is also responsible for osteochondrogenic differentiation of matrix elements and increased VSMC apoptosis, which results in vascular and valvular calcification [9, 23].

Mechanical Stress

In patients with impaired renal function, valvular endothelial microfractures from mechanical stress initiate valvular calcification. Valvular microfractures are more prevalent in patients with renal insufficiency and are particularly apparent in patients on hemodialysis because of the high output state associated with anemia, AV fistulas, hypertension, and volume overload [9, 10]. This increases the mechanical stress on the valves and promotes valvular calcification.

Clinical Impact of Vascular Calcification

Vascular calcification begins in the early stages of CKD and rapidly progresses as renal function decreases. Patients with CKD stage 3 or above are considered to be the highest risk population for subsequent cardiovascular events associated with worsening vascullar/valvular calcification [37]. The most prevalent clinical complications of vascular calcification include coronary artery disease (CAD) and peripheral artery disease (PAD).

In patients with CKD, diagnosis of CAD can be challenging due to atypical clinical presentations. Many commonly used diagnostic tests for CAD, such as single-photon emission computed tomography (SPECT), have a decreased sensitivity and specificity in ESRD patients [38, 39]. In these patients, the determination of coronary artery calcification using electron-beam CT (EBCT) can be a useful, noninvasive tool for the evaluation and diagnosis of CAD. Ultimately, invasive coronary angiography continues to be the gold standard for diagnosis of anatomic CAD burden [40]. However, contrast-induced nephropathy (CIN) during coronary angiography and percutaneous intervention remains a concern in patients with CKD. New research suggests that fluid administration based on LVEDP can reduce the risk of CIN in patients with CKD [41]. Additionally, increased operator experience and improved imaging technology have enabled physicians to reduce the use of contrast in patients with CKD.

The most feared complication of CAD is myocardial infarction (MI). CKD patients presenting with an MI have 3 times higher mortality rates than the general population and ESKD patients with MI have an astounding 15 times higher mortality than the general population [42]. The observed worse outcomes in CKD patients, can in part be explained by a greater frequency of triple vessel or left main disease, increased calcific severity of culprit coronary lesions [43], and uncertainty regarding the optimal treatment strategies for this patient population. Coronary reperfusion with either CABG or PCI is associated with higher rates of operative and long-term mortality in patients with CKD compared to non-CKD patients [44, 45]. In CKD patients undergoing PCI, the widespread vascular calcification can complicate stent implantation due to the presence of complex coronary lesions. In general, the increased calcification of the myocardium and microvasculature of the heart contributes to depressed cardiac function and reserve capacity. This manifests clinically as an increased risk of both surgical and percutaneous procedural complications [45]. The complexity of cardiovascular management in patients with CAD and CKD supports the utilization of a team approach with input from cardiac surgeons, interventional cardiologists, and nephrologists.

Peripheral artery disease is also a common cause for percutaneous intervention or surgical treatment in the CKD population. There is an incremental increase in mortality and morbidity associated with peripheral vascular intervention (PVI) as CKD progresses from mild to severe. CKD is an independent predictor for perioperative re-intervention with no change in perioperative mortality when adjusted for age, CAD, critical limb ischemia (CLI), and diabetes [46]. Severe CKD (stage 4 or 5) has been associated with a decrease in short and long-term survival and an increase in amputation rates. This is possibly due to the presence of small vessel disease and increased multilevel PVI in CKD patients [46].

Medical Strategies to Prevent Calcification

There is currently no medical treatment that can reverse calcification in patients with CKD. Therefore, controlling traditional risk factors such as hypertension, dyslipidemia, smoking, and diabetes is crucial to prevent vascular calcification and associated CVD [47]. Treatment modalities that focus on reducing the calcium phosphorus product (CaXP) to recommended targets (<55, K DIGO) help reduce extra skeletal calcification burden [48].

Treatment options for secondary hyperparathyroidism such as activated vitamin D supplementation and calcimimetics reduce the need for surgical parathyroidectomy and reduce the progression of calcification in patients on dialysis [49]. The application of bisphosphonates, vitamin K supplementation, and sodium thiosulfate in reducing in vascular calcification and mortality are still undetermined and warrant further study [15].

Clinical Impact of Valvular Calcification

In CKD (with or without dialysis), the prevalence of aortic and mitral calcification is significantly higher than in the general population. In CKD, there is a graded relationship between the progressive decrease in GFR and the prevalence of calcification, hospitalizations, cardiovascular events, and death [50]. Complications often associated with valvular calcification include thromboembolism, cardiac arrhythmias, and valvular stenosis.

Thrombotic lesions and ulcers are found on calcified valves and can potentially dispense bursts of calcium-phosphate crystals into the lumen of the heart [11]. Additionally, vegetations that may be present in MAC and aortic valvular calcification (AVC) can embolize and travel through the blood stream to cause ischemia in other organs, most commonly stroke. In patients with MAC, emboli are typically larger and are more likely to cause cerebral ischemia, whereas in patients with AVC, emboli are often smaller and more prone to land in the retinal artery causing monocular blindness [9–11]. In MAC and AVC, calcium can also invade the conduction system of the heart, causing conduction abnormalities such as atrial fibrillation, atrioventricular block, and intraventricular block [10]. Once the calcification begins to impinge on the valvular lumen or restrict the valve leaflets it can cause valvular stenosis.

Aortic Valve

Valvular stenosis is more common in the aortic valve and can lead to severe hemodynamic complications. The progression from asymptomatic aortic disease with calcification to severe symptomatic AS is rapid in patients with renal insufficiency. In patients with CKD, annual reduction in aortic valve area was 0.23 cm^2 as compared to 0.05–0.10 cm^2 in patients without kidney disease [51]. This is a dramatic and rapid decrease in valvular area, given that the aortic valve area is on average 3–4 cm^2. After the onset of symptomatic AS, mean survival in CKD patients is approximately 23 ± 9 months [52].

Valve replacement is the only therapy with survival benefit for severe AS, regardless of whether the patient has CKD. The two main treatment options for AVR are surgical (SAVR) and transcatheter aortic valve replacement (TAVR). In SAVR, CKD is a risk factor for increased 30-day and long-term mortality, with a more than 50% increase in median postsurgical mortality over a span of 15 years [53]. Patients with renal insufficiency have increased complications from SAVR, in part because the technical challenges associated with severe vascular and valvular calcification lead to increased in-hospital mortality, increased hospital length of stay, and increased ICU duration [54].

The less invasive TAVR may be an alternative for valve replacement in patients with advanced CKD, due to the inherent higher surgical risk and the potential to avoid some of the complications observed with SAVR [54]. In patients undergoing TAVR with CKD, femoral access may be limited due to excess vascular calcification (Fig. 2.3), requiring the use of alternative accesses with potentially higher risk of complication such as transapical, transaortic, transcarotid, or transcaval access [55]. The enhancement of technology, technique, and experience has decreased the use of IV contrast and the incidence of complications, suggesting that in the future, TAVR can become the preferred therapeutic choice in patients with advanced CKD (Fig. 2.3)

Despite advances in surgical and percutaneous techniques, valvular calcification is still associated with complications after SAVR and TAVR. Preexisting damage to the heart's conduction system increases the risk of pacemaker requirement after surgical or transcatheter intervention [56]. Porcelain aorta is another risk factor associated with worse outcomes after SAVR and is often considered a nontraditional risk factor for surgical death. This is probably due to the requirement for extensive aortic replacement. Additionally, the degree of annular and left ventricular outflow track calcification is linked to a higher degree of paravalvular regurgitation post-TAVR. Calcification can prevent adequate sealing between the native and bioprosthetic valve after deployment. Evaluation with a preprocedural multidetector computed tomography (MDCT) characterizes the location and severity of calcification and provides critical information necessary to decide the best treatment strategy (TAVR vs. SAVR, Fig. 2.4) [57].

Mitral Valve

Mitral stenosis and/or regurgitation can occur secondary to MAC and may require either surgical or transcatheter intervention. The extensive mitral calcification associated with CKD increases surgical complications such as hemorrhage, atrioventricular disruption, left ventricular rupture, and peri-prosthetic leakage [58]. Ironically, the presence of severe mitral valve disease (MS or MR) associated with severe MAC makes these high-risk patients potential candidates for percutaneous interventions, specifically transcatheter mitral valve replacement. A circumferentially calcified annulus can provide the necessary support and anchoring for a stented transcatheter heart valve deployment and can reduce the risk of embolization [59]. As discussed with TAVR, preprocedural planning for percutaneous intervention with MDCT can help evaluate the MAC distribution in detail (Fig. 2.5). Evidence of transcatheter mitral valve replacement in these situations is limited to case reports and case series [60], with multicenter registries currently being created to better study this treatment strategy.

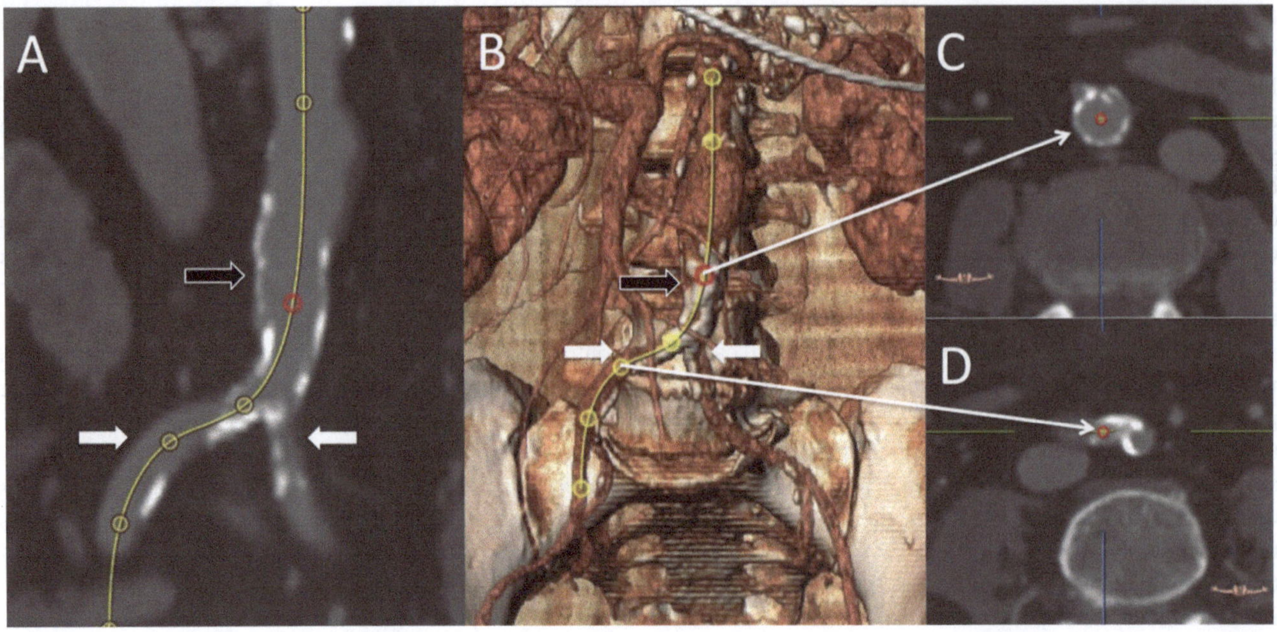

Fig. 2.3 Evaluation of vascular calcification during preprocedural planning for transcatheter aortic valve replacement. Coronal view (**a**) and 3D-reconstruction (**b**) of the abdominal aorta (*black arrows*) and iliac arteries (*white arrows*) allows for visual determination of calcification. The size of the vessels can then be determined from the transverse plane (**c**, **d** transverse plane of locations with severe vessel calcification)

Fig. 2.5 Multidetector cardiac computed tomography for the planning of percutaneous mitral valve intervention, reveals posterior mitral annular calcification (MAC, *white arrows* **a**, **b**) and descending aorta calcification (*gray arrow*, **b**)

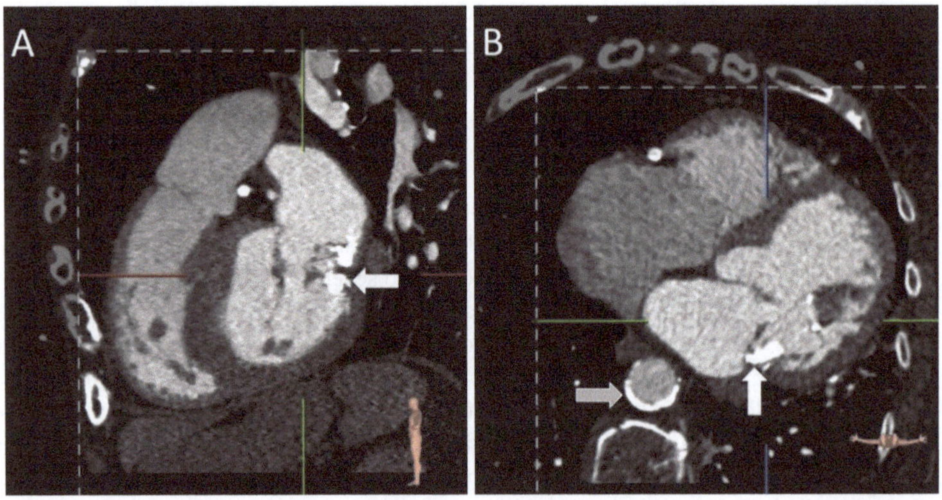

Fig. 2.4 Multidetector cardiac computed tomography revealing severe focal calcification (*arrows*) of the aortic annulus (**a**) and left ventricular outflow track (LVOT, **b**). These calcifications can be related to worse outcomes after surgical or transcatheter aortic valve replacement

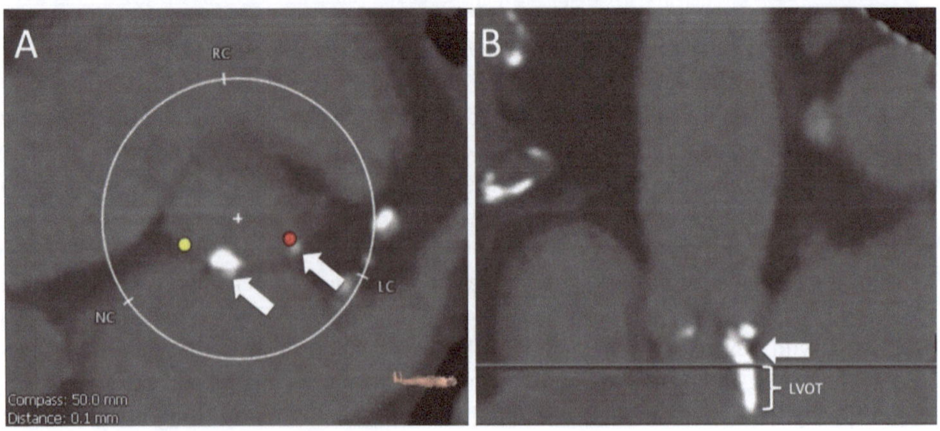

Conclusion

Vascular and valvular calcification in CKD is associated with increase CVD burden, and worse outcomes after coronary reperfusion or valve replacement, respectively. Though calcification in these patients is multifactorial, aggressive control of traditional and nontraditional risk factors can help prevent and slow the progression of disease. However, in those patients requiring intervention for CAD or valvopathy, a multidisciplinary team evaluation is critical to improve outcomes.

Disclosures Vasilis Babaliaros, MD is a consultant and/or has conducted research for Edwards Lifesciences, Medtronic, St. Jude Medical, Boston Scientific, Abbott Medical, and DirectFlow Medical. The other authors have nothing to disclose.

References

1. Gansevoort RT, Correa-Rotter R, Hemmelgarn BR, Jafar TH, Heerspink HJ, Mann JF, et al. Chronic kidney disease and cardiovascular risk: epidemiology, mechanisms, and prevention. Lancet. 2013;382(9889):339–52.
2. Chen NX, Moe SM. Pathophysiology of Vascular Calcification. Curr Osteoporos Rep. 2015;13(6):372–80.
3. Goodman WG, London G, Amann K, Block GA, Giachelli C, Hruska KA, et al. Vascular calcification in chronic kidney disease. Am J Kidney Dis. 2004;43(3):572–9.
4. Shroff R, Long DA, Shanahan C. Mechanistic insights into vascular calcification in CKD. J Am Soc Nephrol. 2013;24(2):179–89.
5. Shroff RC, Shanahan CM. The vascular biology of calcification. Semin Dial. 2007;20(2):103–9.
6. Chen NX, Moe SM. Vascular calcification: pathophysiology and risk factors. Curr Hypertens Rep. 2012;14(3):228–37.
7. Blaha MJ, Budoff MJ, Rivera JJ, Khan AN, Santos RD, Shaw LJ, et al. Relation of aortic valve calcium detected by cardiac computed tomography to all-cause mortality. Am J Cardiol. 2010;106(12):1787–91.
8. Fox CS, Vasan RS, Parise H, Levy D, O'Donnell CJ, D'Agostino RB, et al. Mitral annular calcification predicts cardiovascular morbidity and mortality: the Framingham Heart Study. Circulation. 2003;107(11):1492–6.
9. Senkottaiyan N, Hafidh S, Manian FA, Alpert MA. Valvular and perivalvular involvement in patients with chronic kidney disease. 老年心脏病学杂志 (英文版) ISTIC. 2005;2(3).
10. Umana E, Ahmed W, Alpert MA. Valvular and perivalvular abnormalities in end-stage renal disease. Am J Med Sci. 2003;325(4):237–42.
11. Fulkerson PK, Beaver BM, Auseon JC, Graber HL. Calcification of the mitral annulus: etiology, clinical associations, complications and therapy. Am J Med. 1979;66(6):967–77.
12. Maher ER, Young G, Smyth-Walsh B, Pugh S, Curtis JR. Aortic and mitral valve calcification in patients with end-stage renal disease. Lancet. 1987;2(8564):875–7.
13. Ritschard T, Blumberg A, Jenzer HR. Mitral annular calcification in dialysis patients. Schweiz Med Wochenschr. 1987;117(37):1363–7.
14. Moe SM, Chen NX. Pathophysiology of vascular calcification in chronic kidney disease. Circ Res. 2004;95(6):560–7.
15. Disthabanchong S. Vascular calcification in chronic kidney disease: Pathogenesis and clinical implication. World J Nephrol. 2012;1(2):43–53.
16. Proudfoot D, Shanahan CM. Biology of calcification in vascular cells: intima versus media. Herz. 2001;26(4):245–51.
17. Pai AS, Giachelli CM. Matrix remodeling in vascular calcification associated with chronic kidney disease. J Am Soc Nephrol. 2010;21(10):1637–40.
18. Chung AW, Yang HH, Kim JM, Sigrist MK, Chum E, Gourlay WA, et al. Upregulation of matrix metalloproteinase-2 in the arterial vasculature contributes to stiffening and vasomotor dysfunction in patients with chronic kidney disease. Circulation. 2009;120(9):792–801.
19. Moe SM, Chen NX. Mechanisms of vascular calcification in chronic kidney disease. J Am Soc Nephrol. 2008;19(2):213–6.
20. Schoppet M, Shroff RC, Hofbauer LC, Shanahan CM. Exploring the biology of vascular calcification in chronic kidney disease: what's circulating? Kidney Int. 2008;73(4):384–90.
21. Tyson KL, Reynolds JL, McNair R, Zhang Q, Weissberg PL, Shanahan CM. Osteo/chondrocytic transcription factors and their target genes exhibit distinct patterns of expression in human arterial calcification. Arterioscler Thromb Vasc Biol. 2003;23(3):489–94.
22. Mohler ER 3rd, Gannon F, Reynolds C, Zimmerman R, Keane MG, Kaplan FS. Bone formation and inflammation in cardiac valves. Circulation. 2001;103(11):1522–8.
23. Leskinen Y, Paana T, Saha H, Groundstroem K, Lehtimaki T, Kilpinen S, et al. Valvular calcification and its relationship to atherosclerosis in chronic kidney disease. J Heart Valve Dis. 2009;18(4):429–38.
24. London GM, Guerin AP, Marchais SJ, Metivier F, Pannier B, Adda H. Arterial media calcification in end-stage renal disease: impact on all-cause and cardiovascular mortality. Nephrol Dial Transplant. 2003;18(9):1731–40.
25. Smith JC, Page MD, John R, Wheeler MH, Cockcroft JR, Scanlon MF, et al. Augmentation of central arterial pressure in mild primary hyperparathyroidism. J Clin Endocrinol Metab. 2000;85(10):3515–9.
26. Block GA. Prevalence and clinical consequences of elevated Ca × P product in hemodialysis patients. Clin Nephrol. 2000;54(4):318–24.
27. Andress DL. Adynamic bone in patients with chronic kidney disease. Kidney Int. 2008;73(12):1345–54.
28. Coen G. Adynamic bone disease: an update and overview. J Nephrol. 2005;18(2):117–22.
29. Giachelli CM. The emerging role of phosphate in vascular calcification. Kidney Int. 2009;75(9):890–7.
30. Shanahan CM, Crouthamel MH, Kapustin A, Giachelli CM. Arterial calcification in chronic kidney disease: key roles for calcium and phosphate. Circ Res. 2011;109(6):697–711.
31. Reynolds JL, Skepper JN, McNair R, Kasama T, Gupta K, Weissberg PL, et al. Multifunctional roles for serum protein fetuin-a in inhibition of human vascular smooth muscle cell calcification. J Am Soc Nephrol. 2005;16(10):2920–30.
32. Palaniswamy C, Sekhri A, Aronow WS, Kalra A, Peterson SJ. Association of warfarin use with valvular and vascular calcification: a review. Clin Cardiol. 2011;34(2):74–81.
33. McCabe KM, Booth SL, Fu X, Shobeiri N, Pang JJ, Adams MA, et al. Dietary vitamin K and therapeutic warfarin alter the susceptibility to vascular calcification in experimental chronic kidney disease. Kidney Int. 2013;83(5):835–44.
34. O'Neill WC, Sigrist MK, McIntyre CW. Plasma pyrophosphate and vascular calcification in chronic kidney disease. Nephrol Dial Transplant. 2010;25(1):187–91.
35. Peiskerova M, Kalousova M, Kratochvilova M, Dusilova-Sulkova S, Uhrova J, Bandur S, et al. Fibroblast growth factor 23 and matrix-metalloproteinases in patients with chronic kidney disease: Are they associated with cardiovascular disease? Kidney Blood Press Res. 2009;32(4):276–83.

36. Anand N, Chandrasekaran SC, Alam MN. The malnutrition inflammation complex syndrome-the micsing factor in the perio-chronic kidney disease interlink. J Clin Diagn Res. 2013;7 (4):763–7.
37. Weiner DE, Tighiouart H, Stark PC, Amin MG, MacLeod B, Griffith JL, et al. Kidney disease as a risk factor for recurrent cardiovascular disease and mortality. Am J Kidney Dis. 2004;44(2): 198–206.
38. Marwick TH, Steinmuller DR, Underwood DA, Hobbs RE, Go RT, Swift C, et al. Ineffectiveness of dipyridamole SPECT thallium imaging as a screening technique for coronary artery disease in patients with end-stage renal failure. Transplantation. 1990;49(1):100–3.
39. Holley JL, Fenton RA, Arthur RS. Thallium stress testing does not predict cardiovascular risk in diabetic patients with end-stage renal disease undergoing cadaveric renal transplantation. Am J Med. 1991;90(5):563–70.
40. De Lima JJ, Sabbaga E, Vieira ML, de Paula FJ, Ianhez LE, Krieger EM, et al. Coronary angiography is the best predictor of events in renal transplant candidates compared with noninvasive testing. Hypertension. 2003;42(3):263–8.
41. Brar SS, Aharonian V, Mansukhani P, Moore N, Shen AY, Jorgensen M, et al. Haemodynamic-guided fluid administration for the prevention of contrast-induced acute kidney injury: the POSEIDON randomised controlled trial. Lancet. 2014;383 (9931):1814–23.
42. Wright RS, Reeder GS, Herzog CA, Albright RC, Williams BA, Dvorak DL, et al. Acute myocardial infarction and renal dysfunction: a high-risk combination. Ann Intern Med. 2002;137(7):563–70.
43. Medi C, Montalescot G, Budaj A, Fox KA, Lopez-Sendon J, FitzGerald G, et al. Reperfusion in patients with renal dysfunction after presentation with ST-segment elevation or left bundle branch block: GRACE (Global Registry of Acute Coronary Events). JACC Cardiovasc Interv. 2009;2(1):26–33.
44. Morel O, El Ghannudi S, Jesel L, Radulescu B, Meyer N, Wiesel ML, et al. Cardiovascular mortality in chronic kidney disease patients undergoing percutaneous coronary intervention is mainly related to impaired P2Y12 inhibition by clopidogrel. J Am Coll Cardiol. 2011;57(4):399–408.
45. Cooper WA, O'Brien SM, Thourani VH, Guyton RA, Bridges CR, Szczech LA, et al. Impact of renal dysfunction on outcomes of coronary artery bypass surgery: results from the Society of Thoracic Surgeons National Adult Cardiac Database. Circulation. 2006;113(8):1063–70.
46. Patel VI, Mukhopadhyay S, Guest JM, Conrad MF, Watkins MT, Kwolek CJ, et al. Impact of severe chronic kidney disease on outcomes of infrainguinal peripheral arterial intervention. J Vasc Surg. 2014;59(2):368–75.
47. Saweirs WW, Goddard J. What are the best treatments for early chronic kidney disease? A background paper prepared for the UK Consensus Conference on early chronic kidney disease. Nephrol Dial Transplant. 2007;22(Suppl. 9):ix31–8.
48. Langham RG, Bellomo R, D'Intini V, Endre Z, Hickey BB, McGuinness S, et al. KHA-CARI guideline: KHA-CARI adaptation of the KDIGO Clinical Practice Guideline for Acute Kidney Injury. Nephrology. 2014;19(5):261–5.
49. Raggi P, Chertow GM, Torres PU, Csiky B, Naso A, Nossuli K, et al. The ADVANCE study: a randomized study to evaluate the effects of cinacalcet plus low-dose vitamin D on vascular calcification in patients on hemodialysis. Nephrol Dial Transplant. 2011;26(4):1327–39.
50. Go AS, Chertow GM, Fan D, McCulloch CE, Hsu CY. Chronic kidney disease and the risks of death, cardiovascular events, and hospitalization. N Engl J Med. 2004;351(13):1296–305.
51. Excerpts from the United states renal data system 1998 annual data report. Am J Kidney Dis. 1998;32(2 Suppl 1):S1–162.
52. Urena P, Malergue MC, Goldfarb B, Prieur P, Guedon-Rapoud C, Petrover M. Evolutive aortic stenosis in hemodialysis patients: analysis of risk factors. Nephrologie. 1999;20(4):217–25.
53. Brennan JM, Edwards FH, Zhao Y, O'Brien SM, Douglas PS, Peterson ED, et al. Long-term survival after aortic valve replacement among high-risk elderly patients in the United States: insights from the Society of Thoracic Surgeons Adult Cardiac Surgery Database, 1991 to 2007. Circulation. 2012;126(13):1621–9.
54. Nguyen TC, Babaliaros VC, Razavi SA, Kilgo PD, Guyton RA, Devireddy CM, et al. Impact of varying degrees of renal dysfunction on transcatheter and surgical aortic valve replacement. J Thorac Cardiovasc Surg. 2013;146(6):1399–406 (discussion 13406–13407).
55. Thourani VH, Li C, Devireddy C, Jensen HA, Kilgo P, Leshnower BG, et al. High-risk patients with inoperative aortic stenosis: use of transapical, transaortic, and transcarotid techniques. Ann Thorac Surg. 2015;99(3):817–23 (discussion 23–25).
56. Nazif TM, Dizon JM, Hahn RT, Xu K, Babaliaros V, Douglas PS, et al. Predictors and clinical outcomes of permanent pacemaker implantation after transcatheter aortic valve replacement: the PARTNER (Placement of AoRtic TraNscathetER Valves) trial and registry. JACC Cardiovasc Interv. 2015;8(1 Pt A):60–9.
57. Jilaihawi H, Kashif M, Fontana G, Furugen A, Shiota T, Friede G, et al. Cross-sectional computed tomographic assessment improves accuracy of aortic annular sizing for transcatheter aortic valve replacement and reduces the incidence of paravalvular aortic regurgitation. J Am Coll Cardiol. 2012;59(14):1275–86.
58. Okada Y. Surgical management of mitral annular calcification. Gen Thorac Cardiovasc Surg. 2013;61(11):619–25.
59. Himbert D, Bouleti C, Iung B, Nejjari M, Brochet E, Depoix JP, et al. Transcatheter valve replacement in patients with severe mitral valve disease and annular calcification. J Am Coll Cardiol. 2014;64(23):2557–8.
60. Fassa AA, Himbert D, Brochet E, Depoix JP, Cheong AP, Alkhoder S, et al. Transseptal transcatheter mitral valve implantation for severely calcified mitral stenosis. JACC Cardiovasc Interv. 2014;7(6):696–7.

Sudden Cardiac Death in CKD and ESKD: Risk Factors, Mechanisms, and Therapeutic Strategies

3

Darren Green, Diana Y.Y. Chiu, and Philip A. Kalra

Introduction

Sudden cardiac death (SCD) is thought to be the leading cause of death in end-stage kidney disease (ESKD), accounting for as much as one in four deaths in this population. A comparison of the event rate for leading causes of death in ESKD is found in Fig. 3.1. Evidence is emerging that SCD in ESKD is not predominantly due to atherosclerotic coronary artery disease (CAD), unlike the case in the general population. This chapter details non-atherosclerotic risk factors for SCD in ESKD, and discusses the limitations of this evidence base which derives from differences in how SCD is defined in ESKD compared to the general population. The chapter also outlines mechanistic theories based on these risk factors, and discusses possible therapeutic strategies for population-specific SCD risk reduction in ESKD.

Defining Sudden Cardiac Death and Establishing Risk Factors

Although it is generally agreed that SCD is common in dialysis patients [1, 2] there is less clarity regarding the event rate and associated factors, and thereby also mechanism. Although these vary between studies because of variation in population characteristics and methodology, the terms and definitions used in describing the phenomenon of SCD differ significantly between studies investigating the problem, limiting epidemiological accuracy. Titles of published works have included the terms "sudden death" [3], "sudden cardiac death" [4], "sudden cardiac arrest" [5], "sudden and cardiac death" [6], "cardiac arrest" [7], or "cardiac arrest and sudden death" [8]. Although addressing similar questions, the differences in definition prevent direct comparison. Compounding this is lack of consistency in the definitions of both "sudden" and "cardiac". "Sudden" may refer to death within one or 24 h of onset of symptoms [9, 10], or simply indicate that someone suffered cardiac arrest [11]. "Cardiac" is not always included in the defining term.

As a result, there is uncertainty regarding the true size, nature, and causation of the problem in ESKD. For example, the reported proportion of dialysis patient deaths due to SCD ranges from 19 to 39% [6, 9], with an incredibly wide event rate range of 4–58 deaths per 1000 patient years [12, 13]. There are also differences in the clinical parameters associated with SCD. Whilst some studies concur with the general population finding that CAD and heart failure are associated with SCD, others do not. Left ventricular hypertrophy, inflammation, vitamin D deficiency, hyper- and hypotension have also been found in association with SCD in ESKD. These variations are summarised in Table 3.1, and the mechanistics of the more prominent risk factors are discussed below. Of note, of the 12 studies in Table 3.1, only two specify that SCD needed be due to a cardiac cause, underlining the point about lack of clarity of definition.

Historically, varying definitions of SCD were also used in studies of the general population [14–16]. As epidemiological and pathophysiological understanding improved there was convergence towards a more homogenous definition. SCD is now generally agreed to refer to death or survived cardiac arrest which is due to a cardiac cause, and either occurs within an hour of onset of symptoms, or is unwitnessed in a previously well patient [17].

This definition is based on the findings of Hinkle and Thaler, who, in their landmark paper, compared the duration of terminal acute illnesses in arrhythmic death versus death due to circulatory collapse. Here, 93% of terminal illnesses of <1 h duration resulted in arrhythmic deaths, and 74% that

D. Green (✉) · D.Y.Y. Chiu · P.A. Kalra
Department of Renal Medicine, Salford Royal NHS Foundation Trust, Stott Lane, Salford, M6 8HD, UK
e-mail: darrengreen@doctors.org.uk

D.Y.Y. Chiu
e-mail: diana_y_y_chiu@hotmail.com

P.A. Kalra
e-mail: philip.kalra@srft.nhs.uk

J. Rangaswami et al. (eds.), *Cardio-Nephrology*,
DOI 10.1007/978-3-319-56042-7_3

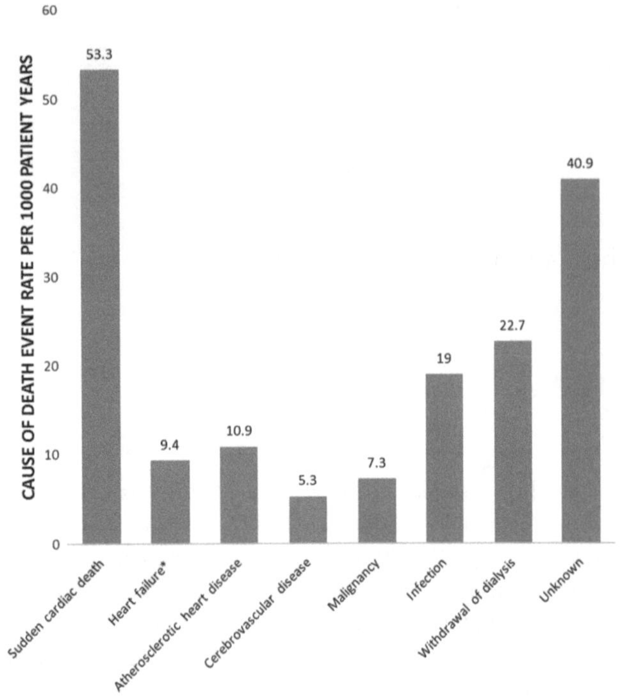

Fig. 3.1 SCD event rate in ESKD compared to other causes of death [12]

lasted >1 day led to death from circulatory failure. 88% of out of hospital deaths were arrhythmic compared with 29% of in-patient deaths. 90% of deaths due to heart disease were arrhythmic, compared with 14% in deaths due to causes other than heart disease. Using the Hinkle and Thaler classification, 11–13% of people in the Western world will die suddenly [15]. SCD, when defined in this way by the speed of onset of terminal illness, is all but synonymous with arrhythmic death and development of interventional strategy can then focus singularly on arrhythmia prevention and management. For example, we know that 80% of SCD in the general population is due to a ventricular tachyarrhythmia. This has led to a proven benefit of implantable cardioverter-defibrillator devices (ICDs) [18–20].

However, although cardiac disease accounts for approximately 80% of SCD, other less common causes include conditions which precipitate death via respiratory arrest such as epilepsy [21], and asthma [22]. This highlights two hurdles faced by nephrologists when investigating SCD in ESKD. Primarily, not specifying that sudden death must be of cardiac origin (Table 3.1) will produce a heterogeneous mix of causes of death and prevent effective single strategy investigation and management. Second, although Hinkle and Thaler used time as a means to differentiate between arrhythmic death and circulatory collapse, using such a definition in ESKD patients may not be able to do this. This is because circulatory collapse in ESKD may be profound and sudden and due to other causes. Any combination of dialysis ultrafiltration, fluid restriction, increased arterial vascular stiffness, loss of autonomic tone, non-ischemic cardiomyopathy, the use of anti-hypertensive agents, anemia, and greater risk of infection and haemorrhage may combine to produce catastrophic circulatory collapse and sudden death which is not of arrhythmic origin. For example, in an analysis of dialysis patient postmortems, 35 of 93 deaths were sudden and the only cause of death more common in those deaths that were sudden compared to those that were not was a ruptured aortic aneurysm [10]. Therefore, to include all ESKD sudden deaths in a single epidemiological model will include a variety of pathological processes which are unlikely to fit into the same risk stratification and management model.

SCD Event Rate in ESKD

The SCD rate in the general population is 1 per 1000 patient years [17]. In post-MI patients with left ventricular ejection fraction <35% the rate is 90–200 per 1000 patient years [15, 17]. Data from the United States Renal Data System (USRDS) place the SCD event rate at 7 per 1000 patient years in pre-dialysis chronic kidney disease (CKD) [23, 24], and 50–200 per 1000 patient years in dialysis patients depending, on comorbidities and duration of dialysis history [12]. A comparison of SCD event rate in ESKD, pre-dialysis CKD, transplantation, and other non-CKD populations is found in Fig. 3.2. Historically, the USRDS defined SCD as death due to either cardiac arrest or primary arrhythmia. The source data is based on diagnosis coding returns from the United States Department of Health and Human Services form 2746: ESRD death notification.

Because of the different definitions, direct comparison between CKD and general populations is difficult. USRDS data suggest that the risk of arrhythmic death in dialysis patients is equivalent to that of a post-MI patient with severe left ventricular dysfunction, but that the risk in CKD patients who are not on dialysis is close to that in the general population. In the general population, SCD accounts for half of all deaths due to coronary artery disease (CAD), and is highest in the 2 years after suffering a myocardial infarction [25].

More recently, the USRDS has revised its definition to specify that SCDs should be due to a primary cardiac cause. However, the newer definition uses the same coding data to determine event rate [26], and this is devoid of independent adjudication. A study that compared the old and new USRDS definitions identified verified, witnessed sudden cardiac deaths. It described sensitivities in correctly identifying any death as being SCD using coding data of 71 versus 84% respectively for the old and new definitions. However, the study did not describe the false positive rate associated

Table 3.1 A comparison of the terms and definition used in different studies of sudden deaths in dialysis patients, and the associated variation in event rate and predictive factors

	Terminology	Definition		Population	Percentage of deaths	Incidence per 1000 pt years	Factors associated with SCD
		Sudden	Cardiac				
Takeda, 1997 [10]	Sudden death	<24 h	Not specified	"Dialysis"	37	N/a	Aortic aneurysm rupture more common in sudden death
Paoletti, 2004 [36]	SCD	Not specified	Not specified	HD > 6 months	19	13% of pp over 10 years	Increasing left ventricular mass index
Bleyer, 2006 [3]	Sudden death	<1 h	Unexpected, non-traumatic	HD	39	N/a	Heart failure or coronary artery disease
Parekh, 2008 [83]	SCD	Not specified	Out of hospital death due to ICD-10 cardiac diseases.	"Dialysis"	22	37	CRP, IL-6, low albumin
USRDS, 2009+ [12]	Cardiac arrest, SCD	Not specified	"Cardiac arrest" or "arrhythmia"	HD	26	58	–
Genovesi, 2009 [9]	Sudden death	<1 h	Unexpected natural death	HD	19	7% over mean 3 years	Atrial fibrillation, diabetes, hyperkalaemia, CRP
Wang, 2010 [84]	SCD	<1 h	Not specified, discounted if aetiology established before death	PD	24	24% of pp over 5 years	Poor LVEF, systolic hypertension, diastolic hypotension
De Lima, 2010 [13]	Unexplained sudden death	<1 h	"Unexplained"	HD on Tx waiting list	20	4	"Any cardiovascular disease" only independent predictor
Dreschler, 2010 [85] & 2011 [4]	SCD	<1 h or "unexpected"	Confirmed arrhythmia or death after onset of cardiac symptoms.	Diabetic HD	27	45	Vitamin D deficiency and low homoarginine
Matsue, 2011 [62]	SCD	<1 h	"Unexpected" or autopsy findings consistent with SCD	HD > 3 months	27	9.5% over mean 4.9 years	BB use associated with lower rate of SCD
Shastri, 2012 [86]	SCD	<24 h or since last HD session if unwitnessed	Arrhythmia, CAD, or other cardiac disease	HD	22	10.4% over median 2.5 years	Age, diabetes, CAD, PVD, creatinine, alkaline phosphatase

Key SCD sudden cardiac death, *HD* haemodialysis, *PD* peritoneal dialysis, *ICD* international classification of diseases, *USRDS* United States Renal Data System, *LVMI* left ventricular mass index, *CAD* coronary artery disease, *CRP* C-reactive protein, *BB* beta-blocker, *PVD* peripheral vascular disease, *LVEF* left ventricular ejection fraction, *Tx* transplant, *IL* interleukin, *pp* prevalent population

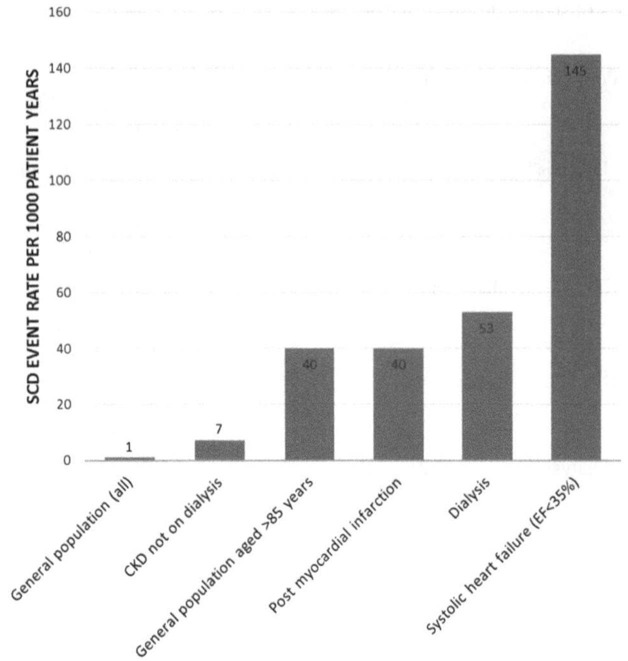

Fig. 3.2 SCD event rate in ESKD compared to other CKD and high-risk population [17]

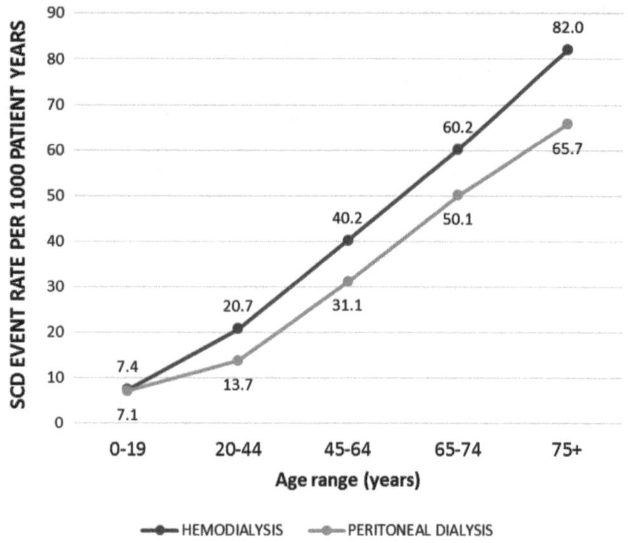

Fig. 3.3 Age and dialysis modality differences in SCD event rate [12]

with either definition. Thus, there is still uncertainty as to whether the rate of true SCD is as high as reports suggest.

Associated Factors and Mechanistic Hypotheses

Age

Older age is an independent risk factor for SCD in all populations. In the general population as a whole, the event rate is 1–2 per 1000 patient years, whereas in people aged >85 years it is 40 per 1000 patient years [17]. According to the USRDS, when using arrhythmia + cardiac arrest as a definition of SCD, the event rate rises from 21 per 1000 patient years in ESKD patients aged 20–44 years to 82 per 1000 patient years in patients aged >75 years (Fig. 3.3) [12]. In a multivariate model of risk prediction for SCD in a haemodialysis population of 1745 (mean age 62 ± 11 years) there was an increase in risk of SCD of 1.31 (1.08–1.59) for every standard deviation increase in age (which was 11 years) [27].

Coronary Artery Disease

SCD in the general population is most often due to CAD, but CAD is not often implicated in ESKD. This is despite up to 38% of the prevalent dialysis population having evidence of CAD [28]. One study noted that CAD was present in 56.3% of hemodialysis patients who died suddenly, but this greater prevalence did not reach statistical significance [29]. Another study of 93 postmortems performed on dialysis patients found that cerebrovascular disease was more common than CAD in sudden death victims (sudden defined as within 24 h of onset) with figures of 26 versus 14% respectively [10]. In that analysis, only four sudden deaths (12%) were deemed to be due to CAD.

Diabetes Mellitus

Diabetes is associated with sudden death independent of its causative association with CAD and CKD. This is often referred to as the "dead in bed" syndrome [30]. It is thought to be arrhythmic in origin, caused by nocturnal hypoglycaemia with consequent prolongation of the QT_c [30]. However, in an analysis of postmortems undertaken in diabetic patients who died suddenly, all cases had evidence of CAD. Perhaps of no surprise, diabetic nephropathy has also been shown to be an independent risk factor for SCD in a diabetic population [31].

The mechanism of SCD in diabetics, particularly those with CKD, may extend beyond CAD and hypoglycaemia. Cardiac autonomic neuropathy is proposed to expose patients to an increased risk of SCD, evidenced indirectly by loss of heart rate variability (HRV) on ECG. Autonomic neuropathy is associated with both diabetes and uremia, and in the former case at least, is a microvascular phenomenon [32]. In a study of 196 haemodialysis patients with left ventricular hypertrophy, SCD-free survival in patients with abnormal HRV was 29%, compared with 98% in those without, over a mean follow up of 4.5 ± 1.9 years [33].

Left Ventricular Hypertrophy

Left ventricular hypertrophy (LVH) is an established risk factor for SCD in the general population [34]. However, treatment algorithms have yet to incorporate this finding other than for inherited hypertrophic cardiomyopathy. The association of LVH with SCD in ESKD is less clear. Indeed, many studies which use multivariate models to determine independent risk factors have failed to show LVH as being one. LVH is associated with greater risk of intra-dialytic ectopy [35], but this phenomenon again does not necessarily indicate increased risk of SCD. The mechanism by which LVH leads to ectopy, arrhythmia, and SCD is likely to be via the abnormal fibrotic myocardial remodelling found in pathological LVH.

In one study of 123 dialysis patients, longitudinal increase in echocardiographic LV mass index was a better predictor of SCD than CAD, but the absolute value of indexed LV mass LVH was not [36]. Conversely, an ECG sub-study of the 4D trial demonstrated that electrocardiographic evidence of LVH does predispose to a greater risk of SCD. This latter study was better powered (1253 patients) and this may go some way to explain the different findings, although the patients in 4D were all diabetic [37].

Factors associated with LVH in ESKD include hypertension, volume overload, and chronic inflammation, i.e. other clinical factors which themselves predispose to increased cardiovascular risk. It is not clear whether it is the pathology of LVH or a specific underlying condition that results in LVH which is causative of SCD, and so it is not certain that any future therapies which may directly inhibit hypertrophic remodelling would benefit ESKD patients. A demonstration of the broad and overlapping pathological contributors to SCD in ESKD is found in Fig. 3.4. Furthermore, as many as 74% of haemodialysis patients have LVH at the initiation of chronic dialysis [38], indicating that any effort geared towards primary prevention of SCD by addressing LVH would actually require much earlier intervention during pre-dialysis CKD or even earlier in the CKD continuum.

Dialysis and Dialysis Modality

Figure 3.3 demonstrates the greater risk of SCD faced by haemodialysis patients compared to peritoneal dialysis patients. For patients aged 45–64 years, the haemodialysis SCD event rate is 40 per 1000 patient years compared to 31 events per 1000 years in peritoneal dialysis [12]. This indicates that there are both common uremic factors which lead to a high risk for both groups, but also that there are haemodialysis specific SCD risk factors.

Cardiac arrest is more common on a dialysis day than a day after dialysis [39]. Echocardiographic and magnetic resonance studies have demonstrated that the process of dialysis itself can induce myocardial ischemia in patients with structural cardiac abnormalities. Dialysis-induced ischemia can contribute to long-term worsening of left ventricular systolic function, and worse prognosis [40]. Intradialytic myocardial ischemia may also manifest as ST-segment depression <1 mm. This has been shown to occur in up to 46% of haemodialysis patients, and arrhythmia are more common in patients who show ST depression during dialysis [41, 42]. There is debate as to whether this is a direct manifestation of underlying CAD and whether intradialytic ST-segment changes translate into greater cardiovascular morbidity [41, 43, 44].

Haemodialysis is also associated with increased frequency of Lown graded ventricular arrhythmia (grades 1–4a)

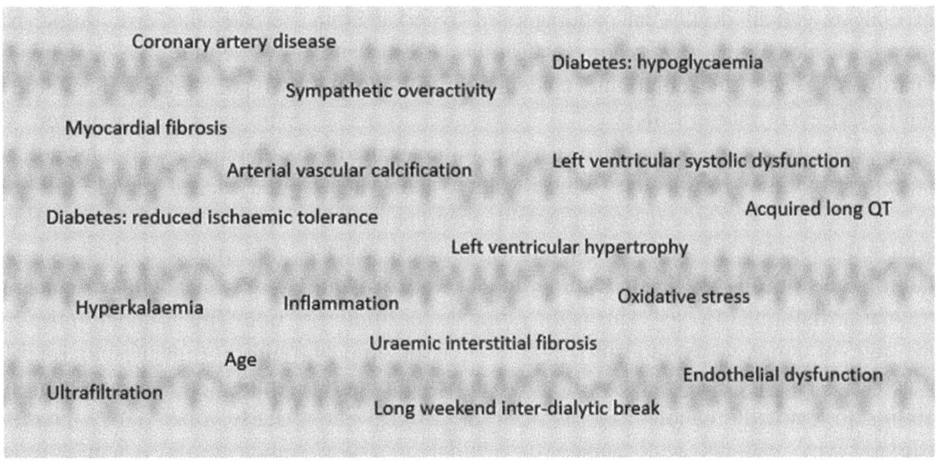

Fig. 3.4 Mechanistic contributions to SCD in ESK

[35]. These grades range from <30 ventricular ectopics per hour to ventricular couplets. However, these grades of arrhythmia are not proven precursors to fatal arrhythmic events.

Although the risk of SCD is high during or immediately after a haemodialysis session, for haemodialysis patients, cardiac arrest, and indeed all-cause mortality, is actually most common at the end of the long weekend inter-dialytic break, i.e. after a prolonged period without dialysis. For example, patients who dialyse on a Monday, Wednesday, Friday regime have an approximately 30% higher risk of cardiac arrest on Sunday compared to all other days [39]. It is likely that greater electrolyte and extracellular fluid accumulation during this time accounts for some of this greater risk.

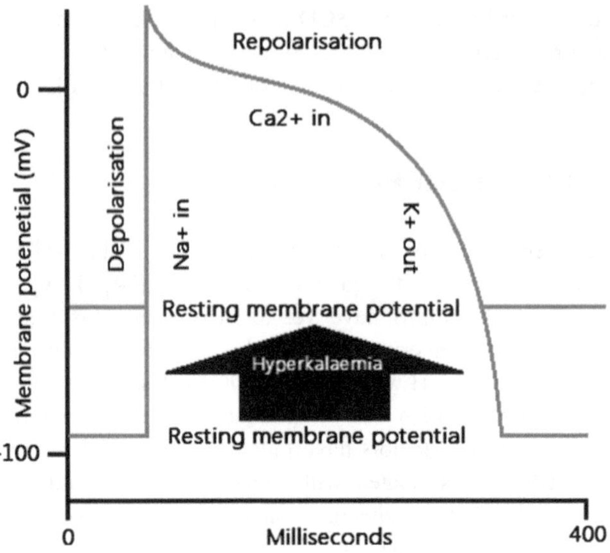

Fig. 3.5 Schematic representation of hyperkalaemia creating arrhythmic vulnerability by potentially destabilising repolarisation by creating a less negative membrane potential

Hyper- and Hypokalemia

Patients with CKD are at increased risk of hyperkalaemia. In a study of SCD in 476 haemodialysis patients, pre-dialytic hyperkalaemia was associated with a 2.7-fold increased risk (95% CI 1.3–5.9) of sudden death [9]. Haemodialysis patients are also at particular risk of post-dialysis hypokalaemia. Potassium is a key component of cardiac conduction given the role of potassium channels in establishing resting membrane potential. It is long established that both hypo- and hyperkalaemia predispose to arrhythmia, with typical ECG appearances for each that begin with changes to the repolarisation wave. The classical tented T-wave of hyperkalaemia is shorter and more peaked than a normal T-wave. This is because high extracellular potassium creates a less negative resting membrane potential and subsequently more rapid repolarisation than when there is a normal, more negative resting potential. Aberrancy of repolarisation is well established as a key period of high risk for onset of ventricular tachyarrhythmia (e.g. R on T phenomenon). The effect of hyperkalaemia on the repolarisation wave is shown in Fig. 3.5. Known hyperkalaemia is responsible for 1–2% of dialysis patient deaths, and undiagnosed hyperkalaemia may be responsible for some of the "cardiac arrest, cause unknown" events that contribute epidemiologically to the high SCD event rate in ESKD.

Importantly, the rate of change of potassium can predispose to arrhythmia, irrespective of the absolute value. This is the paradoxical Zwaardemaker–Libbrecht phenomenon, in which the rapid infusion of potassium to normalise circulating levels in a hypokalaemic animal model leads to ventricular arrhythmia [45, 46]. This is the rationale for limiting the rate of intravenous infusion of potassium in clinical practice. A high dietary intake of potassium without the ability to correctly handle this, as seen in ESKD, may explain why patients with apparently similar measured potassium can have markedly different ECG response. Alternatively, different patients may exhibit differences in vulnerability to the effects of potassium on arrhythmia risk. In one study of 145 ESKD patients, the threshold for developing T-wave abnormalities in hyperkalaemia varied between patients and was shown to be associated with an increased long-term risk of SCD [47].

Hypomagnesemia

Magnesium is necessary for function of the Na^+, K^+-ATPase in cardiac myocytes, and the classical arrhythmic effect of hypomagnesemia is torsades de pointes [48]. Preclinical ECG changes may manifest as QT_c prolongation, and tachycardia. Hypomagnesemia also inhibits effective action of K^+ channels elsewhere, such as in the kidneys, and this may exacerbate the arrhythmic potential of hypomagnesemia by worsening hypokalemia and preventing its treatment. Hypomagnesemia is more common in CKD and ESKD than the general population, and in hemodialysis patients is associated with a hazard ratio for all-cause mortality of 2.06 for each 1 mg/dL fall in serum magnesium [49]. In the hemodialysis setting, observational studies have shown that hypomagnesemia may worsen hyperparathyroidism, and is associated with vascular calcification and atheroma formation. This is underpinned by mechanistic demonstration of an effect of magnesium on calcium homeostasis, particularly by inhibition of calcium from the sarcoplasmic reticulum [50]. Early, open label interventional studies of <100 patients indicate the potential for magnesium supplementation as a therapeutic option in ESKD. For example, oral magnesium supplements given to hemodialysis patients may reduce calcification measured by surrogate endpoints such as carotid intimal medial thickening [51].

The mechanistic role of hypomagnesemia in sudden death is further confounded by how its effect on calcium handling may manifest as neurological as well as cardiac pathologies. In a rat model of magnesium deficient versus control animals, sudden death was not only provoked by rapid cardiac pacing and polymorphic VT, but also by auditory startle stimulus and consequent seizure activity [52].

In summary, hypomagnesemia may therefore be associated with sudden death by way of primary arrhythmia via an effect on myocyte electrolyte handling, ischaemia by provoking vascular calcification and atheroma, or even seizure activity by aberrant calcium homeostasis.

Therapeutic Strategies for SCD Prevention in ESKD

Implantable Cardioverter-Defibrillators (ICD)

First line therapy for both primary and secondary prevention of SCD in the general population is the use of implantable cardioverter-defibrillators (ICD) devices [53]. The indications for ICD target specific high-risk groups, most of whom will have ischemic cardiomyopathy but also including those with inherited or congenital conditions (see Fig. 3.6). In one study, 6.3% of the prevalent haemodialysis population fulfilled these criteria for ICD implantation but none had a device in situ. It is widely acknowledged that dialysis patients have a lower uptake of ICD than other patients groups. This is likely to be because the absolute risk reduction in life years after ICD in ESKD is lower than for other patients. In a meta-analysis of seven studies of ICD therapy in CKD (89 ESKD patients versus 2417 CKD stage 3 and 4 patients) the relative risk of all-cause death in dialysis patients with ICD was 1.62 (0.84–3.14, $p = 0.15$) compared to the CKD group [54].

However, this actually reflects the overall worse survival in ESKD anyway. The relative risk reduction for mortality after ICD in ESKD compared to life expectancy without treatment is 35–42%. Importantly, this is comparable to the relative risk reduction seen in the general population. It is for this reason that current guidelines specify that ESKD patients should not be excluded from consideration of ICD therapy.

The low uptake of ICD in this patient group is likely to be rationalised on the basis of higher complication rates and a reduced cost-effectiveness based on the lower absolute risk reduction discussed above. Haematoma, infection, thrombosis, lead dislodgement, and the need for explantation are higher in ESKD patients with pacing devices compared to the general population [55]. Furthermore, pacing devices require central venous access and in extreme cases will limit dialysis access options, or they will be precluded by occlusion of venous access incurred due to previous catheter use.

As well as worse survival, a different defibrillation threshold is thought to be a further reason for the lower absolute risk reduction after ICD implantation in ESKD [56, 57]. The most common cause of death in patients with ESKD who have an ICD in situ is still arrhythmia [58], and the proportion of arrhythmic deaths is higher than in non-ESKD ICD recipients. In one analysis, arrhythmia accounted for 38.2% of deaths in ESKD ICD patients, compared with 16% in non-dialysis ICD recipients ($n = 822$). It is hypothesised that this difference in defibrillation threshold may relate to the nature of the fibrotic cardiac remodelling in ESKD, or metabolic/electrolyte derangement associated with ESKD, most obviously hyper- and hypokalaemia, which is less often seen outside of this patient group [57].

Indeed, this latter comment highlights the key issue surrounding SCD in ESKD. Namely that the precipitants to arrhythmic death are often likely to be different in ESKD to the general population. We have noted that 6.3% of dialysis patients fulfil criteria for ICD based on conventional guidelines. However, as many as 28% of deaths in dialysis patient with preserved systolic function are due to SCD [59] and so SCD appears as common in dialysis patients who do not fulfil criteria for ICD as those that do. There are two contributory explanations. First, even in the general population, most SCD occurs in low-risk patients, i.e. it is the first presentation of coronary artery disease. Although SCD is relatively more likely in high-risk groups (90–200 events per 1000 patient years in post-MI severe systolic heart failure versus 1 per 1000 patients years in the general population), because so many more people are at low compared to high risk, these patients make for numerically relatively few SCD events. For example, of the approximate 450,000 SCD events per year (depending on exact definition) in the United States, <150,000 (33%) occur in patients who fulfil the criteria for ICD [17].

Second, as discussed above, the mechanism of arrhythmic risk in dialysis patients appears to be different. High-risk patients in the general population are most often those with severe left ventricular systolic function whereas dialysis patients with preserved systolic function have a five-year risk of SCD of up to 28% [59]. The notion that a dialysis patient specific set of criteria for ICD has led to RCT of ICD specifically in these patients outside of general population criteria. However, as yet none have reported their findings [60]. Furthermore, the inclusion criteria for trials such as ICD2 are largely inclusive despite the fact that it appears that the SCD event rate does not justify the global use of ICD

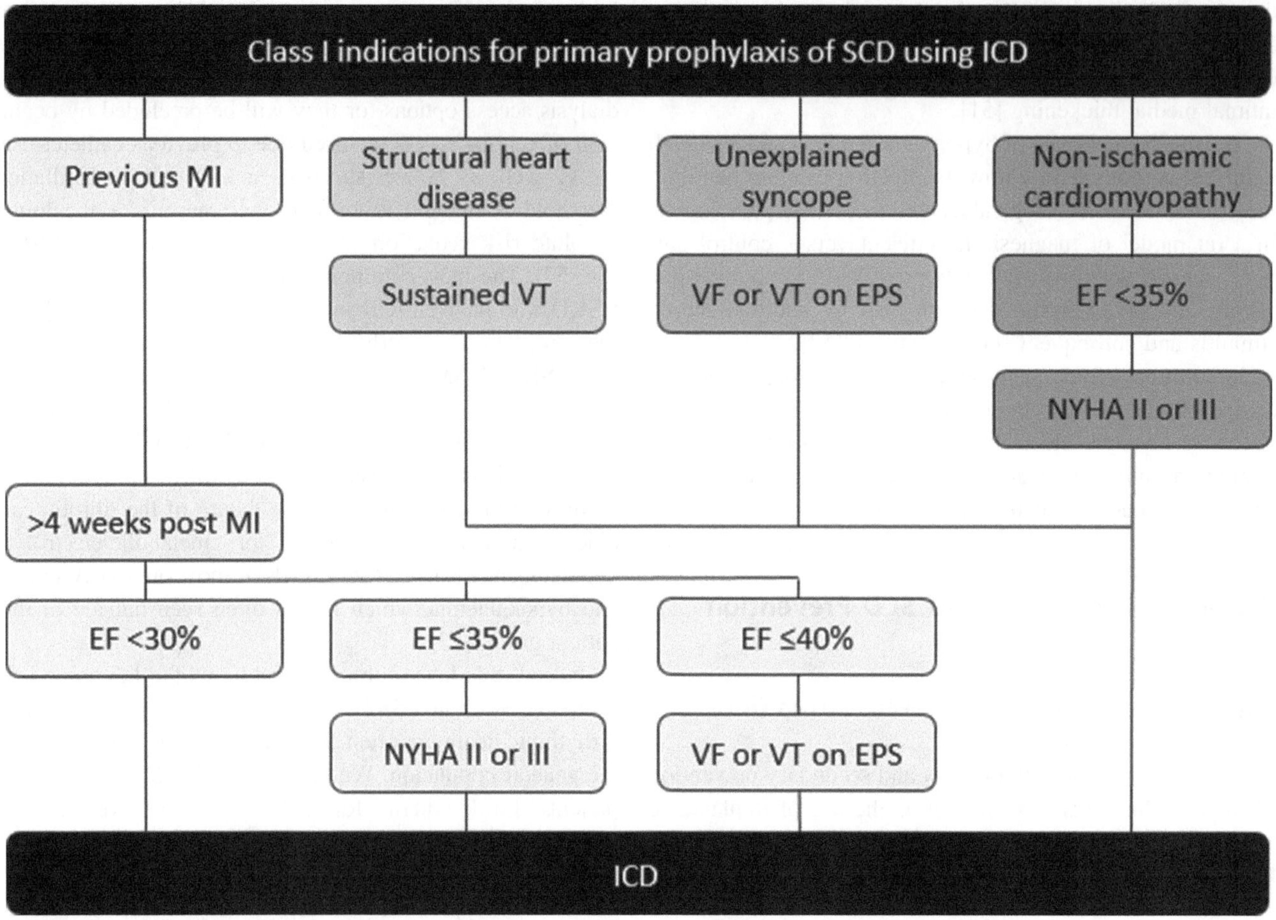

Fig. 3.6 Current guidelines for primary prevention of SCD using ICD in the general population

devices in dialysis patients. After all, these are not used routinely in all post-MI patients despite their comparable risk. Hence, the identification of the higher risk dialysis patients to develop an accurate risk stratification tool is still very much warranted.

Revascularisation for Coronary Atheroma

Coronary artery disease (CAD) is highly prevalent (38–40%) in ESKD but CAD revascularization, much as is the case for ICD therapy, is used less often as a therapeutic strategy in dialysis patients compared to the general population. In one study of 23,262 patients who had suffered non-ST elevation MI, 15% of ESKD patients (n = 278) were treated with PCI/CABG compared to 62% of patients with eGFR $\geq$ 90 mL/min/1.73 m^2 (n = 6064) [61]. In fact, 76% of ESKD patients did not even receive coronary angiography (compared to 18% of those with normal renal function). This is despite CAD having been shown to be the most significant predictor of SCD (HR 1.99, 95% CI 1.43–2.78, $p < 0.001$) in one study [62]. However, this more conservative approach in ESKD has a clinical rationale as there is no proven reduction in early mortality for revascularisation compared to medical management in ESKD (n = 268, HR 1.61, 95% CI 0.84–3.09, $p = 0.15$) [63]. Whether coronary artery bypass grafting (CABG) carries any SCD benefit is less apparent. It has been shown in a survival analysis of 5830 haemodialysis patients who underwent CABG that arrhythmia account for 14% of deaths in the first 2 years post-procedure. The unadjusted event free survival for arrhythmia or cardiac arrests in the first three years after CABG was 0.91, 0.86, and 0.81 for each year, respectively [64].

These data support the view that the mode of arrhythmic risk in ESKD carries components which are unrelated to coronary artery disease, the archetypal cause of SCD in the general population. Furthermore, even coronary artery disease may behave differently and has a different pathogenesis in ESKD compared to the general population with a likely non-atheromatous aetiology relating to factors such as arterial vascular calcification. Outside the limitations of benefit from coronary intervention discussed here, a further effect is noted in the limited benefit of lipid lowering therapy in

ESKD compared to non-dialysis CKD. In a meta-analysis of LLT versus placebo in ESKD, the number needed to treat to prevent 1 atherosclerotic cardiovascular event was 103 [65].

Beta-Blockade

The use of beta-blockers for SCD risk reduction in dialysis patients is underpinned by a small observational study showing a statistically significant reduction in event rate, and also supported by one randomised trial of 114 patients which showed a numerical reduction in SCD and statistical benefit in terms of cardiovascular endpoints [66]. All patients had New York Heart Association class II–III systolic heart failure (LVEF < 35%) for more than 1 year. Patients were randomised to carvedilol or placebo and followed up for 2 years [66]. There were fewer cardiovascular deaths in the carvedilol arm compared to placebo (29.3 vs. 67.9%, relative risk reduction 43.7%). The study was not powered to show a statistical difference in SCD event rate, and SCD events were few. However, there was a numerical benefit to beta-blocker therapy, with 2 versus 6 SCD events in the treatment and placebo arms, respectively ($p = 0.12$). In a retrospective analysis of 316 haemodialysis patients, those prescribed beta-blockers suffered fewer SCD events over a mean of 4.9 ± 1.9 years follow up (4 [$n = 80$] vs. 11% in patients not on beta-blockers [$n = 236$], $p = 0.047$) [67].

The apparent SCD related benefits of beta-blockers in ESKD may actually be by virtue of their effect as an anti-hypertensive agent and in slowing the progression of heart failure rather than due to a direct anti-arrhythmic effect. Nonetheless, beta-blockade would appear to be a sensible first line anti-hypertensive therapy in dialysis patients in the absence of high quality, well powered RCT data.

Despite this potential benefit, beta-blockers are perhaps underused in dialysis patients. In a cross-sectional study, only 40 of 89 (45%) haemodialysis patients with established CAD were prescribed beta-blockade [68]. This is despite the absence of significant evidence that relevant potential side effects of beta-blockers (bradycardia, hyperkalaemia, hypotension) are sufficiently common in haemodialysis patients to preclude their routine use [69].

A noteworthy exception which must be considered is sotalol. Sotalol is a non-selective beta-blocker which also has class III actions and which is primarily used in secondary prevention of ventricular arrhythmia. Sotalol is excreted via the kidneys and is dialysed. It carries a significant risk of causing torsades de pointes in cases of toxicity, in the presence of hypokalaemia, and where QT_c prolongation exists. It is generally advised that sotalol should be avoided in patients with eGFR <15 mL/min/1.73 m^2, although guidelines do specify that it can be considered if dosed at 25% of the dose recommended in cases of normal renal function. Given the risk of fluxes in potassium concentration and hypokalaemia associated with haemodialysis sessions, and of QT_c prolongation with many drugs prescribed in CKD and dialysis patients (macrolide antibiotics, quinines, benzodiazepines, co-trimoxazole, SSRIs, anti-histamines, calcineurin inhibitors), sotalol should perhaps be avoided in this setting.

Other Pharmacotherapeutic Options

In a retrospective study of 729 cardiac arrests suffered by haemodialysis patients, beta-blockers were associated with an adjusted survival benefit with an odds ratio of 0.32 (95% CI 0.17–0.61, $p = 0.0006$) for death at 6 months [7]. The same study showed a similar survival benefit for patients using calcium channel blockers (OR 0.42, 0.23–0.76, $p = 0.004$). Calcium channel blockers are known to be cardioprotective by way of preventing coronary artery spasm after cardiac arrest, potentially reducing ischaemic injury, and by normalising intracellular calcium concentration, potentially preventing life threatening arrhythmia [70]. Renin–angiotensin system blockade was also beneficial (OR 0.51, 0.28–0.95, $p = 0.03$).

A higher circulating aldosterone level is found in CKD [71] and is an independent risk factor for SCD in patients with eGFR <60 mL/min/1.73 m^2 (HR for SCD = 1.32 for each 50 ρg/mL increase in aldosterone, 95% CI 1.15–1.52, $p < 0.001$) [72]. In the general population, RAS blockade is associated with reduced risk of SCD in both primary and secondary prevention for CAD [73]. There are no comparable findings in ESKD, and a clinical trial has not shown any reduction in cardiovascular events and death in dialysis patients with use of ACE inhibitors. The Fosinopril in Dialysis Trial (FOSIDIAL) randomised 397 haemodialysis patients to fosinopril or placebo. After a 2-year follow-up period, the relative risk of cardiovascular events in the treatment arm was 0.93 (0.68–1.26), a non-significant finding [74]. An open label RCT of ARB therapy (candesartan) in 80 haemodialysis patients did show a significant reduction in cardiovascular events and improved survival in the treatment arm [75] after 19.4 ± 1.2 months follow-up [cardiovascular events in treatment arm 16% vs. placebo arm 46% ($p < 0.01$), mortality 0 vs. 19% ($p = 0.01$)]. Only 3 of the end points in this trial were SCD, but all occurred in the placebo arm. Whether the difference in trial findings between ARB and ACE inhibitors is due to a difference in drug class effect or trial design is not evident.

Similar to the effect of RAS blockade in the general population, the aldosterone receptor blocker spironolactone has been shown to reduce SCD. The Randomised Aldactone Evaluation Study (RALES Study) was a randomised trial of 1663 patients with moderate to severe systolic heart failure

(LVEF < 35%) comparing spironolactone with placebo. 48% of participants had CKD stage 3–5, although none were on dialysis. Treatment with spironolactone was associated with a relative risk of sudden death of 0.71 (0.54–0.95, $p = 0.02$) [76]. No comparable trial data exist for ESKD. This is perhaps because of the expectation of high risk for hyperkalaemia. However, a meta-analysis of six studies (7051 patients) of spironolactone use in ESKD showed that mean serum potassium was 4.9 mmol/L and that there were apparently no hyperkalaemic adverse events [77]. An RCT of mineralocorticoid blockade in haemodialysis patients is likely in the future [78], and mineralocorticoid therapy in ESKD may yet have a major beneficial role, provided close monitoring is place.

There is very limited evidence addressing SCD event rate in ESKD when using amiodarone, statins, aspirin, or digoxin and so these agents have not been specifically commented on.

Dialysis Prescription

After the long inter-dialytic weekend break, the next highest risk time point for death in haemodialysis patients is during the 12 h beginning at the start of a dialysis session. Haemodialysis is associated with rapid shifts in electrolytes and fluid, all of which offer a pathway to arrhythmia as discussed above. Amelioration of these dialysis-related changes thereby offers potential pathways to risk reduction.

In an observational study of 81,013 haemodialysis patients which compared mortality between patients based on pre-dialysis serum potassium concentration, the optimal range was found to be 4.6–5.3 mmol/L [79]. There was a J-shaped distribution of the mortality outcome with both hypo- and hyperkalaemia associated with worse cardiovascular survival, more so in hyperkalaemia. However, the approach to reducing risk in hyperkalaemic patients is likely to prove to be more complicated than simply using low potassium dialysate. This is because, in a review of 400 cardiac arrests on haemodialysis units, patients who were dialysed using a low potassium dialysate (0 or 1.0 mmol/L) were more likely to have had a cardiac arrest (17.1 vs. 8.8% for higher potassium dialysate) [8].

Cardiac conduction is also dependent on extracellular calcium. Low calcium dialysate (1.25 mmol/L) has been shown to associate with ECG abnormalities such as prolonged QTc and increased QT dispersion [80, 81]. This has, however, not yet translated into objective evidence of increased SCD risk. A further theoretical benefit of higher dialysate calcium is that higher serum calcium confers a degree of cardio-protection in cases of hyperkalaemia by stabilising the resting membrane potential (hence the established use of intravenous calcium bolus as a therapy in hyperkalaemia). Patients with hyperkalaemia who demonstrate T-wave tenting have been shown to have a numerically lower serum calcium than patients who do not manifest ECG changes (2.20 ± 0.16 vs. 2.27 ± 0.16 mmol/L, $p = 0.147$). It is perhaps therefore of value to avoid low serum calcium and low calcium dialysate for dialysis patients prone to hyperkalaemia.

In a comparison of 502 haemodialysis SCD victims versus age and dialysis duration matched controls, the SCD group were more likely to have high ultrafiltration volumes on dialysis (odds ratio 1.11, 95% CI 1.02–1.33, $p = 0.02$) [82]. Large volume ultrafiltration has been associated with intra-dialytic myocardial ischaemia, hypotension, and RWMA, all of which may reflect the evolving risk of myocardial injury that predisposes to arrhythmic death. In practical terms, severe fluid overload or acute pulmonary oedema may necessitate high volume fluid removal to prevent acute risk of morbidity associated with these. Where this occurs, it may be necessary to move away from the usual 4 h three times a week dialysis regime. Daily dialysis will reduce the daily ultrafiltration requirement, and extended nocturnal haemodialysis can reduce the rate of ultrafiltration. These therapies may reduce the risk of intra-dialytic myocardial injury or circulatory collapse, although the supporting evidence for this rationale is not from randomised interventional trials. Similarly, whether patient support through counselling can avoid excessive intra-dialytic weight gain and salt intake as a means to negate the need for high ultrafiltration volumes has a sound rationale but is objectively unproven.

Summary

ESKD patients face a high risk of SCD. Although the most likely mode of death is arrhythmic, the mechanism underpinning this appears to typically differ from the predominant atherosclerotic pathology seen in the general population. Furthermore, not all sudden deaths in ESKD will be arrhythmic in origin. There persists some uncertainty as to how best to define and categorise sudden deaths in ESKD. These factors necessitate the requirement of a population-specific approach to investigation and management. That said, ESKD patients should not be excluded from preexisting strategies, such as ICD therapy, if they meet criteria for such intervention.

Suggested current strategies for SCD risk reduction in ESKD are summarised in Table 3.2. Unfortunately, these are not based on solid clinical trial evidence and it is unlikely that such evidence will be forthcoming soon. A summary of key points from this chapter is found in Table 3.3.

Table 3.2 Possible therapeutic strategies to prevent SCD in ESKD

Intervention	Comment
Transplantation	Timely transplant work-up imperative given better survival in ESKD after renal transplant versus dialysis, even for most high risk patients
Implantable cardioverter-defibrillators	Patients should not be excluded from primary or secondary prevention using ICD as per current guidelines
Beta-blockade	Appropriate first line anti-hypertensive in view of apparent SCD reduction, and without a preclusive side effect profile
Avoid sotalol	Renal excretion and dialysed but should be avoided due to risk of torsades de pointes associated with toxicity, hypokalaemia, and long QT
Avoid extremes of potassium and potassium shift	Low potassium dialysate and extremes of serum potassium levels have been shown to increase risk of SCD (47)
Avoid hypocalcaemia	Low calcium dialysate may be associated with SCD and relative hypercalcaemia confers cardioprotection in cases of hyperkalaemia
Avoid high hemodialysis ultrafiltration rate: opt for short-hours daily dialysis or overnight haemodialysis	High UF volume during normal hours dialysis associated with higher SCD event rate. Daily dialysis and nocturnal dialysis associated with improved survival

Table 3.3 Key points

SCD appears to be the most common cause of death in ESKD, but not CKD
Variation in definition means SCD epidemiology lacks clarity in ESKD
SCD in ESKD usually has a different mechanism to SCD in the general population
The cardiac structural abnormalities typically found in ESKD are usually present before commencement of dialysis
Therapeutic strategies applicable to the general population should not be ignored but are generally less efficacious in ESKD
Beta-blockade appear the most suitable first line anti-hypertensive but sotalol should be avoided
Haemodialysis can provoke arrhythmia but these are of limited prognostic significance if limited to dialysis sessions
Transplantation is likely to be the most effective therapy for risk reduction in ESKD

References

1. Herzog CA. Don't forget the defibrillator in the dialysis unit. Nephrol Dial Transplant. 2004;19(12):2959–60.
2. Green D, Roberts P, New D, Kalra PA. Sudden cardiac death in hemodialysis patients: an in-depth review. Am J Kidney Dis. 2011;57(6):921–9.
3. Bleyer A, Hartman J, Brannon PC, Satko SG. Characteristics of sudden death in hemodialysis patients. Kidney Int. 2006;88:2268–73.
4. Drechsler C, Meinitzer A, Pilz S, et al. Homoarginine, heart failure, and sudden cardiac death in haemodialysis patients. Eur J Heart Fail. 2011;13:852–9.
5. Pun PH, Lehrich RW, Honeycutt EF, Herzog CA, Middleton JP. Modifiable risk factors associated with sudden cardiac arrest within hemodialysis clinics. Kidney Int. 2010;79(2):1–10.
6. Bleyer AJ, Russell GB, Satko SG. Sudden and cardiac death rates in hemodialysis patients. Kidney Int. 1999;55:1553–9.
7. Pun PH, Lehrich RW, Smith SR, Middleton JP. Predictors of survival after cardiac arrest in outpatient hemodialysis clinics. Clin J Am Soc Nephrol. 2007;2(3):491–500.
8. Karnik JA, Young BS, Lew NL, et al. Cardiac arrest and sudden death in dialysis units. Kidney Int. 2001;60(1):350–7.
9. Genovesi S, Valsecchi MG, Rossi E, et al. Sudden death and associated factors in a historical cohort of chronic haemodialysis patients. Nephrol Dial Transplant. 2009;24(8):2529–36.
10. Takeda K, Harada A, Okuda S, Fujimi S, Oh Y. Sudden death in chronic dialysis patients. Nephrol Dial Transplant. 1997;12:952–5.
11. Lehrich RW, Pun PH, Tanenbaum ND, Smith SR, Middleton JP. Automated external defibrillators and survival from cardiac arrest in the outpatient hemodialysis clinic. J Am Soc Nephrol. 2007;18(1):312–20.
12. Section H-Morbidity and Mortality. In: USRDS 2011 annual data report. National Institute of Health, National Institute of Diabetes and Digestive and Renal Diseases. 2011;129–46.
13. de Lima JJG, Gowdak LHW, de Paula FJ, et al. Unexplained sudden death in patients on the waiting list for renal transplantation. Nephrol Dial Transplant. 2011;26(4):1392–6.

14. Chugh SS, Jui J, Gunson K, et al. Current burden of sudden cardiac death: multiple source surveillance versus retrospective death certificate-based review in a large U.S. community. J Am Coll Cardiol. 2004;44(6):1268–75.
15. Priori SG, Aliot E, Bossaert L, et al. Task force report task force on sudden cardiac death of the European Society of Cardiology. Eur Heart J. 2001;22:1374–450.
16. Thomas AC, Knapman PA, Krikler DM, Davies MJ. Community study of the causes of "natural" sudden death. BMJ. 1988;297 (6661):1453–6.
17. Zipes DP, Camm AJ, Borggrefe M, Buxton AE. ACC/AHA/ESC 2006 guidelines for management of patients with ventricular arrhythmias and the prevention of sudden cardiac death. Circulation. 2006;114:385–484.
18. The AVID Collaborative Group. A comparison of antiarrhythmic-drug therapy with implantable defibrillators in patients resuscitated from near-fatal ventricular arrhythmias. N Engl J Med. 1997;337:1576–83.
19. Moss AJ, Hall WJ, Cannon DS, et al. Improved survival with an implanted defibrillator in patients with coronary disease at high risk for ventricular arrhythmia. Multicenter Automatic Defibrillator Implantation Trial Investigators. N Engl J Med. 1996;335:1933–40.
20. Bardy GH, Lee KL, Mark DB, et al. Amiodarone or an implantable cardioverter-defibrillator for congestive heart failure. N Engl J Med. 2005;352(3):225–38.
21. Langan Y, Nashef L, Sander JWAS, Hill D. Sudden unexpected death in epilepsy: a series of witnessed deaths. J Neurol Neurosurg Psychiatry. 2000;68(2):211–3.
22. Bateman J, Clarke S. Sudden death in asthma. Thorax. 1979;34:40–4.
23. Pun PH, Smarz TR, Honeycutt EF, et al. Chronic kidney disease is associated with increased risk of sudden cardiac death among patients with coronary artery disease. Kidney Int. 2009;76:652–8.
24. Goldenberg I, Moss AJ, McNitt S, et al. Relations among renal function, risk of sudden cardiac death, and benefit of the implanted cardiac defibrillator in patients with ischemic left ventricular dysfunction. J Cardiol. 2006;98:485–90.
25. Gillum R. Geographic variation in sudden coronary death. Am Heart J. 1990;119(2):380–9.
26. Pun PH, Herzog CA, Middleton JP. Improving ascertainment of sudden cardiac death in patients with end stage renal disease. Clin J Am Soc Nephrol. 2012;7(1):116–22.
27. Eknoyan G, Beck G, Cheung A, Daugirdas J, The Hemodialysis (HEMO) Study Group. Effect of dialysis dose and membrane flux in maintenance hemodialysis. N Engl J Med. 2002;347(25): 2010–9.
28. Stack AG, Bloembergen WE. Prevalence and clinical correlates of coronary artery disease among new dialysis patients in the United States: a cross-sectional study. J Am Soc Nephrol. 2001;12 (7):1516–23.
29. Bleyer A, Hartman J, Brannon PC, Satko SG. Characteristics of sudden death in hemodialysis patients. Kidney Int. 2006;88:2268–73.
30. Gill GV, Woodward A, Casson IF, Weston PJ. Cardiac arrhythmia and nocturnal hypoglycaemia in type 1 diabetes—the "dead in bed" syndrome revisited. Diabetologia. 2009;52:42–5.
31. Suarez GA, Clark VM, Norell JE, Kottke TE. Sudden cardiac death in diabetes mellitus: risk factors in the Rochester diabetic neuropathy study. J Neurol Neurosurg Psychiatry. 2005;76:240–5.
32. Hadi HAR, Suwaidi JA. Endothelial dysfunction in diabetes mellitus. Vasc Health Risk Manag. 2007;3(6):853–76.
33. Nishimura M, Tokoro T, Nishida M, Hashimoto T, Kobayashi H, Yamazaki S, et al. Sympathetic overactivity and sudden cardiac death among hemodialysis patients with left ventricular hypertrophy. Int J Cardiol. 2010;142(1):80–6.
34. Haider AW, Larson MG, Benjamin EJ, Levy D. Increased left ventricular mass and hypertrophy are associated with increased risk for sudden death. J Am Coll Cardiol. 1998;32(5):1454–9.
35. Burton JO, Korsheed S, Grundy BJ, McIntyre CW. Hemodialysis-induced left ventricular dysfunction is associated with an increase in ventricular arrhythmias. Ren Fail. 2008;30 (7):701–9.
36. Paoletti E, Specchia C, Di Maio G, et al. The worsening of left ventricular hypertrophy is the strongest predictor of sudden cardiac death in haemodialysis patients: a 10 year survey. Nephrol Dial Transplant. 2004;19(7):1829–34.
37. Krane V, Heinrich F, Meesmann M, et al. Electrocardiography and outcome in patients with diabetes mellitus on maintenance hemodialysis. Clin J Am Soc Nephrol. 2009;4:394–400.
38. Foley RN, Parfrey PS, Harnett JD, Kent GM. The prognostic importance of left ventricular geometry in uremic cardiomyopathy. J Am Coll Cardiol. 1995;5(12):2024–31.
39. Foley RN, Gilbertson DT, Murray T, Collins AJ. Long interdialytic interval and mortality among patients receiving hemodialysis. N Engl J Med. 2011;365(12):1099–107.
40. Burton JO, Jefferies HJ, Selby NM, McIntyre CW. Hemodialysis-induced cardiac injury: determinants and associated outcomes. Clin J Am Soc Nephrol. 2009;4(5):914–20.
41. Conlon P, Krucoff MW, Minda S, Schumm D, Schwab SJ. Incidence and long-term significance of transient ST segment deviation in hemodialysis patients. Clin Nephrol. 1998;49(4):236–9.
42. Narula AS, Jha V, Bali HK, et al. Cardiac arrhythmias and silent myocardial ischaemia during hemodialysis. Ren Fail. 2000;22 (3):355–68.
43. Mohi-ud-din K, Bali HK, Banerjee S, Sakhuja V, Jha V. Silent myocardial ischemia and high-grade ventricular arrhythmias in patients on maintenance hemodialysis. Ren Fail. 2005;27(2):171–5.
44. Kitano Y, Kasuga H, Watanabe M, et al. Severe coronary stenosis is an important factor for induction and lengthy persistence of ventricular arrhythmias during and after hemodialysis. Am J Kidney Dis. 2004;44(2):328–36.
45. Zwaakdemaker H. On physiological radioactivity. J Physiol. 1919–1920;53:274.
46. Libbrecht W. Le paradoxe cardiaque. Arch Intern Physiol. 1921;16:448.
47. Green D, Green HD, New DI, Kalra PA. The clinical significance of hyperkalaemia-associated repolarization abnormalities in end-stage renal disease. Nephrol Dial Transplant. 2012;28(1):99–105.
48. Kieboom BC, Niemeijer MN, Leening MJ et al. Serum magnesium and the risk of death from coronary heart disease and sudden cardiac death. J Am Heart Assoc. 2016;5(1)e002707.
49. Meema HE, Oreopoulos DG, Rapoport A. Serum magnesium level and arterial calcification in end stage renal disease. Kidney Int. 1987;32:388–94.
50. Massy ZA, Drüeke TB. Magnesium and outcomes in patients with chronic kidney disease: focus on vascular calcification, atherosclerosis and survival. Clin Kidney J. 2012;5(S1):i52–61.
51. Turgut F, Kanbay M, Metin MR, et al. Magnesium supplementation helps to improve carotid intima media thickness in patients on hemodialysis. Int Urol Nephrol. 2008;40(4):1075–82.
52. Fiset C, Kargacin ME, Kondo CS, Lester WM, Duff HJ. Hypomagnesemia: characterization of a model of sudden cardiac death. J Am Coll Cardiol. 1996;27(7):1771–6.
53. Connolly SJ, Hallstrom AP, Cappato R, Schron EB, Kuck K, Zipes DP, et al. Meta-analysis of the implantable cardioverter

defibrillator secondary prevention trials. Eur Heart J. 2000;21:2071–8.
54. Sakhuja R, Keebler M, Lai T-S, McLaughlin Gavin C, Thakur R, Bhatt DL. Meta-analysis of mortality in dialysis patients with an implantable cardioverter defibrillator. Am J Cardiol. 2009;103 (5):735–41.
55. Dasgupta A, Montalvo J, Medendorp S, Lloyd-Jones DM, Ghossein C, Goldberger J, et al. Increased complication rates of cardiac rhythm management devices in ESRD patients. Am J Kidney Dis. 2007;49(5):656–63.
56. Hreybe H, Ezzeddine R, Bedi M, Barrington W, Bazaz R, Ganz LI, et al. Renal insufficiency predicts the time to first appropriate defibrillator shock. Am Heart J. 2006;151(4):852–6.
57. Wase A, Basit A, Nazir R, Jamal A, Shah S, Khan T, et al. Impact of chronic kidney disease upon survival among implantable cardioverter defibrillator recipients. J Interv Cardiol Electrophysiol. 2004;11(3):199–204.
58. Charytan D, Patrick A, Liu J, Setoguchi S, Herzog C, Brookhart M, et al. Trends in the use and outcomes of implantable cardioverter-defibrillators in patients undergoing dialysis in the United States. Am J Kidney Dis. 2011;58(3):409–17.
59. Mangrum J, Lin D, Dimarco J, Lake D. Prognostic value of left ventricular systolic function in renal dialysis patients. Heart Rhythm. 2006;3(5s):154.
60. De Bie MK, van Dam B, Gaasbeek A, van Buren M, van Erven L, Bax JJ, et al. The current status of interventions aiming at reducing sudden cardiac death in dialysis patients. Eur Heart J. 2009;30 (13):1559–64.
61. Shastri S, Tangri N, Tighiouart H, Beck GJ, Vlagopoulos P, Ornt D, et al. Predictors of sudden cardiac death: a competing risk approach in the hemodialysis study. Clin J Am Soc Nephrol. 2012;7(1):123–30.
62. Parfrey PS, Foley RN. The clinical epidemiology of cardiac disease in chronic renal failure. J Am Soc Nephrol. 1999;10 (7):1606–15.
63. Szummer K, Lundman P, Jacobson S, Schön S, Lindbäck J, Stenestrand U, et al. Influence of renal function on the effects of early revascularization in non-ST-elevation myocardial infarction. Circulation. 2009;120(10):851–8.
64. Herzog CA, Strief JW, Collins AJ, Gilbertson DT. Cause-specific mortality of dialysis patients after coronary revascularization: why don't dialysis patients have better survival after coronary intervention? Nephrol Dial Transplant. 2008;23(8):2629–33.
65. Green D, Ritchie JP, Kalra PA. Meta-analysis of lipid lowering therapy in maintenance dialysis patients. Nephron Clin Pract. 2014;124(3–4):209–17.
66. Cice G, Ferrara L, D'Andrea A, D'Isa S, Di Benedetto A, Cittadini A, et al. Carvedilol increases two-year survival in dialysis patients with dilated cardiomyopathy. J Am Coll Cardiol. 2003;41 (9):1438–44.
67. Matsue Y, Suzuki M, Nagahori W, Ohno M, Matsumura A, Hashimoto Y. Beta-blocker prevents sudden cardiac death in patients with hemodialysis. Int J Cardiol. 2011;165(3):519–22.
68. Miller LM, Hopman WM, Garland JS, Yeates KE, Pilkey RM. Cardioprotective medication use in hemodialysis patients. Can J Cardiol. 2006;22(9):755–60.
69. Furgeson SB, Chonchol M. Beta-blockade in chronic dialysis patients. Semin Dial. 2008;21(1):43–8.
70. Myerburg R, Kessler K, Mallon S, Cox M, DeMarchena E, Interian A, et al. Life-threatening ventricular arrhythmias in patients with silent myocardial ischemia due to coronary–artery spasm. N Engl J Med. 1992;326(22):1451–5.
71. Greene EL, Kren S, Hostetter TH. Role of aldosterone in the remnant kidney model in the rat. J Clin Investig. 1996;98(4): 1063–8.
72. Tomaschitz A, Pilz S, Ritz E, Grammer T, Drechsler C, Boehm B, et al. Association of plasma aldosterone with cardiovascular mortality in patients with low estimated GFR: the Ludwigshafen Risk and Cardiovascular Health (LURIC) Study. Am J Kidney Dis. 2011;57(3):403–14.
73. Domanski MJ, Exner DV, Borkowf CB, Geller NL, Rosenberg Y, Pfeffer MA. Effect of angiotensin converting enzyme inhibition on sudden cardiac death in patients following acute myocardial infarction. A meta-analysis of randomized clinical trials. J Am Coll Cardiol. 1999;33(3):598–604.
74. Zannad F, Kessler M, Lehert P, Grünfeld JP, Thuilliez C, Leizorovicz A, et al. Prevention of cardiovascular events in end-stage renal disease: results of a randomized trial of fosinopril and implications for future studies. Kidney Int. 2006;70(7): 1318–24.
75. Takahashi A, Takase H, Toriyama T, Sugiura T, Kurita Y, Ueda R, et al. Candesartan, an angiotensin II type-1 receptor blocker, reduces cardiovascular events in patients on chronic haemodialysis—a randomized study. Nephrol Dial Transplant. 2006;21(9): 2507–12.
76. Pitt B, Zannad F, Remme W, Cody R, Castaigne A, Perez A, et al. The effect of spironolactone on morbidity and mortality in patients with severe heart failure. N Engl J Med. 1999;341(10):709–17.
77. Chua D, Lo A, Lo C. Spironolactone use in heart failure patients with end-stage renal disease on hemodialysis: is it safe? Clin Cardiol. 2010;33(10):604–8.
78. Hammer F, Krane V, Störk S, Röser C, Hofmann K, Pollak N, et al. Rationale and design of the Mineralocorticoid Receptor Antagonists in End-Stage Renal Disease Study (MiREnDa). Nephrol Dial Transplant. 2014;29(2):400–5.
79. Kovesdy CP, Regidor DL, Mehrotra R, Jing J, McAllister CJ, Greenland S, et al. Serum and dialysate potassium concentrations and survival in hemodialysis patients. Clin J Am Soc Nephrol. 2007;2(5):999–1007.
80. Näppi SE, Virtanen VK, Saha HH, Mustonen JT. Pasternack a I. QTc dispersion increases during hemodialysis with low-calcium dialysate. Kidney Int. 2000;57(5):2117–22.
81. Pun PH, Horton JR, Middleton JP. Dialysate calcium concentration and the risk of sudden cardiac arrest in hemodialysis patients. Clin J Am Soc Nephrol. 2013;8(5):797–803.
82. Pun PH, Lehrich RW, Honeycutt EF, Herzog CA, Middleton JP. Modifiable risk factors associated with sudden cardiac arrest within hemodialysis clinics. Kidney Int. 2011;79:218–27.
83. Parekh RS, Plantinga LC, Kao WHL, et al. The association of sudden cardiac death with inflammation and other traditional risk factors. Kidney Int. 2008;74(10):1335–42.
84. Wang AY, Lam CW, Chan IH, Wang M, Lui S, Sanderson JE. Sudden cardiac death in end-stage renal disease patients: a 5-year prospective analysis. Hypertension. 2010;56:210–6.
85. Drechsler C, Pilz S, Obermayer-Pietsch B, et al. Vitamin D deficiency is associated with sudden cardiac death, combined cardiovascular events, and mortality in haemodialysis patients. Eur Heart J. 2010;31(18):2253–61.
86. Shastri S, Tangri N, Tighiouart H, et al. Predictors of sudden cardiac death: a competing risk approach in the hemodialysis study. J Am Soc Nephrol. 2012;7(1):123–30.

Coronary Artery Disease in CKD: Traditional and Nontraditional Risk Factors, Diagnosis and Management

4

Christian Witzke, Igor Palacios, and Andre Macedo Dias

Epidemiology of CAD in CKD Patients

The prevalence of chronic kidney disease (CKD) is increasing worldwide and is considered an independent risk factor for the development of coronary artery disease (CAD) [1–5]. Overall, patients with CKD are at significantly higher risk of developing of CAD than those in the general population without CKD [6–8]. The reported 1-year mortality rate of patients with ESKD was approximately 20% in US dialysis population, and the single most important contributor to this high mortality was cardiovascular disease, accounting for over 50% of all mortality [3].

According to data from the National Cardiovascular Data Registry–Acute Coronary Treatment and Intervention Outcomes Network (NCDR-ACTION), the prevalence of CKD among patients presenting with ST segment–elevation myocardial infarction was 30.5% (STEMI) and among patients presenting with non-ST segment–elevation myocardial infarction was 42.9% (NSTEMI) [9].

In addition, the Atherosclerosis Risk in Communities (ARIC) study [10] and Valsartan in Acute Myocardial Infarction Trial (VALIANT) trial [11] demonstrate a strong correlation between the estimated GFR (eGFR) and the rate of cardiovascular mortality in patients with eGFR of ≤ 80 cc/min/1.73 m^2, and increased event rates even with early CKD. Considering the high prevalence of renal disease in the US with approximate 500,000 patients on renal replacement therapy and the even larger number of patients with early CKD, the population at risk for cardiovascular disease may be significantly larger than initially thought.

The relationship between CKD and severity of coronary atherosclerosis has also been assessed in population-based autopsy samples. A significant association between CKD and the presence of diffuse multivessel involvement, vessel calcification, and coronary atherosclerosis has been found in histopathological studies [12]. The degree of renal impairment is also an important predictor of worse clinical outcomes and survival among CAD patients undergoing revascularization, in particular coronary artery bypass graft (CABG) [13]. Higher re-infarction rates and 1- and 2-year mortality was also reported among patients with abnormal renal function in data from acute coronary syndrome trials [14].

Pathophysiology

CKD patients frequently have significant cardiovascular pathology. Two different mechanisms may be responsible for worse survival and clinical outcomes in patients with CKD: atherosclerosis and arteriosclerosis. Atherosclerosis consists of intimal disease characterized by fibroatheromatous plaques, with different level of calcification and intimal/medial thickness [15, 16]. These changes are most commonly seen in small distal coronary arteries, predisposing to chronic myocardial ischemia, that ultimate leads to local inflammation, fibrosis and left ventricular remodeling. It is believed that over time, chronic small vessel ischemia may be responsible of the high incidence of sudden cardiac death seen in patients with CKD (particularly in patients on dialysis) in the absence of macroscopic acute plaque rupture [17].

Arteriosclerosis of moderate size vessels is also an important vascular pathology commonly present in CKD patients. It is characterized by the thickening and calcification of the medial arterial bed, and hyperplasia and

C. Witzke · A.M. Dias (✉)
Einstein Medical Center, 5501 Old York Rd, Philadelphia, PA 19141, USA
e-mail: andremacdias@gmail.com

C. Witzke
e-mail: witzkec@einstein.edu

I. Palacios
Massachusetts General Hospital, 55 Fruit Street, Boston, MA 02114, USA
e-mail: ipalacios@partners.org

J. Rangaswami et al. (eds.), *Cardio-Nephrology*,
DOI 10.1007/978-3-319-56042-7_4

hypertrophy of the vascular smooth muscle cells, leading to increased vessel stiffness and increased collagen deposition in the vessel wall [15].

This vessel stiffening contributes to the hemodynamic alterations frequently observed in these patients such as arterial dampening function, increased left ventricular afterload, increased systolic and pulse pressures, increased myocardial oxygen demand and sub-endocardial blood flow impairment [15, 16].

Epicardial coronary atherosclerosis in CKD patients also has distinctive coronary plaque features than differ them from patients with normal kidney function. In a study from the Massachusetts General Hospital OCT registry, patients with CKD had a larger lipid index with a higher prevalence of calcium, cholesterol crystals, and plaque disruption [18].

Traditional and Nontraditional Risk Factors

Several epidemiological studies have revealed a correlation between the severity of renal impairment and the traditional risk factors in the pathogenesis of atherosclerosis. Age, male gender, hypertension, diabetes mellitus, hyperlipidemia, smoking, and a family history of premature CVD are the most widely studied risk factors for cardiovascular events. Some of these factors can be modified to decrease morbidity and mortality even in patients with overt cardiovascular disease [19].

Even though traditional risks factors are highly prevalent in CKD patients, it is believed that it cannot fully explain the disproportionately increased cardiovascular morbidity and mortality observed in this population. There are several nontraditional risk factors, unique to CKD: uremic toxins, anemia, elevated levels of specific inflammatory cytokines, abnormalities in bone mineral metabolism, endothelial cell dysfunction, hyperhomocysteinemia, and poor nutritional status [20, 21]. The chronic inflammatory state unique to CKD (malnutrition inflammation complex) is associated with increased oxidative stress and has been linked with increased atheromatous burden in patients with CKD [22, 23].

Increased levels of C-reactive protein (CRP) and asymmetric dimethylarginine are commonly detected in the CKD population. Both markers were found to be independently associated with an increased risk of cardiovascular mortality in the Modification of Diet in Renal Disease (MDRD) study [24, 25]. Having said that, this correlation was not confirmed in the Irbesartan for Diabetic Nephropathy trial, making these findings questionable [26].

Post hoc analyses from different studies suggested that moderate increases in albuminuria over time may be also be a significant predictor of cardiovascular risk as it correlates with endothelial dysfunction [27–29]. Other pathways, including activation of the renin-angiotensin-aldosterone and the sympathetic nervous systems have been implicated in the pathogenesis of CVD in CKD patients [30]. Finally, aberrant mineralocorticoid release is becoming increasingly recognized in the development of CVD as it may cause tissue inflammation, remodeling, and fibrosis [30].

Recent studies have also shown vitamin D supplementation with calcitriol appears to be associated with significantly greater cardiovascular survival in patients with CKD [31, 32].

The existence of traditional and nontraditional risk factors has therapeutic implications. Indeed, while it is crucial to treat and control the well-known traditional risk factors in patients with CKD, there is data showing that several of these therapies typically highly effective in the general population, when used in CKD patients, particularly those who are already on renal replacement therapy, are less or minimally effective [22].

Clinical Presentation

Not uncommonly, CKD patients with acute coronary syndrome (ACS) may present differently to patients without CKD. The prevalence of chest pain among patient presenting with ACS appears to be inversely related to the stage of CKD—the lower the eGFR, the less likely to present with chest pain [33–35].

According to the United States Renal Data System (USRDS) and the National Registry of Myocardial Infarction (NRMI) patients with advanced CKD and on dialysis were less prone to present with chest pain upon admission than those without CKD. Patients with severe renal dysfunction were more likely to have heart failure upon presentation. The type of ACS presentation also differed between CKD patients when compared to the general population. Acute plaque rupture with transmural ischemia and ST segment elevation MI are less likely in patients with renal impairment [33–35].

Reduction of CAD Risk in CKD Patients

In the past, the vast majority of clinical trials of patients with coronary artery disease excluded patients with CKD. Meta-analysis of CAD trials published between 2006 and 2010 noted that between 56 and 75% of those studies had excluded CKD patients [36].

More recently, few randomized trials have been conducted specifically in CKD patients, especially regarding statin therapy. The ongoing ISCHEMIA-CKD study, comparing the effectiveness of optimal medical therapy versus invasive therapy in patients with stable ischemic heart disease with GFR < 30 cc/min, including patients on dialysis, is an example of the efforts in the direction of increasing interest in specifically studying optimal CAD management in this high-risk population.

Medical Therapy

Medical therapy consists of statin therapy, antiplatelet therapy, blood pressure management and aggressive lifestyle modification measures such as smoking cessation, weight loss, glycemic control, and physical activity.

Statins

Lipid metabolism abnormalities are frequently present in patients with CKD. The most common abnormalities are an impaired lipid removal from the circulation. The presence of high cholesterol concentration in the blood stream, with an associated with high cholesterol oxidation are the ultimate pathway for the development of atherosclerosis.

The reduction of circulating LDL with statin therapy in patients with CKD not requiring dialysis has shown a significant reduction in cardiovascular events. The Study of Heart and Renal Protection (SHARP) [37] trial specifically evaluated cholesterol lowering with a statin to prevent major vascular events in patients with CKD and concluded that simvastatin plus ezetimibe prevented atherosclerotic events in CKD patients not requiring dialysis.

It is important to mention that the majority of these trials enrolled older patients with several traditional risk factors such as diabetes and hypertension and therefore the extrapolation of statin therapy in younger population with CKD due to a primary kidney disorder is unclear.

Interestingly, recent studies indicate that the benefits of using a statin in CKD patients may be related to both "cholesterol dependent" and, the so called, "pleiotropic" (cholesterol independent) effects. The latter effect involves the improvement of endothelial dysfunction with atherosclerotic plaques stabilization, decreasing inflammation, and preventing thrombogenesis.

Regarding lipid management there are as yet no robust clinical trials comparing cardiovascular outcomes among CKD patients who were assigned to a specific target LDL level, as well as no good evidence on titrating statin therapy. The Kidney Disease Improving Global Outcomes (KDIGO) guidelines on management of dyslipidemia in CKD recommend standard statin dose based upon cardiovascular risk and level of estimated GFR.

In CKD patients requiring renal replacement therapy, there are two large clinical trials worth mentioning: Die Deutsche Diabetes Dialyse (4-D) and A Study to Evaluate the Use of Rosuvastatin in Subjects on Regular Hemodialysis: An Assessment of Survival and Cardiovascular Events (AURORA) [38, 39]. Both studies assessed the effect of statin therapy in dialysis patients and respective outcomes: death from cardiovascular causes, nonfatal myocardial infarction (MI), and stroke. In spite of a significant decrease detected in serum low-density lipoprotein (LDL)-cholesterol levels of CKD patients taking statins, both trials found that the initiation of statin therapy had no cardiovascular benefit [38, 39] except for a possible benefit of statins in reducing cardiovascular events among diabetic CKD patients who were on dialysis (subgroup analysis).

Based on these results the 2013 Kidney Disease: Improving Global Outcomes (KDIGO) guidelines stated that statin therapy should not be routinely initiated in dialysis patients [40]; however they also suggest that statin therapy could be continued in patients who were already on statins or a statin/ezetimibe combination prior or at the time of initiation of dialysis particularly those patients with significantly high LDL levels [40].

Blood Pressure Management

Multiple trials on outcomes with hypertension management have shown that adequate blood pressure control improves cardiovascular outcomes. There are as yet no consistent data on targeting of exact BP and this is still a topic of debate. More recently the SPRINT trial shed some light into this topic. Among patients at higher risk for cardiovascular events but without diabetes, targeting a systolic blood pressure of less than 120 mmHg, as compared with less than 140 mmHg, resulted in lower rates of fatal and nonfatal major cardiovascular events and death from any cause, at the expense of higher rates of some adverse events, including acute kidney injury observed in the intensive-treatment group. [41]. At this time, data from SPRINT cannot fully be extrapolated into the CKD population, especially advanced CKD, and further recommendations of optimal targets in this population are awaited (also refer to Chap. 39).

Several post hoc analyses of CKD subgroups in cardiovascular trials have shown that antihypertensive therapy reduces the risk of cardiovascular events. These observations do not favor any specific antihypertensive drug, particularly in non-proteinuric CKD patients [42–44].

In proteinuric CKD patients there is evidence supporting the use of specific antihypertensive drugs such as ACE inhibitors since it may reduce the progression of renal disease [42–44]. Attention to optimal blood pressure management and avoidance of hypotensive episodes is crucial in CKD patients on dialysis, as intradialytic hypotension may cause subendocardial ischemia with transient myocardial dysfunction and stunning. The effect of repetitive subendocardial ischemic events has been look at in different observational studies. We should also consider ischemic events due to transient hypotension in patients with established epicardial coronary artery disease, as they can also be the source of ischemic events that may ultimate increase the risk for peridialysis MI and sudden cardiac death. Hemodialysis has been associated with repetitive myocardial ischemia, which, in the absence of CAD, may be due to coronary microvascular dysfunction. Functional post stress recovery is consistent with myocardial stunning induced by hemodialysis. This process may be important in the development of heart failure in long-term hemodialysis patients [45].

Antiplatelet Therapy

In the general population, long-term use of aspirin decreases the risk of myocardial infarction (MI), stroke, and improves cardiovascular mortality among those with prior manifestations of CVD. Nevertheless, there is a paucity of data regarding the benefit and efficacy of aspirin in CKD patients, particularly those already on dialysis [46, 47].

As an example, data from the Dialysis Outcomes and Practice Patterns Study (DOPPS) which included 28,320 hemodialysis patients, aspirin was found to be associated with an increased risk of MI whereas the risk of stroke was decreased with aspirin [48].

Similarly, results were reported by an observational study of 41,425 hemodialysis patients where aspirin was associated with an increased risk of mortality [49].

In a more recent Cochrane meta-analysis that included 50 studies and a total of 27,139 CKD patients (non-dialysis and dialysis patients) primary antiplatelet therapy significantly reduced the incidence of myocardial infarction with a significant increased risk of major bleeding [46].

Based on current available data, the decision to start antiplatelet therapy to prevent cardiovascular disease in patients with CKD should be individualized and always taking into account other aspects such as the presence of traditional CVD risk factors and patient's bleeding risk.

Revascularization in CKD Patients

Stable Angina

Data from the COURAGE (Clinical Outcomes Utilizing Revascularization and Aggressive Drug Evaluation) trial has shown that optimal medical therapy (OMT) employed in CKD patients is effective and associated with the same blood pressure and lipid levels as in patients without CKD. In the same trial, PCI plus OMT in CKD patients did not reduce the risk of death or myocardial infarction and was also not associated with worse outcomes in this high-risk group [50].

This supports that medical therapy is well tolerated and highly efficient in the management of patients with CAD and stable angina. In the COURAGE trial, the number of antianginal medication, rate of cross over to PCI to treat ischemic chest pain, impaired quality of life were all higher in the medical arm group, especially in patients with high-risk nuclear stress test (myocardial at risk >8%) [51].

Interesting, the presence of CKD was found to be an independent predictor of death or nonfatal myocardial, while PCI had no effect on these outcomes [51].

STEMI and NSTEMI

There are no randomized clinical trials assessing the benefits of antiplatelet therapy, specifically in CKD patients. Intuitively, patients with CKD require careful drug dose adjustments, and appear to have higher likelihood of drug-related adverse effects given the altered metabolism and clearance of these drugs in the setting of renal impairment. CKD patients are more likely to develop major bleeding episodes in the setting of glycoprotein IIb/IIIa inhibitors or clopidogrel administration [52].

Several studies have reported significant differences between non-CKD and CKD patients with respect to the use of "standard of care" medical therapy: angiotensin-converting enzyme inhibitors, beta-blockers and a GP IIb/IIIa inhibitors are all less likely to be used in CKD patients. As expected, diagnostic angiography and percutaneous coronary intervention (PCI) are underutilized in patients with CKD, most likely due to the potential risk of contrast-induced nephropathy [53–58].

Compared to patients with normal renal function, where there are several randomized controlled trials showing better outcomes with PCI over fibrinolytic therapy in the treatment of STEMI patients [59], however this data is lacking in patients with CKD. The best data addressing the role of PCI in CKD patients arises from the GRACE (Global Registry of Acute Coronary Events) study. In this Registry, reperfusion therapy was used (PCI versus fibrinolysis) in 12,532 patients with renal dysfunction. The overall outcome was poor in CKD patients, mainly due to a low reperfusion success rates and ST segment elevation/left bundle branch block (LBBB). Both STE and LBBB were associated with high mortality, low reperfusion rates, and overall outcomes were poor in CKD patients regardless the type of reperfusion therapy [60, 61].

Revascularization with primary PCI in STEMI patients is associated with an increased risk of CNS bleeding and the risk is even higher when thrombolysis is used in CKD patients [60, 61].

Despite above-mentioned limitations, current guidelines support that fibrinolytic therapy should only be considered first line therapy for CKD patients presenting with STEMI, whenever primary PCI is not available.

Among patients with non-ST elevation ACS the crucial decision frequently oscillates between immediate coronary angiography and medical therapy. In a meta-analysis of seven randomized trials which included more than 8000 NSTEMI patients, early invasive therapy decreased mortality by 25% at a mean of 2 years of follow-up, compared with a more conservative approach. Early invasive therapy was also associated with lower incidence of recurrent unstable angina requiring re-hospitalization [62].

A recent retrospective analysis of all NSTEMI patients in Sweden—SWEDEHEART found that an early invasive strategy was associated with greater 1-year survival in patients with NSTEMI and mild-to-moderate CKD, however the benefit declined with worsening renal function, and could be even harmful for end-stage kidney disease patients [63].

Overall, the survival of patients with CKD who undergo coronary revascularization with PCI or fibrinolytic therapy is worse than those with coronary artery disease without CKD.

CABG Versus PCI in CKD Patients

The ARTS (Arterial Revascularization Therapies Study) trial assigned 1205 participants with and without CKD to CABG or multivessel PCI with bare metal stenting. Among them, 290 participants (25%) had CKD at entry into ARTS [64]. One hundred fifty-one patients received PCI, and 139 received CABG. In patients with multivessel CAD and CKD, treatment with CABG or PCI with multivessel stenting led to similar outcomes of death, MI, or stroke, but CABG was associated with decreased repeat revascularizations. When compared with ARTS participants with normal renal function, those with CKD had substantially higher risk of adverse clinical outcomes after coronary revascularization.

However, the applicability of ARTS findings in clinical practice became unclear with the recent widespread use drug-eluting stents (DES) especially because there is data demonstrating that PCI with sirolimus DES is superior to bare metal stent (BMS) in dialysis patients [65].

Data is still scarce on long-term survival of dialysis patients undergoing CABG versus PCI in the era of DES.

In a retrospective study [66] of 23,033 US dialysis patients who underwent coronary revascularizations (6178 CABG, 5011 BMS, 11,844 DES) from 2004 to 2009, the authors concluded that in-hospital mortality was higher after CABG in comparison to PCI, but long-term survival was superior if internal mammary grafting (IMG) was performed. In-hospital mortality was lower for DES patients, but the probability of repeat revascularization was higher.

More recently [67], in CKD patients, CABG was associated with higher short-term risk of death, stroke, and repeat revascularization, whereas PCI with DES everolimus was associated with a higher long-term risk of repeat revascularization, favoring CABG over PCI in dialysis patients.

In conclusion, revascularization decisions for dialysis patients should always be individualized. CABG should be attempted in dialysis patients if IMG is feasible (Table 4.1) and PCI may be an alternative therapeutic modality if calculated perioperative mortality and morbidity are high or if IMG cannot be performed. Observational data has consistently shown that among CKD patients undergoing CABG, preoperative GFR is an important predictor of operative mortality and morbidities [13].

Table 4.1 Comparison of cardiovascular features between CKD and Non CKD Patients

CVD highlights	CKD patients	Non CKD patients
ACS presentation	Frequently with heart failure	Frequently with chest pain
Acute plaque rupture with transmural ischemia	Less common	Common
Diffuse multivessel involvement and/or vessel calcification	Common	Less common
Re-infarction rates	Higher	Lower
Plaque features	High lipid index with a high prevalence of calcium	Lower lipid index with lower prevalence of calcium
Traditional risk factors	Common	Common
Nontraditional risk factors	Common	Less common
Statins	CKD not requiring dialysis—Significant reduction in cardiovascular events CKD requiring dialysis—Should not be routinely initiated however could be continued in patients who were already on statins	Significant reduction in cardiovascular events
Blood pressure control	Important	Important
Survival after PCI or thrombolysis for ACS	Worse	Better
CABG versus PCI	CABG should probably be attempted in dialysis patients if IMG is feasible	As per guidelines

Traditional risk factors—age, male gender, hypertension, diabetes mellitus, hyperlipidemia, smoking and a family history of premature CVD
Nontraditional risk factors—uremic toxins, anemia, inflammatory cytokines, abnormalities in bone mineral metabolism, endothelial cell dysfunction, hyperhomocysteinemia, and poor nutritional status
CVD Cardiovascular, *ACS* acute coronary syndrome, *PCI* percutaneous coronary intervention, *IMG* internal mammary grafting

References

1. Sarnak MJ, Levey AS, Schoolwerth AC, Coresh J, Culleton B, Hamm LL, McCullough PA, Kasiske BL, Kelepouris E, Klag MJ, Parfrey P, Pfeffer M, Raij L, Spinosa DJ, Wilson PW. Kidney disease as a risk factor for development of cardiovascular disease: a statement from the American Heart Association Councils on Kidney in Cardiovascular Disease, High Blood Pressure Research, Clinical Cardiology, and Epidemiology and Prevention. Circulation. 2003;108:2154.
2. US Renal Data System. USRDS 2009 annual data report: atlas of end-stage renal disease in the United States. Am J Kidney Dis. 2010;55(Suppl 1):S1.
3. Chen J, Muntner P, Hamm LL, Jones DW, Batuman V, Fonseca V, Whelton PK, He J. The metabolic syndrome and chronic kidney disease in U.S. adults. Ann Intern Med. 2004;140:167.
4. Kaysen GA, Eiserich JP. The role of oxidative stress-altered lipoprotein structure and function and microinflammation on cardiovascular risk in patients with minor renal dysfunction. J Am Soc Nephrol. 2004;15:538.
5. Ix JH, Shlipak MG, Liu HH, Schiller NB, Whooley MA. Association between renal insufficiency and inducible ischemia in patients with coronary artery disease: the heart and soul study. J Am Soc Nephrol. 2003;14:3233.
6. Collins AJ, Foley RN, Herzog C. USRDS 2012 annual data report. Am J Kidney Dis. 2013;61(1 Suppl 1):e1–421.
7. Weiner DE, Tabatabai S, Tighiouart H, Elsayed E, Bansal N, Griffith J, Salem DN, Levey AS, Sarnak MJ. Cardiovascular outcomes and all-cause mortality: exploring the interaction between CKD and cardiovascular disease. Am J Kidney Dis. 2006;48:392–401.
8. Go AS, Chetow GM, Fan D, McCulloch CE, Hsu CY. Chronic kidney disease and the risk of death, cardiovascular events, and hospitalization. N Engl J Med. 2004;351:1296–305.
9. Washam JB, Herzog CA, Beitelshees AL, Cohen MG, Henry TD, Kapur NK, Mega JL, Menon V, Page RL 2nd, Newby LK. Pharmacotherapy in chronic kidney disease patients presenting with acute coronary syndrome: a scientific statement from the American Heart Association. Circulation. 2015;131(12):1123–49.
10. Wattanakit K, Coresh J, Muntner P, Marsh J, Folsom AR. Cardiovascular risk among adults with chronic kidney disease, with or without prior myocardial infarction. J Am Coll Cardiol. 2006;48:1183.
11. Anavekar NS, McMurray JJ, Velazquez EJ, Solomon SD, Kober L, Rouleau JL, White HD, Nordlander R, Maggioni A, Dickstein K, Zelenkofske S, Leimberger JD, Califf RM, Pfeffer MA. Relation between renal dysfunction and cardiovascular outcomes after myocardial infarction. N Engl J Med. 2004;351:1285–95.
12. Nakano T, Ninomiya T, Sumiyoshi S. Association of kidney function with coronary atherosclerosis and calcification in autopsy samples from Japanese elders: the Hisayama study. Am J Kidney Dis. 2010;55:21–30.
13. Cooper WA, O'Brien SM, Thourani VH, Guyton RA, Bridges CR, Szczech LA, Petersen R, Peterson ED. Impact of renal dysfunction on outcomes of coronary artery bypass surgery: results from the Society of Thoracic Surgeons National Adult Cardiac Database. Circulation. 2006;113:1063–70.
14. Al Suwaidi J, Reddan DN, Williams K, Pieper KS, Harrington RA, Califf RM, Granger CB, Ohman EM, Holmes DR Jr, Gusto-IIB, Gusto-III, Pursuit. Global use of strategies to open occluded coronary arteries. Platelet glycoprotein IIB/IIIA in unstable angina: receptor suppression using integrilin therapy; Paragon-A

investigators. Platelet Iib/Iiia Antagonism for the reduction of acute coronary syndrome events in a global organization network. Prognostic implications of abnormalities in renal function in patients with acute coronary syndromes. Circulation. 2002; 106:974–80.

15. London GM, Marchais SJ, Guerin AP, Metivier F, Adda H. Arterial structure and function in end-stage renal disease. Nephrol Dial Transpl. 2002;17:1713–24.
16. Schwarz U, Buzello M, Ritz E, Stein G, Raabe G, Wiest G, Mall G, Amann K. Morphology of coronary atherosclerotic lesions in patients with end-stage renal failure. Nephrol Dial Transpl. 2000;15:218–23.
17. Herzog CA. Sudden cardiac death and acute myocardial infarction in dialysis patients: perspectives of a cardiol00 gist. Semin Nephrol. 2005;25:363–6.
18. Kato K, Yonetsu T, Jia H, Abtahian F, Vergallo R, Hu S, Tian J, Kim SJ, Lee H, Mcnulty I, Lee S, Uemura S, Jang Y, Park SJ, Mizuno K, Yu B, Jang IK. Non-culprit coronary plaque characteristics of chronic kidney disease. Circ Cardiovasc Imaging. 2013;6(3):448–56.
19. Shlipak MG, Fried LF, Cushman M, Manolio TA, Peterson D, Stehman-Breen C, Bleyer A, Newman A, Siscovick D, Psaty B. Cardiovascular mortality risk in chronic kidney disease: comparison of traditional and novel risk factors. JAMA. 2005;293:1737.
20. Kaysen GA, Eiserich JP. The role of oxidative stress-altered lipoprotein structure and function and microinflammation on cardiovascular risk in patients with minor renal dysfunction. J Am Soc Nephrol. 2004;15:538.
21. Becker B, Kronenberg F, Kielstein JT, Haller H, Morath C, Ritz E, Fliser D, MMKD Study Group. Renal insulin resistance syndrome, adiponectin and cardiovascular events in patients with kidney disease: the mild and moderate kidney disease study. J Am Soc Nephrol. 2005;16:1091.
22. Wong TY, Coresh J, Klein R, Muntner P, Couper DJ, Sharrett AR, Klein BE, Heiss G, Hubbard LD, Duncan BB. Retinal microvascular abnormalities and renal dysfunction: the atherosclerosis risk in communities study. J Am Soc Nephrol. 2004;15:2469.
23. Hillege HL, Fidler V, Diercks GF, van Gilst WH, de Zeeuw D, van Veldhuisen DJ, Gans RO, Janssen WM, Grobbee DE, de Jong PE. Prevention of Renal and Vascular End Stage Disease (PREVEND) Study Group. Urinary albumin excretion predicts cardiovascular and noncardiovascular mortality in general population. Circulation. 2002;106:1777.
24. Menon V, Greene T, Wang X, Pereira AA, Marcovina SM, Beck GJ, Kusek JW, Collins AJ, Levey AS, Sarnak MJ. C-reactive protein and albumin as predictors of all-cause and cardiovascular mortality in chronic kidney disease. Kidney Int. 2005;68:766.
25. Young JM, Terrin N, Wang X, Greene T, Beck GJ, Kusek JW, Collins AJ, Sarnak MJ, Menon V. Asymmetric dimethylarginine and mortality in stages 3 to 4 chronic kidney disease. Clin J Am Soc Nephrol. 2009;4:1115.
26. Friedman AN, Hunsicker LG, Selhub J, Bostom AG, Collaborative Study Group. C-reactive protein as a predictor of total arteriosclerotic outcomes in type 2 diabetic nephropathy. Kidney Int. 2005;68:773.
27. Chronic Kidney Disease Prognosis Consortium, Matsushita K, van der Velde M, Woodward M, Levey AS, de Jong PE, Coresh J, Gansevoort RT. Association of estimated glomerular filtration rate and albuminuria with all-cause and cardiovascular mortality in general population cohorts: a collaborative meta-analysis. Lancet. 2010;375:2073.
28. Tonelli M, Muntner P, Lloyd A. Sing proteinuria and estimated glomerular filtration rate to classify risk in patients with chronic kidney disease: a cohort study. Using proteinuria and estimated glomerular filtration rate to classify risk in patients with chronic kidney disease: a cohort study. Ann Intern Med. 2011;154:12.
29. Tonelli M, Jose P, Curhan G, Sacks F, Braunwald E, Pfeffer M. Cholesterol and Recurrent Events (CARE) Trial Investigators. Proteinuria, impaired kidney function, and adverse outcomes in people with coronary disease: analysis of a previously conducted randomised trial. BMJ. 2006;332:1426.
30. Fox CS, Larson MG, Keyes MJ, Levy D, Clouse ME, Culleton B, O'Donnell CJ. Kidney function is inversely associated with coronary artery calcification in men and women free of cardiovascular disease: the Framingham Heart Study. Kidney Int. 2004;66:2017.
31. Weiner DE, Tighiouart H, Amin MG, et al. Chronic kidney disease as a risk factor for cardiovascular disease and all-cause mortality: a pooled analysis of community-based studies. J Am Soc Nephrol. 2004;15:1307.
32. Tonelli M, Wiebe N, Culleton B, et al. Chronic kidney disease and mortality risk: a systematic review. J Am Soc Nephrol. 2006;17:2034.
33. Fox CS, Muntner P, Chen AY, Alexander KP, Roe MT, Cannon CP, Saucedo JF, Kontos MC, Wiviott SD. Acute Coronary Treatment and Intervention Outcomes Network Registry. Use of evidence-based therapies in short term outcomes of ST-segment elevation myocardial infarction and non–STsegment elevation myocardial infarction in patients with chronic kidney disease: a report from the National Cardiovascular Data Acute Coronary Treatment and Intervention Outcomes Network registry. Circulation. 2010;121:357–65.
34. Herzog CA, Littrell K, Arko C, Frederick PD, Blaney M. Clinical characteristics of dialysis patients with acute myocardial infarction in the United States: a collaborative project of the United States Renal Data System and the National Registry of Myocardial Infarction. Circulation. 2007;116:1465–72.
35. Szummer K, Lundman P, Jacobson SH, Schön S, Lindbäck J, Stenestrand U, Wallentin L, Jernberg T. Swedeheart. Relation between renal function, presentation, use of therapies and in-hospital complications in acute coronary syndrome: data from the Swedeheart register. J Intern Med. 2010;268:40–9.
36. Coca SG, Krumholz HM, Garg AX, Parikh CR. Underrepresentation of renal disease in randomized controlled trials of cardiovascular disease. JAMA. 2006;296:1377.
37. Baigent C, Landray MJ, Reith C, Emberson J, Wheeler DC, Tomson C, Wanner C, Krane V, Cass A, Craig J, Neal B, Jiang L, Hooi LS, Levin A, Agodoa L, Gaziano M, Kasiske B, Walker R, Massy ZA, Feldt-Rasmussen B, Krairittichai U, Ophascharoensuk V, Fellström B, Holdaas H, Tesar V, Wiecek A, Grobbee D, de Zeeuw D, Grönhagen-Riska C, Dasgupta T, Lewis D, Herrington W, Mafham M, Majoni W, Wallendszus K, Grimm R, Pedersen T, Tobert J, Armitage J, Baxter A, Bray C, Chen Y, Chen Z, Hill M, Knott C, Parish S, Simpson D, Sleight P, Young A, Collins R. Sharp investigators. The effects of lowering LDL cholesterol with simvastatin plus ezetimibe in patients with chronic kidney disease (Study of Heart and Renal Protection): a randomised placebo-controlled trial. Lancet. 2011;377 (9784):2181–92.
38. Fellström BC, Jardine AG, Schmieder RE, Holdaas H, Bannister K, Beutler J, Chae DW, Chevaile A, Cobbe SM, Grönhagen-Riska C, De Lima JJ, Lins R, Mayer G, McMahon AW, Parving HH, Remuzzi G, Samuelsson O, Sonkodi S, Sci D, Süleymanlar G, Tsakiris D, Tesar V, Todorov V, Wiecek A, Wüthrich RP, Gottlow M, Johnsson E, Zannad F. Aurora Study Group. Rosuvastatin and cardiovascular events in patients undergoing hemodialysis. N Engl J Med. 2009;360:1395.

39. Holdaas H, Holme I, Schmieder RE, Jardine AG, Zannad F, Norby GE. Fellström BC; Aurora Study Group. Rosuvastatin in diabetic hemodialysis patients. J Am Soc Nephrol. 2011;22:1335.
40. KDIGO Clinical Practice Guideline for Lipid Management in. Chronic kidney disease. Kidney Int Suppl. 2013;3:263.
41. Wright JT Jr, Williamson JD, Whelton PK, Snyder JK, Sink KM, Rocco MV, Reboussin DM, Rahman M, Oparil S, Lewis CE, Kimmel PL, Johnson KC, Goff DC Jr, Fine LJ, Cutler JA, Cushman WC, Cheung AK, Ambrosius WT. A randomized trial of intensive versus standard blood-pressure control. N Engl J Med. 2015;373(22):2103–16.
42. Mann JF, Gerstein HC, Pogue J, Bosch J, Yusuf S. Renal insufficiency as a predictor of cardiovascular outcomes and the impact of ramipril: the HOPE randomized trial. Ann Intern Med. 2001;134:629.
43. Perkovic V, Ninomiya T, Arima H, Gallagher M, Jardine M, Cass A, Neal B, McMahon S, Chalmers J. Chronic kidney disease, cardiovascular events, and the effects of perindopril-based blood pressure lowering: data from the progress study. J Am Soc Nephrol. 2007;18:2766.
44. Blood Pressure Lowering Treatment Trialists' Collaboration, Ninomiya T, Perkovic V, Turnbull F, Neal B, Barzi F, Cass A, Baigent C, Chalmers J, Li N, Woodward M, McMahon S. Blood pressure lowering and major cardiovascular events in people with and without chronic kidney disease: meta-analysis of randomised controlled trials. BMJ. 2013;347:f5680.
45. Mcintyre CW, Burton JO, Selby NM, Leccisotti L, Korsheed S, Baker CS, Camici PG. Hemodialysis-induced cardiac dysfunction is associated with an acute reduction in global and segmental myocardial blood flow. Clin J Am Soc Nephrol. 2008;3(1):19–26.
46. Palmer SC, Di Micco L, Razavian M, Craig JC, Perkovic V, Pellegrini F, Jardine MJ, Webster AC, Zoungas S, Strippoli GF. Antiplatelet agents for chronic kidney disease. Cochrane Database Syst Rev. 2013;2:CD008834.
47. Palmer SC, Di Micco L, Razavian M, Craig JC, Perkovic V, Pellegrini F, Copetti M, Graziano G, Tognoni G, Jardine M, Webster A, Nicolucci A, Zoungas S, Strippoli GF. Effects of antiplatelet therapy on mortality and cardiovascular and bleeding outcomes in persons with chronic kidney disease: a systematic review and meta-analysis. Ann Intern Med. 2012;156:445.
48. Ethier J, Bragg-Gresham JL, Piera L, Akizawa T, Asano Y, Mason N, Gillespie BW, Young EW. Aspirin prescription and outcomes in hemodialysis patients: the Dialysis Outcomes and Practice Patterns Study (DOPPS). Am J Kidney Dis. 2007;50:602.
49. Chan K, Lazarus J, Thadhani R, Hakim R. Anticoagulant and antiplatelet usage associates with mortality among hemodialysis patients. J Am Soc Nephrol. 2009;20:872.
50. Spertus JA, Maron DJ, Cohen DJ, Kolm P, Hartigan P, Weintraub WS, Berman DS, Teo KK, Shaw LJ, Sedlis SP, Knudtson M, Aslan M, Dada M, Boden WE, Mancini GB. Clinical Outcomes Utilizing Revascularization and Aggressive Drug Evaluation (COURAGE) Trial Investigators and Coordinators. Frequency, predictors, and consequences of crossing over to revascularization within 12 months of randomization to optimal medical therapy in the Clinical Outcomes Utilizing Revascularization and Aggressive Drug Evaluation (COURAGE) trial. Circ Cardiovasc Qual Outcomes. 2013;6(4):409–18.
51. Tonelli M, Muntner P, Lloyd A, Manns BJ, Klarenbach S, Pannu N, James MT, Hemmelgarn BR. Risk of coronary events in people with chronic kidney disease compared with those with diabetes: a population-level cohort study. Lancet. 2012;380:807.
52. Pun PH, Al-Khatib SM, Han JY, Edwards R, Bardy GH, Bigger JT, Buxton AE, Moss AJ, Lee KL, Steinman R, Dorian P, Hallstrom A, Cappato R, Kadish AH, Kudenchuk PJ, Mark DB, Hess PL, Inoue LY, Sanders GD. Implantable cardioverter-defibrillators for primary prevention of sudden cardiac death in CKD: a meta-analysis of patient-level data from 3 randomized trials. Am J Kidney Dis. 2014;64:32.
53. Gibney EM, Casebeer AW, Schooley LM, Cunningham F, Grover FL, Bell MR, McDonald GO, Shroyer AL, Parikh CR. Cardiovascular medication use after coronary bypass surgery in patients with renal dysfunction: a national Veterans Administration study. Kidney Int. 2005;68:826.
54. Newsome BB, Warnock DG, Kiefe CI, Weissman NW, Houston TK, Centor RM, Person SD, Mcclellan WM, Allison JJ. Delay in time to receipt of thrombolytic medication among Medicare patients with kidney disease. Am J Kidney Dis. 2005;46:595.
55. Han JH, Chandra A, Mulgund J, Roe MT, Peterson ED, Szczech LA, Patel U, Ohman EM, Lindsell CJ, Gibler WB. Chronic kidney disease in patients with non-ST-segment elevation acute coronary syndromes. Am J Med. 2006;119:248.
56. Patel UD, Ou FS, Ohman EM, Gibler WB, Pollack CV Jr, Peterson ED, Roe MT. Hospital performance and differences by kidney function in the use of recommended therapies after non-ST-elevation acute coronary syndromes. Am J Kidney Dis. 2009;53:426.
57. Charytan D, Mauri L, Agarwal A, Servoss S, Scirica B, Kuntz RE. The use of invasive cardiac procedures after acute myocardial infarction in long-term dialysis patients. Am Heart J. 2006;152:558.
58. Fox CS, Muntner P, Chen AY, Alexander KP, Roe MT, Cannon CP, Saucedo JF, Kontos MC, Wiviott SD. Acute Coronary Treatment AND Intervention OutcomesNetwork registry. Use of evidence-based therapies in short-term outcomes of ST-segment elevation myocardial infarction and non-ST-segment elevation myocardial infarction in patients with chronic kidney disease: a report from the National Cardiovascular Data Acute Coronary Treatment and Intervention Outcomes Network registry. Circulation. 2010;121:357.
59. O'Gara PT, Kushner FG, Ascheim DD, Casey DE Jr, Chung MK, de Lemos JA, Ettinger SM, Fang JC, Fesmire FM, Franklin BA, Granger CB, Krumholz HM, Linderbaum JA, Morrow DA, Newby LK, Ornato JP, Ou N, Radford MJ, Tamis-Holland JE, Tommaso CL, Tracy CM, Woo YJ, Zhao DX, Anderson JL, Jacobs AK, Halperin JL, Albert NM, Brindis RG, Creager MA, DeMets D, Guyton RA, Hochman JS, Kovacs RJ, Kushner FG, Ohman EM, Stevenson WG, Yancy CW, American College of Cardiology Foundation/American Heart Association Task Force on Practice Guidelines. 2013 ACCF/AHA guideline for the management of ST-elevation myocardial infarction: a report of the American College of Cardiology Foundation/American Heart Association Task Force on Practice Guidelines. Circulation. 2013;127:e362–425.
60. Dragu R, Behar S, Sandach A, Boyko V, Kapeliovich M, Rispler S, Hammerman H. Should primary percutaneous coronary intervention be the preferred method of reperfusion therapy for patients with renal failure and STelevation acute myocardial infarction. Am J Cardiol. 2006;97:1142–55.
61. Medi C, Montalescot G, Budaj A, Fox KA, López-Sendón J, Fitzgerald G, Brieger DB. Reperfusion in patients with renal dysfunction after presentation with ST-segment elevation or left bundle branch block: GRACE (Global Registry of Acute Coronary Events). JACC Cardiovasc Interv. 2009;2:26–33.
62. Bavry A, Kumbhani D, Rassi A, Bhatt D, Askari A. Benefit of early invasive therapy in acute coronary syndromes: a metaanalysis of contemporary randomized clinical trials. J Am Coll Cardiol. 2006;48:1319–25.
63. Szummer K, Lundman P, Jacobson S, Schön S, Lindbäck J, Stenestrand U, Wallentin L, Jernberg T. Influence of renal function on the effects of early revascularization in non-ST-elevation

myocardial infarction: data from the Swedish Web-System for Enhancement and Development of Evidence-Based Care in Heart Disease Evaluated According to Recommended Therapies (SWEDEHEART). Circulation. 2009;120:851–8.

64. Aoki J, Ong AT, Hoye A, van Herwerden LA, Sousa JE, Jatene A, Bonnier JJ, Schönberger JP, Buller N, Bonser R, Lindeboom W, Unger F, Serruys PW. Five year clinical effect of coronary stenting and coronary artery bypass grafting in renal insufficient patients with multivessel coronary artery disease: insights from ARTS trial. Eur Heart J. 2005;26:1488.
65. Schmieder RE, Mann JF, Schumacher H, Gao P, Mancia G, Weber MA, McQueen M, Koon T, Yusuf S. Changes in albuminuria predict mortality and morbidity in patients with vascular disease. J Am Soc Nephrol. 2011;22:1353.
66. Shroff GR, Solid CA, Herzog CA. Long-term survival and repeat coronary revascularization in dialysis patients after surgical and percutaneous coronary revascularization with drug-eluting and bare metal stents in the United States. Circulation. 2013;127:1861–9.
67. Bangalore S, Guo Y, Samadashvili Z, Blecker S, Xu J, Hannan E. Revascularization in patients with multivessel coronary artery disease and chronic kidney disease: everolimus-eluting stents versus coronary artery bypass graft surgery. J Am Coll Cardiol. 2015;66(11):1202–9.

CKD Associated Cardiomyopathy: Molecular Mechanisms, Imaging Modalities, Disease Evolution and Interventions

5

Nicola C. Edwards, Manvir Kaur Hayer, Charles J. Ferro, Jonathan N. Townend, and Richard P. Steeds

Introduction

In patients with end-stage kidney disease (ESKD), cardiovascular deaths account for about half of all mortality. Most are due to sudden cardiac death, heart failure and arrhythmias rather than the atherosclerotic coronary occlusive events commonly seen in the general population [1]. This may be attributable to the near universal prevalence of structural left ventricular (LV) disease, originally termed uremic cardiomyopathy (UC). First described in echocardiographic studies, the characteristic structural and functional features of UC include LV hypertrophy (LVH), LV dilatation, and infrequently, reduced LV ejection fraction. The development of cardiac magnetic resonance (CMR) imaging in the 1990s allowed more accurate and reproducible assessment of UC, with the additional advantage of tissue characterization, allowing the identification of myocardial fibrosis in ESKD [2]. There is now strong evidence that abnormalities of LV structure, function and fibrosis are present much earlier than hitherto expected and are not restricted to advanced 'uremic' states; thus the term CKD-associated cardiomyopathy is a preferred terminology.

Although increased LV mass is the principle structural abnormality seen in CKD-associated cardiomyopathy, myocardial interstitial fibrosis may be the key intermediate phenotype (Fig. 5.1). Animal and human myocardial biopsy studies demonstrate not only cellular hypertrophy but also severe myocyte disarray and extensive, diffuse interstitial fibrosis (DIF), similar to the appearances in hypertrophic cardiomyopathy [3]. The increase of fibrotic tissue impairs LV contractility in two ways: first, increases in the collagen type I: III ratio enhance stiffness; second, changes in collagen alignment relative to cardiomyocytes impairs transmission of force to the LV. As a result, diastolic relaxation is impaired, leading to exercise intolerance, and ultimately to heart failure and ventricular arrhythmias.

Molecular Mechanisms

Numerous possible stimuli to LV hypertrophy and fibrosis are present from the earliest stages of CKD but there are limited data to indicate whether these are causative (Fig. 5.2).

Renin-Angiotensin-Aldosterone System (RAAS)

There is strong evidence from both animal and human studies that activation of the RAAS is important in the development of LVH and fibrosis (Fig. 5.3). Historically, angiotensin II (Ang II) has been viewed as the primary mediator of end-organ fibrosis through its activation of cellular proliferation, inflammatory cytokines and increased production of metalloproteinases and collagen synthesis. The efficacy of angiotensin-converting enzyme (ACE) inhibitors and angiotensin receptor blockers (ARBs) in reducing CV mortality, reproducible in CKD subjects, is testament to the deleterious actions of Ang II [4]. Aldosterone however, is also a key modulator of inflammation and

N.C. Edwards · J.N. Townend · R.P. Steeds
Department of Cardiology, Queen Elizabeth Hospital Birmingham, Mendlesohn Way, Birmingham, B15 2TH, UK
e-mail: nicky.edwards@uhb.nhs.uk

J.N. Townend
e-mail: John.Townend@uhb.nhs.uk

R.P. Steeds
e-mail: rick.steeds@uhb.nhs.uk

M.K. Hayer (✉) · C.J. Ferro
Department of Nephrology, Queen Elizabeth Hospital Birmingham, Mendlesohn Way, Birmingham, B15 2TH, UK
e-mail: mkh242@gmail.com

C.J. Ferro
e-mail: Charles.ferro@uhb.nhs.uk

J. Rangaswami et al. (eds.), *Cardio-Nephrology*,
DOI 10.1007/978-3-319-56042-7_5

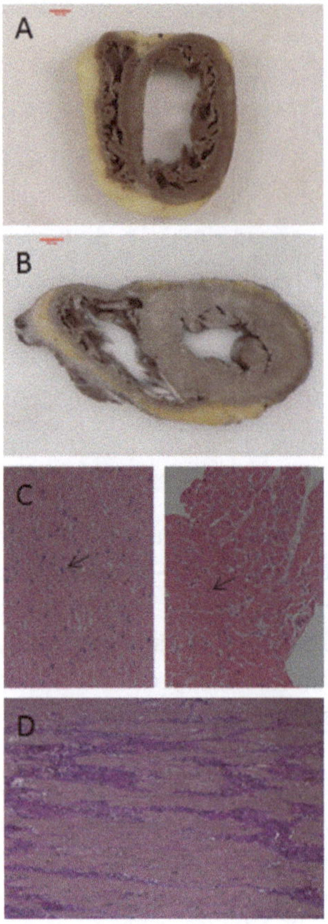

Fig. 5.1 Histopathology images of CKD-associated cardiomyopathy. **a** A dilated left ventricle. The walls of the ventricle get thinner due to the stretching. **b** Cross section through a heart showing mild concentric left ventricular hypertrophy with a normal chamber size. There are no discrete areas of fibrosis within the myocardium. **c** Haematoxylin and eosin stained sections both taken at the same magnification (×20 objective lens). The section on the left shows myocyte hypertrophy as evidenced by the marked enlargement of purple myocyte nuclei within the pink cytoplasm. The section on the right is from a recent cardiac transplant biopsy showing more normal-sized myocytes as demonstrated by comparing the size of the purple nuclei to the hypertrophied ones. **d** Elastic Van Gieson (EHVG) stained section showing diffuse interstitial fibrosis (*bright pink*), myocytes stain brown

fibrosis through both paracrine and autocrine effects, not only by cytokine production and inflammatory cell recruitment but also by increased synthesis of transforming growth factor-1 and plasminogen activator-1 [5]. It is of interest that primary hyperaldosteronism is characterized by DIF and diastolic dysfunction. The cardiac and vascular inflammatory effects of aldosterone are exacerbated and may be dependent on the presence of sodium excess. In sodium retention states such as CKD and heart failure, aldosterone levels are inappropriately elevated (aldosterone escape) due to loss of the normal negative feedback mechanisms relative to sodium and fluid balance and this combination plays a central role in sensitizing the CV system to the deleterious effects of aldosterone. In animal models, 8 weeks of exogenous aldosterone administration and high salt diet resulted in LVH and accumulation of collagen within the interstitial space without myocyte necrosis. Fibrillar collagen was increased in both right and left ventricle, irrespective of hypertrophy and was prevented with the MR antagonist spironolactone without a reduction in blood pressure [6].

Abnormal Calcium and Phosphate Metabolism

Abnormal calcium and phosphate metabolism is a common consequence of CKD and manifests with altered circulating levels of calcium, phosphate, parathyroid hormone (PTH), vitamin D and phosphatonins such as fibroblast growth factor (FGF)-23. The close interplay of these factors is shown in Fig. 5.4a, b.

Phosphate

The ability of the kidneys to excrete phosphate is reduced at a GFR < 60 ml/min/1.73m^2 but serum phosphate remains within the normal range until the GFR < 30 ml/min/1.73m^2 because of increased production of PTH and FGF-23, which promote urinary phosphate excretion. Observational data have demonstrated an association between serum phosphate and CV mortality in patients with CKD, ESKD and after renal transplantation even when serum phosphate levels are within the reference range [7]. Elevated phosphate results in increased vascular calcification but whether it exerts a direct toxic effect on cardiomyocytes is unknown. In animal models of CKD, both high dietary phosphate and hyperphosphatemia induce arterial wall thickening and interstitial cardiac fibrosis.

Fibroblast Growth Factor 23 (FGF-23)

Produced by osteocytes, FGF-23 increases urinary phosphate excretion and reduces gastrointestinal calcium and phosphate absorption by suppressing 1,25 dihydroxyvitamin D synthesis. FGF-23 acts through the membrane-bound FGF receptor (FGFR) and its obligate co-receptor transmembranous Klotho. Levels of FGF-23 rise as early as stage 2 CKD, (before a rise in serum phosphate, PTH and decline in 1,25 dihydroxyvitamin D) and increase logarithmically as GFR falls, reaching levels two- to fivefold normal in early stage disease and more than a 1000-fold normal in ESKD. Expression of Klotho declines in CKD as FGF-23 increases. In observational data from both CKD and ESRD, increases in FGF-23 are associated with greater CV morbidity while reduced levels of circulating soluble Klotho are associated with cardiac hypertrophy and dysfunction [8]. In mouse models of CKD, there is evidence that FGF-23 plays a direct role in the causation of CKD-associated cardiomyopathy via FGFR dependent activation of the calcineurin-NFAT (nuclear factor of activated T cells) signalling pathway (an

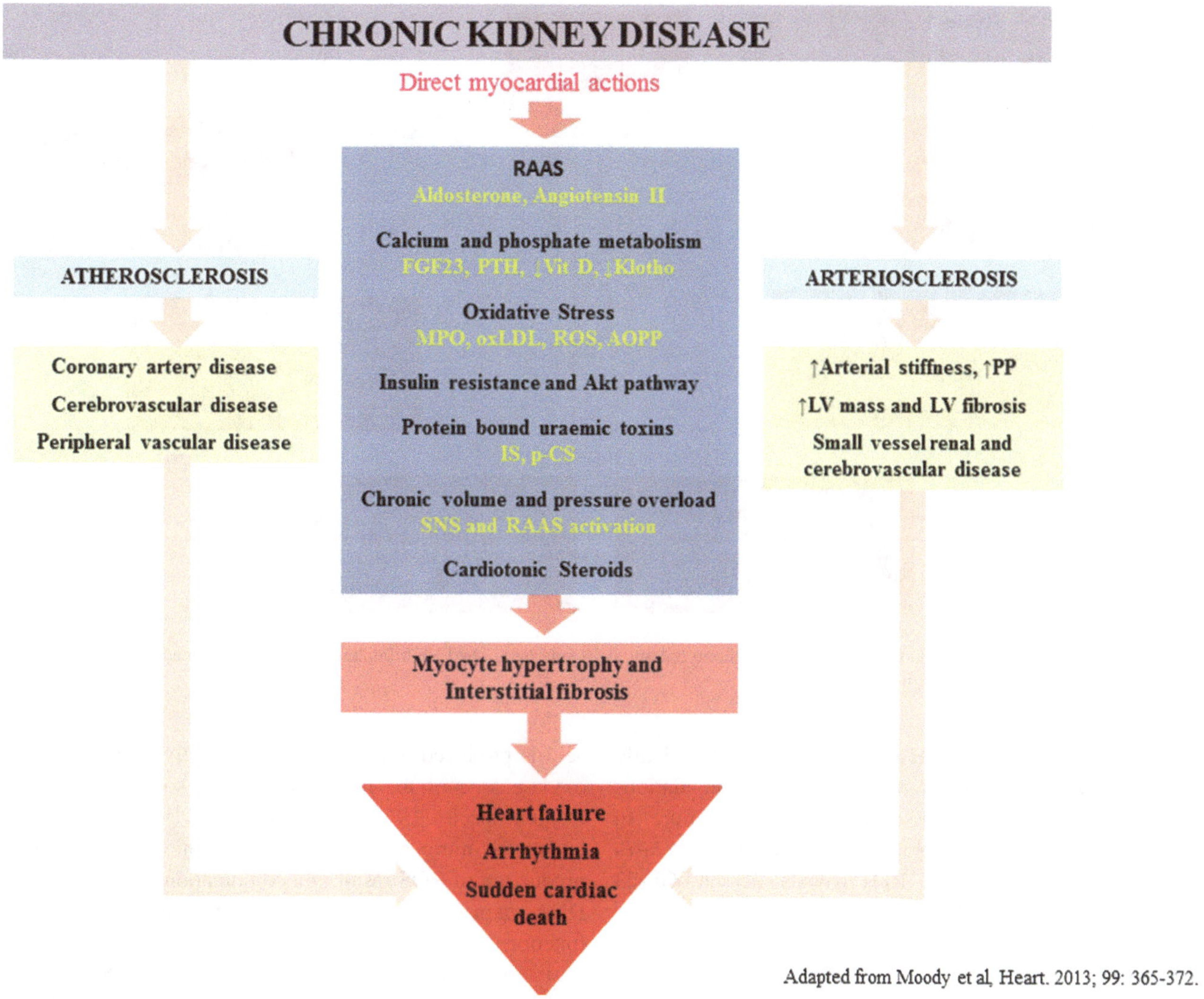

Fig. 5.2 An overview of the various mechanisms contributing towards heart disease in CKD. While there are many pathways resulting in heart disease in CKD, the largest disease burden arises from structural changes to the myocardium including hypertrophy and fibrosis. *AOPP* advanced oxidation protein products, *FGF-23* fibroblast growth factor 23, *LV* left ventricular, *MPO* myeloperoxidase, *oxLDL* oxidised low-density lipoprotein, *PP* pulse pressure, *PTH* parathyroid hormone, *RAAS* renin-angiotensin-aldosterone system, *ROS* reactive oxygen species, *SNS* sympathetic nervous system, *Vitamin D* 1,25 dihydroxyvitamin, *IS* indoxyl sulphate, *p-CS* p-cresyl sulphate. Reprinted with permission from BMJ Publishing Group Ltd: Heart. William E Moody, Nicola C Edwards, Colin D Chue, Charles J Ferro, and Jonathan N Townend. Arterial disease in chronic kidney disease, copyright 2013

important and established pathway in LVH), but does not appear to require Klotho. Furthermore, treatment with an FGF–receptor blocker in both animal and cultured cardiomyocyte models caused attenuation of FGF-23 induced myocyte hypertrophy [9]. Consistent with these animal data, a small human autopsy study reported that in patients with ESKD, cardiac levels of FGF-23 were elevated and were associated with LVH. There was also upregulation of FGFR and reduced levels of soluble (circulation derived) Klotho [10]. Further evidence that FGF-23 may act to cause LVH via the calcineurin-NFAT pathway came from the finding that expression of calcineurin and NFAT mRNA were increased in patients with LVH but not in those without. Myocardial FGF-23 rapidly decreases after renal transplantation mirrored by a reduction in calcineurin–NFAT signalling, providing further support for a role in this cascade in up-regulating FGF-23/FGFR.

Parathyroid Hormone

In animal models, PTH increases entry of calcium into myocytes and promotes hypertrophy through stimulation of protein kinase C while parathyroidectomy attenuates these changes. FGFR receptors are present on the parathyroid gland and FGF-23 can directly increase PTH production. In both primary and secondary hyperparathyroidism, there is a graded relationship between the level of serum PTH and LV

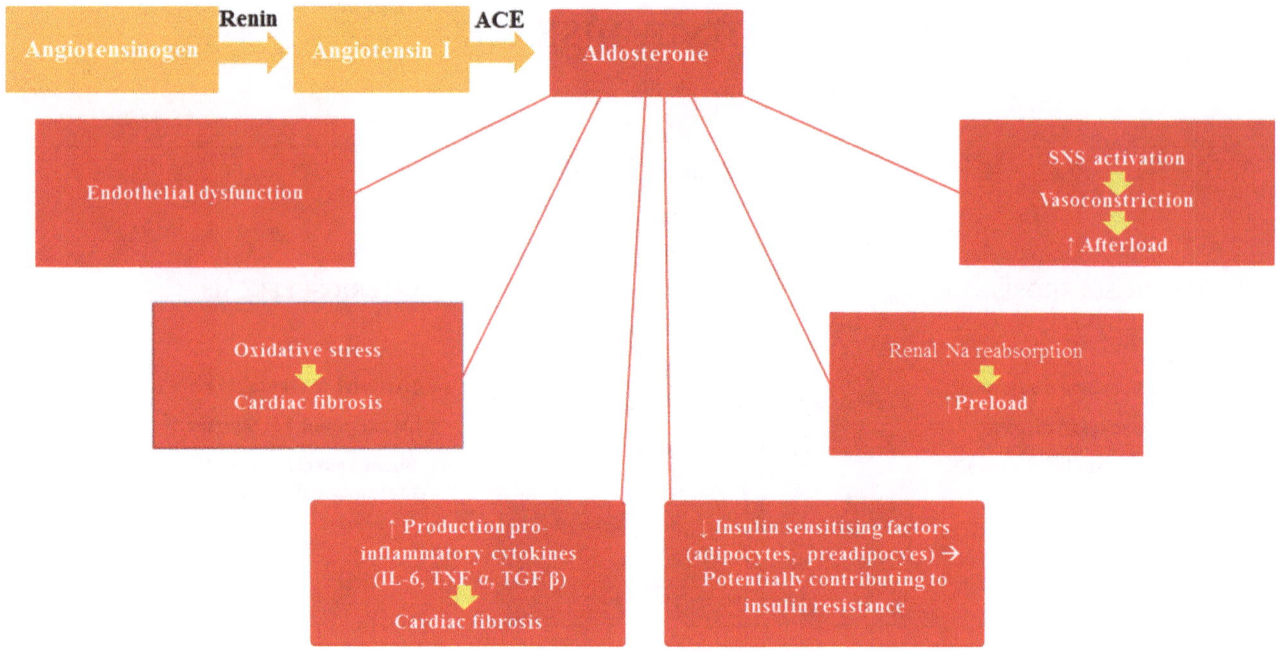

Fig. 5.3 The role of aldosterone in CKD-associated cardiomyopathy. IL-6, interleukin 6; TNF α [alpha], tumour necrosis factor α [alpha]; TGF β [beta], transforming growth factor β [beta]

mass [11]. The level of PTH has also been independently associated with LV mass in community-based populations and excess PTH has been associated with heart failure. In animal models, PTH accelerates LVH and also increases expression of collagen type 1. PTH may also act via FGF-23 by increasing osteocyte FGF-23 secretion [8].

Vitamin D

Several epidemiological observational studies have shown an important association between vitamin D deficiency and cardiovascular mortality but mechanistic data is limited [12]. In animal models of vitamin D receptor knockout mice, hypertension and LVH were observed and postulated to reflect an increase in renin consequent to loss of normal suppression of the renin-angiotensin system by vitamin D. In rats, treatment with vitamin D analogues ameliorated LVH and improved LV diastolic function. The effects of Vitamin D on cardiovascular mortality in CKD are summarized in detail in a separate chapter.

Hyperuricemia

Hyperuricemia is a frequent finding in CKD and may be a risk factor or biomarker for CV outcomes. In heart failure patients, hyperuricaemia is associated with more symptoms, worse exercise capacity and reduced survival. It has been suggested that hyperuricaemia may promote CKD-associated cardiomyopathy via oxidative stress. Uric acid is produced with superoxide by activation of xanthine oxidase, one of the main intracellular sources of reactive oxygen species (ROS), including NAD(P)H oxidase, and uncoupled nitric oxide synthase. Chronic increases in the production of ROS result in a combination of mitochondrial DNA damage, cellular injury and impaired contractile function by modifying proteins central to excitation-contraction coupling. Moreover, ROS activate a broad variety of hypertrophy signalling kinases and transcription factors and mediate apoptosis. They can also stimulate cardiac fibroblast proliferation and activate the matrix metalloproteinases, leading to extracellular matrix remodelling and DIF [13].

Protein Bound Uremic Toxins

The progressive loss of kidney function in CKD leads to the accumulation of protein bound "uremic toxins" (PBUTs). These PBUTs are cardiotoxic and are associated with increased CV mortality. Attention has been focused on indoxyl sulphate (IS) and p-Cresyl sulphate. In health, these molecules are cleared from the systemic circulation by renal tubular secretion but levels rise in early stage CKD [2, 3] and increase up to 100 times in ESKD. Studies in vitro and in vivo have implicated both molecules in direct cardiac injury through potent inflammatory and fibrogenic effects [14–16]. In vitro, IS stimulation of rat cardiomyocytes and fibroblasts induces pro-inflammatory and fibrotic changes. In a

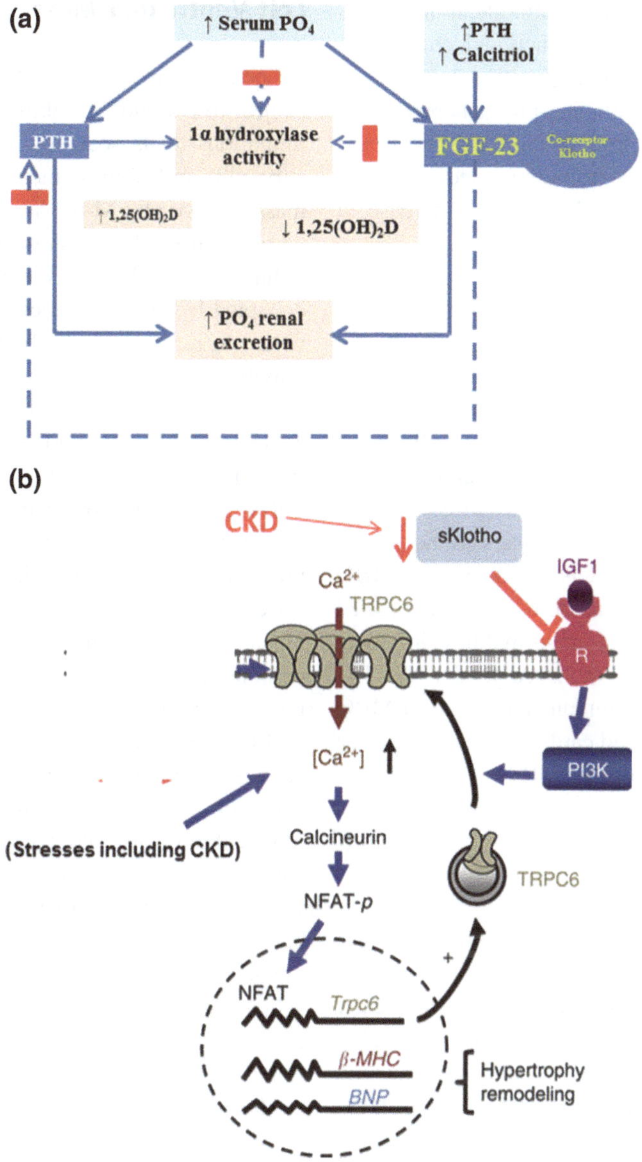

Fig. 5.4 **a** The association between phosphate, parathyroid hormone, vitamin D and FGF-23 and the co-receptor Klotho. Both PTH and FGF-23 are released in response to a high phosphate, and act by reducing renal phosphate re-absorption from urine. PTH increases the production of 1,25 dihydroxyvitamin D, while FGF-23 suppresses synthesis of 1,25 dihydroxyvitamin D, thereby reducing phosphate and calcium absorption from the intestine. FGF-23 acts by binding to the FGF-23 receptor and its obligate co-receptor transmembranous Klotho. Expression of Klotho declines in CKD while FGF-23 expression increases, resulting in cardiac remodelling and dysfunction, and increased cardiovascular morbidity. PTH, Parathyroid hormone; FGF-23, Fibroblast Growth Factor 23; 1,25(OH)2D, 1,25 dihydroxyvitamin D; PO4, Phosphate. Reprinted with permission from Elsevier: American Journal of Kidney Diseases. Ranjani N. Moorthi and Sharon M. Moe. CKD–Mineral and Bone Disorder: Core Curriculum 2011, copyright 2011. **b** The role of soluble Klotho. Stresses (such as those encountered in CKD) cause abnormal intracellular Ca2 + signalling, thereby activating the calcineurin-NFAT signalling cascade. This results in cardiac remodelling and hypertrophy, as well as TRCP6 gene expression. IGF1 activates PI3K to promote exocytosis of TRPC6. Soluble Klotho (sKlotho) inhibits IGF1 activation of PI3K, resulting in downregulation of the TRCP6 receptor, and thus sKlotho protects the heart from stress-induced cardiac hypertrophy. Without stress signal to upregulate TRPC6 expression, soluble Klotho has no effect on the heart at baseline. Reprinted with permission from Nature Publishing Group: Nature Communications. Jian Xie, Seung-Kuy Cha, Sung-Wan An, Makoto Kuro-o, Lutz Birnbaumer et al. Cardioprotection by Klotho through downregulation of TRPC6 channels in the mouse heart, copyright 2012

5/6-subtotal nephrectomy rat model of CKD, serum IS levels increased in association with reduced GFR and detectable diastolic dysfunction on Doppler echocardiography. Treatment to reduce IS levels improved renal function and reduced cardiac fibrosis by 68% independent of blood pressure and renal dysfunction [17]. Furthermore, PBUTs may also cause post-translational protein modifications. Carbamylation promotes structural and functional changes in type I collagen. In addition, altered glycation leads to an accumulation of advanced glycation end-products precursors which have been shown to alter collagen in the vascular and myocardial matrices leading to disordered and defective collagen. This is believed to contribute to the increase in arterial and myocardial stiffening in CKD.

Cardiotonic Steroids

Circulating levels of cardiotonic steroids such as marinobufagenin (MBG) are increased in CKD. In vitro studies have demonstrated their role in initiating an intracellular signal cascade with a resultant increase in oxidant stress activity, genomic modulation and induction of state cardiac hypertrophy. In experimental rat models, infusion of MBG induced comparable levels of cardiac fibrosis with associated structural and functional cardiac abnormalities in sham operated rats as seen with the established model of CKD using partial (5/6) nephrectomy. Immunization against MBG attenuated cardiac hypertrophy and cardiac fibrosis without a significant reduction in blood pressure [18].

Insulin Resistance

Experimental rodent models have shown insulin resistance to be present at very early stages of CKD. Consequent alterations of intracellular signalling pathways, specifically the serine/threonine protein kinase B or Akt pathway lead to changes in pleiotropic and metabolic actions of insulin which play a key role in regulating the development of LVH and in cardiac fibrosis, cellular apoptosis, calcium cycling and metabolic dysfunction [19].

Imaging Modalities in CKD-Associated Cardiomyopathy

The structural and functional changes that typify CKD-associated cardiomyopathy were first documented using transthoracic echocardiography and this remains the first line clinical cardiovascular imaging modality in CKD. Echocardiography is inexpensive, portable and widely available, and ultrasound carries no risk, while delivering much incremental information beyond clinical and electrocardiographic assessment. For a number of reasons however, echocardiography is increasingly being supplanted by CMR in the assessment of CKD-associated cardiomyopathy [2] (See Table 5.1).

Left Ventricular Mass

Echocardiography is a skilled technique and is inherently subject to operator variability. In addition, there are specific limitations to its accuracy in CKD that are exemplified by variability in LV mass measurement. All algorithms for LV mass, whether by M-mode, 2D or 3D echocardiography, are based on the subtraction of the LV cavity volume from the volume enclosed by the LV epicardium to obtain the volume occupied by the LV myocardium. This volume is then converted to mass by multiplying wall volume by the specific gravity of myocardium. Both M-mode and 2D methods make geometric assumptions about LV shape to generate this 'myocardial volume' but these assumptions can be inaccurate in CKD. First, the shape of the LV changes in response to different stimuli—for example, concentric remodelling in hypertension and eccentric remodelling with increased pre-load in chronic anaemia (Fig. 5.5). Second, all methods for calculation of LV mass by echocardiography, including 3D, are dependent on measurement of the LV volume, which exhibits high day-to-day variability in CKD. Echocardiography consistently overestimates LV mass compared to CMR; almost half of those diagnosed with LVH on M-mode echocardiography do not have hypertrophy on CMR [20]. Three-dimensional echocardiography generates a shell volume without using geometric assumptions and so overcomes some of these issues and measures LV mass and volumes with comparable accuracy to CMR. This modality however, is even more susceptible to limitations of acoustic window, image quality, and observer expertise than M-mode and 2D echo as the ultrasound probes tend to be larger and operate at a lower frame rate in 3D. Measurements of LV mass may differ by 8 + 5% between 3D scans and the limits of agreement can be up to 33g using the latest software compared to CMR in non-ischemic cardiomyopathy.

In contrast, CMR measures LV mass without using geometric assumptions, by performing a stack of cine acquisitions from the atrioventricular ring to the apex of the heart, followed by planimetry of the endocardial and epicardial borders to generate volume and mass parameters with greater accuracy (Fig. 5.6). Image quality is usually much better than echocardiography, as the stack is acquired from any angle without requirement for a specific 'window' and can be done equally well in obese subjects and those with lung disease.

Myocardial Fibrosis

Two distinct patterns of collagen accumulation can be distinguished in myocardial fibrosis: focal, to replace dead cardiomyocytes and form scar (replacement fibrosis, seen

Table 5.1 A comparison of imaging modalities in CKD-associated cardiomyopathy

Imaging techniques strengths and limitations

Imaging features	2D echocardiography /ultrasonography	Comment	Cardiac Magnetic Resonance	Comment	Multidetector Computed Tomography	Comment
LV mass	M-mode or 2D	Increased interstudy and operator variability. LV geometric assumptions. Volume dependent image quality.	Short-axis LV contouring.	Reference standard. High reproducibility. No geometric assumptions. Load independent.	Not applicable.	
Myocardial fibrosis	Integrated backscatter	Validation against histological collagen content. Assessment of interstitial fibrosis. Wide availability. Low reproducibility.	Late gadolinium enhancement T1 mapping.	Reference standard. Histological validation. Limited to detection of coarse scarring. Use precluded if eGFR < 30 ml/min/1.73 m^2. Detection of diffuse fibrosis. New non-contrast techniques.	Measured dynamic equilibrium of iodinated contrast.	As good as CMR at calculating extracellular volume. Risks of iodinated contrast. Exposure to radiation.

Adapted from Edwards et al. [2]
2D 2-dimensional, *LV* left ventricular, *ESRD* end stage renal disease, *CMR* cardiac magnetic resonance imaging

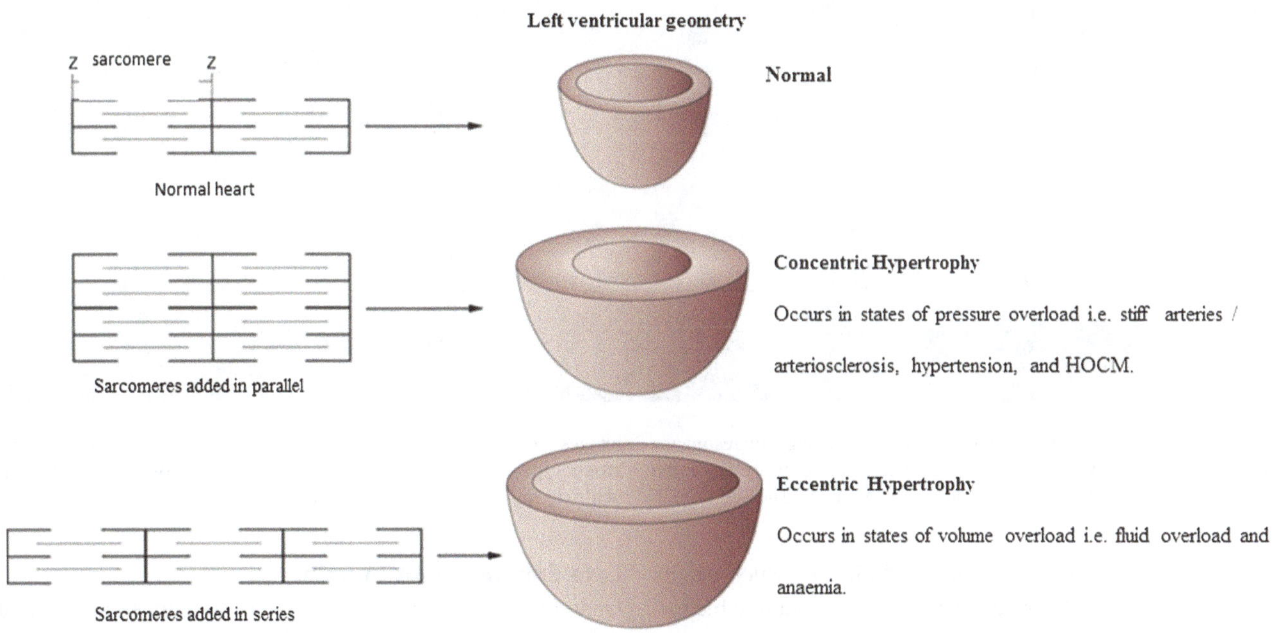

Fig. 5.5 Concentric versus eccentric hypertrophy. In both types of hypertrophy the left ventricular mass is increased. However, the relative wall thickness is preserved in eccentric hypertrophy but it is increased in concentric hypertrophy. Reprinted with permission from Nature Publishing Group: Nature Reviews Cardiology. Ola Gjesdal, David A. Bluemke, and Joao A. Lima. Cardiac remodelling at the population level-risk factors, screening, and outcomes, copyright 2011

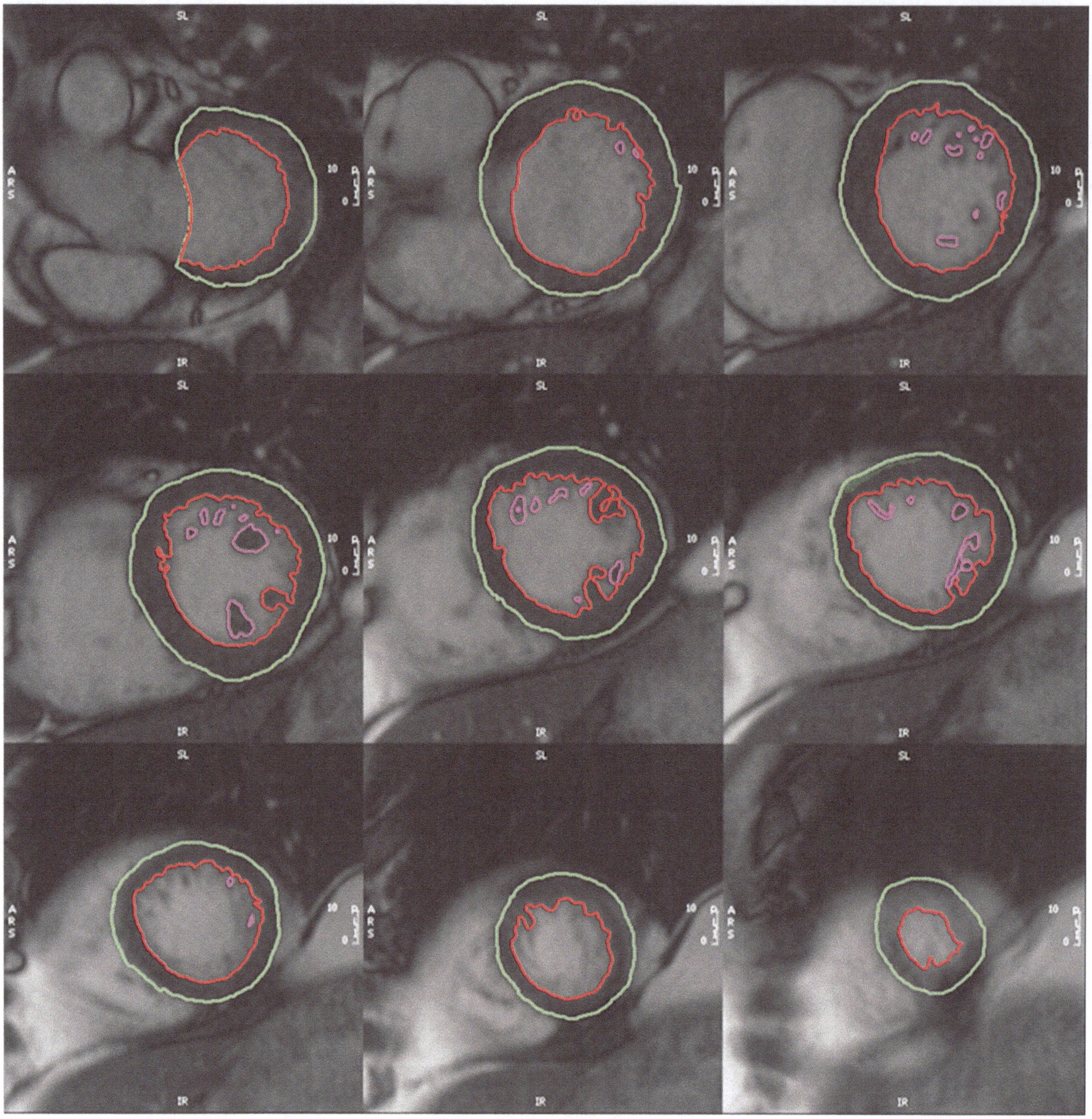

Fig. 5.6 Images from a short-axis stack on cardiac magnetic resonance imaging. A short-axis stack showing slices of the heart from the atrioventricular junction (slice 1) down to the apex (slice 9). These images were taken in diastole. In the diastolic phase, circles are drawn around the endocardium (*red*) and epicardium (*green*) of the left ventricle in order to calculate the LV mass

following myocardial infarction), and diffuse, which occurs in the interstitial and perivascular spaces without notable cell loss (reactive fibrosis, as in most hypertrophic cardiomyopathies). CMR is an effective tool for the identification of focal (replacement) fibrosis using late enhancement and for diagnosis and quantification of DIF using either native T1 mapping or contrast-based extracellular volume quantification.

Late Enhancement Imaging

Gadolinium-DTPA (Gd-DTPA) is a paramagnetic metal that diffuses rapidly from the vasculature into the extravascular tissue fluid but not into cells. When taken up into the extracellular space, Gd-DTPA potently shortens T1 time; making areas with contrast appear bright on inversion recovery imaging compared to areas without contrast. The volume of bright, 'late enhancement' correlates closely to the size of sub-endocardial scar following myocardial infarction but also distinguishes regions of myocyte disarray and replacement fibrosis in conditions such as CKD-associated cardiomyopathy. In a cross-sectional study of 134 patients with ESKD, sub-endocardial 'late enhancement' consistent with myocardial infarction was found in 14% but an equal number were found to have mid-wall 'late enhancement' consistent with non-ischaemic replacement fibrosis [21].

T1 Mapping

After excitation by a radiofrequency pulse, the time (T1 relaxation) taken for protons to 'relax' to their normal state (re-equilibrate) within the local tissue environment is specific to that environment. 'Native' (non-contrast) T1 relaxation time of myocardium also varies with water content and increases with interstitial fibrosis. Using T1 mapping, increased DIF was demonstrated in a case-control study of 129 age and gender-matched subjects with stage II-IV CKD compared to hypertensive and healthy control subjects (Fig. 5.7) [22]. While T1 mapping seems ideal in CKD, since no contrast is required to detect DIF, some issues remain. First, 'native' T1 relaxation values include signals from cells and interstitium. In ESKD, it is not known how variable T1 values may be in the myocardium when there may be variation in water content. Second, native mapping has been most successful where there is a large pathophysiological change, such as with infiltrative accumulation seen in amyloid and Fabry disease. In CKD, the 'native' T1 relaxation times overlap between cases and controls, and it is not yet established whether the difference in the 'signal' from DIF will be large enough to track in individuals over time or in response to treatment. One option that overcomes the issue of signal from cells and interstitium is to measure T1 values before and after Gd-DTPA contrast, which when combined with haematocrit can then be used to derive both an extracellular volume fraction and an intracellular volume fraction for the myocardium.

Gadolinium-Based Contrast Agents in CKD

In patients with advanced kidney disease (and with renal dysfunction due to hepato-renal syndrome, or in the peri-operative period after liver transplantation), the use of Gd-DTPA contrast has been associated with the development of a rare but untreatable and potentially lethal condition

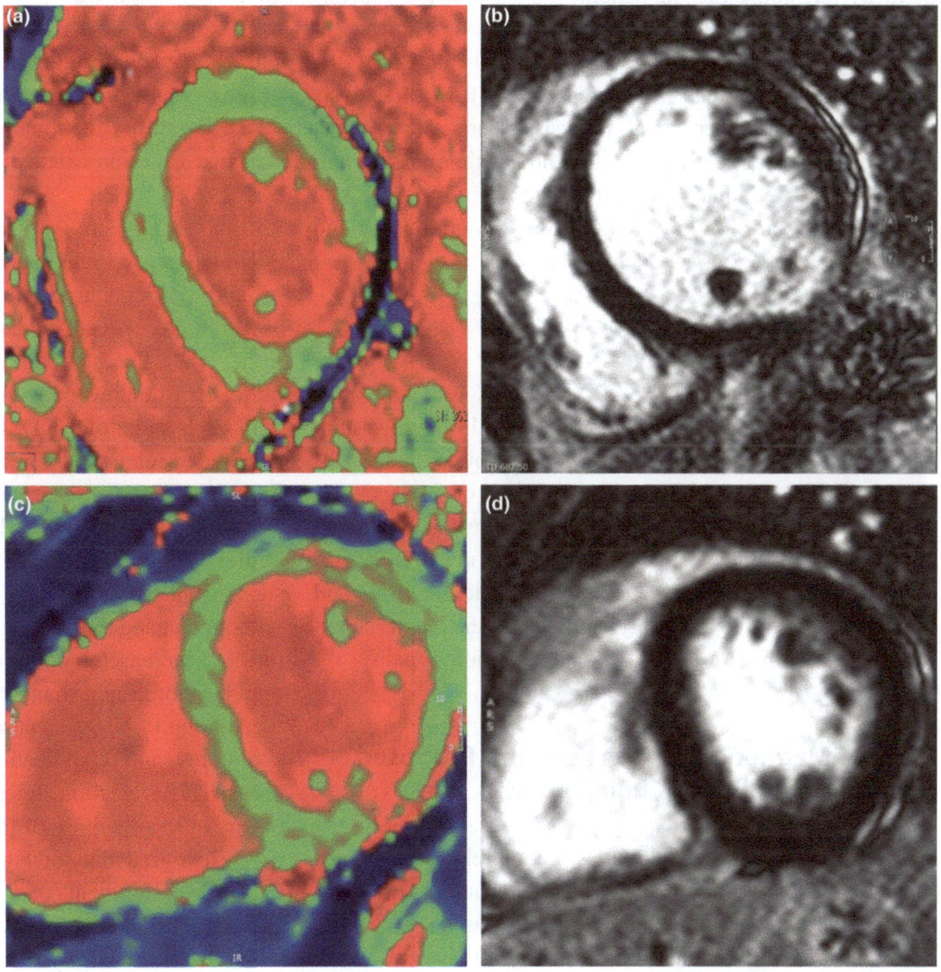

Fig. 5.7 An example of T1 images and late gadolinium enhancement (LGE). **a** Increased T1 time (*red*) within the infero-lateral myocardial segment. Normal myocardium (green). **b** Evidence of LGE (coarse fibrosis) correlating with increased T1 times at an equivilent level. **c** Increased T1 time (*red*) indicative of diffuse interstitial fibrosis not seen with standard LGE imaging. **d** No evidence of LGE. Thus, calculating T1 times can identify both coarse scarring that can also be seen using late gadolinium enhancement (LGE), and it can identify diffuse fibrosis that cannot be detected using LGE

called nephrogenic systemic fibrosis (NSF). Characterized by fibrosis of the skin and connective tissue, onset can occur anytime within the first 3 months following contrast administration. Early symptoms include pain, pruritus, erythema and swelling in the legs, followed by thickening of the skin and subcutaneous tissues and fibrosis of the internal organs [23]. Cases of NSF have mainly been described in patients with chronic severe kidney disease (stage 5 or ESKD), or in individuals with acute kidney injury. A few cases (<5) were initially reported in individuals with CKD stage 4 but on clarification, subjects had been exposed to gadolinium several times or had acute kidney injury. The risk of NSF occurrence depends on the type of gadolinium contrast agent and the dose of contrast used. Most cases of NSF have occurred with nonionic linear chelates of Gadolinuim, as compared to macrocyclic preparations which are more stable and therefore safer. The incidence of NSF is near zero at 0.1 mmol/kg Gd-DTPA regardless of renal function. The most recent FDA advice recommends caution in patients with eGFR < 30 ml/min/1.73m^2, use of a marcocylic preparation of Gd-DTPA at the lowest dose possible and obligatory assessment of renal function. Despite a lack of evidence, the FDA considers a role for "prompt" (not defined) haemodialysis in patients on established dialysis treatment after gadolinium and then for the next 2 consecutive days, based on the assumption that >95% of the gadolinium contrast can be cleared by 12–15 h of dialysis [24]. In contrast, peritoneal dialysis clears Gd contrast poorly and the risk of NSF may be higher than haemodialysis [23, 24]. Similarly, data for rates of Gd associated nephrotoxicity are low in CKD if doses are minimized and intra-arterial injections avoided [23].

Computed Tomography

Multidetector computed tomography (MDCT) offers similar capabilities to CMR in the detection and quantification of microvascular obstruction and calculation of extracellular volume by measuring dynamic equilibrium of iodinated contrast within tissues. At the moment, the negative consequences of MDCT, with the risks of iodinated contrast and radiation exposure, probably outweigh the incremental information gained in CKD-associated cardiomyopathy.

Cardiac Magnetic Resonance as the Proposed Imaging Modality of Choice in CKD

As outlined above, CMR provides a comprehensive assessment of cardiac structure, function and characterization of the myocardial tissue, making it ideally suited to be the principal imaging modality for cardiac assessment in all stages of CKD and work up for renal transplantation. Undoubtedly, improved availability and expertise of CMR over the past 20 years have allowed a better understanding of the cardiac phenotype in CKD, the high prevalence of CKD-cardiomyopathy and an explanation as to why heart failure and sudden death are the primary mode of death in ESKD. Other advantages include safety and high reproducibility for serial studies/response to treatment, assessment of patterns of ventricular wall thickness, right ventricular morphology/function, aortic stiffness and myocardial perfusion. CMR is not limited by "trade offs" seen with other imaging modalities; in CT and nuclear imaging ionizing radiation exposure limits use for serial studies, while echocardiography can be precluded by poor acoustic windows and reliability of serial quantitative assessment.

Evolution of CKD-Associated Cardiomyopathy

Heart failure of any cause is a progressive condition, from often initial asymptomatic structural and functional changes to reduced symptomatic status and ultimately death. Longitudinal data however, specifically relating to the evolution of CKD-associated cardiomyopathy are sparse and the available evidence is mostly limited to cross-sectional studies. The data available suggests however, that there is a probable progression of myocardial disease from the earliest stages of CKD. In a cross-sectional echocardiographic study of 3,487 patients, LVH prevalence rates of 32, 48, 57 and 75% for eGFR categories >60, 45 to 59, 30 to 44, and <30 ml/min/1.73 m^2, respectively were reported [25]. A similar graded relationship was demonstrated using CMR in 2548 participants in the Dallas Heart study, with a close association between increasing level of cystatin C and LV mass, wall thickness and concentric remodelling. While these data demonstrate the increase in frequency of LVH with each stage of CKD, there are obvious confounders to the graded relationship such as the control of hypertension. The time course of these structural changes is also unknown. A recent prospective CMR study of uninephrectomy in kidney donors with a fall in eGFR of 30 mL/min/1.73 m^2 showed an increase in LV mass of 7 + 10 g at 12 months without a change in BP, suggesting that LVH is not simply a result of increased blood pressure and that structural changes may be more rapid than previously considered [26].

Although LVH is a cause of systolic dysfunction, limiting symptoms and CV death in CKD, heart failure with a reduced LV ejection fraction (LVEF) is uncommon and occurs in less than 8% of those with ESKD. Moreover, there is no clear graded association between LVEF and severity of CKD. Measurement of LVEF however, is a load- and geometry-dependent method of assessing LV contractility which lacks sensitivity in the assessment of CKD-associated cardiomyopathy. Other imaging measures of LV contractility suggest that systolic dysfunction in CKD-associated cardiomyopathy is not only common but also manifests early in the course of the disease. The assessment of systolic deformation (strain/strain rate), which may be studied using tissue Doppler echocardiography, speckle tracking echocardiography or CMR methods is a more sensitive, less load-dependent method of measuring LV function. Using these techniques, a reduction in strain (the fractional change in length of a myocardial segment) has been consistently documented in stage II and III CKD. Moreover, there is a graded association between CKD and reduction in global longitudinal strain, which is an independent predictor of all-cause mortality [27]. Using CMR, it has been possible to show that in stage 2 and 3 CKD there is a reduction in strain and strain rate affecting not only longitudinal myocardial shortening but also circumferential contraction, specifically affecting the mid-wall and endocardium. This preferential adverse effect on the endocardium is thought to be the functional consequence of DIF.

It is well known that the strongest predictor of exercise capacity in the general population without myocardial ischaemia is diastolic and not systolic function. Exercise capacity is limited in many patients with CKD and diastolic function is impaired early on in CKD-associated cardiomyopathy and then deteriorates over time. Assessment of diastolic function using blood pool Doppler has not always demonstrated a change in prevalence or incidence of diastolic dysfunction with higher stages of CKD [25]. More recent data however, using multiple methods that included tissue-based measures, including early myocardial relaxation velocity, mitral valve early filling velocity/early myocardial relaxation velocity (E/e′) and left atrial volume have demonstrated not only the highest prevalence of diastolic dysfunction in CKD IV and V but also that there was deterioration over 1-year follow-up. Increased left atrial volume, which is considered a reliable barometer of diastolic dysfunction and increased LV filling pressure, has been confirmed in both early CKD and ESKD as an adverse predictor of CV mortality.

Studies of the interaction between CKD and right ventricular (RV) structure and function are limited to patients with ESRD, in whom reduction in RV contractility has been identified using tissue velocity imaging and tricuspid annular plane systolic excursion on TTE. The difficulty in using these data in CKD is that such measures are load dependent, and the prevalence of pulmonary hypertension in ESKD may be as high as 60%. Assessment of right ventricular structure and function is a unique strength of CMR, and studies are awaited that investigate both cross-sectional change according to severity of CKD and longitudinal outcome. It is not therefore currently clear whether CKD-associated cardiomyopathy affects only the LV.

Interventions for CKD-Associated Cardiomyopathy

While there may be a graded inverse relationship between renal function and the evolution of CKD-associated cardiomyopathy, the reciprocal interaction between cardiac structural and functional improvement following renal transplantation is not so clear. Although CV risk is reduced after successful renal transplantation, morbidity and mortality still remain higher than in the general population. LVH persists in over 50% of renal transplant patients with abnormal LV geometry at 5 years follow-up [28]. Use of anti-hypertensive medication was not a factor in LVH regression, and those with the highest pre-transplant LV mass index were least likely to normalize (<115 g/m^2 in men). This has led to the suggestion that better prevention of CV disease in the earliest phases of CKD might be the best treatment strategy. At present however, treatment of CKD-associated cardiomyopathy relies on use of standard blood pressure and heart failure therapies such as beta blockers, angiotensin-converting enzyme inhibitors and angiotensin receptor antagonists despite the systematic exclusion of patients with moderate-severe CKD from the landmark trials demonstrating the efficacy of these interventions in the general population. The current evidence base in CKD is therefore based on small prospective studies or retrospective analyses of controlled trials and registry data.

Continuous Haemodialysis Regimes

In the ESKD population, patients on CAPD have been found to have a lower prevalence of LVH and LV mass index compared with patients on haemodialysis. It is also now recognized that prolonged and slow haemodialysis regimens, such as short daily dialysis or nocturnal hemodialysis reduce left ventricular mass index. Frequent dialysis also has salutary effects on blood pressure and survival rates [29.] The Frequent Haemodialysis Network Trials was the first prospective randomized control trial to compare cardiovascular outcome in patients undergoing continuous daily haemodiaysis (1.5–2.75 h 6 days in a week) and daily nocturnal haemodialysis (≥ 6 h 6 days in a week) with patients on conventional haemodialysis three times a week. They showed that LV mass index as measured with CMR was significantly reduced with continuous haemodialysis when compared with conventional haemodialysis. The effect of continuous haemodialysis on LV mass was especially pronounced in those patients that had LVH at baseline. Daily nocturnal haemodialysis also reduces LVH and LV mass index compared with conventional haemodialysis, although these results did not reach statistical significance [30]. Similar evidence exists from observational studies of prolonged haemodialysis regimens [29]; initial favourable reductions in LV mass that are obtained during the first year of prolonged haemodialysis regimens persist in the mid- and long term as well, thereby reflecting the more physiologic nature of this dialytic approach. Myocardial stunning refers to the recurrent haemodialysis-induced ischaemic cardiac injury patients experience as a result of high ultrafiltration requirements and intradialytic hypotension. Echocardiographic images acquired during various dialysis regimens have shown that frequent haemodialysis regimens associated with lower ultrafiltration volumes and rates are associated with less dialysis-induced myocardial stunning, which may thus contribute to the improved outcomes associated with these frequent haemodialysis therapies [31].

Aldosterone

Mineralocorticoid receptor antagonists (MRAs) such as spironolactone and eplerenone are highly effective in LV remodelling and reducing CV mortality in patients with heart failure and reduced ejection fraction. Evidence that this may be due to antagonism of aldosterone mediated pro-fibrotic and pro-inflammatory LV remodelling has been gained from studies showing reductions in serological markers of collagen turnover and an association of effects on these markers with outcome. In early stage CKD, treatment with spironolactone 25 mg daily for 40 weeks reduced LV mass and improved LV systolic and diastolic function compared to placebo [32]. These data were matched by reductions in B natriuretic peptide and attenuation of serum collagen turnover markers. In a single centre study of spironolactone in haemodialysis patients, there was a 6% reduction in the primary endpoint of death and hospitalization from cardiovascular and cerebrovascular disease after 3 years compared to controls. Concerns regarding the serious risks of hyperkalaemia with MRAs in CKD continue. There is however, emerging evidence that non-steroidal MRAs appear to have an improved safety and tolerability profile compared with other clinically available steroidal MRAs (spironolactone and eplerenone) in patients with CKD and impaired LVEF [33].

Phosphate

To date, treatment to counteract hyperphosphatemia using non-calcium containing oral phosphate binders in early stage CKD has not been shown to reduce LV mass or improve cardiac function on CMR [34]. In ESKD, clinical studies have been more focused on the effects of coronary and vascular calcification than the direct actions promoting cardiomyopathy.

Parathyroid Hormone (PTH)

An oral calcimimetic agent which lowers PTH, calcium and phosphate was examined in The Evaluation of Cinacalet Hydrochloride Therapy to Lower Cardiovascular Events (EVOVLE) study. This multi-centre, prospective randomized control trial of 3883 patients with ESKD on dialysis over a median follow up of 21 months showed no reduction in the composite primary endpoint of death, MI, hospitalization with angina, heart failure, or vascular events [35].

Vitamin D

In the multi-centre, double-blind, randomized placebo-controlled trial (PRIMO Study) of 227 patients with stage III-IV CKD, treatment with the oral active vitamin D analogue, paricalcitol did not alter LV mass or indices of diastolic function after 48 weeks of therapy despite confirmed PTH suppression and well controlled blood pressure [36].

Hyperuricemia and Oxidative Stress

Recent, randomized studies attempting to modify ROS activation with the xanthine oxidase inhibitor allopurinol have not proven effective in the treatment of patients with heart failure, and specifically in sub-group analysis of those with advanced CKD [37].

Novel Targets and Treatments

FGF Inhibitors

In a 5/6 nephrectomised rats model of CKD, an inhibitor of all FGF isoforms (PD173074) attenuated LVH. Recent extension of this work has shown reductions in LV mass, myocardial fibrosis and cardiac expression of genes associated with LVH independent of changes in blood pressure and renal function with an FGF inhibitor started early after the renal insult [38]. At present there are no commercially available oral FGF inhibitors although this is an area of intense research given the importance of FGF and FGF signalling in over 40 human diseases.

Klotho

In Klotho-deficient CKD mice intravenous delivery of a transgene encoding soluble Klotho ameliorated cardiac hypertrophy. In vitro, Klotho inhibited TGF-β[beta]1-, angiotensin II-, or high phosphate-induced fibrosis and abolished TGF-β[beta]1- or angiotensin II-induced hypertrophy of cardiomyocytes. These data provide mechanistic insights into the recent human myocardial autopsy data showing reduced levels of soluble klotho in myocardium of subjects with CKD [39].

Indoxyl Sulphate

A sixfold increase in IS levels is observed early (2 weeks) in CKD 5/6 nephrectomized rat models. Treatment with the oral gut absorbent AST-120 which reduces gastrointestinal uptake of indole and hence reduced IS synthesis was associated with reductions in cardiac fibrosis, TGF-β[beta] and phosphorylated NF-κ[kappa]B protein expression. Reductions in cardiac fibrosis were evident before a change in LVH or cardiac function and were independent of blood pressure and renal function [17]. AST-120 is available in Asia as an agent to prolong the time to initiation of hemodialysis. However, two double-blind, placebo-controlled trials have failed to demonstrate a benefit of adding AST-120 to prevent the progression of CKD.

Summary

CKD-associated cardiomyopathy is common and is associated with heart failure, arrhythmia and sudden cardiac death. Changes in LV structure and function are present from the earliest stages of CKD and multiple molecular mechanisms are likely to be responsible. Echocardiography may be adequate for diagnosis in the large populations at risk but there are major advantages in serial assessment of volume, mass and tissue characterization with CMR. Evidence of effective treatment is limited to date but there are new options in development with exciting prospects.

References

1. Hage FG, Venkataraman R, Zoghbi GJ, Perry GJ, DeMattos AM, Iskandrian AE. The scope of coronary heart disease in patients with chronic kidney disease. J Am Coll Cardiol. 2009;53 (23):2129–40.
2. Edwards NC, Moody WE, Chue CD, Ferro CJ, Townend JN, Steeds RP. Defining the natural history of uremic cardiomyopathy in chronic kidney disease: the role of cardiovascular magnetic resonance. JACC Cardiovasc Imaging. 2014;7(7):703–14.
3. Aoki J, Ikari Y, Nakajima H, Mori M, Sugimoto T, Hatori M, Tanimoto S, Amiya E, Hara K. Clinical and pathologic characteristics of dilated cardiomyopathy in hemodialysis patients. Kidney Int. 2005;67(1):333–40.
4. Mann JF, Gerstein HC, Pogue J, Bosch J, Yusuf S. Renal insufficiency as a predictor of cardiovascular outcomes and the impact of ramipril: the HOPE randomized trial. Ann Intern Med. 2001;134(8):629–36.
5. Brown NJ. Aldosterone and vascular inflammation. Hypertension. 2008;51(2):161–7.
6. Brilla CG, Weber KT. Reactive and reparative myocardial fibrosis in arterial hypertension in the rat. Cardiovasc Res. 1992;26 (7):671–7.
7. Chue CD, Edwards NC, Moody WE, Steeds RP, Townend JN, Ferro CJ. Serum phosphate is associated with left ventricular mass in patients with chronic kidney disease: a cardiac magnetic resonance study. Heart. 2012;98(3):219–24.
8. Silver J, Naveh-Many T. FGF-23 and secondary hyperparathyroidism in chronic kidney disease. Nat Rev Nephrol. 2013;9 (11):641–9.
9. Faul CAA, Oskouei B, Hu MC, Sloan A, Isakova T, et al. FGF23 induces left ventricular hypertrophy. J Clin Invest. 2011;121 (11):4393–408.
10. Leifheit-Nestler M, Grosse Siemer R, Flasbart K, Richter B, Kirchhoff F, Ziegler WH, Klintschar M, Becker JU, Erbersdobler A, Aufricht C, et al. Induction of cardiac FGF23/FGFR4 expression is associated with left ventricular hypertrophy in patients with chronic kidney disease. Nephrol Dial Transplant. 2016;31(7):1088–99.
11. Palmer SC, Hayen A, Macaskill P, Pellegrini F, Craig JC, Elder GJ, Strippoli GF. Serum levels of phosphorus, parathyroid hormone, and calcium and risks of death and cardiovascular disease in individuals with chronic kidney disease: a systematic review and meta-analysis. JAMA. 2011;305(11):1119–27.
12. Drechsler C, Pilz S, Obermayer-Pietsch B, Verduijn M, Tomaschitz A, Krane V, Espe K, Dekker F, Brandenburg V, Marz W, et al. Vitamin D deficiency is associated with sudden cardiac death, combined cardiovascular events, and mortality in haemodialysis patients. Eur Heart J. 2010;31(18):2253–61.
13. Tsutsui H, Kinugawa S, Matsushima S. Oxidative stress and heart failure. Am J Physiol Heart Circ Physiol. 2011;301(6):H2181–90.
14. Lekawanvijit SAA, Kelly DJ, Kompa AR, Wang BH, Krum H. Does indoxyl sulfate, a uraemic toxin, have direct effects on cardiac fibroblasts and myocytes? Eur Heart J. 2010;31:1771–9.
15. Meijers BKVKS, Verbeke K, Dehaen W, Vanrenterghem Y, Hoylaerts MF, Evenepoel P. The uremic retention solute p-cresyl sulfate and markers of endothelial damage. Am J Kidney Dis. 2009;54:891–901.
16. Mann DL. Inflammatory mediators and failing heart: past, present, and the foreseeable future. Circ Res. 2002;91:988–98.
17. Lekawanvijit S, Kompa AR, Wang BH, Kelly DJ, Krum H. Cardiorenal syndrome: the emerging role of protein-bound uremic toxins. Circ Res. 2012;111(11):1470–83.
18. Kennedy DJ, Vetteth S, Periyasamy SM, Kanj M, Fedorova L, Khouri S, Kahaleh MB, Xie Z, Malhotra D, Kolodkin NI, et al. Central role for the cardiotonic steroid marinobufagenin in the pathogenesis of experimental uremic cardiomyopathy. Hypertension. 2006;47(3):488–95.
19. Thomas SS, Zhang L, Mitch WE. Molecular mechanisms of insulin resistance in chronic kidney disease. Kidney Int. 2015;88 (6):1233–9.
20. Stewart GA, Foster J, Cowan M, Rooney E, McDonagh T, Dargie HJ, Rodger RS, Jardine AG. Echocardiography overestimates left ventricular mass in hemodialysis patients relative to magnetic resonance imaging. Kidney Int. 1999;56(6):2248–53.
21. Mark PB, Johnston N, Groenning BA, Foster JE, Blyth KG, Martin TN, Steedman T, Dargie HJ, Jardine AG. Redefinition of uremic cardiomyopathy by contrast-enhanced cardiac magnetic resonance imaging. Kidney Int. 2006;69(10):1839–45.
22. Edwards NC, Moody WE, Yuan M, Hayer MK, Ferro CJ, Townend JN, Steeds RP. Diffuse interstitial fibrosis and myocardial dysfunction in early chronic kidney disease. Am J Cardiol. 2015;115(9):1311–7.
23. Perazella M. Current status of gadolinium toxicity in patients with kidney disease. Clin J Am Soc Nephrol. 2009;4:461–9.

24. Penfield JRR. What nephrologists need to know about gadolinium. Nat Rev Nephrol. 2007;3:654–68.
25. Park M, Hsu CY, Li Y, Mishra RK, Keane M, Rosas SE, Dries D, Xie D, Chen J, He J, et al. Associations between kidney function and subclinical cardiac abnormalities in CKD. J Am Soc Nephrol. 2012;23(10):1725–34.
26. Moody WE, Ferro CJ, Edwards NC, Chue CD, Lin EL, Taylor RJ, Cockwell P, Steeds RP, Townend JN. Cardiovascular effects of unilateral nephrectomy in living kidney donors. Hypertension. 2016;67(2):368–77.
27. Krishnasamy R, Isbel NM, Hawley CM, Pascoe EM, Leano R, Haluska BA, Stanton T. The association between left ventricular global longitudinal strain, renal impairment and all-cause mortality. Nephrol Dial Transplant. 2014;29(6):1218–25.
28. An JN, Kim YH, Park JB, Hwang JH, Yoo KD, Park JY, Kim CT, Kim HL, Kim YJ, Han DJ, et al. The reciprocal interaction between LV remodelling and allograft outcomes in kidney transplant recipients. Heart. 2015;101(22):1826–33.
29. Mishra R, Dublin R. The effects of frequent haemodialysis on left ventricular mass, volumes, and geometry. Clin J Am Soc Nephrol. 2013;8(12):2025–7.
30. Chan C, Greene T, Chertow G, Kliger A, Stokes J, Beck G, Daugirdas J, Kotanko P, Larive B, Levin N, et al. Determinants of left ventricular mass in patients on haemodialysis: Frequent Haemodialysis Network (FHN) Trials. Circ Cardiovasc Imaging. 2012;5:251–61.
31. Jefferies H, Virk B, Schiller B, Morran J, McIntyre C. Frequent hemodialysis schedules are associated with reduced levels of dialysis-induced cardiac injury (myocardial stunning). Clin J Am Soc Nephrol. 2011;6(6):1326–32.
32. Edwards NC, Steeds RP, Stewart PM, Ferro CJ, Townend JN. Effect of spironolactone on left ventricular mass and aortic stiffness in early-stage chronic kidney disease: a randomized controlled trial. J Am Coll Cardiol. 2009;54(6):505–12.
33. Pitt B, Kober L, Ponikowski P, Gheorghiade M, Filippatos G, Krum H, Nowack C, Kolkhof P, Kim SY, Zannad F. Safety and tolerability of the novel non-steroidal mineralocorticoid receptor antagonist BAY 94-8862 in patients with chronic heart failure and mild or moderate chronic kidney disease: a randomized, double-blind trial. Eur Heart J. 2013;34(31):2453–63.
34. Chue CD, Townend JN, Moody WE, Zehnder D, Wall NA, Harper L, Edwards NC, Steeds RP, Ferro CJ. Cardiovascular effects of sevelamer in stage 3 CKD. J Am Soc Nephrol. 2013;24(5):842–52.
35. Chertow GM, Block GA, Correa-Rotter R, Drueke TB, Floege J, Goodman WG, Herzog CA, Kubo Y, London GM, Mahaffey KW, et al. Effect of cinacalcet on cardiovascular disease in patients undergoing dialysis. N Engl J Med. 2012;367(26):2482–94.
36. Thadhani R, Appelbaum E, Pritchett Y, Chang Y, Wenger J, Tamez H, Bhan I, Agarwal R, Zoccali C, Wanner C, et al. Vitamin D therapy and cardiac structure and function in patients with chronic kidney disease: the PRIMO randomized controlled trial. JAMA. 2012;307(7):674–84.
37. Givertz MM, Anstrom KJ, Redfield MM, Deswal A, Haddad H, Butler J, Tang WH, Dunlap ME, LeWinter MM, Mann DL, et al. Effects of xanthine oxidase inhibition in hyperuricemic heart failure patients: the xanthine oxidase inhibition for hyperuricemic heart failure patients (EXACT-HF) study. Circulation. 2015;131(20):1763–71.
38. Di Marco GS, Reuter S, Kentrup D, Grabner A, Amaral AP, Fobker M, Stypmann J, Pavenstadt H, Wolf M, Faul C, et al. Treatment of established left ventricular hypertrophy with fibroblast growth factor receptor blockade in an animal model of CKD. Nephrol Dial Transplant. 2014;29(11):2028–35.
39. Hu MC, Shi M, Cho HJ, Adams-Huet B, Paek J, Hill K, Shelton J, Amaral AP, Faul C, Taniguchi M, et al. Klotho and phosphate are modulators of pathologic uremic cardiac remodeling. J Am Soc Nephrol. 2015;26(6):1290–302.

Part II

Chronic Kidney Disease and CAD: Two Sides of the Same Coin

CKD as CAD Equivalent: Inflammatory Milieu and Vascular Oxidative Stress

6

Shien Wen Sheryl Gan and Christopher T. Chan

Inflammation and Chronic Kidney Disease

Chronic kidney disease (CKD) is recognized as an independent risk factor for cardiovascular disease (CVD). Cardiovascular disease related morbidity and mortality account for a huge part of the disease burden of CKD. Higher than expected CVD related mortality rates are seen in the CKD population compared to that of the general population [1, 2]. Manifestations of CVD in CKD can be broadly divided as those affecting the myocardium and those affecting the blood vessels. These processes are not mutually exclusive. Traditional risk factors for atherosclerotic CVD are insufficient to explain this vastly increased risk. Hence, the contribution of CKD specific cardiac risk factors have been postulated including anemia, proteinuria, abnormal bone mineral metabolism, and chronic inflammation. Raised inflammatory, oxidative stress, and pro-coagulant biomarkers, such as C-reactive protein (CRP) and interleukin-6 (IL-6), have been shown to be strong predictors of all-cause mortality and cardiovascular outcomes in patients with end stage renal disease (ESKD).

Overview of Inflammation in CKD

The etiology of chronic inflammation in CKD is not entirely elucidated and is likely multifactorial including elevated levels of uremic toxins, circulating pro-inflammatory cytokines, oxidative stress, carbonyl stress, protein-energy wasting, and increased incidence of infections (Fig. 6.1).

C.T. Chan (✉)
University Health Network, University of Toronto, 200 Elizabeth Street, 8N Room 846, Toronto, ON M5G 2C4, Canada
e-mail: christopher.chan@uhn.ca

S.W.S. Gan
Department of Renal Medicine, Singapore General Hospital, Academia Building, Level 3, 20 College Road, Singapore, 169856, Singapore

J. Rangaswami et al. (eds.), *Cardio-Nephrology*,
DOI 10.1007/978-3-319-56042-7_6

Chronic Kidney Disease

Decline in renal function may increase inflammation by reduction in renal clearance of inflammatory factors. Levels of tumor necrosis factor-alpha (TNF-α[alpha]) and IL-1, for example, are higher in animals with impaired renal function, compared to controls with normal renal function [4, 5]. In humans, CRP, IL-6 and hyaluronan levels increase with worsening renal function. There is no consensus with regards to optimal levels of inflammatory markers in CKD patients. Interestingly, patients with CKD also have abnormal cellular and humoral immunity. Impaired T-cell proliferation and function, poor antibody response and defective antigen presentation by monocytes contributes to increased infections and malignancies in dialysis patients [6].

Volume overload is another possible cause of inflammation in CKD. Vascular congestion of the gastrointestinal tract may alter its permeability causing, endotoxins such as lipopolysaccharides and bacteria to accumulate. This in turn stimulates monocytes and the release of proinflammatory cytokines. The progression of CKD in itself is associated with metabolic alterations of the bacterial flora in the lumen of the intestinal tract. In healthy individuals, the phyla Bacteriodetes and Firmicutes contribute to more than 90% of all species that colonize the gastrointestinal tract (*Bacteroides* spp., *Alistipes* spp., *Prevotella* spp. *Faecalibacterium* spp. and *Lactobacillus* spp. are examples of these). In uremic patients, certain species of the normal gut microbacterial flora, with pathogenic potential, are increasedsuch as Helicobacter, *Bacteriodes* and *Prevotella* spp. In addition, there is a loss of mucosal barrier integrity and increased bacterial translocation in uraemic patients, resulting in gastrointestinal malabsorption, protein-energy wasting and systemic inflammation [7].

Periodontal disease is a contributor to local and chronic systemic inflammation in CKD. Gram-negative bacteria causing periodontitis interact with toll-like receptors expressed on surface of neutrophils and monocytes. These complexes activate signal transduction pathways, leading to the production of cytokines and acute phase proteins [8].

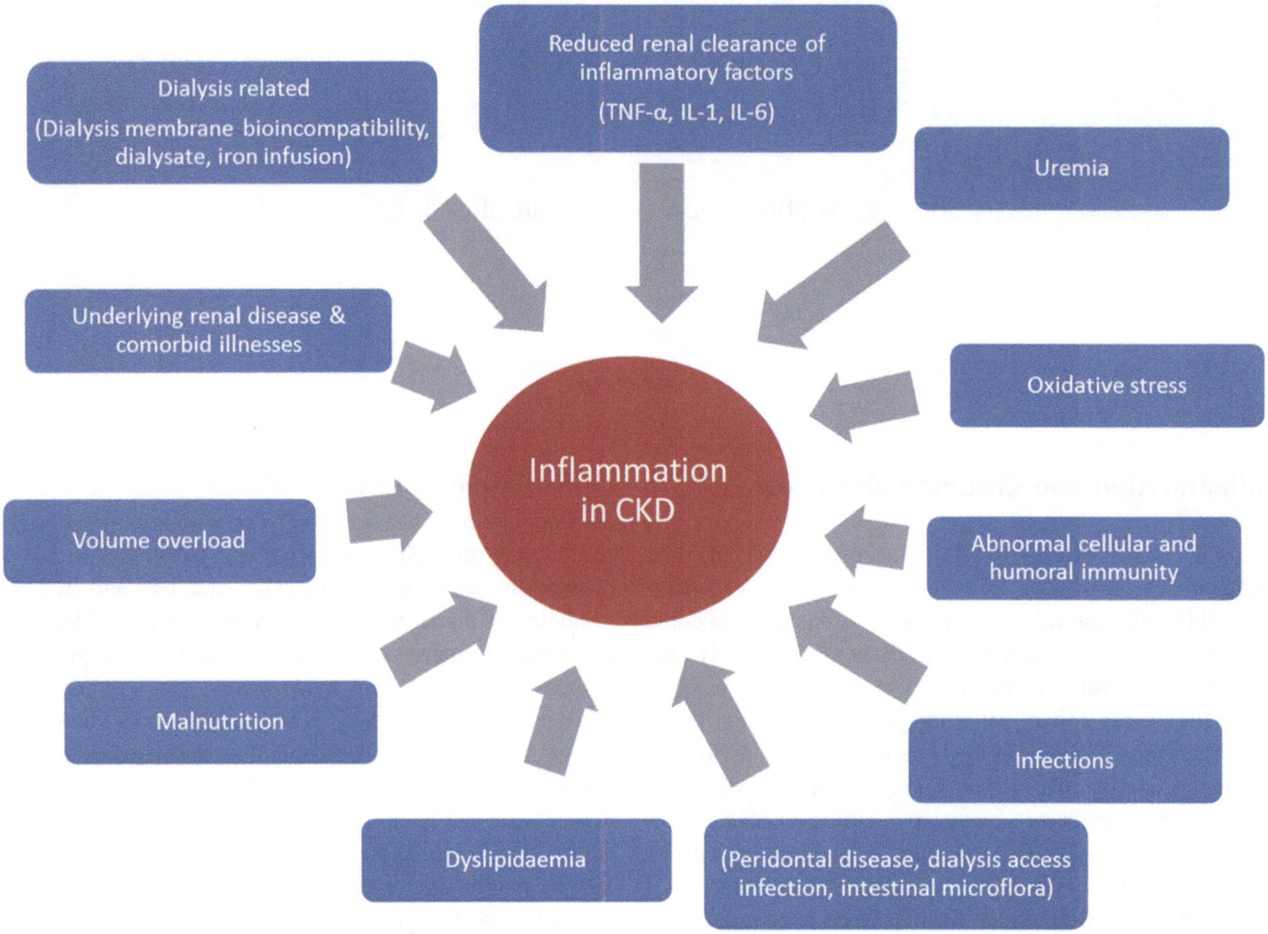

Fig. 6.1 Causes of inflammation in CKD. Adapted from Filiopoulos et al. [3]

Multiple comorbid illnesses in CKD also contribute towards a hypercatabolic state and the development of inflammation. Systemic autoimmune diseases, which may be the etiology of CKD, genetic factors, recurrent or unrecognized persistent infections may also drive the inflammation seen in CKD patients.

Hemodialysis

The hemodialysis (HD) process itself may enhance inflammation by exposure of patients to dialysis tubing and dialysis membranes (especially less biocompatible membranes such as cuprophane). This cellular response may lead to acute symptoms such as fever or hypotension, or chronic symptoms such as anemia, malnutrition, immunological dysfunction, and dialysis-related amyloidosis [9]. There are two potential mechanisms by which hemodialysis-induced inflammation may occur: (1) the generation of complement fragments due to plasma protein-membrane contact and (2) via contact of immunocompetent cells with dialysis system material.

Poor-quality dialysis water and back-filtration of contaminants may also lead to exposure to endotoxins. The widespread use of ultrapure dialysate fluid has resulted in improved nutritional status, decrease in levels of inflammatory markers and slower decline in residual renal function.

Finally, the HD patient may have foreign materials in situ, such as vascular grafts and intravenous dialysis catheters, which may act as another source of chronic inflammation.

Peritoneal Dialysis

Peritoneal dialysis (PD) patients are constantly exposed to a milieu of chronic inflammation. Causative factors include episodes of peritonitis or PD catheter related infections and chronic exposure to less biocompatible PD solutions [10].

Cytokines and Markers of Inflammation in CKD

Inflammation is a complex chain of events that involve numerous mediators and cells. While there is currently no single gold standard test to assess for inflammation in CKD, several biomarkers of inflammation are elevated even in early CKD, such as TNFα[alpha], IL1β[beta], IL-6, IL-10 and C reactive protein (CRP).

High CRP levels are a strong predictor for cardiovascular events and mortality. CRP in itself may contribute directly to the pathogenesis of atherosclerosis. It does so via three mechanisms. First, CRP binds to damage cells and activates the complement system. Second, it also displays calcium-dependent in vitro binding and aggregation of low density lipoprotein (LDL) and very-low-density lipoprotein (VLDL). Finally, it is a potent stimulator of tissue factor production by monocytes, and the effect is augmented in the presence of other inflammatory mediators [11].

Uremic Toxins

Uremic toxins consist of heterogeneous substances with proinflammatory effects that induce cytokine release, including several organic compounds and peptides. The European Uremic Toxin Work group have identified multiple compounds in their classification of these toxins [12]. They can be divided into three major groups—small water-soluble compounds, middle molecules, and protein-bound compounds.

Small water-soluble compounds have a molecular weight (MW) of <500 Da. Examples include urea and phosphorous. They are generally removed readily by conventional dialysis.

Middle molecules have a MW > 500 Da. B2-microglobulin and advanced glycosylation end products are such examples. Their clearance is limited in conventional HD, but more effective in PD. Higher permeability HD membranes and hemofiltration improve their clearance as well. A reduction in their accumulation is associated with reduced mortality risk [13].

Protein-bound compounds account for approximately 27% of the uremic compounds [12]. Removal of these molecules by conventional dialysis is limited. Dialysis with protein-leaking membranes may offer better clearance of these molecules. However, albumin loss and hypoalbuminemia tend to occur with high cut-off dialysis membranes. There is an emerging body of the literature which suggests that protein-bound uremic solutes are associated with detrimental cardiac effects [14]. Specifically, *p*-cresyl sulfate increases collagen synthesis in cardiac fibroblasts and protein synthesis in cardiac myocytes. Another compound, phenylacetic acid increases protein synthesis in cardiac myocytes. Phenol also suppresses contractility of cardiac muscle [15].

Of interest, Indoxyl sulfate is a protein-bound uremic solute which is currently under active investigation [16]. It is produced in the liver from indole, a tryptophan derivative generated by bacteria in the large intestines. It has poor urinary clearance and has a high affinity to albumin and is poorly cleared by conventional hemodialysis. Indoxyl sulfate is reported to stimulate vascular smooth muscle cell proliferation and vascular calcification [17].

Oxidative Stress in CKD

Oxidative stress occurs when there is excessive free-radical production often in the context of low antioxidant levels. Reactive oxygen species (ROS) are constantly produced in physiological conditions, as a part of the host defense mechanism against infectious organisms and malignant cells. An improper maladaptive activation of the oxidative process, such as in uremia, contributes to cell and tissue injury [18].

Exaggerated 02- Generation

High homocysteine (HC) level is a risk factor for CVD via enhancement of atherosclerosis and other thrombotic events. Levels of HC increases with declining glomerular filtration rate (GFR), possibly due to reduced HC clearance by the kidneys. In vitro/vivo studies suggest that high HC levels lead to an increased production of ROS and decreased endothelial nitric oxide (NO). Thus, increasing the oxidative damage at the vascular interface. High HC level may also cause proliferation of smooth muscle cells, leading to increased oxidation of low-density lipoproteins [19].

During oxidative stress, there is an imbalance between NO and ROS. Numerous studies have demonstrated that lower levels of NO leads to endothelial cell injury and dysfunction, platelet aggregation and potentiate atherosclerosis. Endogenous NO synthase (NOS) inhibitor—asymmetric dimethylarginine (ADMA) is associated with oxidative stress process via its inhibition of NO. ADMA is a strong and independent predictor of death and incident CVD complications in CKD and non-CKD patients [20]. The renin angiotensin aldosterone system also activates nicotinamide adenine dinucleotide phosphate oxidase, which lead to increase ROS production. This is associated with uremic cardiomyopathy, intramyocardial capillary loss, endothelial damage and atherosclerosis

Deficient 02- Scavenging Capacity

Protection against reactive species can be achieved by prevention of free radical formation or by repairing damaged molecules. Intracellular enzymatic antioxidants convert substrates to less reactive forms. Superoxidase dismutase (SOD), catalase, and glutathione peroxidase are examples. The main non-enzymatic cellular antioxidant is reduced glutathione (GSH). Oxidized glutathione (GSSG) and glutathione redox status (GSSG/GSH) are markers of severe cellular oxidative stress. Patients with CKD have a higher level of conjugated dienes and lipid hydroperoxides, increased levels of GSSG, increased redox status GSSG/GSH and decreased resistance to oxidation of LDL. In addition, serum urea and creatinine correlate with the amount of GSSG and redox ratio GSSG/GSH. suggesting that CKD patients may have reduced antioxidant potency [21].

Dyslipidemia

Patients with CKD have a secondary form of dyslipidemia consisting of both quantitative and qualitative abnormalities in serum lipoproteins resulting from alterations in lipoprotein metabolism and composition. Generally, uremic patients have an increase in serum triglyceride levels due to elevated VLDL remnants and intermediate-density lipoprotein, and low high-density lipoprotein (HDL) cholesterol. LDL cholesterol is often normal, but abnormal deposition of cholesterol may arise from the atherogenic small and dense LDL subclasses [22].

The release of lipoprotein lipase from extrahepatic vascular surfaces during heparin administration is another possible mechanism whereby triglyceride levels increase and VLDL levels decrease. Heparin may also modify the properties of LDL, which lead to aggregation and fusion of LDL and eventual atherogenesis [23].

Uremic patients also have increased levels of oxidized LDL (ox–LDL). These modifications occur at the level of apolipoprotein B (apoB)-100, surface phospholipids or within the core region. The ox-LDL in turn triggers a cascade of cytokine and growth factor expression and release, increase endothelial cell activation and dysfunction and alterations in mediators such as NO.

Malnutrition

In patients with advanced CKD, reduced total cholesterol is a biomarker of malnutrition and inflammation. The prevalence of malnutrition and inflammation in the CKD population ranges from 30 to 70% [24]. Inflammatory cytokines disrupt cholesterol-mediated LDL receptor feedback regulation, leading to intracellular accumulation of unmodified LDL, foam cell formation and eventual atherosclerosis. This may explain in part the U-shaped relationship between cholesterol levels and cardiovascular events and mortality in the CKD population.

The malnutrition-inflammation-atherosclerosis (MIA) syndrome describes the high correlation of these three significant separate clinical entities that coexist in dialysis patients. Several cytokines have been identified to be involved in this process Such as TNFα[alpha], IL-1 and IL-6. Their effects lead to enhanced resistance to insulin, increased protein catabolism, endothelial dysfunction, and anorexia [25].

The Effects of Inflammation and Oxidative Stress

In this section, we will focus on the effects on inflammation and oxidative stress on CVD (Fig. 6.2). However, it is worth noting that inflammation and oxidative stress simultaneously promotes renal injury and worsening of CKD [26].

Blood Vessels

Both atherosclerosis and arteriosclerosis are common in CKD and are associated with endothelial dysfunction [27]. Atherosclerosis is a disease of the intima characterized by calcified fibro-atheromatous plaques, which ultimately rupture causing vaso-occlusive events. Arteriosclerosis affects the media of large and middle size arteries with an increased collagen:elastin ratio with concurrent calcification, hyperplasia, and hypertrophy of vascular smooth muscle cells. The resultant decrease in vessel wall elasticity and compliance, leads to increased afterload, left ventricular hypertrophy and fibrosis.

A normal healthy endothelium balances appropriate anti-clotting, anti-adhesion and vasodilatory mediators. Normal dynamic changes within the endothelium are mediated by oxidized lipoproteins, shear stress, endothelial cell production of cytokines, and inhibitors that interfere with NO production.

Under the exposure to modified LDL, endothelial cells undergo complex interaction generating the release of cytokines, inflammatory mediators, growth factors and reactive oxygen species. In contrast, under exposure to oxidized-LDL, vascular smooth muscle cells and monocyte-macrophages proliferate. This is largely postulated to be due to lysophosphatidylcholine (lysoPC), and other bioactive lipid products. These compounds induce expression and release of growth factors and apoptotic factors, which in turn lead to variable responses from different vascular cells. Nuclear factor-κ[kappa]B (NF-κ[kappa]B), the ox-LDL receptor LOX-1, NADPH oxidase and vascular endothelial growth factor (VEGF) all play a role in this complex pathway.

Inhibitors of NOS may also accelerate the pathogenesis of CVD in CKD. Asymmetric dimethylarginine (ADMA) is one such example of the many proposed inhibitors. Urea itself can inhibit inducible NOS, which lead to the accumulation of macrophages, enhanced NF-κ[kappa]B-dependent expression of vascular cell adhesion molecule-1 (VACM-1), macrophage-colony stimulating factor (MCSCP) and monocyte chemoattractant protein-1 expression. Oxidized-LDL can reduce NO production by a few possible mechanisms—the

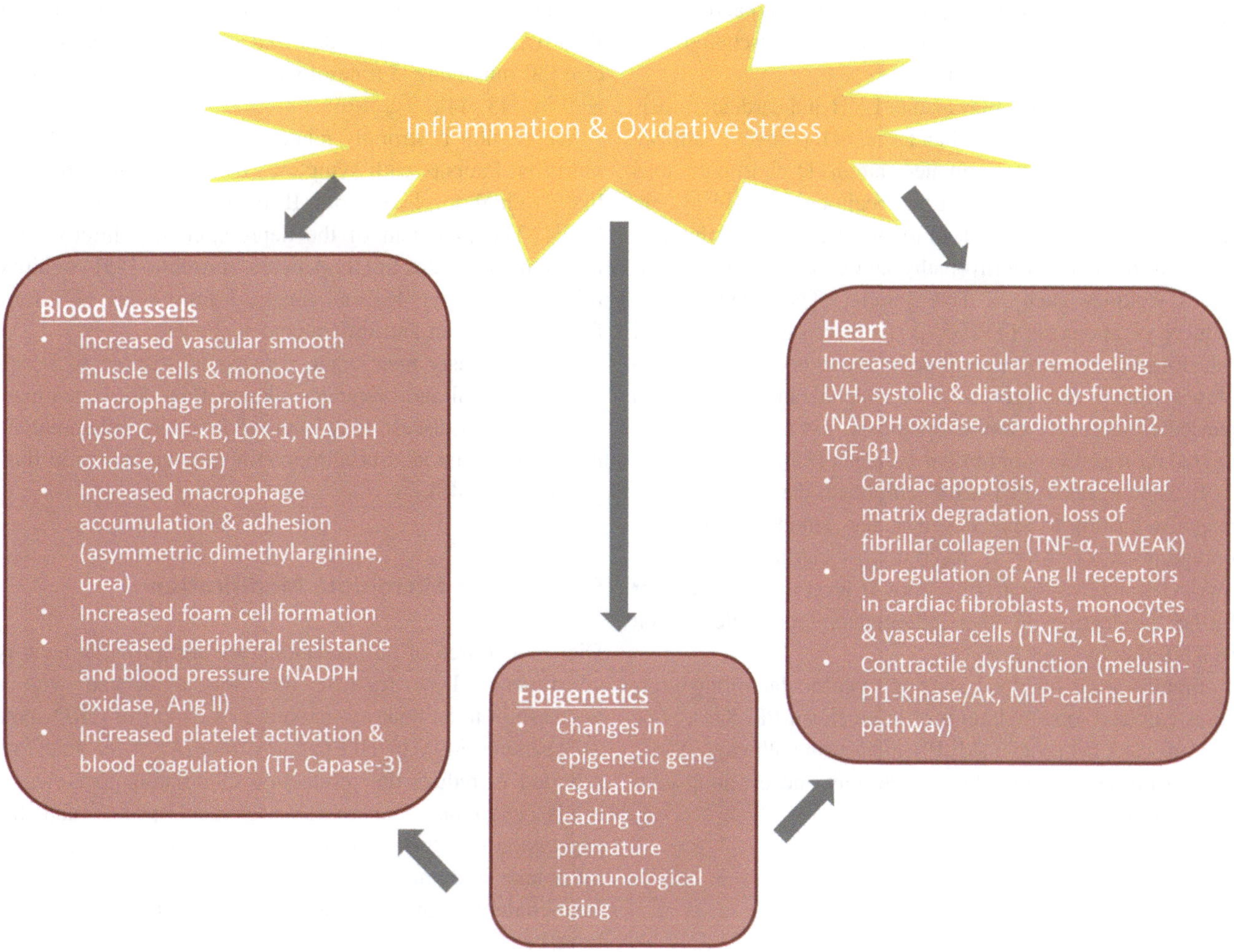

Fig. 6.2 Effects of inflammation and oxidative stress on the cardiovascular system

LOX receptor, and depletion of caveolae of cholesterol that displaces endothelial NOS (eNOS) [28].

Scavenger receptors recognize modified forms of LDL. This in turn leads to an excessive update of cholesterol and lipids and the eventual formation of foam cells. These receptors may also play a role in adhesion, differentiation, host defence and phagocytosis of damaged cells. Apart from modified LDL, uremia dose-dependently enhances these receptors activities.

ROS is increased in hypertension, which is highly prevalent in patients with CKD. Oxidative stress induces blood pressure elevation and the raised blood pressure in itself increases ROS generation. This vicious cycle leads to increased peripheral resistance and blood pressure elevation. NADPH oxidase and angiotensin II (Ang II) have been identified to play a part in this pathway.

Finally, the tissue factor (TF) pathway may also increase atherosclerosis risk. TF is a regulator of blood coagulation which exists latently on cell surfaces, and it can be activated by oxidized lipids. Activated TF in turn leads enhanced platelet activation, which is encountered frequently in uremic patients [29].

Heart

Structural alterations of the myocardium in CKD include ventricular remodeling that may lead to eccentric or concentric left ventricular hypertrophy (LVH), systolic and diastolic dysfunction and eventual clinical symptoms of heart failure. In various studies [30], the prevalence of LVH varies according to the stage of CKD: 30% in stages 3 and 4 [31], 5–21% in stage 3 to 4 [32] and 55% in stages 3 to 5 [33]. It is widely recognized that increased oxidative stress in the heart leads to oxidation and damage of macromolecules, membranes, DNA and enzymes involved in energy production. Ultimately, sustained elevation of oxidative stress is associated with cellular damage, energetic deficit and cell death [34].

NADPH oxidases, which are a major source of ROS, contribute to the pathogenesis of cardiac remodeling, hypertrophy, and fibrosis [35]. Its expression and activity are increased in the myocardium of patients with ischemic and non-ischemic cardiomyopathy.

Other processes that may lead to LVH and cardiac fibrosis are activation of the mammalian target of rapamycin pathway (mTOR), parathyroid hormone-vitamin D-phosphate axis and activation of the intracardiac renin-angiotensin system (RAAS). Clinically, these lead to systolic and diastolic dysfunction, dilated cardiomyopathy and congestive heart failure. Cytokines such as TNFα[alpha], TNF-related weak inducer of apoptosis (TWEAK), IL-6, cardiotrophin 1 and transforming growth factor β[beta]1 have been identified to play a role in this process. TNFα[alpha] and TWEAK in particular increases cardiac apoptosis, extracellular matrix degradation and loss of fibrillar collagen [35].

It is suggested that CRP amplifies the inflammatory response leading to adverse ventricular remodeling. There is upregulation of Ang II receptors in cardiac fibroblasts, myocytes and vascular cells. Ang II receptors may trigger further production of other inflammatory molecules—such as TNFα[alpha] and IL-6.

Finally, fluid overload and high ventricular filling pressures can lead to stimulations of the melusin-PI3-Kinase/Ak and muscle LIM protein (MLP)-calcineurin pathways. These in turn promote ventricular hypertrophy and eventual contractile dysfunction and CHF [36].

Epigenetics

Epigenetics refers to the modification of gene expression which is not explained by changes in DNA sequence [37]. In CKD, several factors such as uremia, hyperhomocysteinemia and inflammation contribute to changes in the epigenetic gene regulation. This in turn leads to alternations in DNA methylation, histone modification, and RNA interference. Abnormal epigenetic modification has been associated with premature immunological aging [38], increase in CVD prevalence, and cardiovascular mortality. Some studies in this field, looking at these effects [39, 40] and searching for epigenetic biomarkers [41] have been promising. We wait for more data in this field to emerge in the future.

Therapeutic Interventions

Physical Activity and Lifestyle Modification

Exercise training in CKD patients shows favorable although inconsistent effect on the catabolic state in uremic muscles and on inflammatory markers [42]. Most studies confirm that dialysis patients have poor physical activity and high CRP levels. In addition, there is a downregulation in T-lymphocytes and monocyte activation, reduction in IL-6/IL-10 ratio when randomized to regular walking exercise (30 min a day, 5 times a week) compared to usual daily activity [43, 44].

Depression is strongly related to inflammation and malnutrition. Patients with symptoms of depression were more likely to high levels of serum IL-6 and lower serum albumin levels. The treatment of the depression may improve the inflammatory state. In HD patients, sertraline [45] cognitive behavior therapy [46] and omega-3 fatty acids [47] were found to have an anti-inflammatory effect.

As previously mentioned, periodontal disease is associated with local and systemic inflammation. Thus, treatment of periodontal disease may improve systemic inflammation, nutritional status and erythropoietin responsiveness in dialysis patients [48].

Dietary and Microbiota Modification

Diet is a source of anti-inflammatory and proinflammatory constituents. Low fructose diet was associated with a decrease in inflammatory markers in a cohort of CKD stage 2–3 patients [49]. In HD patients, omega-3 fatty acids are reported to reduce the production of inflammatory eicosanoids, cytokines and reactive oxygen species and the expression of adhesion molecules [50]. Lowering saturated fat intake and increased polyunsaturated fat intake—like long-chain n-3 polyunsaturated fatty acids (PUFA) may also have beneficial effect on inflammation [51].

Decrease in inflammatory biomarkers in HD patients has been demonstrated with the consumption of decaffeinated green tea [52], pomegranate juice [53] and soy-derived isoflavones [54]. Measures to alter the intestinal microbiota may alsoreduce systemic inflammation [55].

Increasing Hemodialysis Frequency

Prevention of chronic micro-inflammation in HD should incorporate a comprehensive strategy such as biocompatible dialytic membranes, ultrapure water, adjustments of vitamin deficiencies and optimizing nutrition, anemia correction, optimal fluid balance, and efficient removal of uremic toxins.

Daily nocturnal HD (DNHD) has also demonstrated improvement in ejection fraction and peripheral arterial blood flow, despite no change in extracellular fluid volume [56, 57]. Thus, suggesting other mechanisms such as inflammation reduction may be involved.

Endothelial progenitor cells (EPC) play a role in angiogenesis and repair of the ischemic myocardium [58]. Reduced number of EPC has been associated with an elevated cardiovascular risk. CKD patients have a reduced number and function of EPCs. In a matched cohort of DNHD patients, EPC number and function [59] approximate those of normal controls, making this an attractive option in optimizing CVD risk in these patients.

Antioxidants

The role of anti oxidant supplementation with the goal of improving CVD outcomes, especially in CKD remains controversial. Several antioxidants have been explored to reduce the cardiovascular impact of inflammation. L-arginine, a precursor of NO, has been shown to improve endothelial function in coronary vessels and lowers endothelin levels [60–62]. *N*-acetylcysteine (600 mg twice daily) has been studied in PD and HD patients. It has been shown to decrease IL-6 levels [63] and reduce primary composite cardiovascular end points respectively [64]. Vitamin E supplementation [65] reduced composite CVD endpoints and myocardial infarction in a secondary prevention trial in patients with ESKD.

In contrast, tocopherol—a thiol-containing antioxidant, did not show a significant reduction in inflammatory and oxidative stress biomarkers or surrogate outcomes (erythropoietin responsiveness) [66]. Other large clinical trials, such as CHAOS [67] and the GISSI prevention trial [68], did not demonstrate a reduction in CVD or atherosclerosis with antioxidant supplementation. It is postulated that the reasons for the negative results is that is a lack of bioavailability at specific locations where the oxidative stress occurs, and antioxidant supplementation is unlikely to provide a significant increase in oxidant defence in well-nourished patients. In addition, these two trials were conducted in the non-CKD population. Further studies are needed to confirm the role of antioxidants in the CKD-CVD spectrum.

Lowering Homocysteine Level

Two studies have explored the effects of lowering homocysteine levels—the Homocysteine study (HOST) [69] and Heart Outcomes Prevention Evaluation-2 (HOPE-2) [70]. Unfortunately, neither trial demonstrated any significant benefit on CVD risk or all-cause mortality with HC lowering interventions with folic acid, vitamin B6, and vitamin B12.

Statins

Hydroxymethylgluaryl-coenzyme A inhibitors (Statins) are commonly used to lower blood cholesterol level and possess anti-inflammatory effects. Some investigators suggest that Statins may reduce inflammatory cell adhesion via inhibition of β[beta] integrin lymphocyte function-associated antigen (LFA)-1. Indeed, observational studies using statins were associated with a decreased in CRP levels in PD [71] and CKD patients [72].

Although statins may exert an anti-inflammatory effect in patients with CKD or ESRD, large-scale trials confer conflicting results. The Study of Heart and Renal Protection (SHARP) demonstrated the use of simvastatin with ezetimibe lowers the annual incidence of major vascular events (defined as non-fatal myocardial infarction or any cardiac death, any stroke, or any arterial revascularisation, excluding dialysis access procedures) in CKD patients [73]. However, other studies specifically in HD patients on statin, failed to demonstrate a reduction in cardiovascular events compared to placebo [74, 75].

AST-120

AST-120 is an oral charcoal adsorbent that reduces the levels of circulating uremic toxins. It prevents progression of LVH, vascular calcification and atherosclerosis, possibly via the reduction of oxidative stress by removing uremic toxins such as indoxyl sulfate. So far most studies have been conducted on animal models, with short-term, promising human studies recently confirming this effect [76–78].

Other Medical Therapies that Influence Vascular Inflammation

Megestrol acetate is a synthetic derivate of progesterone that is mainly used as an appetite stimulant, which was found to improve appetite, energy, protein intake, quality of life and increase body weight. In addition, it was found to inhibit the activity of proinflammatory cytokines such as IL-1, IL-6 and TNF-α.

Pentoxifylline is a nonspecific phosphodiesterase inhibitor that inhibits the production of TNF, IL-6 and IL-10. A recent trial demonstrated reduction in TNF, IL-6 and CRP in HD patients [79].

Sevelamer hydrochloride and bicarbonate are used as phosphate binders in CKD patients. Sevelamer hydrochloride reduced CRP levels [80] and improved endothelial dysfunction [81]. It is proposed that reduction in calcium phosphate microcrystal deposition in vessel walls may decrease macrophage activation and cytokine production. Alternatively, changes in gastrointestinal milieu may stabilize intimal plaques or ameliorate atherosclerotic plaque size [82].

Conclusion

CKD patients are at high risk of premature cardiovascular complications. Conventional CVS risk factors do no fully account for the CVD burden in CKD. Nontraditional risk factors such as uremia and chronic inflammation impact the unique cardiovascular risk burden of patients with chronic kidney disease. Novel strategies directly addressing these CKD specific risks, may mitigate the inappropriate cardiovascular risk burden of this patient population.

References

1. Alani H, Tamimi A, Tamimi N. Cardiovascular co-morbidity in chronic kidney disease: current knowledge and future research needs. World J Nephrol. 2014;3(4):156–68.
2. Hajhosseiny R, Khavandi K, Goldsmith DJ. Cardiovascular disease in chronic kidney disease: untying the Gordian knot. Int J Clin Pract. 2013;67(1):14–31.
3. Filiopoulos V, Vlassopoulos D. Inflammatory syndrome in chronic kidney disease: pathogenesis and influence on outcomes. Inflamm Allergy Drug Targets. 2009;8(5):369–82.
4. Bemelmans MH, Gouma DJ, Buurman WA. Influence of nephrectomy on tumor necrosis factor clearance in murine model. J Immunol. 1993;150(5):2007–17.
5. Poole S, et al. Fate of injected interleukin 1 in rats: sequestration and degradation in the kidney. Cytokine. 1990;2(6):416–22.
6. Hamlett L, Haraqsim L. Quotidian hemodialysis and inflammation associated with chronic kidney disease. Adv Chronic Kidney Dis. 2007;14(3):e35–42.
7. Anders HJ, Andersen K, Stetcher B. The intestinal microbiota, a leaky gut, and abnormal immunity in kidney disease. Kidney Int. 2013;83(6):1010–6.
8. Linden GJ, et al. Persistently raised C-reactive protein levels are associated with advanced periodontal disease. K Clin Periodontol. 2008;35:741–7.
9. Walter R, Mischak H, Haller H. Haemodialysis, atherosclerosis and inflammation-identifying molecular mechanisms of chronic vascular disease in ESDR patients. Nephrol Dial Transpl. 2002;17 (Suppl 3):24–9.
10. Krediet RT, Balafa O. Cardiovascular risk in the peritoneal dialysis patient. Nat Rev Nephrol. 2010;6(8):451–60.
11. Aric M, Walls J. End-stage renal disease, atherosclerosis, and cardiovascular mortality: is C-creative protein the missing link? Kidney Int. 2001;59(2):407–14.
12. Vanholder R, et al. European Uremic Toxin Work Group (EUTox). Review on uremic toxins: classification, concentration and interindividual variability. Kidney Int. 2003;63(5): 1934–43.
13. Peters SA, et al. HDF Pooling Project Investigators. Haemodiafiltration and mortality in end-stage kidney disease patients: a pooled individual participant data analysis from four randomized controlled trials. Nephrol Dial Transpl. 2015;31:978–84.
14. Lekawanvijit S, et al. Cardiorenal syndrome: the emerging role of protein-bound uremic toxins. Circ Res. 2012;111(11):1470–83.
15. Lee JC, Downing SE. Negative inotropic effects of phenol on isolated cardiac muscle. Am J Pathol. 1981;102(3):367–72.
16. Fujii H, Nakai K, Fukagawa M. Role of oxidative stress ad indoxyl sulfate in progression of cardiovascular disease in chronic kidney disease. Ther Apher Dial. 2011;15(2):125–8.
17. Adijiang A, et al. Indoxyl sulphate promotes aortic calcification with expression of osteoblast-specific proteins in hypertensives rats. Nephrol Dial Transpl. 2008;23(6):1892–901.
18. Del Vecchio L, Locatelli F, Carini M. What we know about oxidative stress in patients with chronic kidney disease on dialysis—clinical effects, potential treatment, and prevention. Semin Dial. 2011;24(1):56–64.
19. Utpal S, Paras KM, Neetu T, Suresh CT. Homocysteine to hydrogen sulfide or hypertension. Cell Biochem Biophys. 2010;57 (2–3):49–58.
20. Locatelli F, et al. Oxidative stress in end-stage renal disease: an emerging threat to patient outcome. Nephrol Dial Transpl. 2003;18 (7):1272–80.
21. Annuk M, Zilmer M, Fellstrom B. Endothelium-dependent vasodilation and oxidative stress in chronic renal failure: impact on cardiovascular disease. Kidney Int Suppl. 2003;84:S50–3.
22. Wratten ML, et al. Evolution of oxidative stress and inflammation during hemodialysis and their contribution to cardiovascular disease. Antioxid Redox Signal. 2002;4(6):935–44.
23. Wunder A, et al. The injection of heparin prolongs the plasma clearance of oxidized low density lipoprotein in the rat. Thromb Res. 1995;78(2):139–49.
24. Peev V, Nayer A, Contreras G. Dyslipidemia, malnutrition, inflammation, cardiovascular disease and mortality in chronic kidney disease. Curr Opin Lipidol. 2014;25(1):54–60.
25. Zyga S, Christopoulou G, Malliarou M. Malnutrition-inflammation-atherosclerosis syndrome in patients with end-stage renal disease. J Ren Care. 2011;37(1):12–5.
26. Tucker PS, Scanlan AT, Dalbo VJ. Chronic kidney disease influences multiple systems: describing the relationship between oxidative stress, inflammation, kidney damage, and concomitant disease. Oxid Med Cell Longev. 2015;2015:806358 doi: 10.1155/2015/806358. Epub 2015 Mar 15.
27. Moody WE, et al. Endothelial dysfunction and cardiovascular disease in early-stage chronic kidney disease: cause or association? Atherosclerosis. 2012;233(1):86–94.
28. Pirillo A, Norata GD, Catapano AL. LOX-1, OxLDL, and atherosclerosis. Mediators Inflamm. 2013;2013:152786.
29. Moarndi H, Sica DA, Kalantar-Zadeh K. Cardiovascular burden associated with uremic toxins in patients with chronic kidney disease. Am J Nephrol. 2013;38(2):136–48.
30. Menon V, Ul A, Sarnak MJ. Cardiovascular risk factors in chronic kidney disease. Kidney Int. 2005;68(4):1413–8.
31. McMahon LP, Roger SD, Levin A, Slimheart Investigators Group. Development, prevention, and potential reversal of left ventricular hypertrophy in chronic kidney disease. J Am Soc Nephrol. 2004;15(6):1640–7.
32. Go AS, et al. Chronic kidney disease and the risks of death, cardiobascular events, and hospitalization. N Engl J Med. 2004;351(13):1296–305.
33. McAlister FA, et al. Renal insufficiency and heart failure: prognostic and therapeutic implications from a prospective cohort study. Circulation. 2004;109(8):1004–9.
34. Popolo A, Autore G, Pinto A, Marzocco S. Oxidative stress in patients with cardiovascular disease and chronic renal failure. Free Radic Res. 2013;47(5):346–56.
35. Fuji H, Nakai K, Fukagawa M. Role of oxidative stress and indoxyl sulfate in progression of cardiovascular disease in chronic kidney disease. Ther Apher Dial. 2011;15(2):125–8.
36. Colombo PC, et al. Inflammatory activation: cardiac, renal and cardio-renal interactions in patients with the cardiorenal syndrome. Heart Fail Rev. 2012;17(2):177–90.
37. Zawada AM, Roacev KS, Heine GH. Clinical relevance of epigenetic dysregulation in chronic kidney disease-associated cardiovascular disease. Nephrol Dial Transpl. 2013;28(7):1663–71.

38. Betjes MG. Immune cell dysfunction and inflammation in end-stage renal disease. Nat Rev Nephrol. 2013;9(5):255–65.
39. Stenvinkel P, et al. Impact of inflammation on epigenetic DNA methylation—a novel risk factor for cardiovascular disease? J Intern Med. 2007;261:488–99.
40. Geisel J, et al. Decreased p66Shc promoter methylation in patients with end-stage renal disease. Clin Chem Lab Med. 2007;45:1764–70.
41. Sapienza C, et al. DNA methylation profiling identifies epigenetic differences between diabetes patients with ESRD and diabetes patients without nephropathy. Epigenetics. 2011;6:20–8.
42. Machowska A, et al. Therapeutics targeting persistent inflammation in chronic kidney disease. Transl Res. 2016;167(1):204–13
43. Cobo G, et al. Clinical Determinants of reduced physical activity in hemodialysis and peritoneal dialysis patients. J Nephrol. 2015;28(4):503–10.
44. Viana JL, et al. Evidence for anti-inflammatory effects of exercise in CKD. J Am Soc Nephrol. 2014;25:2121–30.
45. Taraz M, et al. Sertraline decreases serum level of interleukin-6 I hemodialysis patients with depression: results of a randomized double-blind, placebo-controlled clinical trial. Int Immunopharmacol. 2013;70:655–65.
46. Chen HY, et al. Cognitive behavioral therapy for sleep disturbances decreased inflammatory cytokines and oxidative stress in hemodialysis patients. Kidney Int. 2011;80:415–22.
47. Gharekhani A, et al. The effect of omega-3 fatty acids on depressive symptoms and inflammatory markers in maintenance hemodialysis patients: a randomized, placebo-controlled clinical trial. Eur J Clin Pharmacol. 2014;70:655–65.
48. Yazdi FK, et al. Effect of nonsurgical periodontal treatment on C-reactive protein levels in maintenance hemodialysis patients. Ren Fail. 2013;35:711–7.
49. Brymora A, et al. Low-fructose diet lowers blood pressure and inflammation in patients with chronic kidney disease. Nephrol Dial Transpl. 2012;27:608–12.
50. Friedman A, Moe S. Review of the effects of omega-3 supplementation in dialysis patients. Clin J Am Soc Nephrol. 2006;1:182.
51. Huang X, et al. Serum fatty acid patterns, insulin sensitivity and the metabolic syndrome in individuals with chronic kidney disease. J Intern Med. 2014;275:71–83.
52. Hsu SP, et al. Chronic green tea extract supplementation reduces hemodialysis-enhanced production of hydrogen peroxide and hypochlorous acid, atherosclerotic factors, and proinflammatory cytokines. Am J Clin Nutr. 2007;86:1539–47.
53. Shema-Didi L, et al. One year of pomegranate juice intake decreases oxidative stress, inflammation, and incidence of infections in hemodialysis patients: a randomized placebo-controlled trial. Free Radic Biol Med. 2012;53:297–304.
54. Fanti P, et al. Positive effect of dietary soy in ESRD patients with systemic inflammation—correlation between blood levels of the soy isoflavones and the acute phase reactants. Nephrol Dial Transpl. 2006;21:2239–46.
55. Anders HJ, Andersen K, Stecher B. The intestinal microbiota, a leaky gut and abnormal immunity in kidney disease. Kidney Int. 2013;83(6):1010–6.
56. Chan CT, Floras JS, Miller JA, Pierratos A. Improvement in ejection fraction by nocturnal hemodialysis in end stage renal failure patients with coexisting heart failure. Nephrol Dial Transpl. 2002;17(8):1518–21.
57. Chan CT, Mardirossian S, Faratro R, Richardson RM. Improvement of lower-extremity peripheral arterial disease by nocturnal hemodialysis. Am J Kidney Dis. 2003;41(1):225–9.
58. Hamlett L, Haragsim L. Quotidian hemodialysis and inflammation associated with chronic kidney disease. Adv Chronic Kidney Dis. 2007;14(3):e35–42.
59. Chan CT, Li SH, Verma S. Nocturnal hemodialysis is associated with restoration of impaired endothelial progenitor cell biology in end-stage renal disease. Am J Physiol Renal Physiol. 2005;289(4):F679–84.
60. Lerman A, et al. Long-term L-arginine supplementation improved small-vessel coronary endothelial function in humans. Circulation. 1998;97(21):213–8.
61. Adams MR, et al. Oral L-arginine improved endothelium-dependent dilatation and reduces monocyte adhesion to endothelial cells tin young men with coronary artery disease. Atherosclerosis. 1997;129(2):261–9.
62. Rector, et al. Randomized, double-blind, placebo-controlled study of supplemental oral L-arginine in patients with heart failure. Circulation 1996;93(12):2135–41.
63. Nascimento MM, et al. Effect of Oral *N*-acetylcysteine treatment on plasma inflammatory and oxidative stress markers in peritoneal dialysis patients: a placebo-controlled study. Perit Dial Int. 2010;30:336–42.
64. Tepel M, et al. The antioxidant acetylecysteine reduces cardiovascular events in patients with end-stage renal failure: a randomized, controlled trial. Circulation. 2003;107:992–5.
65. Boaz M, et al. Secondary prevention with antioxidants of cardiovascular disease in endstage renal disease (SPACE): randomized placebo-controlled trial. Lancet. 2000;356(9237):1213–8.
66. Himmelfarb J, et al. Provision of antioxidant therapy in hemodialysis (PATH): a randomized clinical trial. J Am Soc Nephrol. 2014;25:623–33.
67. Stephens NG, et al. Randomized controlled trial of vitamin E in patients with coronary disease: Cambridge Heart Antioxidant Study (CHAOS). Lancet. 1996;347(9004):781–6.
68. GISSI-Prevenzione Investigators (Gruppo Italiano per lo Studio della Sopravvivenza nell'Ifarto miocardico) Dietary supplementation with n-3 polyunsaturated fatty acids and vitamin E after myocardial infarction: results of the GISSI-Prevenzione trial. Lancet. 1999;354(9177):447–55.
69. Jamison RL, et al. Veterans Affairs Site Investigators. Effects of homocysteine lowering on mortality and vascular disease in advanced chronic kidney disease and end-stage renal disease: a randomized controlled trial. JAMA. 2007;298(10):1163–70.
70. Mann JF, et al. HOPE-2 investigators. Homocysteine lowering with folic acid and B vitamins in people with chronic kidney disease—results of the renal Hope-2 study. Nephrol Dial Transpl. 2008;23(2):546–53.
71. Cucto-Manzano AM, et al. Anti-inflammatory interventions in end-stage kidney disease: a randomized, double-blinded controlled and crossover clinical trial on the use of pravastatin in continuous ambulatory peritoneal dialysis. Arch Med Res. 2013;44:633–7.
72. Ridker PM, et al. Efficacy of rosuvasatin among men and women with moderate chronic kidney disease and elevated high-sensitivity C-reactive protein: a secondary analysis from the JUPITER (Justification for the use of statins in prevention-an intervention trial evaluating rosuvastatin) trial. J Am Soc Nephrol. 2010;21:353–61.
73. Baigent C, et al. SHARP investigators. The effects of lowering LDL cholesterol with simvastatin plus ezetimibe in patients with chronic kidney disease (Study of Heart and Renal Protection): a randomized placebo-controlled trial. Lancet. 2011;377(9784):2181–92.
74. Wanner C, et al. German Diabetes and Dialysis Study Investigators. Atorvastatin in patients with type 2 diabetes mellitus undergoing hemodialysis. N Engl J Med. 2005;353(3):238–48.
75. Fellstrom BC, et al. AURORA Study Group. Rosuvastatin and cardiovascular events in patients undergoing hemodialysis. N Engl J Med. 2009;360(14):1395–407.

76. Lee CT, et al. Effects of AST-120 on blood concentrations of protein-bound uremic toxins and biomarkers of cardiovascular risk in chronic dialysis patients. Blood Purif. 2014;37(1):76–83.
77. Wu IW, et al. Oral adsorbent AST-120 potentiates the effect of erythropoietin-stimulating agents on Stage 5 chronic kidney disease patients: a randomized crossover study. Nephrol Dial Transpl. 2014;29(9):1719–27.
78. Yamamoto S, et al. Continuous reduction of protein-bound uraemic toxins with improved oxidative stress by during the oral charcoal adsorbent AST-120 in hemodialysis patients. Sci Rep. 2015;23(5):14381.
79. Gonzalez-Espinoza L, et al. Pentoxifylline decreases serum levels of tumor necrosis factor alpha, interleukin 6 and C-reactive protein in hemodialysis patients: results of a randomized double-blind, controlled clinical trial. Nephrol Dial Transpl. 2012;27:2023–8.
80. Navarro-Gonzalez JF, et al. Mineral metabolism and inflammation in chronic kidney disease patients: a cross sectional study. Clin J Am Soc Nephrol. 2009;4:1646–54.
81. Caglar K, et al. Short-term treatment with sevelamer increases serum fetuin-a concentration and improves endothelial dysfunction in chronic kidney disease stage 4 patients. Clin J Am Soc Nephrol. 2008;3:61–8.
82. Brandenburg VM, Jahnen-Dechent W, Ketteler M. Sevelamer and the bone-vascular axis in chronic kidney disease: bone turnover, inflammation, and calcification regulation. Kidney Int Suppl. 2009;114:S26–33.

7 Phosphorus and Mortality: Do We Have the Panacea?

Tatsuo Shimosawa and Rika Jimbo

Introduction

Normal kidney function is central to maintaining calcium–phosphorus homeostasis. As glomerular filtration rate (GFR) declines, the ability to maintain tight regulation of these minerals, by the renal tubular epithelium is impaired. The calcium–phosphorus product (CaP) is regulated by the interplay of baseline GFR, vitamin D levels and PTH. This chapter focuses on altered phosphate metabolism and the cascade of events triggered by declining GFR, and its impact on cardiovascular outcomes.

Dietary phosphorus intake is around 1–1.5 g/day with typical Western diets, and 60–80% of this is absorbed in the small intestine. The rate limiting step for phosphorus absorption is mediated by the sodium–phosphorus cotransporter type II(NaPi-II)b [1]. NaPi-III (PIT-1) is another phosphate cotransporter that plays a key role in absorption of dietary phosphorus phosphorous into the bone [2–4]. PTH, vitamin D and acidosis independently regulate phosphorus release and deposition from and into the bone. The proximal tubule of the kidney reabsorbs 60–70% of filtered phosphorus, and the rest is reabsorbed in the distal tubules. NaPi-IIa, c and PIT-2 located in the proximal tubule tightly regulate phosphorus resorption, as illustrated (Fig. 7.1).

In CKD, early and progressive increases in PTH levels lead to suppression of phosphate reabsorption, with resultant phosphaturia. Moreover, intestinal absorption of phosphorus is decreased due to reduced levels of vitamin D, which are reversible with vitamin D replacement [5, 6]. Recently in addition to role of the vitamin D and PTH axis, the role of fibroblast growth factor 23 (FGF23) in regulating vitamin D, PTH, calcium and phosphorus was clarified. Since then, the relationship between FGF23 and cardiovascular events has been widely studied and both basic and clinical research implicates this axis as an evolving target to reduce cardiovascular morbidity and mortality in patients with CKD.

FGF23 and Its Effect on Phosphorus Metabolism

FGF23 is a 251-amino-acid protein (26 kDa) composed of a 24 amino-terminal signal peptide, an FGF-like sequence (residues 25–180) and a unique carboxyl-terminal sequence (residues 181–251) [7]. FGF23 is synthesized and secreted by osteoblasts and osteocytes [8, 9], and its production and actions are stimulated by vitamin D, high phosphate levels, calcium intake, and PTH [10, 11]. FGF23 reduces NaPi-II a and c in the proximal tubular epithelial cells to increase phosphorus excretion as well as inhibiting NaPi-IIb and 25-hydroxyvitamin D-1α[alpha]-hydroxylase (1α[alpha]-hydroxylase) activity to reduce phosphorus absorption in the gut [12–16]. In addition to 1α[alpha]-hydroxylase deactivation, FGF23 increases the activity of 25-hydroxyvitamin D-24 hydroxylase and promote degradation of vitamin D [16]. NaPi-IIa and c are also controlled by PTH which acutely reduce those activity of these transporters, when compared to FGF-23 [17]. These above-mentioned effect of FGF23 are mediated through its receptor and its co-receptor Klotho [18, 19] (Fig. 7.1). Klotho is a 130-kDa transmembrane β[beta]-glucuronidase [20]. That is predominantly expressed in the distal tubule. In addition to affecting the process of aging, it appears to have some modulatory effects on insulin sensitivity. The name of the gene comes from Klotho, one of the Fates in Greek mythology. When Klotho is deleted specifically in distal tubule, the metabolic effects

T. Shimosawa (✉)
Department of Clinical Laboratory, Faculty of Medicine, International University of Health and Welfare, 4-3 Kozu-no-Mori, Narita, Chiba 286-8686, Japan
e-mail: tshimo-tky@umin.ac.jp

T. Shimosawa
Department of Clinical Laboratory, Mita Hospital, IUHW, 1-4-3, Mita, Minatoku, Tokyo 108-8329, Japan

R. Jimbo
Department of Internal Medicine, Tohto Bunkyo Hospital, 3-5-7, Yushima, Bunkyo-ku, Tokyo 113-0034, Japan
e-mail: rikajimbo1211@hotmail.com

J. Rangaswami et al. (eds.), *Cardio-Nephrology*,
DOI 10.1007/978-3-319-56042-7_7

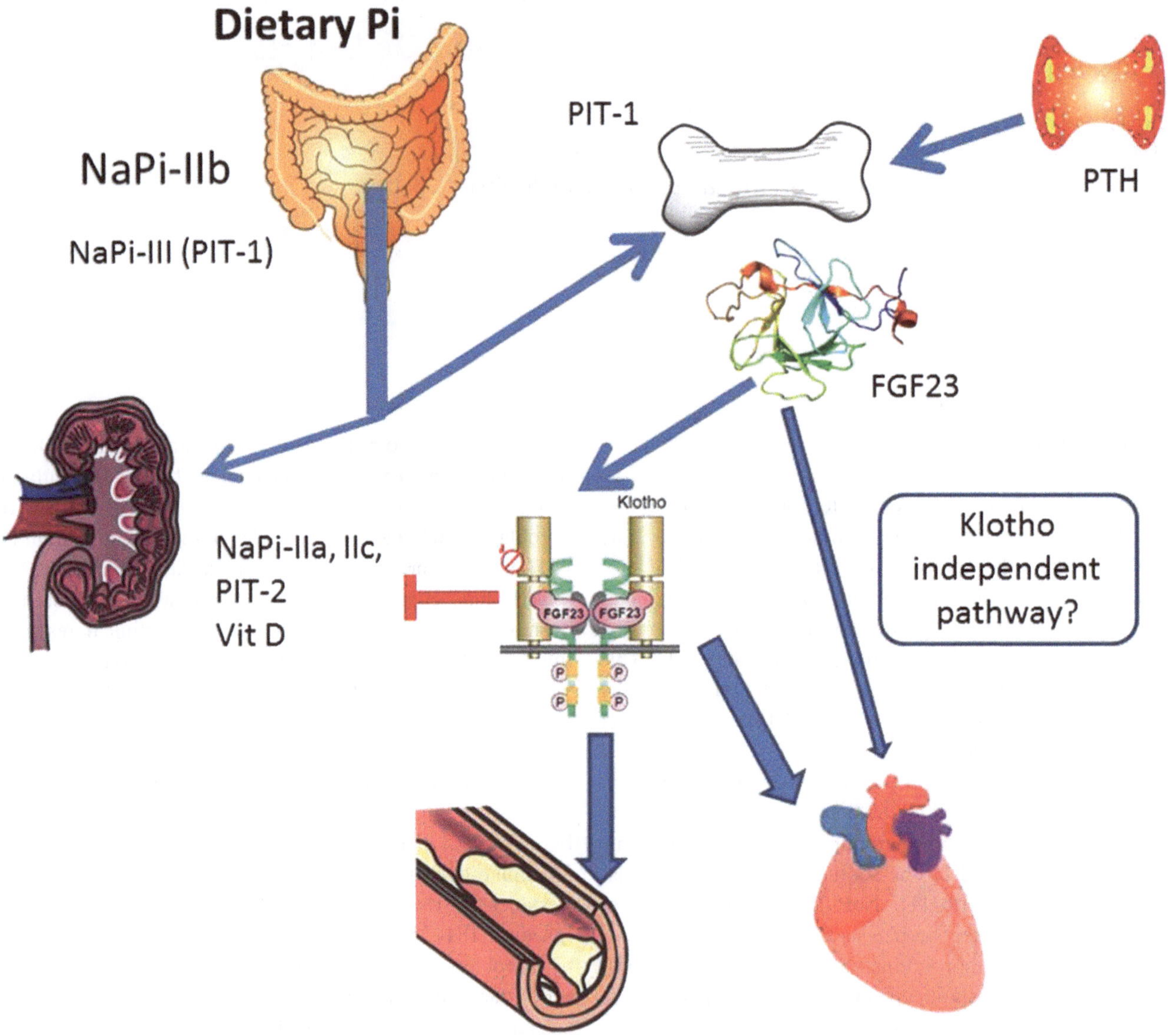

Fig. 7.1 Dietary phosphorus is absorbed in the small intestine by NaPi-IIb and NaPi-III (Pit-1) plays minor role. Pit-1 plays key role in storing phosphorus in the bone. PTH and vitamin D regulate release of phosphorus from the bone stores. In the kidney, NaPi-IIa, c, and PIT-2 locate in the proximal tubules and reabsorb filtered phosphorus. FGF23 is major phosphorus regulating hormone that synthesized mainly in the bone. FGF23 suppresses NaPi-IIa, b, c and vitamin D activation to reduce serum phosphorus. These physiological activities are through its receptor complex (FGFR-Klotho). On the other hand, high in FGF23 promotes vascular calcification and cardiac hypertrophy. These effects may via FGFR-Klotho complex or possibly independent pathway

of FGF23 on phosphorus and vitamin D are disrupted [21, 22].

In Klotho deficient mice, decrease in Klotho expression and activity induces early senescence and high inflammation [23] and accelerates CKD progression. There is also evidence of accelerated atherosclerosis, impaired endothelium dependent vasodilation and angiogenesis suggesting that Klotho may be cardioprotective through endothelium derived NO production [23].

The mechanism of action of Klotho is not fully understood, but it changes cellular calcium homeostasis, by both increasing the expression and activity of TRPV5 and decreasing that of TRPC6. Additionally, klotho increases membrane expression of the inward rectifier channel ROMK [23]. In CKD, Klotho expression decreases with declining GFR, and is being strongly considered key the pathogenesis of accelerated atherosclerosis in the context of declining GFR [10].

Phosphorus Level and CVD

Epidemiological observations has shown that higher serum phosphorus is an independent risk factor for cardiovascular disease (CVD) [24]. CKD is also a risk for cardiovascular event, partially due to vascular calcification. In addition to vitamin D deficiency in CKD [25], hyperphosphatemia in CKD leads to calcification in the intima and media of vasculature thereby contributing to atherosclerosis and vascular stiffness [26]. Besides ectopic calcification, phosphorus promote phonotypical transformation of vascular smooth muscle cells (VSMC) into osteoblast-like cells [27].

FGF23 and CVD: A New Window into Vascular Calcification

In every stages of CKD, high levels of serum FGF23 have been associated with cardiac hypertrophy [28, 29], vascular calcification [30], arterial stiffness, plaque formation [31] stroke [32] and all-cause CVD mortality [33]. Although Klotho is not expressed in the heart, FGF23 stimulate PLC-γ[gamma] independent from Klotho to induce cardiomyocyte hypertrophy [29]. There is controversial discussion if Klotho exists in the VSMCs [34]. We showed that Klotho is expressed in the aorta in vivo [35], and in ex vivo experiments, showed that explanted aortic tissue from a uremic rat model in which Klotho was detectable, FGF 23 aggravated vascular calcification. Moreover, when Klotho is induced into cultured cells, high phosphorus levels with high FGF23 activity promote osteoblastic transformation of VSMC via ERK1/2 pathway [35].

In targeting CVD risk, maintaining endothelial function is critical. Both alternative splicing and ectodomain shedding by ADAM 10 and 17 produce soluble Klotho [36]. This soluble Klotho has sialidase activity and modulates several channels on cell surface. For example, NaPi-IIa is modified by soluble Klotho to increase it endocytosis and inactivate it [37]. On the other hand, endocytosis of transient receptor potential cation channel, subfamily V member 5(TRPV5) is reduced and results in an increase in calcium currents [38]. In addition, Soluble Klotho, FGF23 and phosphorus deteriorate NO production and increase oxidative stress in endothelial cells [39, 40].

In addition to these observational studies, recent data illustrates that FGF23 can be a new target for therapy to reduce CVD in CKD patients [41]. The EVOLVE trial was done in patients undergo hemodialysis who were on conventional therapy with phosphate binders and vitamin D. 2985 samples were randomized either placebo or the calcimimetic, cinacalcet. Although cinacalcet failed to reduce mortality in end-stage kidney disease (ESKD) [42], in the EVOLVE trial, cinacalcet reduced FGF23 more than 30% than placebo by indirectly modifying the calcium-phosphate PTH axis. Besides cinacalcet, recent data shows that β[beta]-blockers can directly reduce FGF23 levels [43]. β[beta]-blockers are widely used for stable congestive heart failure patients, and reduce cardiovascular mortality. Direct inhibition of FGF23 or its signaling may be on the mechanisms through which this effect is realized, although larger data are needed to confirm this.

Non-Pharmacologic Reduction of Serum Phosphate

Observational data suggests that serum phosphate concentration >3.5 mg/dL is independently associated with mortality [44, 45]. Even in patients with eGFR > (60 mL/min)/(1.73 m^2), elevated phosphate concentration is a risk for mortality [46, 47]. For non-pharmacologic prevention of CVD, it is critical to reduce dietary intake of phosphorus to reduce FGF-23 levels. Reduction of protein intake and subsequent decrease in dietary phosphorus intake which is abundant in highly processed foods, have been associated with reduced mortality [48, 49]. After dietary sodium, sugar and overall calorie reduction efforts, phosphorus is the next target to reduce mortality on a large population basis.

Conclusion

Phosphorus is an independent risk factor for cardiovascular mortality in healthy people as well as in CKD. Modulating the FGF-Klotho complex through dietary phosphorus restriction is a promising approach to reduce the strong link with CV mortality, for the future.

Conflict of interest The authors declare that they have no conflict of interest.

References

1. Sabbagh Y, O'Brien SP, Song W, Boulanger JH, Stockmann A, Arbeeny C, et al. Intestinal npt2b plays a major role in phosphate absorption and homeostasis. J Am Soc Nephrol. 2009;20(11):2348–58.
2. Giral H, Caldas Y, Sutherland E, Wilson P, Breusegem S, Barry N, et al. Regulation of rat intestinal Na-dependent phosphate transporters by dietary phosphate. Am J Physiol Renal Physiol. 2009;297(5):F1466–75.
3. Lederer E, Miyamoto K. Clinical consequences of mutations in sodium phosphate cotransporters. Clin J Am Soc Nephrol. 2012;7(7):1179–87.
4. Forster IC, Hernando N, Biber J, Murer H. Phosphate transporters of the SLC20 and SLC34 families. Mol Aspects Med. 2013;34(2–3):386–95.
5. Evenepoel P, Wolf M. A balanced view of calcium and phosphate homeostasis in chronic kidney disease. Kidney Int. 2013;83(5):789–91.
6. Davis GR, Zerwekh JE, Parker TF, Krejs GJ, Pak CY, Fordtran JS. Absorption of phosphate in the jejunum of patients with chronic renal failure before and after correction of vitamin D deficiency. Gastroenterology. 1983;85(4):908–16.

7. Fukumoto S, Yamashita T. FGF23 is a hormone-regulating phosphate metabolism—unique biological characteristics of FGF23. Bone. 2007;40(5):1190–5.
8. Riminucci M, Collins MT, Fedarko NS, Cherman N, Corsi A, White KE, et al. FGF-23 in fibrous dysplasia of bone and its relationship to renal phosphate wasting. J Clin Investig. 2003; 112(5):683–92.
9. Pereira RC, Juppner H, Azucena-Serrano CE, Yadin O, Salusky IB, Wesseling-Perry K. Patterns of FGF-23, DMP1, and MEPE expression in patients with chronic kidney disease. Bone. 2009;45(6):1161–8.
10. Hu MC, Shiizaki K, Kuro-o M, Moe OW. Fibroblast growth factor 23 and Klotho: physiology and pathophysiology of an endocrine network of mineral metabolism. Annu Rev Physiol. 2013;75: 503–33.
11. Rodriguez-Ortiz ME, Lopez I, Munoz-Castaneda JR, Martinez-Moreno JM, Ramirez AP, Pineda C, et al. Calcium deficiency reduces circulating levels of FGF23. J Am Soc Nephrol. 2012;23(7):1190–7.
12. Shimada T, Urakawa I, Yamazaki Y, Hasegawa H, Hino R, Yoneya T, et al. FGF-23 transgenic mice demonstrate hypophosphatemic rickets with reduced expression of sodium phosphate cotransporter type IIa. Biochem Biophys Res Commun. 2004; 314(2):409–14.
13. Segawa H, Kawakami E, Kaneko I, Kuwahata M, Ito M, Kusano K, et al. Effect of hydrolysis-resistant FGF23-R179Q on dietary phosphate regulation of the renal type-II Na/Pi transporter. Pflugers Arch. 2003;446(5):585–92.
14. Shimada T, Kakitani M, Yamazaki Y, Hasegawa H, Takeuchi Y, Fujita T, et al. Targeted ablation of Fgf23 demonstrates an essential physiological role of FGF23 in phosphate and vitamin D metabolism. J Clin Investig. 2004;113(4):561–8.
15. Miyamoto K, Ito M, Kuwahata M, Kato S, Segawa H. Inhibition of intestinal sodium-dependent inorganic phosphate transport by fibroblast growth factor 23. Ther Apher Dial. 2005;9(4):331–5.
16. Shimada T, Hasegawa H, Yamazaki Y, Muto T, Hino R, Takeuchi Y, et al. FGF-23 is a potent regulator of vitamin D metabolism and phosphate homeostasis. J Bone Miner Res. 2004;19(3):429–35.
17. Vervloet MG, van Ittersum FJ, Buttler RM, Heijboer AC, Blankenstein MA, ter Wee PM. Effects of dietary phosphate and calcium intake on fibroblast growth factor-23. Clin J Am Soc Nephrol. 2011;6(2):383–9.
18. Urakawa I, Yamazaki Y, Shimada T, Iijima K, Hasegawa H, Okawa K, et al. Klotho converts canonical FGF receptor into a specific receptor for FGF23. Nature. 2006;444(7120):770–4.
19. Kurosu H, Ogawa Y, Miyoshi M, Yamamoto M, Nandi A, Rosenblatt KP, et al. Regulation of fibroblast growth factor-23 signaling by klotho. J Biol Chem. 2006;281(10):6120–3.
20. Kuro-o M, Matsumura Y, Aizawa H, Kawaguchi H, Suga T, Utsugi T, et al. Mutation of the mouse klotho gene leads to a syndrome resembling ageing. Nature. 1997;390(6655):45–51.
21. Olauson H, Lindberg K, Amin R, Jia T, Wernerson A, Andersson G, et al. Targeted deletion of Klotho in kidney distal tubule disrupts mineral metabolism. J Am Soc Nephrol. 2012;23(10): 1641–51.
22. Farrow EG, Davis SI, Summers LJ, White KE. Initial FGF23-mediated signaling occurs in the distal convoluted tubule. J Am Soc Nephrol. 2009;20(5):955–60.
23. Zhao Y, Banerjee S, Dey N, LeJeune WS, Sarkar PS, Brobey R, et al. Klotho depletion contributes to increased inflammation in kidney of the db/db mouse model of diabetes via RelA (serine)536 phosphorylation. Diabetes. 2011;60(7):1907–16.
24. Osuka S, Razzaque MS. Can features of phosphate toxicity appear in normophosphatemia? J Bone Miner Metab. 2012;30(1):10–8.
25. Pillar R, Lopes MG, Rocha LA, Cuppari L, Carvalho AB, Draibe SA, et al. Severe hypovitaminosis D in chronic kidney disease: association with blood pressure and coronary artery calcification. Hypertens Res. 2013;36(5):428–32.
26. Giachelli CM. Vascular calcification mechanisms. J Am Soc Nephrol. 2004;15(12):2959–64.
27. Giachelli CM, Jono S, Shioi A, Nishizawa Y, Mori K, Morii H. Vascular calcification and inorganic phosphate. Am J Kidney Dis. 2001;38(4 Suppl 1):S34–7.
28. Gutierrez OM, Januzzi JL, Isakova T, Laliberte K, Smith K, Collerone G, et al. Fibroblast growth factor 23 and left ventricular hypertrophy in chronic kidney disease. Circulation. 2009;119(19): 2545–52.
29. Faul C, Amaral AP, Oskouei B, Hu MC, Sloan A, Isakova T, et al. FGF23 induces left ventricular hypertrophy. J Clin Investig. 2011;121(11):4393–408.
30. Lee YT, Ng HY, Chiu TT, Li LC, Pei SN, Kuo WH, et al. Association of bone-derived biomarkers with vascular calcification in chronic hemodialysis patients. Clin Chim Acta. 2016;15(452):38–43.
31. Shah NH, Dong C, Elkind MS, Sacco RL, Mendez AJ, Hudson BI, et al. Fibroblast growth factor 23 is associated with carotid plaque presence and area: the Northern Manhattan Study. Arterioscler Thromb Vasc Biol. 2015;35(9):2048–53.
32. Wright CB, Dong C, Stark M, Silverberg S, Rundek T, Elkind MS, et al. Plasma FGF23 and the risk of stroke: the Northern Manhattan Study (NOMAS). Neurology. 2014;82(19):1700–6.
33. Parker BD, Schurgers LJ, Brandenburg VM, Christenson RH, Vermeer C, Ketteler M, et al. The associations of fibroblast growth factor 23 and uncarboxylated matrix Gla protein with mortality in coronary artery disease: the Heart and Soul Study. Ann Intern Med. 2010;152(10):640–8.
34. Jimbo R, Shimosawa T. Cardiovascular risk factors and chronic kidney disease-FGF23: a key molecule in the cardiovascular disease. Int J Hypertens. 2014;2014:381082.
35. Jimbo R, Kawakami-Mori F, Mu S, Hirohama D, Majtan B, Shimizu Y, et al. Fibroblast growth factor 23 accelerates phosphate-induced vascular calcification in the absence of Klotho deficiency. Kidney Int. 2014;85(5):1103–11.
36. Imura A, Iwano A, Tohyama O, Tsuji Y, Nozaki K, Hashimoto N, et al. Secreted Klotho protein in sera and CSF: implication for post-translational cleavage in release of Klotho protein from cell membrane. FEBS Lett. 2004;565(1–3):143–7.
37. Hu MC, Shi M, Zhang J, Pastor J, Nakatani T, Lanske B, et al. Klotho: a novel phosphaturic substance acting as an autocrine enzyme in the renal proximal tubule. FASEB J. 2010;24(9):3438–50.
38. Cha SK, Ortega B, Kurosu H, Rosenblatt KP, Kuro OM, Huang CL. Removal of sialic acid involving Klotho causes cell-surface retention of TRPV5 channel via binding to galectin-1. Proc Natl Acad Sci USA. 2008;105(28):9805–10.
39. Silswal N, Touchberry CD, Daniel DR, McCarthy DL, Zhang S, Andresen J, et al. FGF23 directly impairs endothelium-dependent vasorelaxation by increasing superoxide levels and reducing nitric oxide bioavailability. Am J Physiol Endocrinol Metab. 2014; 307(5):E426–36.
40. Six I, Okazaki H, Gross P, Cagnard J, Boudot C, Maizel J, et al. Direct, acute effects of Klotho and FGF23 on vascular smooth muscle and endothelium. PLoS ONE. 2014;9(4):e93423.
41. Moe SM, Chertow GM, Parfrey PS, Kubo Y, Block GA, Correa-Rotter R, et al. Cinacalcet, fibroblast growth factor-23, and cardiovascular disease in hemodialysis: the evaluation of Cinacalcet HCl therapy to lower cardiovascular events (EVOLVE) trial. Circulation. 2015;132(1):27–39.
42. Ballinger AE, Palmer SC, Nistor I, Craig JC, Strippoli GF. Calcimimetics for secondary hyperparathyroidism in chronic kidney disease patients. Cochrane Database Syst Rev. 2014;12:CD006254.

43. Fajol A, Chen H, Umbach AT, Quarles LD, Lang F, Foller M. Enhanced FGF23 production in mice expressing PI3K-insensitive GSK3 is normalized by beta-blocker treatment. FASEB J. 2015 Nov 2.
44. Kestenbaum B, Sampson JN, Rudser KD, Patterson DJ, Seliger SL, Young B, et al. Serum phosphate levels and mortality risk among people with chronic kidney disease. J Am Soc Nephrol. 2005;16(2):520–8.
45. Palmer SC, Hayen A, Macaskill P, Pellegrini F, Craig JC, Elder GJ, et al. Serum levels of phosphorus, parathyroid hormone, and calcium and risks of death and cardiovascular disease in individuals with chronic kidney disease: a systematic review and meta-analysis. JAMA. 2011;305(11):1119–27.
46. Tonelli M, Sacks F, Pfeffer M, Gao Z, Curhan G. Relation between serum phosphate level and cardiovascular event rate in people with coronary disease. Circulation. 2005;112(17): 2627–33.
47. Sim JJ, Bhandari SK, Smith N, Chung J, Liu IL, Jacobsen SJ, et al. Phosphorus and risk of renal failure in subjects with normal renal function. Am J Med. 2013;126(4):311–8.
48. Kasiske BL, Lakatua JD, Ma JZ, Louis TA. A meta-analysis of the effects of dietary protein restriction on the rate of decline in renal function. Am J Kidney Dis. 1998;31(6):954–61.
49. Hansen HP, Tauber-Lassen E, Jensen BR, Parving HH. Effect of dietary protein restriction on prognosis in patients with diabetic nephropathy. Kidney Int. 2002;62(1):220–8.

Inhibition of the Renin–Angiotensin System: How Far Have We Come?

8

Jay Ian Lakkis and Matthew R. Weir

The Renin–Angiotensin–Aldosterone System in Health

The renin–angiotensin–aldosterone system (RAAS) plays a vital role in both health and disease states, most importantly in the cardiovascular system and in the kidneys. This system is best viewed as the sum total of its complementary and coordinated branches: a systemic branch and a multitude of local tissue-specific paracrine and autocrine branches. The systemic RAAS plays a key role in maintaining blood pressure homeostasis and vascular tone, while each local RAAS serves functions more customized to the tissue in which it is present. For example, the kidney RAAS is responsible for maintaining fluid as well as sodium and potassium balance in the distal nephron, while prevention of aberrant and excessive activation of cardiac RAAS halts its vital pathological role in the genesis of cardiac hypertrophy and myocardial fibrosis, and brain RAAS influences the central control of blood pressure [1].

To understand the full complexity of the RAAS, it is essential to be familiar with its individual components (Table 8.1; Fig. 8.1). The circulating hepatic 14-amino acid glycopeptide angiotensinogen is converted by renin to angiotensin I (decapeptide, AngI), which in turn is converted predominantly by pulmonary vascular endothelial angiotensin converting enzyme (ACE) to angiotensin II (AngII). AngII binds the transmembrane angiotensin II type 1 (AT1) and angiotensin II type 2 (AT2) receptors; in the zona glomerulosa of the adrenal cortex. Such binding stimulates the secretion of aldosterone, an end product of cholesterol metabolism. Aldosterone binds the cytosolic mineralocorticoid receptor (MR), a ligand-dependent transcription factor that has been localized to epithelial and non-epithelial tissues; epithelial sites include the principal cells and the alpha-intercalated cells in the cortical collecting duct of the nephron, and non-epithelial sites include the myocardial cells, vascular endothelial, and smooth muscle cells. Under physiologic conditions, the effects of systemic and local RAASs converge to maintain a steady state of fluid balance and normal blood pressure as well as a healthy steady state in specific tissues. Multiple agents that interrupt the aforementioned series of reactions are clinically available.

Not all AngII is produced via the ACE-dependent pathway; other ACE-independent pathways have been described. Of significance is a local RAAS serine protease chymase, which catalyzes production of the bulk of AngII in the heart and the blood vessels and this same chymase has been noted to be upregulated in the kidneys in some forms of CKD [2]. No pharmacological interventions that interrupt the actions of chymase are available to this date.

Angiotensin III (AngIII) and Angiotensin IV (AngIV) are end products of AngII metabolism; AngIII exerts effects similar to AngII and binds the same AT1 and AT2 receptor albeit with a lower affinity for AT1 and a higher affinity for AT2. AngIV binds angiotensin receptor 4 (AT4), an insulin-regulated aminopeptidase, in renal proximal and convoluted tubular cells as well as endothelial cells but its clinical relevance is not certain [3].

Vascular endothelial angiotensin-converting enzyme 2 (ACE2) converts AngI into Angiotensin 1–9; it also converts AngII into Angiotensin 1–7. Angiotensin 1–9 simulates the vasoconstrictive effects of AngII and promotes the actions of bradykinin. Angiotensin 1–9 is then converted by ACE to Angiotensin 1–7, a heptapeptide with counter-regulatory effects to AngII in the cardiovascular system. Angiotensin 1–7 binds to its Mas receptor, and this active complex binds the AT1 receptor thereby blocking its availability to AngII,

J.I. Lakkis
Department of Medicine, John A. Burns School of Medicine, University of Hawaii at Manoa, Maui Memorial Medical Center, 21 Kamaiki Cir, Kahului, HI 96732-3153, USA
e-mail: jay.lakkis@gmail.com

M.R. Weir (✉)
Division of Nephrology, Department of Medicine, University of Maryland School of Medicine, N3W 143 Nephrology, UMMC, Baltimore, MD 21201, USA
e-mail: mweir@medicine.umaryland.edu

J. Rangaswami et al. (eds.), *Cardio-Nephrology*,
DOI 10.1007/978-3-319-56042-7_8

Table 8.1 Elements of the renin–angiotensin–aldosterone system

Substrate	Characteristics
Renin	Structure: 337 amino acid monomeric aspartyl protease enzyme Molecular weight: 38,000 g/mol Human renin gene has been localized to chromosome 1q42 Precursors: preprorenin and prorenin (inactive) Sites of production: juxtaglomerular cells of cortical nephrons in the kidney in response to reduced NaCl distal delivery to the macula densa, heart Sites of action: substrate angiotensinogen Functions: catalyzes the enzymatic hydrolysis of an N-terminal peptide bond of angiotensinogen 1–14 to produce the Angiotensin I decapeptide
Angiotensin-converting enzyme (ACE)	Structure: a kinase Molecular weight: 480,000 g/mol Precursors: none Sites of production: vascular endothelium in the lungs, kidneys, blood vessels Sites of action: substrate angiotensin I Functions: (1) catalyzes the conversion of angiotensin I decapeptide to an angiotensin II octapeptide by the cleavage of two amino acids from its carboxy terminal. (2) Converts angiotensin 1–9 to angiotensin 1–7. (3) Inactivates the vasodilator peptide bradykinin
Angiotensin-converting enzyme 2 (ACE2)	Structure: carboxypeptidase Sites of production: vascular endothelial cells, heart, kidneys Sites of action: binds angiotensin receptor 4 (AT4) in the renal proximal and convoluted tubular cells as well as endothelial cells Functions: (a) converts angiotensin I to angiotensin 1–9. (b) Hydrolysis of AngII and its conversion to angiotensin 1–7
Angiotensinogen	Structure: about 453-amino acid circulating hepatic glycopeptide which contains the sequence for the alpha-globulin angiotensinogen 1–14 (C85H123N21020) Molecular weight: 56,800 g/mol; angiotensinogen 1–14: 1759.01482 g/mol Precursors: none. Sites of production: liver, kidneys Sites of action: inactive Functions: inactive
Angiotensin I	Structure: 10-amino acid decapeptide (C62H89N17014) Molecular weight: 1296.47556 g/mol Precursors: angiotensinogen 1–14 Sites of production: systemic Sites of action: mostly inactive Functions: mostly inactive
Angiotensin II	Structure: 8-amino acid octapeptide Asp-Arg-Val-Tyr-Ile-His-Pro-Phe (C50H71N13012) that is produced after the cleavage of two amino acids -His-Leu from the C-terminal of angiotensin I by ACE Molecular weight: 1046.17864 g/mol Precursors: angiotensin I Sites of production: lungs Sites of action: binds the angiotensin II type 1 (AT1) and angiotensin II type 2 (AT2) receptors in the zone glomerulosa of the adrenal cortex Functions: (a) AT1R binding: (a1) stimulates the adrenal cortex zona glomerulosa to release aldosterone. (a2) Increases BP via its short term actions as a potent but labile arteriolar (and less so venous) vasoconstrictor. (a3) Increases BP and extracellular fluid volume (ECFV) in the longterm via decreasing renal salt and water excretion both directly and via aldosterone secretion. (a4) Stimulates angiogenesis. (a5) Prothrombotic effect. (a6) Profibrotic effect. (a7) Promotes production of reactive oxygen species (ROS) and enhances vascular remodeling. (b) Role of AT2 receptor is less clear: (b1) enhances NO production, produces vasodilatation and decreases BP. (b2) inhibits growth and induces differentiation (b3) plays a role in apoptosis

(continued)

Table 8.1 (continued)

Substrate	Characteristics
Angiotensin 1–9	Structure: 9-amino acid nanopeptide Precursors: angiotensin I Sites of production: ACE 2 converts AngI to angiotensin 1–9 Sites of action: cardiovascular system Functions: (a) vasoconstrictor (b) prothrombotic effect (c) Enhances effects of bradykinin
Angiotensin 1–7	Structure: 7-amino acid heptapeptide Precursors: angiotensin 1–9 Sites of production: ACE converts angiotensin 1–9 to angiotensin 1–7. ACE2 converts AngII to angiotensin 1–7 Sites of action: cardiovascular system Functions: (a) counter-regulatory to AngII, (b) vasodilator, (c) anti-inflammatory effects, (d) anti-fibrotic effects, (e) enhances platelet recovery after myelosuppression
Angiotensin III	Structure: 7-amino acid heptapeptide. C46H66N1209 Molecular weight: 931.09124 g/mol Precursors: angiotensin II Sites of action: cardiovascular system Functions: similar effects to angiotensin II via AT1 and AT2 receptor albeit with lower affinity with AT1 and higher affinity with AT2
Angiotensin IV	Structure: 6-amino-acid hexapeptide. C40H54N808, angiotensin 3–8 Molecular weight: 774.90556 g/mol Precursors: angiotensin III Sites of action: binds angiotensin receptor 4 (AT4) in the renal proximal and convoluted tubular cells as well as endothelial cells, brain, heart, bladder, spleen, prostate, adrenals, colon Functions: unknown
Aldosterone	Structure: C12H2805 is the principal physiologic mineralocorticoid, a steroid hormone formed as one of the end products of cholesterol metabolism via the enzymatic actions of aldosterone synthase (corticosterone methyloxidase) on 18-hydroxycorticosterone Molecular weight: 360.44402 g/mol Precursors: 18-hydroxycorticosterone Sites of production: adrenal cortex zona glomerulosa, blood vessels, mycoardium, brain Sites of action: binds the cytosolic mineralocorticoid receptor (MR), a ligand-dependent transcription factor, that has been localized to epithelial and non-epithelial tissues. Epithelial sites include the principal cells + alpha-intercalated cells in the cortical collecting duct of the nephron, colon, salivary glands, sweat glands, retina and its pigment epithelium, urinary bladder, and rectal mucosa. Non-epithelial sites include the myocardial cells in the heart, vascular endothelial and smooth muscle cells, and the brain Functions: (a) increases ECFV and BP and (b) determines the final concentration of potassium in the urine: this is achieved by enhancing electrogenic sodium reabsorptive transport via the apical epithelial sodium channel (ENaC) and by increasing the density of the Na–K ATPase in the basolateral membrane of the principal cells; to maintain luminal electroneutrality sodium reabsorption is coupled with potassium secretion via ROMK1, the expression of which is also increased by aldosteone. (c) Augments activity of apical membrane H^+-ATPase in the alpha-intercalated cells thus enhancing hydrogen ion secretion

and promoting vasodilatory, anti-inflammatory, anti-angiogenic, anti-proliferative, and anti-fibrotic effects [2].

In summary, our understanding of the RAAS and its clinical relevance continues to evolve. In the following section we will discuss the role of RAAS, mainly AngII and Aldosterone, in cardiovascular and kidney disease and the interruption of such effects with RAAS inhibition; however, it is worth emphasizing that Angiotensin 1–7 and ACE2 seem to play a counter-regulatory protective role in both organ systems.

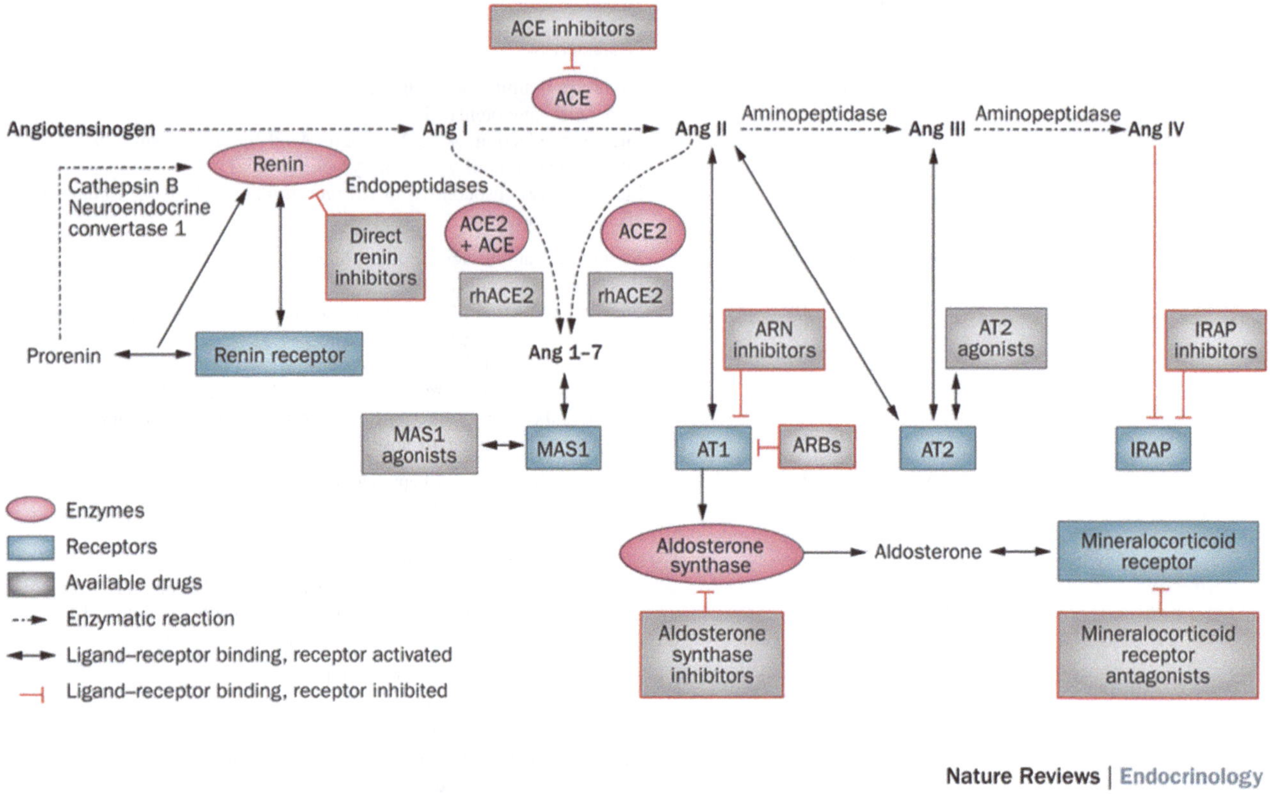

Fig. 8.1 Prorenin can be activated proteolytically in the kidneys (by neuroendocrine convertase 1 or cathepsin B) or nonproteolitically by the renin receptor in many tissues. Circulating renin can also bind to the renin receptor, which increases its enzymatic activity. Renin converts angiotensinogen to Ang I, which can then enter three main pathways. These three axes, ACE–Ang II–AT1–aldosterone, ACE2–Ang 1–7–MAS1 and Ang IV–IRAP, are highlighted. Activation of the AT1 receptor in the adrenal gland results in production of aldosterone, which can then bind to the mineralocorticoid receptor. *Abbreviations*: *ACE* angiotensin-converting enzyme, *ACE2* angiotensin-converting enzyme 2, *Ang* angiotensin, *ARB* angiotensin receptor blocker, *ARN* angiotensin receptor–neprilysin, *AT1* type-1 Ang II receptor, *AT2* type-2 Ang II receptor, *IRAP* leucyl–cystinyl aminopeptidase (also known as insulin-regulated membrane aminopeptidase or insulin-responsive aminopeptidase), *MAS1* proto-oncogene Mas, *rh* recombinant human. Reprinted with authorization from: Romero et al. Nat Rev Endocrinol. 2015 Apr;11(4):242–52

The RAAS in Kidney and Heart Disease

RAAS in Kidney Disease

The major etiologies of chronic kidney disease (CKD) worldwide are diabetes mellitus (DM) and systemic arterial hypertension (HTN); furthermore, cardiovascular disease has been associated with increased risk of CKD [United States Renal Data System (USRDS) 2015 Annual Data Report]. CKD and abnormal urinary albumin excretion are risk factors for end-stage kidney disease (ESKD) and mortality [4, 5]. Albuminuria has been validated as a surrogate end point for the progression of CKD and it is estimated that a 30% reduction in the urinary albumin excretion results in a 23.7% reduction in the risk of progression to ESKD [6].

There is a growing body of evidence that blockade of the RAAS in the CKD patient population reduces the rate of albumin excretion, decelerates the progression of CKD, and thus the development of ESKD; and while observational studies also report a resultant reduction in all-cause and cardiovascular mortality rate, a systematic review detected such a trend but the benefits did not meet statistical significance [7]. Some of the mechanisms by which RAAS inhibition protects against kidney disease are hereby described.

AngII promotes oxidative stress, inflammation, proliferative effects, fibrosis, and atrophy in the tubulointerstitum, and thus accelerates progression of CKD; it also impairs endothelial structure as well as function and suppresses nitric oxide (NO) bioactivity, stimulates vascular endothelial growth factor (VEGF) and vascular smooth muscle cell as well as endothelial proliferation, triggers synthesis of extracellular matrix proteins, impairs the integrity of the glomerular basement membrane, promotes podocyte apoptosis and augment's urinary protein excretion. AngII augments albumin proximal tubular reabsorption and endocytosis, a process which stimulates proximal tubular RAAS and a self-perpetuating vicious cycle in which the albumin uptake further enhances inflammation and fibrosis [2]. Aldosterone has similar deleterious effects, which may amplify those of AngII [8].

CKD, irrespective of the specific underlying etiology, is invariably associated with a reduction in renal mass. Hemodynamically, this decrease in nephron mass triggers a series of adaptive mechanisms to restore kidney function (glomerular filtration rate GFR), the major mechanism being glomerular hyperfiltration. However, such persistent hyperfiltration and increased intraglomerular capillary pressure promotes immune activation and an inflammatory state, eventually leading to injury and damage in all the kidney compartments, namely glomerular, vascular endothelial, and tubulointerstitial. Similarly, glomerular podocyte injury, and the resultant micro- and macroalbuminuria, results in a proinflammatory state and tubulointerstitial disease [9, 10].

AngII is a potent vasoconstrictor with preferential vasoconstrictive effects on the glomerular efferent arteriole; this effect plays a physiologic role in maintaining normal hydrostatic and glomerular filtration pressures. RAAS inhibition with an ACE inhibitor (ACEi) or an AngII AT1 receptor antagonist (AIIT1RA, angiotensin receptor blocker ARB), results in a more marked glomerular efferent arteriolar dilatation, which in turn, reversibly reduces the hydrostatic and glomerular filtration pressures. Thus, it is quite expected, as well as desirable, that such RAAS inhibition may result in a reversible rise in the serum creatinine and subsequently a decline in the GFR; it is widely acceptable that such a change is not to exceed 30% from baseline within the first 2–4 weeks after initiation of therapy, especially when optimal BP goals are achieved. The magnitude of such a change in GFR and serum creatinine becomes more prominent clinically in patients with [1] decreased effective arterial blood volume due to conditions such as excessive diuresis, or low forward cardiac output due reduced left ventricular ejection fraction (LVEF), valvular disease, or heart failure (HF), and [2] adaptive glomerular hyperfiltration due to CKD or diabetic nephropathy where this compensatory effect is blunted by glomerular afferent arteriolar vasodilatation [11]. Clinically, significant renal artery stenosis is another condition which may be associated with more substantial reductions in GFR with RAAS inhibition and associated blood pressure reduction.

In summary, RAAS inhibition is kidney protective through its effects on lowering intraglomerular capillary pressure, and decreasing production of AngII and Aldosterone, thereby mitigating their role in the progression of CKD (pro-fibrogenic, pro-proliferative, pro-inflammatory, etc.).

RAAS in Cardiovascular Risk and Disease

Cardiovascular disease is the major cause of mortality in the United States of America (USA) [12], but its risk gains an alarming momentum in patients with CKD and ESKD. CKD, like DM, is a coronary artery disease (CAD) risk equivalent, which implies shared underlying risk factors as well as accelerated pathophysiologic atherogenic pathways in the two disease clusters [13].

In patients with EKSD on renal replacement therapy (RRT), cardiovascular disease accounts for 53.1% of mortality and is attributed to sudden cardiac death (cardiac arrest, arrhythmia) in 37%, acute myocardial infarction (AMI) and atherosclerotic heart disease (AHD) in 6.7%, congestive HF in 5.8%, cerebrovascular accident (CVA) in 3.1%, and other cardiac causes in 0.5% (USRDS 2015 Annual Data Report). It is worth noting that a unique and atypical cardiovascular risk profile (e.g., intermittent and/or chronic volume overload, aberrant mineral metabolism, cardiovascular including valvular and coronary calcifications, chronic inflammation and malnutrition) in patients with ESKD on RRT with dialysis outcompetes the traditional cardiovascular risk factors responsible for cardiovascular disease in non-dialysis CKD and non-CKD patients; in other words, the pretest probability of cardiovascular risk one routinely quantitates based on, or associates with, risk factors such as tobacco use, systemic arterial hypertension, dyslipidemia is no longer a reliable tool in this patient population.

Aberrations in the systemic or local RAAS accelerate AHD, HTN, inflammation, and promote the development of metabolic syndrome at the center of which are insulin resistance and obesity [14].

AngII has numerous cardiovascular effects, some of which are hereby described. AngII is a potent physiologic vascoconstrictor; local tissue AngII has been associated with vascular endothelial dysfunction due to promoting endothelial nitric oxide synthase (eNOS) uncoupling, and enhancing NAD(P)H oxidase (NOX) and xanthine oxidoreductase activity, all of which create a state of oxidative stress with the production of reactive oxygen species (ROS) and superoxide free radicals which degrade nitric oxide, prevent endothelial regeneration, arrest growth, promote apoptosis and eventually result in vascular remodeling. Furthermore, AngII has proliferative and proangiogenic properties; it stimulates certain growth factors (e.g., VEGF), which in turn trigger vascular smooth muscle cell as well as endothelial proliferation. AngII has prothrombotic effects, which clinically manifests as an accelerated atherogenic effect. AngII has profibrogenic effects [2, 15]. In patients with endothelial dysfunction, ACEi or AIIT1RA monotherapy has been shown to improve markers of endothelial function [16].

Angiotensin 1–7 has antagonistic cardiovascular effects to AngII and plays a physiologic counter-regulatory role to reverse the aforementioned effects of AngII. Parenteral Angiotensin 1–7 is currently undergoing trials for its anti-proliferative and anti-angiogenic effects in cancer patients [17, 18].

ACE2 infusions have been shown to decrease SBP in animal models thought to be due to enhanced AngII degradation and subsequent decreasing in AngII levels [19].

Aldosterone shares many of the pathogenic properties of AngII in animal and human models. Local tissue as well as adrenal aldosterone promote tissue fibrosis after ischemia, impair endothelial cell function, inhibit NO synthesis, increase oxidative stress, and decrease the number of endothelial progenitor cells [15].

Finally, reduced insulin sensitivity or Insulin resistance, is a precursor to DM, a major risk factor for both cardiovascular and kidney diseases, and is promoted by a series of effects mediated by AngII and Aldosterone in autocrine and paracrine RAAS. Examples of such effects include the previously mentioned increased oxidative stress, accelerated pancreatic beta cell apoptosis, aberrant insulin signaling and diminished glucose transport [20]. Hypothetically, RAAS blockade should restore insulin sensitivity and reduce the incidence of type 2 DM (T2DM) through various mechanisms, such as enhanced skeletal muscle perfusion with subsequent improved tissue insulin signaling and uptake and glucose transport as well as pancreatic beta cell insulin production [21]. However, the clinical evidence to prove or disprove the aforementioned hypothesis is conflicting and is discussed later.

In summary, this vital role of local and systemic RAAS in the pathogenies of atherosclerosis and cardiovascular disease in animal and human models has paved the way to the clinically established role of RAAS inhibition as an essential therapy for secondary prevention of cardiovascular disease and possibly its BP-independent benefits.

RAAS in Cardiorenal Diseases

Injury in one organ triggers a chain of events that reverberates in distant organs; as mentioned earlier, there is accumulating evidence that kidney disease is a risk factor for cardiovascular disease and vice versa [22]. This bidirectional organ cross talk is essential to maintain homeostasis in health, and its disruption is best represented by the cardiorenal syndromes (CRS). CRS has been classified into five subtypes [23]:

- Type 1 CRS or acute CRS refers to acute kidney injury (AKI) as a result of acute rapidly worsening heart disease.
- Type 2 or chronic CRS refers to progressive CKD as a result of chronic heart disease.
- Type 3 CRS or acute renocardiac syndrome refers to acute heart disease due to AKI.
- Type 4 CRS or chronic renocardiac syndrome refers to heart disease (functional as well as structural) as a result of CKD.
- Type 5 or secondary CRS refers to heart and kidney disease as a result of a systemic illness.

Inhibitors of the Renin Angiotensin Aldosterone System

- Four main classes of drugs inhibit the RAAS (Table 8.2).

Direct Renin Inhibitors (DRI)

The only DRI available to this date in the United States (US) is Aliskiren and it was approved by the US Food and Drug Administration (FDA) in 2007 for the treatment of hypertension. This approval is rooted in many trials in different patient populations.

The beneficial effects of direct renin inhibition seem to mirror those of ACEi and AIIT1RA, namely:

- blood pressure control.
- reduction in albuminuria in patients with hypertension [24].
- renoprotective effects as reflected by reduction in albuminuria in patients with diabetic nephropathy [25].

Angiotensin Converting Enzyme Inhibitors (ACEi)

ACEi were introduced into clinical practice with the FDA approval of captopril in 1981. Currently, there are ten ACI approved for clinical use in the USA by the FDA (Table 8.2). Their clinical effects are similar to other forms of RAAS inhibitors, mainly as BP lowering agents, renoprotective and anti-proteinuric agents, treatment of HF and secondary prevention of cardiovascular disease.

Angiotensin II AT1 Receptor Blockers (AIIT1RA)

Losartan was the first AIIT1RA to be approved by the FDA in 1995 and since then nine more AIIT1RA have been in clinical use (Table 8.2). Their renoprotective and cardioprotective effects are almost identical to ACEi and the two classes are used interchangeably in clinical practice. Their safety profile is more favorable than that of ACEi.

Table 8.2 Inhibitors of the renin angiotensin aldosterone system approved by the United States food and drug administration

Class	Drug	Indications for use
Direct renin inhibitors	Aliskiren	Lowers blood pressure No reduction in renal or cardiorenal endpoints when added to AIIT1RA or ACE-i in patients with type 2 DM and CKD. Statistically significant higher rates of hyperkalemia were noted in the Aliskiren group
Angiotensin converting enzyme inhibitors	Benazepril, captopril, enalapril/enalaprilat, fosinopril, lisinopril, moexipril, perindopril, quinapril, ramipril, trandolapril	Lower blood pressure Micro- and macroalbuminuria/proteinuria HF and reduced left ventricular ejection fraction Acute coronary syndrome Diabetes mellitus induced CKD ESKD on PD with residual kidney function
Angiotensin II T1 (AT1) Receptor Blockers	Azilsartan, candesartan, eprosartan, irbesartan, losartan, olmesartan, telmisartan, valsartan	Lower blood pressure. Micro- and macroalbuminuria/proteinuria. Acute coronary syndrome. ESKD on PD with residual Kidney Function
Selective Aldosterone receptor antagonists	Eplerenone, spironolactone	Lower blood pressure Micro- and macroalbuminuria/proteinuria Reduced left ventricular ejection fraction <35% and NYHA class II–IV CHF Acute myocardial infarction complicated by left ventricular dysfunction and heart failure: STEMI + LVEF $\leq$ 40% + (symptomatic CHF or DM) Block the local effects of RAAS and Aldosterone in the myocardium such as hypertrophy and fibrosis

Aldosterone Receptor Antagonists

The two FDA approved aldosterone receptor antagonists are eplerenone (approved in 2002), a selective aldosterone receptor antagonist (SARA), and spironolactone (approved in 1985), a nonselective aldosterone receptor antagonist and a potassium sparing diuretic. Both agents are indicated as adjunctive therapy in patients with treatment-resistant hypertension and/or primary hyperaldosteronism and like other RAAS inhibitors, reduce urinary protein excretion. Both agents decrease mortality rates in patients with symptomatic HF and reduced LVEF when added to standard therapy.

Clinical Relevance of RAAS Inhibition in Kidney and Heart Disease

Perturbations in systemic or paracrine RAAS contribute to elevations in blood pressure, heart and kidney disease, and thus interruption of this system at different levels has been the subject of heavy research for more than three decades and has proved to be protective in different ways. However, such benefits may be forestalled by other factors, such as non-ACE dependent AngII production, such as through chymase, as well as aldosterone synthesis escape, which continue to be a challenge even when using multilevel RAAS blockade [1].

Stage 1–5 Chronic Kidney Disease

One of the cornerstones of slowing down the progression of kidney disease, whether diabetic or non-diabetic in etiology, is achieving goal BP, which in itself is a more important and renoprotective end point than the choice of the BP lowering class or agent. Non-pharmacological lifestyle modifications and pharmacological interventions should target a BP less than 140/90 mmHg in patients with stage 1–5 CKD or DM according to JNC8 (Eighth Joint National Committee 2014 evidence-based guideline for the management of high blood pressure) [26] and to levels less than 130/80 mmHg in the presence of micro- or macroalbuminuria as per the 2012 Kidney Disease: Improving Global Outcomes (KDIGO) Clinical Practice Guideline for the Management of Blood Pressure in Chronic Kidney Disease [27]. A 2014 European Renal Best Practice (ERBP) position statement endorsed the KDIGO guidelines for the management of BP in CKD patients [28].

This focus on BP control is highly relevant in the stage 1–5 CKD patient population, in whom the prevalence of systemic arterial hypertension exceeds 70–80% and varies proportionately with the degree of kidney disease with as many as 84.1% of patients with stages 4–5 CKD having systemic arterial hypertension [29]. While, the optimal level of blood pressure control in different patient populations continues to evolve, it is widely acceptable that controlling blood pressure (BP) to levels <140/90 mmHg has kidney as well as cardiovascular protective effects; lower target BP levels have been recommended for patients with CKD, microalbuminuria, proteinuria >1 g/day, and cardiovascular disease. With the recent publication of the SPRINT trial results, many guidelines will likely adopt lower SBP goals for optimal reduction of cardiovascular events [30]. However, this trial did not have enough power to examine the influence of BP goals on renal disease progression. More discussion about optimal BP goals would occur in another chapter in this book.

Direct renin inhibition with Aliskiren in patients with albuminuric stage 1–3 CKD (diabetic and non-diabetic) and HTN over a period of 24 weeks successfully reduced SBP and DBP, significantly decreased albuminuria and preserved GFR [31].

RAAS inhibition with an ACEi or an AIIT1RA is recommended by the JNC 8 [26], KDIGO [27], National Kidney Foundation (NKF) K/DOQI [32], American College of Physicians (ACP) [33], and ERBP [28] guidelines for treatment of systemic arterial hypertension in CKD. Such inhibition reduces albuminuria and slows down progression of CKD, with a BP-independent effect which offers more protection than can be accounted for by BP lowering alone. However, the bulk of clinical evidence at the core of these guidelines applies to patients with Stages 1–3 CKD or with micro- or macroalbuminuria; evidence is scarce regarding its role in stages 4–5 CKD or patients with normal urinary albumin excretion rate [34].

A meta-analysis of eleven randomized trials (RCTs) identified the slowest rate of CKD progression over a period over 2.2 years in patients whose systolic blood pressure (SBP) was 110–129 mmHg and whose daily urine protein excretion was <2.0 g; therapy with an ACEi provided an additional 33% risk reduction even after accounting for the beneficial effects of the blood pressure control and reduction in urinary protein excretion. Higher SBP was associated with a worse progression of CKD when the daily urinary protein excretion rate exceeded 1 g [35].

A meta-analysis of twelve RCTs evaluated the effect of ACEi therapy in patients with pre-existing CKD (diabetic and non-diabetic) over a mean duration of 3 years, and reported a 55–75% risk reduction in the progression of CKD when compared to patients with normal baseline kidney function treated with an ACEi; furthermore, the magnitude of the acute reduction in GFR after initiation of therapy is a prognostic factor for the protection to be expected, provided it does not exceed the 30% ceiling [11].

Proteinuria and its magnitude are independent risk factors for progression of CKD, and for cardiovascular morbidity and mortality [36]. Reduction in proteinuria with RAAS inhibition slows down the progression of CKD independent of blood pressure reductions.

In a meta-analysis (2000) of 119 RCTs, which included 64,768 patients with CKD, treatment with an ACEi improved the odds of kidney failure to 0.61 and of a major cardiovascular event to 0.82 when compared to placebo; these respective odds were consistently better than those offered by AIIT1RA, calculated at 0.70 and 0.76 [37].

A Cochrane systematic review identified four RCTs, which evaluated 2177 non-diabetic adult patients with stage 1–3 CKD; treatment with either an ACEi or an AIIT1RA offered no benefit over placebo when the primary end point was all-cause mortality, cardiovascular death and cardiovascular events, or progression to ESKD. Based on one single-study data included in the review, only patients with underlying glomerular disease, as opposed to other renal pathologies, who were treated with ACEi had a lower risk of doubling their serum creatinine at 36 months when compared to placebo. The same study reported a 29% reduction in proteinuria and a 4.5–8.0 mmHg reduction in SBP at 36 months in patients treated with an ACEi compared to a 9% and a 1.0–3.7 mmHg increase in the same measures in the placebo group [38].

In summary, RAAS inhibition plays an essential role in slowing down the progression of CKD and reducing urinary protein excretion, with the evidence being scarce in stages 4–5 or advanced CKD due to exclusion of these patients in most major clinical trials. This renoprotective effect is both BP dependent and BP-independent.

Microalbuminuria and Proteinuria

A Cochrane Database Systematic Review of 27 RCTs (2014) evaluated the impact of aldosterone receptor antagonists (ARA, spironolactone and eplerenone) with or without further RAAS inhibition on cardiovascular and renal outcomes in patients with proteinuric stage 1–3 CKD (diabetic and non-diabetic, proteinuria 0.5–3.6 g/day) over a period of 2–20 months. When compared to an ACEi or an AIIT1RA or both, the addition of spironolactone significantly reduced the degree of proteinuria and SBP but had no effect on cardiovascular outcomes or on the rate of progression to ESKD; it had a less well-defined effect on glomerular filtration rate but it increased the risk of hyperkalemia and gynecomastia. The authors could not obtain adequate data regarding the effect of adding eplerenone to an ACEi or an AIIT1RA on the magnitude of proteinuria, SBP, GFR but individual trials reported effects similar those of spironolactone; addition of eplerenone, too, increased risk of hyperkalemia but there was no risk of gynecomastia [39]. Another meta-analyses from 2009 yielded similar results [40].

In summary, ACEi as well as AIIT1RA, DRI and aldosterone receptor antagonists reduce levels of prtoeinuria. Combination RAAS blockade has the benefit of additional reduction in urinary protein excretion but is associated with increased risks of hyperkalemia, AKI, and hypotension depending on the agents chosen.

Diabetic Kidney Disease

Kidney disease complicates DM in 25–40% after a course of 20–25 years, and around one third of those patients develop ESKD requiring RRT but the majority will die of cardiovascular causes before progression to ESKD [41]. Microalbuminuria in diabetic patients is a predictor of early cardiovascular mortality [42] with a two to fourfold increase in such risk with microalbuminuria, and an even higher risk in patients who have HTN and macroalbuminuria [43].

A Cochrane Database Systemic review of 50 RCTs highlighted the important concept that neither ACEi nor AIIT1RA had a significant effect on all-cause mortality in patients with diabetic CKD unless full-dose or maximum-tolerable dose was used with ACEi; three RCT compared ACEi to AIIT1RA and found no difference in all-cause mortality between the two forms of therapy in diabetic kidney disease. Both forms of therapy resulted in a statistically significant reduction in the risk of ESKD and of progression from micro- to macroalbuminuria with a significant increase in regression from micro- to norma-albuminuria [43].

In summary, full-dose RAAS blockade decelerates the progression of diabetic CKD and attenuates the degree of albuminuria.

Insulin Sensitivity and Diabetic Kidney Disease

The clinical evidence to prove or disprove the effect of RAAS inhibition on insulin sensitivity in nondiabetic subjects is conflicting. On the one hand, restoring tissue insulin sensitivity, at least partially, with ACEi has been reported in various clinical trials such as the HOPE trial (Heart Outcomes Prevention Evaluation) where ramipril, compared to placebo, reduced the incidence of T2DM (RR 0.66 and $p < 0.001$) after a mean followup of 5 years. On the other hand, the DREAM Trial Investigators (Effect of Ramipril on the Incidence of Diabetes) reported no change in the incidence of T2DM after 3 years of therapy with ramipril in patients with impaired fasting glucose compared to placebo, despite a significant restoration of normoglycemia in the Ramipril group [44].

Similar benefits were published with AIIT1RA trials such as the NAVIGATOR Study Group (Effect of valsartan on the incidence of diabetes and cardiovascular events) reported that non-pharmacological lifestyle modifications and pharmacological therapy with AIIT1RA valsartan resulted in a 14% relative reduction in the incidence of T2DM among patients with pre-DM and established cardiovascular disease or risk factors [45].

To address this question, several meta-analyses have been conducted over the past several years:

- in a meta-analysis (2004) of ten RCTs whose secondary end point was the incidence of T2DM in patients with HTN or HF, RAAS inhibition with either an ACEi or an AIIT1RA offered a 22% relative risk reduction of incident T2DM after a mean follow-up of 1–6 years; the number needed to treat (NNT) to prevent one incident case of T2DM was 45 patients over 4–5 years [21];
- a meta-analysis (2005) of 12 RCTs, showed a 27% reduction in incident T2DM with ACEi and 23% with AIIT1RA [46];
- a meta-analysis (2007) of 13 RCTs showed a 26% relative risk reduction of incident T2DM with RAAS inhibition, 28% with ACEi and 27% with AIIT1RA [47]; a meta-analysis (2010) of 18 RCTs showed that therapy with an ACEi or an AIIT1RA decreased the incidence of new-onset T2DM by 22% (RR 0.78, $p = 0.003$) and by 20% (RR 0.8, $p < 0.0001$) respectively [48];
- a meta-analysis (2011) of 11 RCTs similarly revealed that both ACEi [OR 0.8, (0.7–1.0), $p = 0.07$] and AIIT1RA [OR 0.8, (0.8–0.9), $p < 0.01$], reduced the incidence of new-onset T2DM [49]; a meta-analysis (2012) of eleven RCTs show that AIIT1RA therapy reduced the incidence of new-onset T2DM [OR 0.79, (0.74–0.84)] [50]; a meta-analysis (2013) of nine RCTs showed that therapy with an ACEi reduced the risk of new onset T2DM [OR 0.80, (0.71–0.91)] in patients with HTN or CAD or HF [51];
- a meta-analysis (2015) of four RCTs showed that ACEi were more effective at improving insulin sensitivity than AIIT1RA in hypertensive patients (standard mean difference SMD 0.45, 95% CI 0.17–0.73) [52].

In summary, all the above meta-analyses reproduced the same results, namely that RAAS inhibition with an ACEi or an AIIT1RA in nondiabetic patients with HTN or HF reduces the risk of incident T2DM.

Autosomal Dominant Polycystic Kidney Disease (ADPKD)

The management of ADPKD, the most common hereditary kidney disease, focuses largely on supportive measures including BP control. A Cochrane Database Systematic Review analyzed the efficacy of 11 interventions at preventing the progression of ADPKD and reported mixed effects on kidney function (no significant effect of ACEi or

AIIT1RA on serum creatinine or GFR when they were compared to each other or to no treatment; however, GFR was significantly better with calcium channel blocker CCB compared to ACEi) and total kidney volume (no significant difference with ACEi versus no treatment; AIIT1RA alone, but not ACEi, was associated with a significant increase in total kidney volume (TKV) when compared to an AIIT1RA combined with mTOR inhibitor); however, both forms of therapy significantly decreased urinary protein excretion but only when compared to CCBs (no significant difference with ACEi vs. no treatment). Effects of RAAS inhibition on BP were similarly non-convulsive and there was no significant difference in SBP with ACEi versus no treatment or ACEi versus AIIT1RA; however, ACEi, was associated with significantly reduced diastolic blood pressure (DBP) and mean arterial pressure (MAP) when compared to no treatment but there were no differences when compared to AIIT1RA. In the RCTs pooled into the systematic review, none of the interventions which evaluated cardiovascular events or all-cause mortality showed any benefit [53].

Stage 5D CKD Renal Replacement Therapy (RRT) with Dialysis

There is a scarcity of evidence-based medical literature to guide the management of patients with ESKD; the majority of RCTs exclude patients with advanced stage 4–5 CKD and patients with ESKD on dialysis (stage 5D CKD), be it hemodialysis (HD) or peritoneal dialysis (PD). As mentioned earlier, cardiovascular mortality accounts for 53.1% of deaths in this patient population; yet the role of RAAS inhibition in this subgroup is the least studied in the CKD population.

RAAS inhibition, with either an ACEi or an AIIT1RA, results in a progressive regression in left ventricular hypertrophy (LVH), as assessed by left ventricular mass index (LVMI), in patients with ESKD receiving RRT with dialysis; dual therapy with ACEi and AIIT1RA had no added benefit when compared to each agent alone [54, 55].

In patients with ESKD on HD, HTN and LVH, atenolol-based antihypertensive therapy was associated with a lower rate of serious cardiovascular events (AMI, stroke, hospitalization for HF, cardiovascular death) and all-cause hospitalization when compared to lisinopril-based antihypertensive therapy [56].

In a cohort of 1800 adult Taiwanese patients with ESKD receiving RRT with HD or PD and with no history of a major cardiovascular event or AIIT1RA therapy for 6 months prior to enrollment, and followed over a period over 5 years, long-term use of AIIT1RA (>365 days) significantly reduced the incidence of major cardiovascular events (including AMI, CAD requiring coronary stenting or percutaneous transluminal coronary angioplasty (PTCA), peripheral arterial disease (PAD) requiring percutaneous transluminal coronary angioplasty (PTCA), and acute CVA/stroke)) and their protective effect was directly proportional to the cumulative prescription days of AIIT1RA [57].

A Cochrane Database Systematic Review of six RCTs evaluated the impact of ACEi or AIIT1RA on residual kidney function in ESKD patients receiving RRT with continuous ambulatory PD (CAPD), and reported a significant and similar benefit on preserving residual kidney function with long-term therapy ($\geq$12 months) with an AIIT1RA or ACEi; however, one RCT pooled in this meta-analysis evaluated the effect of ACEi therapy on cardiovascular events and mortality when compared with other antihypertensive agents and reported no significant differences [58]. The results of this meta-analysis are concordant with prior published literature [59].

Erythropoietin deficiency and anemia in CKD are common findings in patients with ESKD on dialysis. AngII may play a minor physiological role in stimulating erythropoietin production in humans [60–62]. ACEi may reduce the response to recombinant human erythropoietin therapy and contribute to erythropoietin hyporesponsiveness or resistance [63, 64].

In conclusion, in patients with ESKD on HD and who have HTN and LVH, beta blockers may be first line agents for antihypertensive therapy. In addition to beta-blocker therapy and when needed, we recommend the initiation of RAAS inhibition with an ACEi or an AIIT1RA in patients with ESKD receiving HD or PD for antihypertensive therapy, prevention of major cardiovascular events, and preservation of residual kidney function. An aldosterone receptor antagonist may also be added for patients with treatment-resistant hypertension (TRH) or with symptomatic HF and reduced LVEF (<35%).

Stage 5T CKD Kidney Transplantation

The use of RAAS inhibition is usually preserved for the intermediate (1–4 months) and late ($\geq$4 months) post-transplant period and avoided in the early post-transplant period (first month) due to the increased risk of hyperkalemia and worsening kidney allograft function [29, 65, 66]. A systematic review of 21 trials reported that therapy with an ACEi or an AIIT1RA over a period of 27 months was associated with significant reductions in GFR, hematocrit and urinary protein excretion [66] but there was a paucity of evidence evaluating the long-term effect of RAAS inhibition on allograft survival, cardiovascular events or all-cause mortality.

Therapy with AIIT1RA in patients with Interstitial fibrosis/tubular atrophy (IF/TA), a major cause of kidney transplant allograft loss, resulted in a significant decrease in the volume of the cortical interstitium when compared to placebo, but this pathological benefit failed to translate into any clinical endpoints on secondary analysis, namely time to a composite endpoint of doubling of serum creatinine, ESKD or death. However, there was a trend towards decreased incidence of all-cause ESKD with AIIT1RA therapy [67].

In conclusion, we suggest the use of RAAS inhibition with an ACEi or an AIIT1RA in kidney transplant recipients in the late post-transplant period, and in the intermediate post-transplant period if a compelling indication arises, for antihypertensive therapy, prevention of major cardiovascular events, slowing down progression of CKD, and proteiuria. ARA may be added for patients with TRH or with symptomatic HF and reduced LVEF (<35%).

Post-kidney Transplantation Erythrocytosis

Post-transplant erythrocytosis complicates around 10–15% of kidney transplants and occurs 8–24 months post-transplantation with a spontaneous remission rate of 25% at 2 years. This is clinically relevant because 10–30% develop arterial or venous thrombotic complications (including CVA and pulmonary embolism) with a 1–2% mortality rate. Treatment with an ACEi or an AIIT1RA is the mainstay of treatment [68].

Systemic Arterial Hypertension

A comparative analysis showed that Aliskiren has similar BP lowering effects to hydrochlorothiazide and AIIT1RA, was equal to ACEi for lowering SBP but was superior in lowering DBP [30].

Both ACEi and AIIT1RA are considered first line therapy for HTN in patients with CKD, micro- or macroalbuminuria, and secondary prevention of cardiovascular disease such as HF and CAD. A Cochrane systematic review pooled nine RCTs to evaluate the impact of ACEi and AIIT1RA therapy in patients with primary HTN on all-cause and cardiovascular mortality and found no difference between either form of RAAS inhibition on all-cause mortality or cardiovascular mortality [69].

The ideal BP goal that maximizes cardiovascular and kidney protection and minimizes mortality and morbidity remains elusive and not well defined, and has been the subject of heavy scrutiny over the past few years. To address this question, the SPRINT research group evaluated the impact of two different systolic BP (SBP) goals on 9361 high cardiovascular risk non-diabetic patients over a period of 3.26 years and reported that the group with more intensive SBP control (121.4 vs. 136.2 mmHg) had a significantly lower all-cause mortality and a lower rate of the primary composite end point of AMI, other acute coronary syndromes, CVA, HF and death from cardiovascular disease. However, there was a significantly higher rate of hypotension, syncope, AKI, electrolyte abnormalities in the intensive treatment group [70].

In summary, RAAS inhibition, especially with an ACEi or an AIIT1RA, is recommended by most best practice guidelines as first line antihypertensive therapy.

Cardiac Disease

Coronary Artery Disease and Acute Coronary Syndromes

The role of direct renin inhibition in the prevention and treatment of atherosclerotic heart disease has not been evaluated in randomized controlled trials in humans, although there is evidence to that effect in animal models [71, 72].

The use of an ACEi (Captopril) within 3–16 days after an AMI in patients whose LVEF was $\leq 40\%$ and whose serum creatinine was <2.5 mg/dL reduced risk of future cardiovascular events [73].

The European Renal Best Practice (ERBP) clinical practice guidelines for managing patients with diabetic CKD and a GFR >45 mL/min/1.73 m^2 BSA provide the following recommendations for primary and secondary prevention and treatment of cardiovascular disease:

- A clinically indicated coronary angiogram should not be delayed for concerns over contrast-induced nephropathy.
- Medical therapy for stable CAD should be optimized and is the preferred choice of therapy unless there is significant myocardial ischemia, proximal left anterior descending (LAD), or left main coronary disease is present.
- In patients with multi-vessel CAD or complex lesions, coronary artery bypass graft is preferred over percutaneous coronary interventions for revasularization.
- Neither the presence of DM nor that of CKD should impact the therapy of acute coronary syndrome.
- Maximal dose ACEi, and not an AIIT1RA, is the treatment of choice for secondary prevention of cardiovascular disease in patients with HF or CAD; combination RAAS inhibition should be avoided.
- Goal BP is <140/90 mmHg and in the absence of microalbuminuria all antihypertensive agents are equal to lower BP [74].

In summary, ACEi are essential for secondary prevention and decrease mortality in patients with post-myocardial infarction left ventricular dysfunction.

Reduced Left Ventricular Systolic Function and or Heart Failure (HF)

Lower LVEF is an independent predictor of cardiovascular death and all-cause mortality in patients with heart failure (HF) [75].

In patients with HF due to decreased LVEF or valvular disease, there is a state of chronic renal hypoperfusion in the setting of an increased overall extracellular fluid volume; counter-regulatory adaptive mechanisms to restore perfusion result in neurohormonal activation of the RAAS, sympathetic nervous system and anti-diuretic hormone, the end result being more sodium and water retention and further volume expansion.

In patients with HF, kidney dysfunction portends a worse long-term prognosis with higher hospitalization rate [75] and a higher cardiovascular as well as all-cause mortality and the risk rises with the severity of the kidney disease [76, 77], with a 7% increase in mortality for every eGFR decrement of 10 mL/min/1.73 m^2 of body surface area [78]. The renal impairment is a more powerful predictor of mortality in patients with advanced HF than the LVEF or New York Heart Association (NYHA) class [79] and its validity as a prognosticator does not change whether the HF is due to systolic or diastolic dysfunction [80]. Similarly, renal impairment predicts a higher all-cause mortality and cardiovascular mortality as well as recurrent myocardial infarction in patients who had an AMI [73, 81] especially with an eGFR <45/1.73 m^2 of body surface area [73].

In adult patients with cardiorenal syndrome, defined by a left ventricular ejection fraction $\leq 45\%$ and NYHA class II–IV chronic heart failure and an estimated GFR 30–75 mL/min/1.73 m^2 of body surface area, the addition of Aliskiren therapy for 26 weeks, on top of standard therapy consisting of ACEi (or AIIT1RA) and β-blocker, did not change renal blood flow but significantly decreased GFR and filtration fraction when compared to placebo [82].

In patients with clinically diagnosed HF and angiographic evidence of coronary artery disease (CAD), ACEi reduced mortality at 12 months in patients with creatinine clearance ≥ 60 mL/min/1.73 m^2 of body surface area but not in those whose creatinine clearance was <60 mL/min/1.73 m^2 of body surface area [83]. However, other trials have shown a survival benefit with ACEi in patients with HF across all strata of creatinine clearance [80].

In summary, ACEi are essential for secondary cardiovascular prevention in patients with HF and/or reduced LVEF; they help optimize cardiac function, decrease mortality as well as hospitalization rate. Furthermore, evidence from the RALES trials supports adjunctive aldosterone receptor antagonist therapy with spironolactone to decrease mortality and morbidity in patients with severe HF and a LVEF <35% [84]; similarly, the EMPHASIS-HF Study Group reported that adjunctive eplerenone therapy decreased mortality and morbidity in patients with NYHA class II HF and LVEF <35% [85].

Sudden Cardiac Death

As mentioned earlier, sudden cardiac death accounts for 37% of mortality seen in patients with ESKD on HD.

A meta-analysis of seven RCTs (2867 patients) evaluated the benefits of primary prevention implantable cardioverter-defibrillator (ICD) in CKD and found that the survival benefit attributed to ICDs is GFR dependent and retained its statistical significance for a GFR ≥ 60 mL/min/1.73 m^2 but not lower [86].

Although RAAS inhibition plays an important role in reducing cardiovascular mortality, we are not aware of any trials that evaluate its direct role in the prevention of sudden cardiac death.

Coronary Angiogram and Contrast-Induced Nephropathy (CIN)

CIN is the end result of contrast-induced tubular toxicity, intense vasoconstriction and tubular as well as medullary ischemia, and oxidative stress [87].

ERBP clinical practice guidelines for managing patients with diabetic CKD and a GFR >45 mL/min/1.73 m^2 BSA recommend that a clinically indicated coronary angiogram should not be delayed for concerns over contrast-induced nephropathy.

Risk factors for CIN include pre-existing CKD, DM, effective arterial volume depletion especially in patients on diuretics, HF and reduced LVEF, hypotension, and age. Prevention of contrast nephropathy after a coronary angiogram is a constant cause for nephrology consultations. Thus, several prediction models have been devised and validated but none reported their impact on clinical decision making or patient outcomes [88]. Strategies to prevent contrast-induced nephropathy include isotonic fluid resuscitation to maintain optimal effective arterial volume and avoid volume depletion with sodium bicarbonate or normal saline, using iso-osmolal contrast agents, minimizing the volume of contrast used and avoiding repetitive administration over a short time-frame, oral *N*-acetylcysteine, and oral statin [89]. Furthermore, it may be advisable to stop RAAS inhibition 1–3 days before the administration of the contrast. A pilot study (CAPTAIN trial) in patients with moderate CKD (serum creatinine ≥ 1.7 mg/dL within 3 months or creatinine ≥ 1.5 mg/dL within 1 week prior to angiogram) demonstrated a nonsignificant reduction in CIN and a significantly lower rise in serum creatinine after the angiogram [90].

Cardiorenal Syndromes

The main challenge in types 1 and 2 cardiorenal syndromes is to achieve the optimal balance between successive diuresis and the maximal benefit of RAAS inhibition to avoid the fluctuation from one extreme and another, namely between acuter decompensated heart failure on the one hand and AKI due to excessive diuresis and effective arterial volume depletion on the other. Furthermore, worsening kidney function may predispose to hyperkalemia and deprive patients with symptomatic HF and reduced LVEF from the survival benefits associated with dual aldosterone receptor antagonist therapy and ACEi or AIIT1RA therapy.

A meta-analysis evaluated the impact of worsening kidney function (WRF) after initiation of RAAS inhibition in patients with HF and left ventricular systolic dysfunction, and included five clinical trials (SOLVD—Studies of Left Ventricular Dysfunction, SAVE Survival and Ventricular Enlargement Trial, RALES—the Randomized Aldactone Evaluation Study, Val-HeFT—Valsartan Heart Failure Trial, and EPHESUS—Eplerenone Post-Acute Myocardial Infarction Heart Failure Efficacy and Survival Study) and showed a survival benefit with RAAS inhibition irrespective of whether the patients experienced WRF (Relative Risk RR 0.72, $p < 0.001$) or not (RR 0.91, $p = 0.04$). More patients in the RAAS treatment group developed WRF and WRF was a predictor of increased mortality (RR 1.22, $p = 0.0003$) when compared to the RAAS treatment group with no WRF. However, when the mortality rates in the RAAS treatment group with WRF were compared to the placebo group with WRF, RAAS inhibition was associated with a reduction in mortality; the magnitude of this protective effect was greatest in patients in the treatment subgroup with WRF [81].

Combination Therapy Using Different Classes of RAAS Inhibitors

Dual Blockade

Direct Renin Inhibitor Plus ACEi or AIIT1RA

Dual RAAS blockade with a regimen including DRI has been evaluated with mixed results.

In adult patients with hypertension, type 2 diabetes mellitus, diabetic nephropathy with macroalbuminuria and a GFR $\geq$ 30 mL/min/1.73 m^2 of body surface area, the addition of Aliskiren to maximal dose Losartan had renoprotective effects independent of its blood pressure lowering effects, and was reflected by 20% reduction in the magnitude of albuminuria at 6-months of follow-up; there was also a statistically non-significant trend to a slower decline in GFR ($p = 0.07$) [25].

A meta-analysis of ten RCTs evaluated the safety of dual RAAS blockade with Aliskiren and an AIIT1RA or an ACEi versus monotherapy with any of the three agents for at least 4 weeks, demonstrated that dual therapy was associated with a significantly increased risk of hyperkalemia but not of AKI [91].

The ALTITUDE investigators (Cardiorenal end points in a trial of Aliskiren for type 2 diabetes) evaluated the impact of adjunctive Aliskiren therapy added to ACEi or AIIT1RA on cardiovascular and renal outcomes in patients with systemic arterial hypertension, DMT2 and with diabetic nephropathy (micro- or macroalbuminuria) or cardiovascular disease or both, GFR $\geq$ 30 < 60 mL/min/1.73 m^2 of body surface area, aged 35 years or older, and reported that addition of Aliskiren resulted in a (statistically non-significant) trend with an increase in adverse primary composite outcome of cardiorenal events, secondary composite outcome of cardiovascular and renal events, and all-cause mortality; more patients in the treatment group experienced an adverse event and subsequently discontinued the DRI ($p < 0.001$) with the most encountered complications being hyperkalemia, acute kidney injury, and hypotension. Dual therapy was associated with lower BP and urinary protein excretion rate [92].

ACEi Plus AIIT1RA

The ONTARGET investigators (Renal outcomes with telmisartan, ramipril, or both, in people at high vascular risk) showed a significant increase in the primary renal outcome (dialysis, doubling of serum creatinine, death) and secondary renal outcomes (dialysis, doubling of serum creatinine) and a significant decline in GFR (−6.11 mL/min, $p < 0.0001$) [93, 94].

In patients with HF or acute myocardial infarction and symptomatic left ventricular dysfunction, dual therapy with ACEi and AIIT1RA was associated with high rate of withdrawal due to a significant rise in the rates of AKI and symptomatic hypotension as well as an increase in hyperkalemia [95].

A meta-analysis of 33 RCTs evaluated the impact of long-term (>1 year) dual RAAS blockade versus monotherapy on all-cause as well as cardiovascular mortality, and concluded that there was no benefit of dual blockade over monotherapy for either endpoint. Dual therapy resulted in a significant decrease in HF hospitalization rate (18% reduction), but there was a significantly higher risk of hyperkalemia (55% increase), hypotension (66% increase), AKI (41%) and adverse events leading to withdrawal of therapy (27% increase). Subgroup analysis showed a significantly higher risk of AKI with dual therapy in patients with HF as compared to those without HF, and a higher all-cause mortality in patients without HF when compared to those with HF [96].

Similarly, the risk–benefit of dual versus single RAAS blockade in patients with albuminuria or stage 3–5 CKD was evaluated in a meta-analysis of 59 RCTs, and reported a statistically significant reduction in urinary albumin excretion rate with dual blockade, as well as a higher success rate at achievement of blood pressure goal; however, dual blockade was associated with a statistically significant reduction in GFR and a higher rate of hypotension and hyperkalemia and had no effect on mortality rates [97].

Aldosterone Receptor Antagonist Plus ACEi or AIIT1RA

The addition of spironolactone to an ACEi or an AIIT1RA, in patients with proteinuric stage 1–3 CKD, over a period of 2–20 months, reduced the degree of proteinuria and SBP but had no effect on cardiovascular outcomes or on the rate of progression to ESKD; it had a less well-defined effect on GFR but it increased the risk of hyperkalemia and gynecomastia. Individual trials report similar results with eplerenone; addition of eplerenone, too, increased risk of hyperkalemia but there was no risk of gynecomastia [39].

The addition of a DRI or an AIIT1RA or and aldosterone receptor antagonist to ACEi-based conventional therapy in patients with HF and its impact on mortality and cardiovascular event rate was evaluated in a meta-analyses of 16 RCTs (31,429 patients) over a period of 3 months. Only additional aldosterone receptor antagonists, and not DRI or an AIIT1RA, significantly reduced the risk of all-cause mortality, cardiovascular mortality, HF hospitalization but there was an increase in the rate of hyperkalemia. The addition of an AIIT1RA increased the rate of hyperkalemia, AKI and hypotension; additional DRI increased risk of hypotension [98].

Beyond Dual Blockade

The ASTRONAUT investigators evaluated the effect of adjunctive Aliskiren therapy versus placebo in patients hospitalized with HF (LVEF < 40%) and fluid overload when added to standard therapy on cardiovascular death and hospitalizations over a median follow-up period of 11.3 months and reported no benefit on either endpoint. With standard therapy, 84.2% patients were receiving ACEi or AIIT1RA and 57% were receiving mineralocorticoid receptor antagonist. Patients who received Aliskiren had a higher rate of hyperkalemia, hypotension and AKI [99].

In summary, while most trials report reduction in BP and urinary excretion rates, and in view of the increased risks of AKI, hyperkalemia, and hypotension associated with multilevel RAAS blockade, dual RAAS blockade should be preserved for clinical use where evidence rather than theory exists. Its major use is in patents with HF and reduced LVEF where aldosterone receptor antagonists offer a survival benefit [100].

RAAS Inhibition and Variability by Race

Systemic arterial hypertension is more prevalent and more severe in blacks than in whites; furthermore, it is associated with higher rates of morbidity and mortality from cardiovascular and cerebrovascular as well as ESKD. Blacks with primary hypertension, compared to whites, may have low renin and salt-sensitive hypertension and achieve the best blood pressure lowering with diuretics and CCBs [101]. These observations may have disfavored RAAS inhibition as a first line mono therapy in blacks with systemic arterial hypertension but no microalbuminuria or heart disease, but their use in combination with diuretics and CCBs exerts a synergistic effect and is highly recommended if BP goals are not met (<140/90 mmHg) [102, 103]. In the AASK investigators reported that ramipril therapy decreased the progression of CKD in patients with systemic arterial hypertension and non-diabetic proteinuric CKD [104]. RAAS inhibition remains first line therapy whenever a compelling indication arises such as, micro- or macroalbuminuria, HF or reduced LVEF.

RAAS and Genetics

The search for and identification of RAAS related single nucleotide polymorphisms (SNPs) that may alter the disease risk or responsiveness to RAAS inhibition has yielded inconsistent results. For example, analysis of insertion/deletion (I/D) SNPs of the ACE gene, which determines the concentrations of ACE, and by proxy of AngII and response to ACEi therapy, identified genotypes that have been associated with pathogenesis and progression of CKD, as well as cardiovascular disease. The DD genotype promotes a wide array of deleterious effects in the cardiovascular system in certain patients [105]. In contrast, the DD genotype has also been associated with a favorable response to AIIT1RA in patients with more advanced diabetic nephropathy. The II genotype has been associated with a milder course of diabetic nephropathy as well as non-diabetic proteinuric CKD and with the best effective response to ACEi therapy in the early stages of diabetic CKD [106].

In summary, the role of RAAS SNPs in identifying cardiovascular and renal risk and predicting therapy with best outcomes is still in a development phase and its clinical impact remains quite limited.

Adverse Events and Safety

Aliskiren (prescribed at doses of once daily 150 mg, 300 mg or 600 mg) has a safety profile similar to placebo and to Irbesartan 150 mg; the most frequent side effects reported were headache, dizziness, and diarrhea [107].

Cough is a common cause of withdrawal of ACEi therapy and is thought to be bradykinin mediated; therapy with ACEi, but not AIIT1RA, is associated with an increased risk of cough as high as 5–35% [43, 94, 108]. In a Cochrane meta-analysis, AIIT1RA were associated with a lower rate of withdrawal due to adverse events than ACEi after a mean followup of 4.1 years with 43% of the ACEi withdrawal being due to cough as opposed to a mere 4% with AIIT1RA [69].

ACEi therapy is the leading cause of drug-induced angioedema, also associated with high levels of bradykinin. While the angioedema usually occurs within days after initiating therapy, it may occur at any time during therapy. Therapy is based on discontinuation of the ACEi and use of a selective bradykinin beta-2 receptor antagonist [109, 110]. Patients who develop angioedema with ACEi have a 10% chance of developing angioedema with an AIIT1RA, this counseling the patient is essential when a compelling indication for use arises. DRI have similar rates of angioedema as ACEi.

The ONTARGET investigators reported a significantly higher risk of angioedema with ACEi when compared to an AIIT1RA (0.3 vs. 0.1%) as well as cough (4.2 vs. 1.1%) but less hypotension (1.7 vs. 2.6%) and no difference in the rate of syncope [94].

Spironolactone disturbs the balance of androgens and estrogens in favor of the latter with enhanced peripheral conversion of testosterone to estradiol, and at higher doses may result in male gynemomastia [111]. Eplerenone is less likely to cause gynecomastia.

All forms of RAAS inhibition are contraindicated in pregnancy.

RAAS Inhibition and Hyperkalemia

Increase in serum potassium on 0.4–0.5 meq/L are common with RAAS inhibition. This change in serum potassium can be more substantial in patients with CKD and/or CHF. The presence of hyperkalemia often limits the dose or even the use of RAAS inhibitors. As a consequence, patients with CKD and/or CHF may not derive the clinical benefits from their appropriate use. The only available chronic therapies for hyperkalemia were until recently loop diuretics and poorly tolerated sodium polystyrene sulfonate (kayexalate). Patiromer is a non-absorbed polymer which was designed to exchange potassium for calcium. This action predominately occurs in the distal colon where the free concentration of potassium is the highest [112, 113]. The net result is an increase in secretion and reduction of serum potassium levels of about meq/L [70]. It has been well studied in clinical trials up to 1 year in duration [114]. It is well tolerated and safe with only minor gastrointestinal side effects. It was recently approved by the FDA. The FDA has recommended separating patiromer and kayexalate dosing from other medicines by 6 h until more clinical testing is done to be sure there are no drug binding interactions. Another new medication in development for hyperkalemia is sodium zirconium cyclosilicate [115, 116], known as ZS-9. This is a highly selective inorganic cation exchange that entraps potassium in the intestinal tract in exchange for sodium and hydrogen. It has been demonstrated to be efficacious, with an approximate 1 meq/L reduction in serum potassium [115, 116]. Like patiromer, it is an insoluble compound which needs to be dissolved in a small amount of water before consumption. It is well tolerated with only minor gastrointestinal complaints, and some pedal edema if used in higher doses €. Thus, both patiromer and ZS-9 appear to be important new, well-tolerated, and predictable medication to consistently and safely reduce potassium levels. They will likely permit greater use and appropriate dosing of RAAS inhibitors.

Summary and Conclusions

RAAS inhibition has provided an important opportunity to slow the progression of cardiovascular and renal disease progression in patients with established disease. This benefit is consistent and reproducible. The future will focus on strategies to improve upon this benefit with novel therapies, and ensure greater opportunity for safety and efficacy through better control of hyperkalemia, and other potential adverse effects. We have come a long way in our understanding about this important catalytic pathway, and have much more to learn about how best to modulate its effects on the circulation and target organs.

References

1. Lakkis J, Lu WX, Weir MR. RAAS escape: a real clinical entity that may be important in the progression of cardiovascular and renal disease. Curr Hypertens Rep. 2003;5(5):408–17.
2. Rüster C, Wolf G. Renin–angiotensin–aldosterone system and progression of renal disease. J Am Soc Nephrol JASN. 2006;17 (11):2985–91.
3. Wright JW, Krebs LT, Stobb JW, Harding JW. The angiotensin IV system: functional implications. Front Neuroendocrinol. 1995;16(1):23–52.
4. Fox CS, Matsushita K, Woodward M, Bilo HJG, Chalmers J, Heerspink HJL, et al. Associations of kidney disease measures with mortality and end-stage renal disease in individuals with and

without diabetes: a meta-analysis. Lancet Lond Engl. 2012;380 (9854):1662–73.
5. Hallan SI, Matsushita K, Sang Y, Mahmoodi BK, Black C, Ishani A, et al. Age and association of kidney measures with mortality and end-stage renal disease. JAMA. 2012;308 (22):2349–60.
6. Heerspink HJL, Kröpelin TF, Hoekman J, de Zeeuw D. Reducing albuminuria as surrogate endpoint (REASSURE) consortium. Drug-induced reduction in albuminuria is associated with subsequent renoprotection: a meta-analysis. J Am Soc Nephrol JASN. 2015;26(8):2055–64.
7. Khan UA, Garg AX, Parikh CR, Coca SG. Prevention of chronic kidney disease and subsequent effect on mortality: a systematic review and meta-analysis. PLoS ONE. 2013;8(8):e71784.
8. Remuzzi G, Perico N, Macia M, Ruggenenti P. The role of renin–angiotensin–aldosterone system in the progression of chronic kidney disease. Kidney Int Suppl. 2005;99:S57–65.
9. Remuzzi G, Bertani T. Pathophysiology of progressive nephropathies. N Engl J Med. 1998;339(20):1448–56.
10. Remuzzi G, Ruggenenti P, Perico N. Chronic renal diseases: renoprotective benefits of renin–angiotensin system inhibition. Ann Intern Med. 2002;136(8):604–15.
11. Bakris GL, Weir MR. Angiotensin-converting enzyme inhibitor-associated elevations in serum creatinine: is this a cause for concern? Arch Intern Med. 2000;160(5):685–93.
12. Centers for Disease Control and Prevention (CDC). National Vital Statistics Report (NVSR). Deaths: final data for 2013. Atlanta, GA: US Department of Health and Human Services, Centers for Disease Control and Prevention; 2013.
13. Briasoulis A, Bakris GL. Chronic kidney disease as a coronary artery disease risk equivalent. Curr Cardiol Rep. 2013;15(3):340.
14. Favre GA, Esnault VLM, Van Obberghen E. Modulation of glucose metabolism by the renin–angiotensin–aldosterone system. Am J Physiol Endocrinol Metab. 2015;308(6):E435–49.
15. Becher UM, Endtmann C, Tiyerili V, Nickenig G, Werner N. Endothelial damage and regeneration: the role of the renin–angiotensin–aldosterone system. Curr Hypertens Rep. 2011;13 (1):86–92.
16. Shahin Y, Khan JA, Samuel N, Chetter I. Angiotensin converting enzyme inhibitors effect on endothelial dysfunction: a meta-analysis of randomised controlled trials. Atherosclerosis. 2011;216(1):7–16.
17. Gallagher PE, Arter AL, Deng G, Tallant EA. Angiotensin-(1–7): a peptide hormone with anti-cancer activity. Curr Med Chem. 2014;21(21):2417–23.
18. Trask AJ, Ferrario CM. Angiotensin-(1–7): pharmacology and new perspectives in cardiovascular treatments. Cardiovasc Drug Rev. 2007;25(2):162–74.
19. Batlle D, Wysocki J, Soler MJ, Ranganath K. Angiotensin-converting enzyme 2: enhancing the degradation of angiotensin II as a potential therapy for diabetic nephropathy. Kidney Int. 2012;81(6):520–8.
20. Luther JM, Brown NJ. The renin–angiotensin–aldosterone system and glucose homeostasis. Trends Pharmacol Sci. 2011;32 (12):734–9.
21. Scheen AJ. Prevention of type 2 diabetes mellitus through inhibition of the renin–angiotensin system. Drugs. 2004;64 (22):2537–65.
22. Grams ME, Rabb H. The distant organ effects of acute kidney injury. Kidney Int. 2012;81(10):942–8.
23. Ronco C, Haapio M, House AA, Anavekar N, Bellomo R. Cardiorenal syndrome. J Am Coll Cardiol. 2008;52(19):1527–39.
24. Spanos G, Kalaitzidis RG, Karasavvidou DP, Zikou X, Siamopoulos KC. Aliskiren in an alternate-day administration schedule in hypertensive albuminuric patients. Blood Press Monit. 2014;19(6):359–65.
25. Parving H-H, Persson F, Lewis JB, Lewis EJ, Hollenberg NK. AVOID Study Investigators. Aliskiren combined with losartan in type 2 diabetes and nephropathy. N Engl J Med. 2008;358 (23):2433–46.
26. James PA, Oparil S, Carter BL, Cushman WC, Dennison-Himmelfarb C, Handler J, et al. 2014 evidence-based guideline for the management of high blood pressure in adults: report from the panel members appointed to the Eighth Joint National Committee (JNC 8). JAMA. 2014;311(5):507–20.
27. Kidney Disease: Improving Global Outcomes (KDIGO) Blood Pressure Work Group: KDIGO clinical practice guideline for the management of blood pressure in chronic kidney disease. Kidney Int Suppl. 2012;Suppl 2:337–414.
28. Verbeke F, Lindley E, Van Bortel L, Vanholder R, London G, Cochat P, et al. A European Renal Best Practice (ERBP) position statement on the Kidney Disease: improving Global Outcomes (KDIGO) clinical practice guideline for the management of blood pressure in non-dialysis-dependent chronic kidney disease: an endorsement with some caveats for real-life application. Nephrol Dial Transplant Off Publ Eur Dial Transpl Assoc Eur Ren Assoc. 2014;29(3):490–6.
29. Lakkis JI, Weir MR. Treatment-resistant hypertension in the transplant recipient. Semin Nephrol. 2014;34(5):560–70.
30. Chen Y, Meng L, Shao H, Yu F. Aliskiren vs. other antihypertensive drugs in the treatment of hypertension: a meta-analysis. Hypertens Res Off J Jpn Soc Hypertens. 2013;36(3):252–61.
31. Abe M, Suzuki H, Okada K, Maruyama N, Inoshita A, Baba S, et al. Efficacy analysis of the renoprotective effects of aliskiren in hypertensive patients with chronic kidney disease. Heart Vessels. 2013;28(4):442–52.
32. National Kidney Foundation. KDOQI clinical practice guideline for diabetes and CKD: 2012 Update. Am J Kidney Dis Off J Natl Kidney Found. 2012;60(5):850–86.
33. Qaseem A, Hopkins RH, Sweet DE, Starkey M, Shekelle P. Clinical Guidelines Committee of the American College of Physicians. Screening, monitoring, and treatment of stage 1 to 3 chronic kidney disease: a clinical practice guideline from the American College of Physicians. Ann Intern Med. 2013;159 (12):835–47.
34. Taler SJ, Agarwal R, Bakris GL, Flynn JT, Nilsson PM, Rahman M, et al. KDOQI US commentary on the 2012 KDIGO clinical practice guideline for management of blood pressure in CKD. Am J Kidney Dis Off J Natl Kidney Found. 2013;62 (2):201–13.
35. Jafar TH, Stark PC, Schmid CH, Landa M, Maschio G, de Jong PE, et al. Progression of chronic kidney disease: the role of blood pressure control, proteinuria, and angiotensin-converting enzyme inhibition: a patient-level meta-analysis. Ann Intern Med. 2003;139(4):244–52.
36. Keane WF. Proteinuria: its clinical importance and role in progressive renal disease. Am J Kidney Dis Off J Natl Kidney Found. 2000;35(4 Suppl 1):S97–105.
37. Xie X, Liu Y, Perkovic V, Li X, Ninomiya T, Hou W, et al. Renin–angiotensin system inhibitors and kidney and cardiovascular outcomes in patients with CKD: a bayesian network meta-analysis of randomized clinical trials. Am J Kidney Dis Off J Natl Kidney Found. 2015.
38. Sharma P, Blackburn RC, Parke CL, McCullough K, Marks A, Black C. Angiotensin-converting enzyme inhibitors and angiotensin receptor blockers for adults with early (stage 1 to 3) non-diabetic chronic kidney disease. Cochrane Database Syst Rev. 2011;10:CD007751.

39. Bolignano D, Palmer SC, Navaneethan SD, Strippoli GFM. Aldosterone antagonists for preventing the progression of chronic kidney disease. Cochrane Database Syst Rev. 2014;4:CD007004.
40. Navaneethan SD, Nigwekar SU, Sehgal AR, Strippoli GFM. Aldosterone antagonists for preventing the progression of chronic kidney disease: a systematic review and meta-analysis. Clin J Am Soc Nephrol CJASN. 2009;4(3):542–51.
41. Ritz E, Orth SR. Nephropathy in patients with type 2 diabetes mellitus. N Engl J Med. 1999;341(15):1127–33.
42. Dinneen SF, Gerstein HC. The association of microalbuminuria and mortality in non-insulin-dependent diabetes mellitus. A systematic overview of the literature. Arch Intern Med. 1997;157 (13):1413–8.
43. Strippoli GFM, Bonifati C, Craig M, Navaneethan SD, Craig JC. Angiotensin converting enzyme inhibitors and angiotensin II receptor antagonists for preventing the progression of diabetic kidney disease. Cochrane Database Syst Rev. 2006;4:CD006257.
44. DREAM Trial Investigators, Bosch J, Yusuf S, Gerstein HC, Pogue J, Sheridan P, et al. Effect of ramipril on the incidence of diabetes. N Engl J Med. 2006;355(15):1551–62.
45. NAVIGATOR Study Group, McMurray JJ, Holman RR, Haffner SM, Bethel MA, Holzhauer B, et al. Effect of valsartan on the incidence of diabetes and cardiovascular events. N Engl J Med. 2010;362(16):1477–90.
46. Abuissa H, Jones PG, Marso SP, O'Keefe JH. Angiotensin-converting enzyme inhibitors or angiotensin receptor blockers for prevention of type 2 diabetes: a meta-analysis of randomized clinical trials. J Am Coll Cardiol. 2005;46(5):821–6.
47. Andraws R, Brown DL. Effect of inhibition of the renin–angiotensin system on development of type 2 diabetes mellitus (meta-analysis of randomized trials). Am J Cardiol. 2007;99 (7):1006–12.
48. Al-Mallah M, Khawaja O, Sinno M, Alzohaili O, Samra ABA. Do angiotensin converting enzyme inhibitors or angiotensin receptor blockers prevent diabetes mellitus? A meta-analysis. Cardiol J. 2010;17(5):448–56.
49. Tocci G, Paneni F, Palano F, Sciarretta S, Ferrucci A, Kurtz T, et al. Angiotensin-converting enzyme inhibitors, angiotensin II receptor blockers and diabetes: a meta-analysis of placebo-controlled clinical trials. Am J Hypertens. 2011;24(5):582–90.
50. Geng D, Jin D, Wu W, Xu Y, Wang J. Angiotensin receptor blockers for prevention of new-onset type 2 diabetes: a meta-analysis of 59,862 patients. Int J Cardiol. 2012;155 (2):236–42.
51. Geng D, Jin D, Wu W, Liang Y, Wang J. Angiotensin converting enzyme inhibitors for prevention of new-onset type 2 diabetes mellitus: a meta-analysis of 72,128 patients. Int J Cardiol. 2013;167(6):2605–10.
52. Yang Y, Wei R-B, Wang Z-C, Wang N, Gao Y-W, Li M-X, et al. A meta-analysis of the effects of angiotensin converting enzyme inhibitors and angiotensin II receptor blockers on insulin sensitivity in hypertensive patients without diabetes. Diabetes Res Clin Pract. 2015;107(3):415–23.
53. Bolignano D, Palmer SC, Ruospo M, Zoccali C, Craig JC, Strippoli GFM. Interventions for preventing the progression of autosomal dominant polycystic kidney disease. Cochrane Database Syst Rev. 2015;7:CD010294.
54. Yang L-Y, Ge X, Wang Y-L, Ma K-L, Liu H, Zhang X-L, et al. Angiotensin receptor blockers reduce left ventricular hypertrophy in dialysis patients: a meta-analysis. Am J Med Sci. 2013;345 (1):1–9.
55. Kanno Y, Kaneko K, Kaneko M, Kotaki S, Mimura T, Takane H, et al. Angiotensin receptor antagonist regresses left ventricular hypertrophy associated with diabetic nephropathy in dialysis patients. J Cardiovasc Pharmacol. 2004;43(3):380–6.
56. Agarwal R, Sinha AD, Pappas MK, Abraham TN, Tegegne GG. Hypertension in hemodialysis patients treated with atenolol or lisinopril: a randomized controlled trial. Nephrol Dial Transplant Off Publ Eur Dial Transpl Assoc Eur Ren Assoc. 2014;29 (3):672–81.
57. Yang C-W, Tzeng N-S, Yin Y-J, Li C-H, Chen H-A, Chiu S-H, et al. Angiotensin receptor blockers decrease the risk of major adverse cardiovascular events in patients with end-stage renal disease on maintenance dialysis: a nationwide matched-cohort study. PloS One. 2015;10(10):e0140633.
58. Zhang L, Zeng X, Fu P, Wu HM. Angiotensin-converting enzyme inhibitors and angiotensin receptor blockers for preserving residual kidney function in peritoneal dialysis patients. Cochrane Database Syst Rev. 2014;6:CD009120.
59. Akbari A, Knoll G, Ferguson D, McCormick B, Davis A, Biyani M. Angiotensin-converting enzyme inhibitors and angiotensin receptor blockers in peritoneal dialysis: systematic review and meta-analysis of randomized controlled trials. Perit Dial Int J Int Soc Perit Dial. 2009;29(5):554–61.
60. Gossmann J, Burkhardt R, Harder S, Lenz T, Sedlmeyer A, Klinkhardt U, et al. Angiotensin II infusion increases plasma erythropoietin levels via an angiotensin II type 1 receptor-dependent pathway. Kidney Int. 2001;60(1):83–6.
61. Freudenthaler SM, Schenck T, Lucht I, Gleiter CH. Fenoterol stimulates human erythropoietin production via activation of the renin angiotensin system. Br J Clin Pharmacol. 1999;48(4):631–4.
62. Freudenthaler S, Benöhr P, Grenz A, Selzer T, Schmidt T, Mörike K, et al. Do alterations of endogenous angiotensin II levels regulate erythropoietin production in humans? Br J Clin Pharmacol. 2003;56(4):378–87.
63. Matsumura M, Nomura H, Koni I, Mabuchi H. Angiotensin-converting enzyme inhibitors are associated with the need for increased recombinant human erythropoietin maintenance doses in hemodialysis patients. Risks of Cardiac Disease in Dialysis Patients Study Group. Nephron. 1997;77(2):164–8.
64. Navarro JF, Mora C, Rivero A. Effect of angiotensin-converting enzyme inhibitors on hematological parameters and recombinant human erythropoietin doses in peritoneal dialysis patients. Nephron. 1998;80(2):239.
65. Curtis JJ, Laskow DA, Jones PA, Julian BA, Gaston RS, Luke RG. Captopril-induced fall in glomerular filtration rate in cyclosporine-treated hypertensive patients. J Am Soc Nephrol JASN. 1993;3(9):1570–4.
66. Hiremath S, Fergusson D, Doucette S, Mulay AV, Knoll GA. Renin angiotensin system blockade in kidney transplantation: a systematic review of the evidence. Am J Transplant Off J Am Soc Transplant Am Soc Transpl Surg. 2007;7(10):2350–60.
67. Ibrahim HN, Jackson S, Connaire J, Matas A, Ney A, Najafian B, et al. Angiotensin II blockade in kidney transplant recipients. J Am Soc Nephrol JASN. 2013;24(2):320–7.
68. Vlahakos DV, Marathias KP, Agroyannis B, Madias NE. Post-transplant erythrocytosis. Kidney Int. 2003;63(4):1187–94.
69. Li ECK, Heran BS, Wright JM. Angiotensin converting enzyme (ACE) inhibitors versus angiotensin receptor blockers for primary hypertension. Cochrane Database Syst Rev. 2014;8:CD009096.
70. SPRINT Research Group, Wright JT, Williamson JD, Whelton PK, Snyder JK, Sink KM, et al. A randomized trial of intensive versus standard blood-pressure control. N Engl J Med. 2015;373(22):2103–16.
71. Lu H, Rateri DL, Feldman DL Jr, Chamigo RJ, Fukamizu A, Ishida J, et al. Renin inhibition reduces hypercholesterolemia-induced atherosclerosis in mice. J Clin Investig. 2008;118(3): 984–93.
72. Wu H, Cheng XW, Hu L, Hao C-N, Hayashi M, Takeshita K, et al. Renin inhibition reduces atherosclerotic plaque neovessel

formation and regresses advanced atherosclerotic plaques. Atherosclerosis. 2014;237(2):739–47.

73. Tokmakova MP, Skali H, Kenchaiah S, Braunwald E, Rouleau JL, Packer M, et al. Chronic kidney disease, cardiovascular risk, and response to angiotensin-converting enzyme inhibition after myocardial infarction: the Survival And Ventricular Enlargement (SAVE) study. Circulation. 2004;110(24): 3667–73.
74. Guideline Development Group. Clinical Practice Guideline on management of patients with diabetes and chronic kidney disease stage 3b or higher (eGFR <45 mL/min). Nephrol Dial Transplant Off Publ Eur Dial Transpl Assoc Eur Ren Assoc. 2015;30(Suppl 2):ii1–142.
75. Hillege HL, Nitsch D, Pfeffer MA, Swedberg K, McMurray JJV, Yusuf S, et al. Renal function as a predictor of outcome in a broad spectrum of patients with heart failure. Circulation. 2006;113(5):671–8.
76. Damman K, Navis G, Voors AA, Asselbergs FW, Smilde TDJ, Cleland JGF, et al. Worsening renal function and prognosis in heart failure: systematic review and meta-analysis. J Card Fail. 2007;13(8):599–608.
77. Shlipak MG, Smith GL, Rathore SS, Massie BM, Krumholz HM. Renal function, digoxin therapy, and heart failure outcomes: evidence from the digoxin intervention group trial. J Am Soc Nephrol JASN. 2004;15(8):2195–203.
78. Smith GL, Lichtman JH, Bracken MB, Shlipak MG, Phillips CO, DiCapua P, et al. Renal impairment and outcomes in heart failure: systematic review and meta-analysis. J Am Coll Cardiol. 2006;47 (10):1987–96.
79. Hillege HL, Girbes AR, de Kam PJ, Boomsma F, de Zeeuw D, Charlesworth A, et al. Renal function, neurohormonal activation, and survival in patients with chronic heart failure. Circulation. 2000;102(2):203–10.
80. McAlister FA, Ezekowitz J, Tonelli M, Armstrong PW. Renal insufficiency and heart failure: prognostic and therapeutic implications from a prospective cohort study. Circulation. 2004;109 (8):1004–9.
81. Clark H, Krum H, Hopper I. Worsening renal function during renin–angiotensin–aldosterone system inhibitor initiation and long-term outcomes in patients with left ventricular systolic dysfunction. Eur J Heart Fail. 2014;16(1):41–8.
82. Schroten NF, Damman K, Hemmelder MH, Voors AA, Navis G, Gaillard CAJM, et al. Effect of additive renin inhibition with Aliskiren on renal blood flow in patients with chronic heart failure and renal dysfunction (additive renin inhibition with Aliskiren on renal blood flow and neurohormonal activation in patients with chronic heart failure and renal dysfunction). Am Heart J. 2015;169(5):693–701.e3.
83. Ezekowitz J, McAlister FA, Humphries KH, Norris CM, Tonelli M, Ghali WA, et al. The association among renal insufficiency, pharmacotherapy, and outcomes in 6,427 patients with heart failure and coronary artery disease. J Am Coll Cardiol. 2004;44(8):1587–92.
84. Pitt B, Zannad F, Remme WJ, Cody R, Castaigne A, Perez A, et al. The effect of spironolactone on morbidity and mortality in patients with severe heart failure. Randomized Aldactone Evaluation Study Investigators. N Engl J Med. 1999;341(10):709–17.
85. Zannad F, McMurray JJV, Krum H, van Veldhuisen DJ, Swedberg K, Shi H, et al. Eplerenone in patients with systolic heart failure and mild symptoms. N Engl J Med. 2011;364(1):11–21.
86. Pun PH, Al-Khatib SM, Han JY, Edwards R, Bardy GH, Bigger JT, et al. Implantable cardioverter-defibrillators for primary prevention of sudden cardiac death in CKD: a meta-analysis of patient-level data from 3 randomized trials. Am J Kidney Dis Off J Natl Kidney Found. 2014;64(1):32–9.
87. Azzalini L, Spagnoli V, Ly HQ. Contrast-induced nephropathy: from pathophysiology to preventive strategies. Can J Cardiol. 2015.
88. Silver SA, Shah PM, Chertow GM, Harel S, Wald R, Harel Z. Risk prediction models for contrast induced nephropathy: systematic review. BMJ. 2015;351:h4395.
89. Zhang B, Liang L, Chen W, Liang C, Zhang S. The efficacy of sodium bicarbonate in preventing contrast-induced nephropathy in patients with pre-existing renal insufficiency: a meta-analysis. BMJ Open. 2015;5(3):e006989.
90. Bainey KR, Rahim S, Etherington K, Rokoss ML, Natarajan MK, Velianou JL, et al. Effects of withdrawing vs continuing renin–angiotensin blockers on incidence of acute kidney injury in patients with renal insufficiency undergoing cardiac catheterization: results from the angiotensin converting enzyme inhibitor/angiotensin receptor blocker and contrast induced nephropathy in patients receiving cardiac catheterization (CAPTAIN) trial. Am Heart J. 2015;170(1):110–6.
91. Harel Z, Gilbert C, Wald R, Bell C, Perl J, Juurlink D, et al. The effect of combination treatment with aliskiren and blockers of the renin–angiotensin system on hyperkalaemia and acute kidney injury: systematic review and meta-analysis. BMJ. 2012;344:e42.
92. Parving H-H, Brenner BM, McMurray JJV, de Zeeuw D, Haffner SM, Solomon SD, et al. Cardiorenal end points in a trial of aliskiren for type 2 diabetes. N Engl J Med. 2012;367 (23):2204–13.
93. Mann JFE, Schmieder RE, McQueen M, Dyal L, Schumacher H, Pogue J, et al. Renal outcomes with telmisartan, ramipril, or both, in people at high vascular risk (the ONTARGET study): a multicentre, randomised, double-blind, controlled trial. Lancet Lond Engl. 2008;372(9638):547–53.
94. ONTARGET Investigators, Yusuf S, Teo KK, Pogue J, Dyal L, Copland I, et al. Telmisartan, ramipril, or both in patients at high risk for vascular events. N Engl J Med. 2008;358(15):1547–59.
95. Phillips CO, Kashani A, Ko DK, Francis G, Krumholz HM. Adverse effects of combination angiotensin II receptor blockers plus angiotensin-converting enzyme inhibitors for left ventricular dysfunction: a quantitative review of data from randomized clinical trials. Arch Intern Med. 2007;167(18):1930–6.
96. Makani H, Bangalore S, Desouza KA, Shah A, Messerli FH. Efficacy and safety of dual blockade of the renin–angiotensin system: meta-analysis of randomised trials. BMJ. 2013;346:f360.
97. Susantitaphong P, Sewaralthahab K, Balk EM, Eiam-ong S, Madias NE, Jaber BL. Efficacy and safety of combined vs. single renin–angiotensin–aldosterone system blockade in chronic kidney disease: a meta-analysis. Am J Hypertens. 2013;26(3):424–41.
98. Bangalore S, Kumar S, Messerli FH. When conventional heart failure therapy is not enough: angiotensin receptor blocker, direct renin inhibitor, or aldosterone antagonist? Congest Heart Fail Greenwich Conn. 2013;19(3):107–15.
99. Gheorghiade M, Böhm M, Greene SJ, Fonarow GC, Lewis EF, Zannad F, et al. Effect of aliskiren on postdischarge mortality and heart failure readmissions among patients hospitalized for heart failure: the ASTRONAUT randomized trial. JAMA. 2013;309 (11):1125–35.
100. Arici M, Erdem Y. Dual blockade of the renin–angiotensin system for cardiorenal protection: an update. Am J Kidney Dis Off J Natl Kidney Found. 2009;53(2):332–45.
101. Brewster LM, van Montfrans GA, Kleijnen J. Systematic review: antihypertensive drug therapy in black patients. Ann Intern Med. 2004;141(8):614–27.

102. Jamerson KA. Rationale for angiotensin II receptor blockers in patients with low-renin hypertension. Am J Kidney Dis Off J Natl Kidney Found. 2000;36(3 Suppl 1):S24–30.
103. Flack JM, Mensah GA, Ferrario CM. Using angiotensin converting enzyme inhibitors in African-American hypertensives: a new approach to treating hypertension and preventing target-organ damage. Curr Med Res Opin. 2000;16(2):66–79.
104. Agodoa LY, Appel L, Bakris GL, Beck G, Bourgoignie J, Briggs JP, et al. Effect of ramipril vs amlodipine on renal outcomes in hypertensive nephrosclerosis: a randomized controlled trial. JAMA. 2001;285(21):2719–28.
105. Pinto YM, van Gilst WH, Kingma JH, Schunkert H. Deletion-type allele of the angiotensin-converting enzyme gene is associated with progressive ventricular dilation after anterior myocardial infarction. Captopril and Thrombolysis Study Investigators. J Am Coll Cardiol. 1995;25(7):1622–6.
106. Ruggenenti P, Bettinaglio P, Pinares F, Remuzzi G. Angiotensin converting enzyme insertion/deletion polymorphism and renoprotection in diabetic and nondiabetic nephropathies. Clin J Am Soc Nephrol CJASN. 2008;3(5):1511–25.
107. Gradman AH, Schmieder RE, Lins RL, Nussberger J, Chiang Y, Bedigian MP. Aliskiren, a novel orally effective renin inhibitor, provides dose-dependent antihypertensive efficacy and placebo-like tolerability in hypertensive patients. Circulation. 2005;111(8):1012–8.
108. Bezalel S, Mahlab-Guri K, Asher I, Werner B, Sthoeger ZM. Angiotensin-converting enzyme inhibitor-induced angioedema. Am J Med. 2015;128(2):120–5.
109. Bas M, Greve J, Strassen U, Khosravani F, Hoffmann TK, Kojda G. Angioedema induced by cardiovascular drugs: new players join old friends. Allergy. 2015;70(10):1196–200.
110. Craig TJ, Bernstein JA, Farkas H, Bouillet L, Boccon-Gibod I. Diagnosis and treatment of bradykinin-mediated angioedema: outcomes from an angioedema expert consensus meeting. Int Arch Allergy Immunol. 2014;165(2):119–27.
111. Rose LI, Underwood RH, Newmark SR, Kisch ES, Williams GH. Pathophysiology of spironolactone-induced gynecomastia. Ann Intern Med. 1977;87(4):398–403.
112. Buysse JM, Huang I-Z, Pitt B. PEARL-HF: prevention of hyperkalemia in patients with heart failure using a novel polymeric potassium binder, RLY5016. Future Cardiol. 2012;8(1):17–28.
113. Weir MR, Bakris GL, Bushinsky DA, Mayo MR, Garza D, Stasiv Y, et al. Patiromer in patients with kidney disease and hyperkalemia receiving RAAS inhibitors. N Engl J Med. 2015;372(3):211–21.
114. Bakris GL, Pitt B, Weir MR, Freeman MW, Mayo MR, Garza D, et al. Effect of patiromer on serum potassium level in patients with hyperkalemia and diabetic kidney disease: the AMETHYST-DN randomized clinical trial. JAMA. 2015;314(2):151–61.
115. Packham DK, Rasmussen HS, Lavin PT, El-Shahawy MA, Roger SD, Block G, et al. Sodium zirconium cyclosilicate in hyperkalemia. N Engl J Med. 2015;372(3):222–31.
116. Kosiborod M, Rasmussen HS, Lavin P, Qunibi WY, Spinowitz B, Packham D, et al. Effect of sodium zirconium cyclosilicate on potassium lowering for 28 days among outpatients with hyperkalemia: the HARMONIZE randomized clinical trial. JAMA. 2014;312(21):2223–33.

Vitamin D and Its Role in CKD and CAD: A Novel Therapeutic Target

9

Kenneth Lim, Thomas F Hiemstra, and Ravi Thadhani

Introduction

Vitamin D deficiency is potentially a significant global public health problem. It is estimated that over 1 billion people worldwide are vitamin D deficient. Vitamin D is indispensible for skeletal health, and its deficiency results in rickets in children and osteomalacia in adults. Effective treatment of rickets in children by sunlight was first described by Sniadeki in 1822, and later by diet through the use of cod liver oil by Trousseau in 1868. However, vitamin D was only isolated and its structure identified in the 1930s, after Askew and colleagues described vitamin D_2 (ergocalciferol).

Through a series of experiments, Nobel Laureaute Adolf Windaus identified the chemical structure of vitamin D produced in the skin as cholecalciferol (vitamin D_3) as well as its parent molecule, 7-dehydrocholesterol. It was at this time in the 1930s that the fortification of milk with 100 IU vitamin D_2 per 8 oz began, effectively eradicating rickets in the United States and Europe. However, this over fortification was thought to be the cause of an outbreak of hypercalcemia, leading to the forbidding of fortification of dairy products with vitamin D in Europe.

Over recent decades, it has become evident that vitamin D is not important only for calcium homeostasis and skeletal health. The vitamin D endocrine system is ubiquitously expressed, and vitamin D deficiency has been linked to a variety of health problems including cardiovascular disease, cancers, autoimmune diseases, and infectious diseases. The importance of vitamin D in health is reflected by the fortification of vitamin D in a variety of staple foods. Today, almost all the milk supply in the United States is fortified with 100 IU vitamin D/cup and in Canada, milk is fortified by law with 35–40 IU/100 ml. Both the United States and Canada mandate the fortification of infant formulas with vitamin D.

Production and Metabolism of Vitamin D

The major source of vitamin D in humans is exposure to sunlight, while most natural food sources contain little inactive vitamin D. Vitamin D_3 is the natural derivative of vitamin D formed by irradiation of 7-dehydrocholesterol in the skin, but can also be derived from dietary sources. Few naturally occurring foods contain vitamin D, including oily fish such as wild salmon, mackerel, herring, and oils from fish such as cod liver oil, egg yolk (raw), cheddar cheese and mushrooms. Vitamin D_2 is the artificial form of vitamin D derived from irradiation of ergosterol, a sterol found in cell membranes of fungi and protozoa, and is often used in food fortification and in high-potency pharmaceutical preparations. Nutritional deficit in addition to the safe sun lobby leading to reduced exposure to sunlight and the use of sunscreens, may paradoxically have led to the persisting vitamin D insufficiency globally, extending across the western civilization today.

7-dehydrocholesterol is converted by ultraviolet B radiation (295–310 nm wavelength) into cholecalciferol (vitamin D_3). Cholecalciferol is biologically inert and is hepatically 25-hydroxylated in a substrate-dependent manner to yield 25-hydroxyvitamin D (calcidiol). 25-hydroxyvitamin D is also largely biologically inactive, and its blood concentration has historically been used as a measure of vitamin D status. 25-hydroxyvitamin D is 1α [alpha]-hydroxylated by CYP2R1 (a cytochrome P450 enzyme) to the highly calcitropic active steroid hormone

K. Lim · R. Thadhani (✉)
Massachusetts General Hospital, Harvard Medical School, 55 Fruit Street, GRB-1008C, Boston, MA 02114, USA
e-mail: rthadhani@mgh.harvard.edu

K. Lim
e-mail: KJLIM@partners.org

T.F. Hiemstra
Cambridge Clinical Trials Unit, University of Cambridge, Box 401Addenbrooke's Hospital, Hills Road, CB2 0QQ Cambridge, UK
e-mail: tfh24@cam.ac.uk

J. Rangaswami et al. (eds.), *Cardio-Nephrology*,
DOI 10.1007/978-3-319-56042-7_9

1,25-dihydroxyvitamin D (calcitriol). 1α[alpha]-hydroxylase was initially identified in proximal tubular cells of the kidney, however, the enzyme is also found in other parts of the nephron including the distal tube and collecting duct. Renal 1α[alpha]-hydroxylase appears to account for the majority of circulating 1,25-dihydroxyvitamin D.

The false belief that 1,25-dihydroxyvitamin D synthesis occurs only in the kidneys has led to the widespread use of 1,25-dihydroxyvitamin D or analogs such as paricalcitol in patients with kidney disease, primarily for the treatment of secondary hyperparathyroidism [these 1α[alpha]-hydroxylated compounds are hereafter referred to as Vitamin D Receptor Activators (VDRAs)]. However, following the discovery of ubiquitous expression of the 1α[alpha]-hydroxylase in extrarenal tissue, it is now recognized that extrarenal synthesis of 1,25-dihydroxyvitamin D occurs outside the kidney and contributes to its circulating concentration. Further, similar to other steroid hormone receptors, the vitamin D receptor (VDR) is ubiquitously expressed. Therefore, autocrine and paracrine synthesis of 1,25-dihydroxyvitamin D occurs in target organs, and in health, the activation of the VDR in these tissues depends on VDR expression and adequate vitamin D concentrations.

Extrarenal production of 1,25-dihydroxyvitamin D was originally identified in studies investigating the pathogenesis of hypercalcemia in sarcoidosis. Cloning of the 1α[alpha]-hydroxylase gene revealed identical cDNA sequences in a variety of extrarenal tissues. 1α[alpha]-hydroxylase expression has been found in skin (basal keratinocytes, hair follicles), lymph nodes (granulomata), colon (epithelial cells and parasympathetic ganglia), brain (cerebellum and cerebral cortex), prostate, breast, testes, and placenta (decidual and trophoblastic cells), pancreas (islets), adrenal medulla, myocardium and in vasculature (endothelial and vascular smooth muscle cells). The extent to which extrarenal 1α[alpha]-hydroxylase activity contributes to circulating vitamin D levels is unclear. However, in reports of anephric individuals who had been given large doses of inactive vitamin D_3, these patients exhibited measurable blood levels of a metabolite(s) that displaced 1,25-dihydroxyvitamin D in receptor binding assays [1]. These findings suggest the existence of significant extrarenal 1α[alpha]-hydroxylase activity.

1,25-dihydroxyvitamin D is a steroid hormone, and exerts its actions through the vitamin D receptor (VDR), a member of the steroid hormone superfamily of nuclear receptors. The VDR has been found to regulate approximately 3% of human genes via its endocrine effects. Binding of calcitriol to VDR causes heterodimerization with retinoid X receptor (RXR) and allows the binding of the heterodimer to vitamin D response elements (VDREs). VDREs are located in the promoter regions of calcitriol responsive genes. Ligand binding triggers recruitment of transcription factors to the pre-initation complex to regulate the rate of gene transcription.

The enzyme 24-hydroxylase (CYP24A1) is responsible for the catabolic inactivation of 1,25-dihydroxyvitamin D and catabolizes both 25-hydroxyvitamin D and 1,25-dihydroxyvitamin D into inactive 24,25-hydroxyvitamin D.

Regulation of Vitamin D Synthesis

1,25-dihydroxyvitamin D is potently calcitropic, and its production is tightly regulated by parathyroid hormone (PTH), serum calcium, phosphorus and the bone-derived hormone, fibroblast growth factor (FGF)-23 (Fig. 9.1). Dietary calcium can regulate the 1α[alpha]-hydroxylase enzyme both directly through changes in serum calcium concentrations or indirectly by altering levels of PTH produced by the parathyroid gland. In vitro studies have shown that calcium can directly suppress 1α[alpha]-hydroxylase activity and mRNA production. Additionally, the stimulation of 1α[alpha]-hydroxylase by low calcium is significantly blunted by parathyroidectomy. In proximal tubular cells, PTH has been shown to directly stimulate 1α[alpha]-hydroxylase gene transcription via changes in cAMP [2].

Restriction of dietary phosphate also increases 1α[alpha]-hydroxylase activity and mRNA production, indirectly by changes in PTH and calcium. Interestingly, phosphate does not appear to directly regulate 1α[alpha]-hydroxylase activity in cell culture and its effects may be mediated by a systemic hormone. Phosphatonins including fibroblast growth factor (FGF-23), frizzled-related protein 4 (FRP-4) and matrix extracellular phosphoglycoprotein (MEPE) are involved in the regulation of phosphate homeostasis. Of these, both FGF-23 and MEPE play an important role in regulating 1α[alpha]-hydroxylase activity of which FGF-23 has been the most studied.

FGF-23 is a 30 kDa hormone produced by bone and functions as an important regulator of mineral balance. FGF-23 directly suppresses 1α[alpha]-hydroxylase activity at the kidney, leading to decreased synthesis of active 1,25-dihydroxyvitamin D (Fig. 9.2). FGF-23 function is dependent on an anti-aging protein called α[alpha]-Klotho, named after the Greek Goddess *Klotho,* who spins the thread of life. α[alpha]-Klotho has two known human isoforms, a full-length 130 kDa transmembrane form and a secreted soluble form that arises from alternative splicing. In proximal and distal tubular cells of the kidney, Klotho functions as a co-receptor with fibroblast growth factor receptor (FGFR)-1 for FGF-23. It was Yo-ichi Nabeshima and colleagues who in 1997 first identified Klotho expression predominantly at the kidney. α[alpha]-Klotho is widely expressed in extrarenal tissues in humans, including arterial, epithelial, endocrine, reproductive and neuronal tissues. This suggests that FGF23 may act on a variety of Klotho expressing extra renal tissues and potentially regulate extrarenal 1,25-dihydroxyvitamin D synthesis.

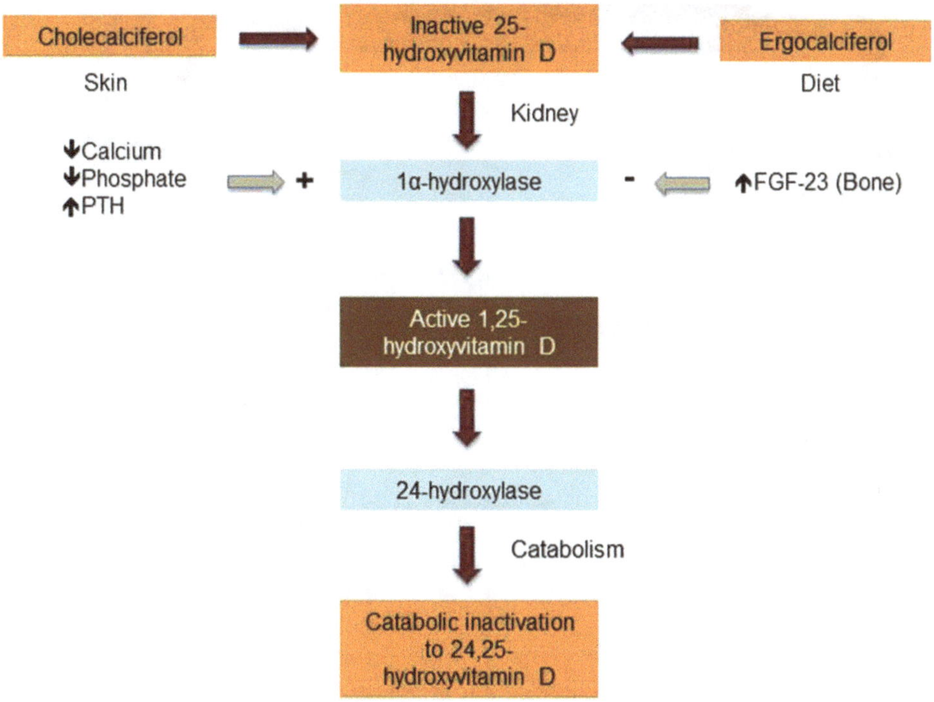

Fig. 9.1 Synthesis and regulation of Vitamin D Synthesis: Cholecalciferol (vitamin D3) is synthesized in the skin from 7-dehydrocholesterol via the action of ultraviolet B (UVB) light. Ergocalciferol (vitamin D2) is the form of vitamin D commonly found in food products. Both cholecalciferol and ergocalciferol are inactive forms that require activation by 1α[alpha]-hydroxylase. Activity of 1α[alpha]-hydroxylase at the kidney is stimulated by low calcium and phosphate levels, and high PTH while its activity is suppressed by FGF-23 produced from bone. Catabolic inactivation of 1,25-dihydroxyvitamin D into inactive 24,25-hydroxyvitamin D is mediated by 24-hydroxylase

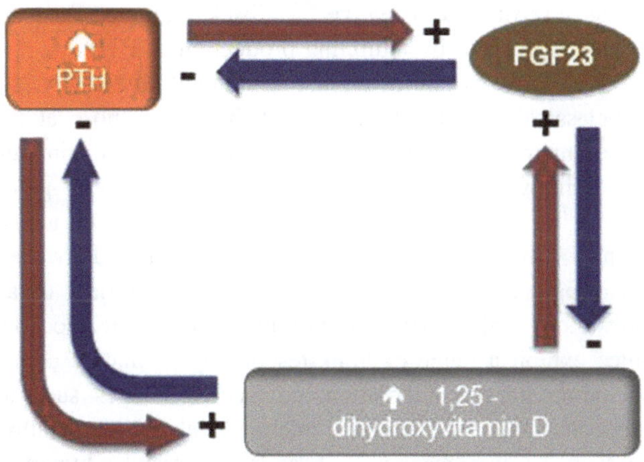

Fig. 9.2 Regulation of vitamin D synthesis: PTH functions to stimulate 1α[alpha]-hydroxylase activity at the kidney, increasing circulating 1,25-dihydroxyvitamin D levels. FGF-23, a phosphaturic hormone released from bone inhibits 1α[alpha]-hydroxylase activity and stimulates phosphate wasting at the kidney. As CKD progresses, FGF-23 levels increase thereby lowering circulating 1,25-dihydroxyvitamin D levels

Feedback regulation by 1,25-dihydroxyvitamin D limits the development of vitamin D intoxication. Experimental studies have shown that 1,25-dihydroxyvitamin D treatment suppresess 1α[alpha]-hydroxylase activity and mRNA production. However, this effect is not mediated through a direct effect of 1,25-dihydroxyvitamin D and its receptor on 1α[alpha]-hydroxylase, rather via the inhibition of PTH production. Furthermore, 24-hydroxylase activity (catabolic pathway) is increased by 1,25-dihydroxyvitamin D and is decreased by PTH.

Functions of Vitamin D

Vitamin D effects can be largely divided into *endocrine* or "classical" actions mediated by circulating vitamin D produced by the kidney, and *autocrine/paracrine* "nonclassical" functions by locally produced extrarenal vitamin D (Fig. 9.3). Endocrine functions of vitamin D mediate a complex interplay between the kidney, bone, parathyroid gland and intestine to regulate mineral metabolism.

Endocrine actions of 1,25-dihydroxyvitamin D play an important role in the regulation of calcium and phosphate homeostasis; the overall effect is to increase calcium and phosphate plasma concentrations. This is achieved by exerting effects on several organs: In the small intestine, 1,25-dihydroxyvitamin D stimulates calcium and phosphate

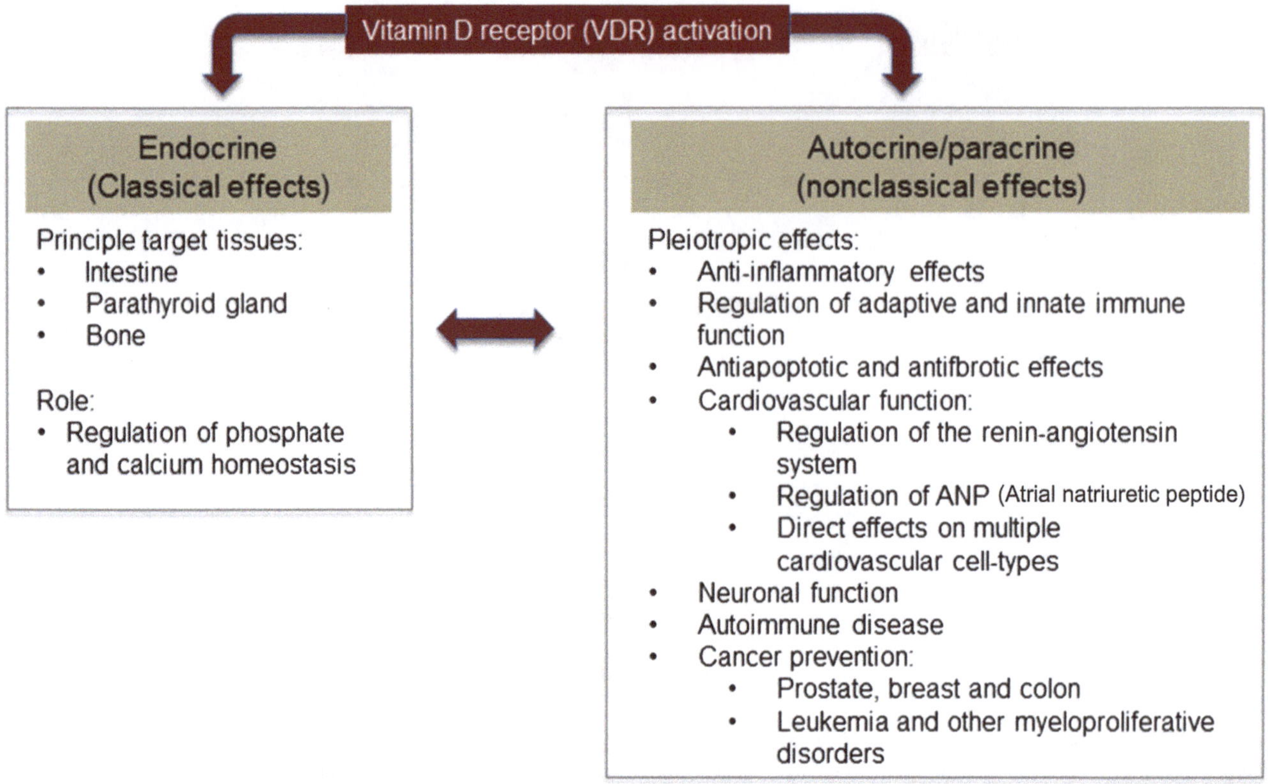

Fig. 9.3 Vitamin D Endocrine and Autocrine/Paracrine Hormonal Systems: The effects of vitamin D can be broadly divided into either endocrine (or "classical") effects that are mediated by circulating vitamin D, and autocrine/paracrine (or "nonclassical") effects mediated by locally produced extrarenal vitamin D

absorption. Active cellular calcium uptake is stimulated by 1,25-dihydroxyvitamin D by inducing expression of TRPV5 and TRPV6 calcium channels. 1,25-dihydroxyvitamin D also increases active phosphate transport by inducing expression of the NaPi-IIb co-transporter. There is evidence that changes in the composition of the enterocyte plasma membrane induced by vitamin D results in increased fluidity and phosphate uptake.

In concert with PTH, vitamin D stimulates bone resorption to release calcium and phosphate into extracellular fluid. 1,25-dihydroxyvitamin D interacts directly with the VDR in osteoblasts to increase the plasma membrane expression of RANKL (Receptor Activator for Nuclear Factor kB Ligand). RANK on preosteoblasts binds to RANKL on osteoblasts stimulating the conversion of preosteoclasts to osteoclasts. This results in the release of chemicals such as hydrochloric acid to metabolize calcium stores from the bone into the circulation.

While 1,25-dihydroxyvitamin D functions to reduce calcium and phosphate loss at the kidney, PTH exerts a phosphate wasting effect in renal tubular cells. PTH therefore primarily functions to raise plasma calcium levels. As mentioned earlier, 1,25-dihydroxyvitamin D functions to raise both calcium and phosphate plasma concentrations while exerting a negative feedback response at the parathyroid gland by inhibiting production of PTH.

Outside of its role in regulating mineral physiology, the nonclassical actions of vitamin D, including those at the bone marrow, immune system, muscle and skin are increasingly being recognized [3]. Given the widespread expression of 1α[alpha]-hydroxylase and the VDR across many organ systems, vitamin D has been found to exert pleiotropic effects in the regulation of both normal organ physiology and influence disease processes. VDR knockout mice exhibit a range of traits resembling premature aging, including growth retardation, cutaneous changes such as alopecia, abnormal blood mineral levels, hyperparathyroidism, cardiac changes such as left ventricular hypertrophy, and defective T cell and macrophage function. These multisystem changes highlight the pleiotropic effects of vitamin D as summarized in Fig. 9.3.

The beneficial effects of nonclassical functions of vitamin D replacement therapy may not be as easily measurable with outcomes such as changes in mineral levels and mortality. Observational studies indicate an increased risk of colon, breast and prostate cancer with reduced 25-hydroxyvitamin D levels, and randomized trial evidence suggests reduced risk of colon cancer with supplementation. A number of translational studies have shown benefits of vitamin D in regulation of immune and inflammatory pathways as discussed in further detail below. In addition, correcting mineral disturbances with agents that modulate the parathyroid gland axis, such as calcimimetics in the absence of vitamin D replacement therapy negate nonclassical benefits of vitamin D and could mask other consequences of vitamin D deficiency.

Vitamin D Deficiency in CKD

Vitamin D Deficiency is a Prevalent Condition in CKD

Vitamin D deficiency is a highly prevalent condition in CKD patients, with estimates as high as 70–80% in some studies. Despite the introduction of international and European guidelines to supplement vitamin D in the dialysis population, reports over the past decade consistently show vitamin D deficiency in this population. Both active 1,25-dihydroxyvitamin D and inactive 25-hydroxyvitamin D are deficient in the majority of patients with CKD. Vitamin D concentrations decrease early in CKD before PTH levels start to increase. Plasma 25-hydroxyvitamin D declines when the glomerular filtration rate (GFR) falls below 45 ml/min/1.73 m^2. Active 1,25-dihydroxyvitamin D levels decline to the lower limits of normal when patients reach the advanced stages of CKD stage 2, with evidently low levels by CKD stage 4.

Many clinicians define vitamin D deficiency as <20 ng/ml, vitamin D insufficiency as 20–29.9 ng/ml and $\geq$ 30 ng/ml as sufficient. In a 2011 report by the Institute of Medicine (IOM), recommendations for dietary allowances for healthy adults and children were made based on health outcomes suggesting the serum 25-hydroxyvitamin D threshold for health is >20 ng/ml. However, the UK Department of Health and Scientific Advisory Committee on Nutrition (SACN) define vitamin D deficiency as <25 nmol/l (10 ng/ml), consistent with the observation that lower levels were associated with rickets and osteomalacia. Additionally, controversy exists regarding the upper limit of normal and different cutoffs have been proposed ranging from 50 to 150 ng/ml. Although the thresholds for defining sufficiency have historically been based on skeletal, health, there is increasing recognition that nonskeletal disease outcomes should also be taken into account. For example, while levels >10 ng/ml are optimal to prevent rickets and osteomalacia, levels >30 ng/ml may be needed to prevent both secondary hyperparathyroidism and osteoporosis.

Various mechanisms have been implicated in the development of vitamin D deficiency in CKD, including loss of renal mass, hyperparathyroidism, hyperphosphatemia, metabolic acidosis, and accumulation of uremic toxins. Not surprisingly, low substrate levels of 25-hydroxyvitamin D are associated with low active 1,25-dihydroxyvitamin D levels, independent of stage of CKD progression. In fact, substrate availability is an important determinant of circulating 1,25-dihydroxyvitamin D levels. Studies have shown that as GFR declines, low substrate levels may limit the delivery of 25-hydroxyvitamin D to the 1α[alpha]-hydroxylase enzyme and therefore impede the generation of 1,25-dihydroxyvtiamin D at the kidney.

In the circulation, 99% of 25-hydroxyvitamin D is bound to Vitamin D Binding Protein (DBP). In the kidney, DBP and its cargo is filtered by the glomerulus, and is reabsorbed in the proximal tubule via megalin-mediated endocytosis. Megalin is a multi-ligand receptor that mediates the active process of vitamin D-DBP endocytosis. As CKD progresses, expression of megalin is reduced and this likely results in reduced reuptake of filtered 25-hydroxyvitamin D, and hence reduced substrate for active 1,25-dihydroxyvitamin D synthesis. 25-hydroxylase production in the liver may also be reduced in uremic environments and may contribute to decreased available 25-hydroxyvitamin D substrate. Additionally, development of proteinuria may be accompanied by high urinary losses of DBP resulting in increased losses of vitamin D metabolites; this is evidenced by the association between nephrotic range proteinuria with vitamin D deficiency. In addition to reduced substrate for 1,25-dihydroxyvitamin D synthesis, several findings indicate that the uremic environment results in reduced affinity of the 1α[alpha]-hydroxylase enzyme for 25-hidroxyvitamin D: Porcine hepatic 1α[alpha]-hydroxylase has reduced affinity for 25-hydroxyvitamin D in uremia, and in a study investigating 1,25-dihydroxyvitamin D deficiency in hemodialysis patients, impaired uptake of 25-hydroxyvitamin D and low affinity of the 1α[alpha]-hydroxylase enzyme to its substrate all determined the need for higher 25-hydroxyvitamin D levels to normalize serum 1,25-dihydroxyvitamin D levels [4]. Further, acidemic and hyperuricemic milieus also reduce 1α[alpha]-hydroxylase enzyme activity.

Over the past 10 years, emerging evidence has implicated FGF-23 as a significant contributing factor behind vitamin D deficiency in CKD. FGF-23 levels begin to rise in the early stages of CKD and directly suppress 1α[alpha]-hydroxylase activity leading to reduced 1,25-dihydroxyvitamin D synthesis at the kidney. FGF-23 also induces 24-hydroxylase which degrades both 1,25-dihydrovitamin D and 25-hidroxyvitamin D. As mentioned earlier, Klotho is widely expressed in extrarenal tissues with an expression profile resembling 1α[alpha]-hydroxylase. It is possible that FGF-23 may suppresses extrarenal vitamin D synthesis through a similar mechanism at the kidney, although this remains unknown.

In addition to increasing vitamin D deficiency with advancing CKD, progressive loss of VDR expression with declining GFR has been demonstrated, leading to vitamin D resistance. Furthermore, the use of therapies such as plasma exchange, a commonly used therapy for the treatment of diseases mediated by circulating pathogenic proteins and in renal transplant patients, induces an acute reversible decrease in 1,25-dihydroxyvitamin D, DBP, calcium, and a sustained decrease in 25-hydroxyvitamin D levels [5].

Targeting Proteinuria with Vitamin D

Proteinuria is a well-known risk factor for adverse cardiorenal outcomes in patients with CKD. Proteinuria is associated with GFR independently of baseline renal function in the general population. In patients with established CKD, the presence of proteinuria is associated with increased risk for the development of ESRD, independently of diabetes and hypertension. Additionally, proteinuria is strongly associated with both cardiovascular and non-cardiovascular mortality in the general population [6]. Conversely, reduction of proteinuria has been shown to have beneficial effects in both renal and cardiovascular end points. An increasing body of evidence indicates that VDRAs ameliorate proteinuria and partially restore nephrin and podocin expression in a rat model of nephrotic syndrome, downregulate renin expression and slow progression in a 5/6th nephrectomy model of CKD, as well as reduce renal fibrosis and scarring in animal models [7].

Several randomized clinical trials have evaluated the effects of active vitamin D therapy on albuminuria. In a small single-center study involving 61 patients, paricalcitol was shown to lower urine protein to creatinine ratios and lower PTH levels compared to placebo [8]. A smaller single-center study that recruited 24 patients showed lower high-sensitivity C-reactive protein concentrations and lower rates of 24-hour albumin excretion in the paricalcitol group compared to placebo [9]. The Vitamin D and Omega-3 (VITAL) trial, published in 2010, was a double-blind multicenter study that enrolled 281 type 2-diabetic patients who were receiving a renin–angiotensin–aldosterone (RAAS) inhibitor [10]. Patients were assigned to receive either 1-μ[mu]g or 2-μ[mu]g paricalcitol or placebo. The results showed a significant reduction in the urinary albumin/creatinine ratio in participants taking the 2-μ[mu]g dose compared with placebo. This was also associated with a reduction of estimated GFR (eGFR), as estimated from serum creatinine of 2 or 4 ml/min per 1.73 m^2, in patients taking 1-μ[mu]g or 2-μ[mu]g paricalcitol respectively twelve weeks after randomization. This latter finding reversed following discontinuation of the intervention, while others have shown that directly measured GFR does not change with paricalcitol therapy. Lastly, in a recent meta-analysis that included six studies representing 688 patients, active vitamin D analogs, which in most cases were given on top of RAAS blockade, resulted in an additional proteinuria reduction of 16% [11].

Regulation of Immunity by Vitamin D

A large body of evidence supports a role for vitamin D in immune modulation. Active vitamin D plays a role in regulating both the innate and adaptive immune system. VDR is expressed widely on many immune cells, including macrophages, T cells, B cells, and dendritic cells. Additionally, monocytes and macrophages carry their own inducible 1α [alpha]-hydroxylase suggesting both an endocrine and autocrine/paracrine vitamin D regulatory system within immune cells. The role of vitamin D in host defense was recently confirmed in a seminal paper by Liu et al., demonstrating that the production of the antimicrobial peptide cathelicidin in macrophages was vitamin D-dependent, and that vitamin D augmented antimicrobial killing in vitro [12]. Indeed, individuals who carry polymorphisms in the VDR gene, or in the gene encoding the vitamin D binding protein (DBP), have increased susceptibility to tuberculosis. Low levels of cathelicidin have been shown to predict increased infectious disease mortality in patients undergoing hemodialysis [13]. In a small study involving 60 patients, vitamin D supplementation was shown to increase cathelicidin levels in patients without kidney disease [14]. In another study involving 95 patients receiving antimicrobial therapy for pulmonary tuberculosis who were randomized to receive adjunctive high-dose vitamin D or placebo, vitamin D supplementation was found to accelerate sputum clearance and enhanced treatment-induced resolution of lymphopenia, monocytosis, hypercytokinemia, and hyperchemokinemia. In a small randomized, double-blinded placebo-controlled trial conducted in India, 247 participants with pulmonary tuberculosis were randomized to receive standard active tuberculosis treatment with either high-dose vitamin D3 or placebo. The study however, found that vitamin D supplementation did not reduce time to sputum culture conversion.

Viral respiratory tract infections have long been understood to follow a seasonal course, with peak incidences during the winter months and a nadir during the summer months. Many studies have suggested an association between vitamin D deficiency and the incidence and duration of viral respiratory tract infections. Vitamin D deficiency is also associated with the severity of community acquired pneumonia, bacterial infections in patients with chronic liver disease, opportunistic viral infections after renal transplantation, risk of Clostridium difficile infections, and orthopedic prosthetic infections. However, the recent Dialysis Infection and Vitamin D In New England (DIVINE) trial was a placebo-controlled, parallel-group multicenter trial that compared two doses of ergocalciferol with placebo. The study enrolled 105 participants who were randomly assigned to either ergocalciferol 50,000 IU weekly or monthly, or placebo for a 12-week treatment period. The study did not find any difference to changes in 25-hydroxyvitamin D levels, hospitalizations, or infectious events [15].

Vitamin D Therapy in Cardiovascular Disease

Cardiovascular disease is the leading cause of death in patients with CKD. Dialysis patients have a 10- to 30-fold higher cardiovascular mortality rate than the general population despite stratification for sex, gender, and race. The 5-year survival for patients on dialysis remains only 31%, and the mortality rate for patients on dialysis for longer than 5 years exceeds 250 per 1000 patient years. Cardiovascular causes are attributed to 40% of deaths in patients receiving dialysis.

The pattern of cardiovascular disease in CKD patients differs substantially from general patient populations, involving complex disease processes driven synergistically by both traditional and novel or CKD-related risk factors, such as uremia, mineral disorders and volume overload

Robust epidemiologic, clinical, and experimental evidence implicates vitamin D deficiency as an important proponent in the pathogenesis of cardiovascular disease. The Framingham Offspring Study that included 1739 Caucasian subjects showed that vitamin D deficiency was associated with incident cardiovascular disease. In participants who had a 25-hydroxyvitamin D level below 15 ng/ml, the study showed a multivariable-adjusted hazard ratio of 1.62 (95% CI 1.11–2.36) for incident Cardiovascular events (including myocardial infarction, coronary insufficiency, angina, stroke, transient ischemic attacks, peripheral claudication or heart failure) compared with participants whose 25-hydroxyvitamin D levels were ≥ 15 ng/ml. In fact, each 10 ng/ml increment in serum 25-hydroxyvitamin D has been shown to be associated with a 14% reduction in mortality (relative risk, 0.86; 95% CI 0.82–0.91).

Signaling components of the vitamin D hormonal system are widely expressed across the various cell types of the cardiovascular system, including myocardial cells, endothelial cells, vascular smooth muscle, fibroblasts, and pericytes. VDR knockout mice exhibit upregulation of the renin–angiotensin–aldosterone (RAAS) system, hypertension, left ventricular hypertrophy, and heart failure. Conversely, supplementation with vitamin D has been shown to abrogate these effects [16]. In vitro, 1,25-dihydroxyvitamin D directly suppresses renin expression, and regulates the proliferation of vascular smooth muscle cells (VSMC) and cardiac myocytes. In addition to decreasing vascular tone, activated vitamin D therapy has been shown to decrease cyclooxygenase-1 expression and production of reactive oxygen species radicals in spontaneously hypertensive rats [17].

Vitamin D and Arterial Calcification

CKD patients exhibit development of progressive vascular calcification, a major contributor to arterial hardening, cardiac strain, and sudden cardiac death. Observational human studies have demonstrated that serum calcitriol levels are inversely correlated with coronary artery calcification in the general population. However, both basic and clinical studies have demonstrated conflicting results as to whether vitamin D is protective or harmful against vascular calcification. In rodents, administration of pharmacological doses of calcitriol or doxercalciferol resulted in increased aortic calcification, while paricalcitol had no effect. Interestingly, calciphylaxis, a severe form of vascular calcification associated with significant morbidity, was found to be more prevalent in patients treated with calcitriol, but not with selective vitamin D analogs including paricalcitol and doxercalciferol. These results suggest that various analogs of vitamin D may exert different properties on the arterial wall.

In another study that conducted dose-dependent experiments in rodents, both active vitamin D analogs calcitriol and paricalcitol were found to be protective against vascular calcification at dosages sufficient to correct secondary hyperparathyroidism [18]. However, higher dosages of both these analogs were however found to induce aortic calcification. These results point to a dose–response relationship with a vasculoprotective role of vitamin D at a currently undefined therapeutic dose, while higher dosages can be vasculotoxic.

Active vitamin D has been shown to directly stimulate the expression of endogenous calcification inhibitors, including Klotho [19] and osteopontin in the vascular wall. Additionally, there is evidence that vitamin D can render arteries susceptible to anti-calcific effects of FGF-23 by reversing arterial Klotho deficiency [19]. However, these beneficial local molecular effects in the vessel wall are likely to at least partly offset pro-calcific systemic increases in calcium and phosphate concentrations.

Vitamin D and Hypertension

Since the 1980s, a large number of observational studies have shown an association between low 25-hydroxyvitamin D levels and hypertension. One systematic review that included 14 cross-sectional and 4 prospective studies representing 78,028 participants reported an inverse relationship between 25-hydroxyvitamin D levels and hypertension. In a large mendelian randomisation study ($n = 49{,}363$), a genetically determined increment of 10 nmol/l in circulating

25-hydroxyvitamin D was associated with a small but statistically significant reduction in systolic BP of 0.37 mmHg [20]. Randomized clinical trials so far have shown discrepant results, but adequately powered trials utilizing meaningful doses of vitamin D are lacking.

Several small interventional studies have specifically assessed the effects of vitamin D on blood pressure, while a number of larger studies have looked at other primary outcomes, but have reported results on blood pressure. In a small clinical trial that included 18 patients, ultraviolet B (UVB) light therapy in untreated hypertensive patients increased 25-hydroxyvitamin D level by 162% and significantly decreased SBP (−6 mmHg, 95% CI −14 to −1 mmHg) and DBP (−6 mmHg, 95% CI −12 to −2) compared to ultraviolet A (UVA) therapy with SBP (0 mmHg, 95% CI −1 to −10 mmHg) and DBP (2 mmHg, 95% CI −1 to −3). In the VITAL trial previously discussed above, the study showed a dose-dependent decrease in SBP in the paricalcitol arm compared to placebo as a secondary outcome [10]. In this study, almost 100% of participants had hypertension at baseline.

Conversely, in the Women's Health Initiative trial, 36,282 post-menopausal women were randomly assigned to received 100 mg of calcium and 400 IU of cholecalciferol daily or placebo with a median follow-up of 7 years [21]. The study showed no significant SBP change (0.22 mmHg, 95% CI −0.05 to 0.49) or DBP change (0.11 mmHg, 95% CI −0.04 to 0.27) after 7 years of therapy with a low dose of vitamin D. These results did not change after adjusting for nonadherence. The study however was confounded by several factors: firstly, the low dose of 400 IU provided of which 75% of patients had a 25-hydroxyvitamin D level below 25 ng/ml at baseline; more than half of the patients in the placebo arm took similar over-the-counter vitamin D doses; and only women were included in this study given observational data of a stronger association between 25-hydroxyvitamin D level and blood pressure in men. In the Paricalcitol Capsule Benefits in Renal Failure-Induced Cardiac Morbidity (PRIMO) trial (discussed below), the study randomized 227 patients to 2μ[mu]g of paricalcitol daily or matching placebo and did not show any difference in blood pressure between the two groups [22].

Vitamin D Therapy for the Treatment of Heart Failure

A strong association exists between vitamin D deficiency and pathogenic processes underlying the development of cardiac failure, including impaired coronary flow, endothelial dysfunction and subclinical atherosclerosis in patients with normal, or near-normal coronary arteries. Vitamin D deficiency is associated with overt coronary heart disease and myocardial infarction, and is a negative prognostic marker for major post-infarction adverse events including, heart failure hospitalizations, recurrent acute myocardial infarction and death. Observational studies have shown a relationship between low vitamin D levels and impaired left ventricular function in a cross-sectional study of patients referred for coronary angiography.

The PRIMO trial revealed significant insights into the effects of VDRA administration on cardiac structure and function [22]. The PRIMO study was a multinational double-blinded placebo-controlled trial that included 227 patients designed to examine the effects of paricalcitol on left ventricular mass index (LVMI) over a period of 48 weeks in stage 3 and 4 CKD patients with mild-to-moderate left ventricular hypertrophy (LVH) at baseline. Cardiac magnetic resonance (CMR) imaging was used to determine changes in LVMI while echocardiography was used to determine left ventricular diastolic function. The study showed that paricalcitol did not alter LVMI, prespecified measures of diastolic function, or SBP compared to placebo. However, an attenuated B-type natriuretic peptide (BNP) and a lower number of cardiovascular hospitalizations in the paricalcitol group was found. In a post hoc analysis of data from the PRIMO study, paricalcitol treatment in all subgroups was found to reduce left atrial volume index, a marker for diastolic dysfunction that is associated with significant cardiovascular risk [23].

Animal studies support beneficial cardiovascular effects of paricalcitol, despite CKD status. Although the failure of PRIMO to demonstrate a significant effect of paricalcitol on LVMI may be due to the absence of an effect in humans, there are several other possible explanations. First, LVH may have been too advanced, blood pressure too well controlled, or treatment duration too short to detect a difference. Another possibility is that the beneficial effects of paricalcitol are overridden by elevated FGF-23 concentrations in CKD, since studies in both animals and humans have shown that FGF-23 can induce LVH.

Clinical trials to-date assessing the role of vitamin D have mainly focused on morphological endpoints such as LVH, and such single surrogate markers may be poorly reflective of cardiovascular performance. In the recent Paricalcitol and Endothelial Function in Chronic Kidney Disease (PENNY) study, the investigators examined vascular endothelial function as measured in the brachial artery by nitric oxide (NO)-dependent flow-mediated dilation (FMD) response to increased shear stress by forearm ischemia, a recognized surrogate endpoint that predicts incident risk for cardiovascular events in patients with CKD. In this double-blinded randomized controlled trial including 88 patients with stage 3 and 4 CKD randomized to receive paricalcitol 2μ[mu] g/day or placebo, flow-mediated dilation increased in the paricalcitol group (mean proportional change of 61%) but not in the placebo group after 12 weeks. These effects were abolished 2 weeks after stopping the treatment.

Emerging evidence suggest that impaired functional cardiovascular reserve as assessed by cardiopulmonary exercise testing (CPET) is a robust, reproducible and sensitive measure of cardiovascular performance. CPET provides a significantly more robust marker for assessment of cardiovascular function compared to conventional static imaging by echocardiography or CMR, which focuses mainly on morphological alterations such as LVH as mentioned above. In a study that recruited 200 healthy adults subjected to CPET, serum vitamin D levels were found to predict maximal aerobic exercise capacity (VO_2Max) which is a CPET index of cardiac functional reserve.

Taken together, the above findings support the need for further clinical trials that will test the effects of vitamin D and its analogs on cardiovascular health across different stages of CKD.

Vitamin D Therapy in the Prevention of Arrhythmia

Large observational studies have shown that the incidence of atrial fibrillation (AF) is higher in the winter than in the summer correlating with seasonal variations in 25-hydroxyvitamin D levels. Patients with nonvalvular AF have been found to have significantly lower 25-hydroxyvitamin D levels. In fact, patients with 25-hydroxyvitamin D levels <50 ng/ml have a twofold higher incidence of nonvalvular AF compared with patients with levels >75 ng/ml. One observational study showed that vitamin D deficiency is associated with new onset AF in hypertensive patients [24]. However, these observational studies do not imply causality. On the contrary, no association between 25-hydroxyvitamin D levels and AF of any type were found in the Framingham Heart Study.

Interestingly, vitamin D treatment of hemodialysis patients was associated with a reduction of QTc dispersion, which is a risk factor for sudden cardiac death (SCD). In a large cross-sectional study that included 3299 Caucasian patients who were routinely referred to coronary angiography, investigators found that low 25-hydroxyvitamin D and 1,25-dihydroxyvitamin D levels were associated with sudden cardiac death. Vitamin D deficiency is also associated with sudden cardiac death in hemodialysis patients [25]. Interventional trials are needed to determine the utility of vitamin D therapy for the management and prevention of arrhythmia.

Vitamin D Replacement and Vitamin D Receptor Activator (VDRAs) Therapy

Vitamin D compounds have been commercially available for many years and include calcitriol (1,25-dihydroxyvitamin D_3), its prodrug alfacalcidol (1α[alpha]-hydroxyvitamin D_3) and calcidiol (25-hydroxyvitamin D_3). The group of newer vitamin D analogs already in use remains quite small, including paricalcitol, 22-oxacalcitriol or maxacalcitriol and doxercalciferol (Fig. 9.4). Paricalcitol and 22-oxacalcitriol are active vitamin D analogs that bind directly to the VDR.

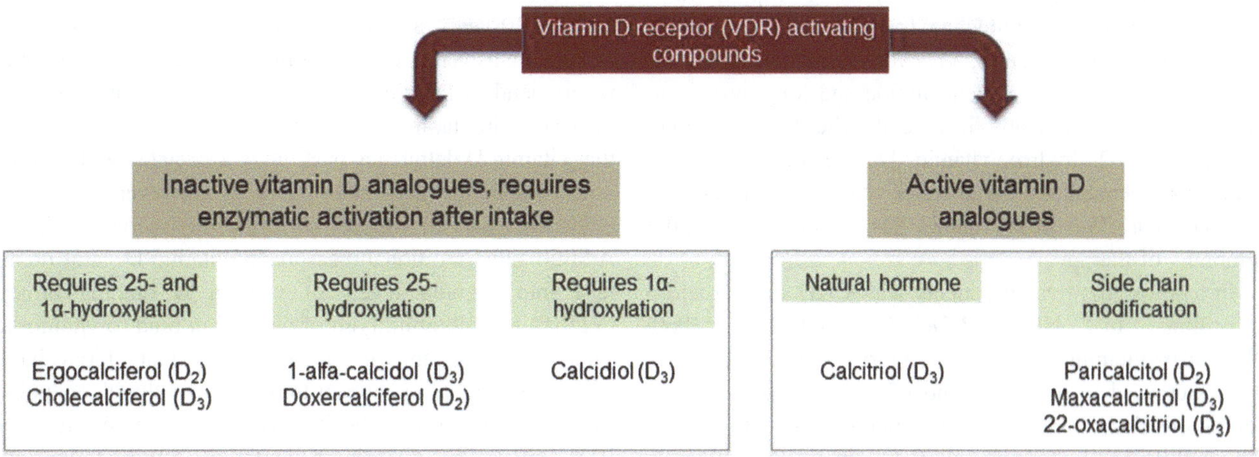

Fig. 9.4 Active and inactive formulations in clinical use: Pharmacological treatment with VDR-activating compounds can be broadly divided into two main groups: inactive vitamin D analogs that are prodrugs requiring hydroxylation after intake and already active vitamin D analogs

Doxercalciferol is analogous to alfacalcidol, a prodrug for 1,25-hydroxyvitamin D that requires enzymatic activation by 25-hydroxyation in the liver.

The National Kidney Foundation (NKF) Kidney Disease Outcomes and Quality Initiative (KDOQI) guidelines published in 2003 facilitated the development of clinical practice guidelines for the management of complications associated with kidney disease for stages earlier than ESRD. In this publication, guideline 7 described the prevention and treatment of vitamin D insufficiency and deficiency in patients with CKD. The guidelines suggested measurement of 25-hydroxyvitamin D levels in patients with CKD stages 3–4 in the setting of secondary hyperparathyroidism in order to identify patients who would benefit from supplementation. These guidelines were opinion based, given the absence of clinical trial data to support inactive vitamin D supplementation.

More recently, the Kidney Disease: Improving Global Outcomes (KDIGO) guidelines published in 2009 also provided opinion-based recommendations for the management of vitamin D supplementation in CKD patients, those receiving dialysis and in kidney transplant recipients. The KDIGO guidelines recommends monitoring serum levels of calcium, phosphorus, PTH, and bone-specific alkaline phosphatase activity beginning in CKD stage 3, similar to the NKF KDOQI guidelines. However, the KDIGO guidelines recommend commencing treatment with calcitriol or vitamin D analogs in patients with CKD stages 3–5 not on dialysis, in whom serum PTH is progressively rising and remains persistently above the upper limit of normal despite correction of modifiable factors (hyperphosphatemia, hypocalcemia and vitamin D deficiency). The KDIGO guidelines did not provide any specific 25-hydroxyvitamin D level for initiating vitamin D supplementation, but discussed the lack of consensus for the definition of 25-hydroxyvitamin D adequacy.

The European Renal Best Practice Group (ERBG) endorsed the KDIGO guideline for 25-hydroxyvitamin D testing and supplementation, however, stated that targets for 25-hydroxyvitamin D supplementation and long-term treatment would be clinically beneficial. The ERBG recommended that 25-hydroxyvitamin D <12.5 ng/ml should indicate supplementation with either vitamin D_2 and vitamin D_3 and that 25-hydroxyvitamin D be remeasured after 6 months of therapy.

In a study that treated patients with CKD stage 3 and 4 according to NKF KDOQI guidelines, both 25-hydroxyvitamin D and 1,25-hydroxyvitamin D levels were increased to the lower end of normal and PTH concentrations decreased by 20% in patients with CKD stage 3. Although PTH levels decreased, they remained significantly elevated above normal limits [26].

Studies using calcitriol in patients with CKD stage 3 and 4 demonstrated a significant decrease in PTH levels. The effectiveness of calcitriol was limited by the development of hypercalcemia and hypercalciuria. Alfacalcidiol and doxercalciferol, vitamin D prohormones also decrease PTH levels in CKD stage 3 and 4 with some degree of hypercalcemia and hypercalciuria. Paricalcitol is a VDR-specific agonist that significantly decreases PTH levels in CKD with minimal effects on serum calcium and phosphate levels, and does not increase urinary calcium. Of note, in a recent randomized crossover trial in hemodialysis patients, no difference between alfacaldiol or paricalcitol was found in the development of hypercalcemia or hyperphosphatemia [27]. Interestingly, there is convincing evidence that vitamin D therapy of any type is correlated with lower mortality in CKD patients [28].

A number of studies have provided evidence that vitamin D2 is several fold less effective than vitamin D3 in raising and/or maintaining 25-hydroxyvitamin D levels while other studies have shown no difference. In a recent meta-analysis that included 10 randomized controlled trials, the results showed that vitamin D3 was more efficacious at raising 25-hydroxyvitamin D concentrations compared to vitamin D2 [29].

Future Directions

Many controversial issues surrounding active vitamin D therapy in CKD and CAD are apparent and subject to debate within the Nephrology, Cardiology, and Vascular communities. Observational studies involving vitamin D therapy in CKD are currently limited through confounding by indication and selection bias. In addition, our current knowledge from clinical trials with vitamin D in CKD is limited by the absence of placebo-controlled mortality trials.

A wealth of information on vitamin D has emerged over the past 20 years, although a number of important questions remain unanswered. Contemporary treatment guidelines now recommend measuring and supplementing vitamin D to achieve a circulating concentration of 75 ng/ml, on the basis that vitamin D deficiency is strongly associated with adverse outcomes in the general population. However, no current evidence exists to support or refute this recommendation. Additionally, traditional measures of vitamin D status do not take into account levels of vitamin D binding protein (VDBP) and albumin, both of which can bind to vitamin D. This is important given evidence that bioavailable 25-hydroxyvitamin D appear to be associated with endpoints such as bone density in healthy individuals, and calcium and PTH levels in dialysis patients as opposed to total 25-hydroxyvitami D levels. With the emerging role of

Table 9.1 Ongoing clinical trials

Trial name	Country	Population	Dose	Main outcomes	Results expected
DOHealth (Vitamin D3—Omega3—Home Exercise—Healthy Aging and Longevity Trial)	Europe	2150 adults aged >70 years	2000 IU D2 or placebo	Bone fractures, infection, blood pressure, cognition and lower extremity function	2017
VIDA (Vitamin D Add-on Therapy Enhances Corticosteroid Responsiveness in Asthma)	New Zealand	18,000 adults aged >50 years	200,000 D3 once (and every June) and 100,000 D3 monthly or placebo	Cardiovascular disease, respiratory disease in COPD, bone fractures	2017
FIND (Finnish Vitamin D Trial)	Finland	18,000 adults, men >60 years and women >65 years	3200 D3 daily, 1600 D3 daily or placebo	Cardiovascular disease, cancer and diabetes mellitus	2019
VIDAL (Vitamin D and Longevity trial)	United Kingdom	20,000 adults, 65–85 years old	100,000 IU D3 monthly, placebo or open control	Mortality, morbidity (infections, doctor's visits, cancer) and vitamin D levels	2020
SIMPLIFIED (Survival Improvement with Cholecalciferol in Patients on Dialysis)	United Kingdom	4200 adults, aged >18 years	Cholecalciferol 60,000 IU fortnightly	Mortality, health-related quality of life, hospital admission, cardiovascular events, cancer incidence	2023

nonclassical effects of vitamin D, involving novel actions of vitamin D metabolites on cardiomyocytes and vascular cells, immune modulation and cytoprotection

Several clinical trials are currently ongoing and summarized in Table 9.1. These trials are critical given the biological significance of vitamin D and the many unanswered questions that remain. We will also need these clinical trials to accurately define the precise therapeutic agent, timing, dosage, and indications of vitamin D therapy. Given the important nonclassical actions of vitamin D, it appears that simple supplementation with native vitamin D in the interim is justified.

Acknowledgements Ravi Thadhani consults for Fresenius Medical Care North America and is funded by NIH Grants NIH K24 DK094872 and NIDDK R01 DK094486. T.F.H. is funded by the National Institute for Health Research (NIHR) award to the Cambridge Biomedical Research Centre and by NIHR Grant 14/49/147. K.L received an Early Clinical Investigator (ECI) grant from the Medical Research Foundation of Oregon.

References

1. Jongen MJ, van der Vijgh WJ, Lips P, Netelenbos JC. Measurement of vitamin D metabolites in anephric subjects. Nephron. 1984;36(4):230–4.
2. Brenza HL, Kimmel-Jehan C, Jehan F, Shinki T, Wakino S, Anazawa H, et al. Parathyroid hormone activation of the 25-hydroxyvitamin D3–1alpha-hydroxylase gene promoter. Proc Natl Acad Sci USA. 1998;95(4):1387–91.
3. Holick MF. Vitamin D deficiency. N Engl J Med. 2007;357 (3):266–81.
4. Gallieni M, Kamimura S, Ahmed A, Bravo E, Delmez J, Slatopolsky E, et al. Kinetics of monocyte 1 alpha-hydroxylase in renal failure. Am J Physiol. 1995;268(4 Pt 2):F746–53.
5. Hiemstra TF, Casian A, Boraks P, Jayne DR, Schoenmakers I. Plasma exchange induces vitamin D deficiency. QJM. 2014;107 (2):123–30.
6. Hillege HL, Fidler V, Diercks GF, van Gilst WH, de Zeeuw D, van Veldhuisen DJ, et al. Urinary albumin excretion predicts cardiovascular and noncardiovascular mortality in general population. Circulation. 2002;106(14):1777–82.
7. Hiemstra TF. Vitamin D in renal disease. Br J Renal Med. 2013;17 (4):23–7.
8. Fishbane S, Chittineni H, Packman M, Dutka P, Ali N, Durie N. Oral paricalcitol in the treatment of patients with CKD and proteinuria: a randomized trial. Am J Kidney Dis. 2009;54(4): 647–52.
9. Alborzi P, Patel NA, Peterson C, Bills JE, Bekele DM, Bunaye Z, et al. Paricalcitol reduces albuminuria and inflammation in chronic kidney disease: a randomized double-blind pilot trial. Hypertension. 2008;52(2):249–55.
10. de Zeeuw D, Agarwal R, Amdahl M, Audhya P, Coyne D, Garimella T, et al. Selective vitamin D receptor activation with paricalcitol for reduction of albuminuria in patients with type 2 diabetes (VITAL study): a randomised controlled trial. Lancet. 2010;376(9752):1543–51.
11. de Borst MH, Hajhosseiny R, Tamez H, Wenger J, Thadhani R, Goldsmith DJ. Active vitamin D treatment for reduction of residual proteinuria: a systematic review. J Am Soc Nephrol. 2013;24 (11):1863–71.
12. Liu PT, Stenger S, Li H, Wenzel L, Tan BH, Krutzik SR, et al. Toll-like receptor triggering of a vitamin D-mediated human antimicrobial response. Science. 2006;311(5768):1770–3.
13. Gombart AF, Bhan I, Borregaard N, Tamez H, Camargo CA Jr, Koeffler HP, et al. Low plasma level of cathelicidin antimicrobial peptide (hCAP18) predicts increased infectious disease mortality in patients undergoing hemodialysis. Clin Infect Dis. 2009;48 (4):418–24.

14. Bhan I, Camargo CA Jr, Wenger J, Ricciardi C, Ye J, Borregaard N, et al. Circulating levels of 25-hydroxyvitamin D and human cathelicidin in healthy adults. J Allergy Clin Immunol. 2011;127(5):1302–4 e1.
15. Bhan I, Dobens D, Tamez H, Deferio JJ, Li YC, Warren HS, et al. Nutritional vitamin D supplementation in dialysis: a randomized trial. Clin J Am Soc Nephrol. 2015;10(4):611–9.
16. Chen S, Law CS, Grigsby CL, Olsen K, Hong TT, Zhang Y, et al. Cardiomyocyte-specific deletion of the vitamin D receptor gene results in cardiac hypertrophy. Circulation. 2011;124(17):1838–47.
17. Wong MS, Delansorne R, Man RY, Svenningsen P, Vanhoutte PM. Chronic treatment with vitamin D lowers arterial blood pressure and reduces endothelium-dependent contractions in the aorta of the spontaneously hypertensive rat. Am J Physiol Heart Circ Physiol. 2010;299(4):H1226–34.
18. Mathew S, Lund RJ, Chaudhary LR, Geurs T, Hruska KA. Vitamin D receptor activators can protect against vascular calcification. J Am Soc Nephrol. 2008;19(8):1509–19.
19. Lim K, Lu TS, Molostvov G, Lee C, Lam FT, Zehnder D, et al. Vascular Klotho deficiency potentiates the development of human artery calcification and mediates resistance to fibroblast growth factor 23. Circulation. 2012;125(18):2243–55.
20. Vimaleswaran KS, Cavadino A, Berry DJ, LifeLines Cohort Study i, Jorde R, Dieffenbach AK, et al. Association of vitamin D status with arterial blood pressure and hypertension risk: a mendelian randomisation study. Lancet Diabetes Endocrinol. 2014;2(9):719–29.
21. Margolis KL, Ray RM, Van Horn L, Manson JE, Allison MA, Black HR, et al. Effect of calcium and vitamin D supplementation on blood pressure: the Women's Health Initiative Randomized Trial. Hypertension. 2008;52(5):847–55.
22. Thadhani R, Appelbaum E, Pritchett Y, Chang Y, Wenger J, Tamez H, et al. Vitamin D therapy and cardiac structure and function in patients with chronic kidney disease: the PRIMO randomized controlled trial. JAMA. 2012;307(7):674–84.
23. Tamez H, Zoccali C, Packham D, Wenger J, Bhan I, Appelbaum E, et al. Vitamin D reduces left atrial volume in patients with left ventricular hypertrophy and chronic kidney disease. Am Heart J. 2012;164(6):902–9 e2.
24. Ozcan OU, Gurlek A, Gursoy E, Gerede DM, Erol C. Relation of vitamin D deficiency and new-onset atrial fibrillation among hypertensive patients. J Am Soc Hypertens. 2015;9(4):307–12.
25. Drechsler C, Pilz S, Obermayer-Pietsch B, Verduijn M, Tomaschitz A, Krane V, et al. Vitamin D deficiency is associated with sudden cardiac death, combined cardiovascular events, and mortality in haemodialysis patients. Eur Heart J. 2010;31 (18):2253–61.
26. Zisman AL, Hristova M, Ho LT, Sprague SM. Impact of ergocalciferol treatment of vitamin D deficiency on serum parathyroid hormone concentrations in chronic kidney disease. Am J Nephrol. 2007;27(1):36–43.
27. Hansen D, Rasmussen K, Danielsen H, Meyer-Hofmann H, Bacevicius E, Lauridsen TG, et al. No difference between alfacalcidol and paricalcitol in the treatment of secondary hyperparathyroidism in hemodialysis patients: a randomized crossover trial. Kidney Int. 2011;80(8):841–50.
28. Teng M, Wolf M, Ofsthun MN, Lazarus JM, Hernan MA, Camargo CA Jr, et al. Activated injectable vitamin D and hemodialysis survival: a historical cohort study. J Am Soc Nephrol. 2005;16(4):1115–25.
29. Tripkovic L, Lambert H, Hart K, Smith CP, Bucca G, Penson S, et al. Comparison of vitamin D2 and vitamin D3 supplementation in raising serum 25-hydroxyvitamin D status: a systematic review and meta-analysis. Am J Clin Nutr. 2012;95(6):1357–64.

Association of Catalytic (Labile) Iron with Cardiovascular Morbidity and Mortality

10

Mohan Rajapurkar, Suhas S. Lele, Nasim Khan, and Sudhir V. Shah

Introduction

Definition of Catalytic (Labile) Iron and Its Importance in Tissue Injury

Iron is the most abundant transitional metal in the body. The term "labile iron pool" was first used to denote a transient pool of weakly chelated iron of low molecular weight that passes through the cell [1]. Critical to iron's importance in biological processes is its ability to cycle reversibly between its ferrous and ferric oxidation states. This precise property, which is essential for its functions, also makes it very dangerous, because free iron can catalyze the formation of free radicals that can damage the cell. Thus, from a pathophysiological standpoint, the broadest definition of a labile iron pool is that it consists of chemical forms that can participate in redox cycling, and is therefore often referred to as catalytic iron [2].

The catalytic iron pool [2, 3] is estimated to be less than 100 mg compared to the total iron in the body, which is approximately 4 g. In most cells iron homeostasis consists of iron uptake, utilization, and storage. The process of iron uptake is carried out by a transferrin receptor (TFR) and a divalent metal transporter 1 (DMT1, also called DCT1 or NRAMP2), whereas ferritin is an intracellular, iron-sequestering protein. Studies are beginning to yield information on the pathways of iron transport, its export from the cell via the divalent iron ion exporter ferroportin-1 [4] and its regulatory mechanisms including hepcidin. Since uptake and storage of iron is carried out by different proteins, the pool of accessible iron ions constitutes a crossroad of metabolic pathways of iron-containing compounds.

Studies using a variety of methods have begun to define intracellular distribution of labile iron (for reviews see Kruszewski) [1]. Using several techniques including laser scanning microscopy, the concentration and distribution of chelatable iron has been estimated to be about 5.0 to 15 μ [mu]M in the cytoplasm and subcellular organelles including mitochondria and nuclei [1]. In vivo, most of the iron is bound to heme or nonheme protein and does not directly catalyze the generation of hydroxyl radicals or a similar oxidant [2]. The bleomycin-detectable iron assay measures catalytic iron and is based on the observation that the anti-tumor antibiotic bleomycin, in the presence of catalytic iron, binds to and degrades DNA with the formation of a product that reacts with thiobarbituric acid to form a chromogen. Thus the assay detects iron complexes capable of catalyzing free radical reactions in biological samples [5]. The binding of the bleomycin-iron complex to DNA makes the reaction site-specific and antioxidants rarely interfere. The bleomycin assay detects only "free" iron and not iron bound to specific transport proteins or to enzymes. In several studies the labile iron pool is measured and described as non-transferrin-bound iron (NTBI) [6, 7].

The ability of iron to participate in redox cycling makes it potentially hazardous by enabling it to participate in the generation of powerful oxidant species such as hydroxyl radical (metal-catalyzed Haber-Weiss reaction, below) and/or reactive iron-oxygen complexes such as ferryl or perferryl ion [2]. In several systems, the amount of free radical generation is related to the amount of labile iron present [8].

M. Rajapurkar · S.S. Lele · N. Khan · S.V. Shah (✉)
Department of Internal Medicine Division of Nephrology, University of Arkansas for Medical Sciences and Central Arkansas Veterans Healthcare System, 4301 West Markham Street Slot 501, Little Rock, AR, USA
e-mail: shahsudhirv@uams.edu

M. Rajapurkar
e-mail: mmrajapurkar@mpuh.org

S.S. Lele
e-mail: lelesuhas@yahoo.com

N. Khan
e-mail: NAKhan@uams.edu

M. Rajapurkar
Department of Nephrology, Muljibhai Patel Urological Hospital, Dr. Virendra Desai Road, Nadiad, Gujarat 387001, India

J. Rangaswami et al. (eds.), *Cardio-Nephrology*,
DOI 10.1007/978-3-319-56042-7_10

$$Fe^{3+} + O_2^{\bullet-} \longrightarrow Fe^{2+} + O_2$$

$$Fe^{2+} + H_2O_2 \longrightarrow Fe^{3+} + OH^- + OH^\bullet$$

$$O_2^{\bullet-} + H_2O_2 \longrightarrow O_2 + OH^- + OH^\bullet$$

Iron also has a major role in lipid peroxidation, either directly or indirectly (through hydroxyl radicals or forming a perferryl ion) in which there is oxidative reaction of polyunsaturated lipids by removing hydrogen atoms from polyunsaturated fatty acids [2].

A major advancement in understanding the important role of iron in the pathophysiology of tissue injury is the recognition that iron plays a role even in the absence of systemic iron overload. It is now known that specific defects in cellular iron metabolism and/or an increase in catalytic iron may be important in several disease processes not associated with iron overload [4, 9]. In Friedreich's ataxia, there is an improper processing of iron because of the deficiency of the iron-chaperone protein frataxin, resulting in accumulation of iron in the mitochondria. Deficiencies in pantothenate kinase, a key enzyme in coenzyme A synthesis, leads to iron depositions and brain damage [9]. In addition to these specific defects in cellular iron, there is now overwhelming evidence that increased catalytic iron from subcellular or other sources participates in tissue injury in a wide variety of common disease states. This has been demonstrated in many disease states including acute and chronic kidney disease [10], neurodegenerative disorders [11], and systemic inflammatory diseases such as rheumatoid arthritis [12, 13]. In large part, the evidence consists of demonstrating an increase in catalytic iron and the ability of iron chelators to provide a protective effect, thus establishing a cause–effect relationship.

Catalytic Iron in Acute Coronary Syndrome

There have been a number of animal studies evaluating the changes in catalytic iron and the effect of an iron chelator on myocardial injury. In addition, there have been several recent human studies that have examined the utility of catalytic iron in the diagnosis and prognosis of acute coronary syndrome.

Catalytic Iron in Ischemia-Reperfusion Injury in Animals

Chevion et al. measured metals capable of free radical reactions in an animal model of cardiac ischemia and reperfusion injury. They reported that, in the first fraction of reperfusion after 35 min of ischemia, the level of copper and iron was eight- to ninefold higher than the pre-ischemic value [14]. In another study there was a 30-fold increase in catalytic iron during experimental cardiac ischemic injury [15]. This increase in the cellular catalytic iron pool is associated with severe oxidative stress [15].

There are limited studies on the effect of an iron chelator in myocardial ischemia/reperfusion injury. In a randomized study of ischemia/reperfusion in dogs, Reddy et al. [16] demonstrated that administration of a potent iron chelator, deferoxamine, reduced the extent of myocyte necrosis, presumably due to the lesser availability of Fenton reaction catalysts. Two iron chelators, deferiprone and deferoxamine, have been demonstrated to protect against experimental cardiac ischemia-reperfusion injury [17–19], and iron loading has been demonstrated to further increase cardiac ischemia-reperfusion injury [17].

Catalytic Iron in the Diagnosis and Prognosis of Acute Coronary Syndrome in Humans

Lele et al. [20] measured catalytic iron in patients with suspected acute coronary syndrome (ACS) and healthy volunteers to evaluate its utility in early detection of patients with acute myocardial infarction (MI) and predicting major adverse cardiac events (MACE). Catalytic iron was measured on admission and 24 h later in 127 patients with acute MI, 51 patients with suspected ACS without MI, and 250 healthy volunteers. Catalytic iron levels at presentation were 1.5 + 2.0, 0.2 + 0.16, and 0.1 + 0.06 μ[mu]mol/L for acute MI, suspected ACS without MI, and normals, respectively ($P < 0.0001$). Catalytic iron was elevated in all patients with MI at presentation. At a cutpoint of 0.30 μ[mu]mol/L, the sensitivity, specificity, and diagnostic accuracy for identifying MI was 84, 95, and 92%, respectively. Increase in catalytic iron at 24 h compared to baseline was associated with MACE at 30 days. Serial evaluation of catalytic iron was independently associated with MACE. This study suggests that, in patients who present with chest pain, increased catalytic iron indicates a high probability that the patient has acute coronary syndrome, whereas normal catalytic iron would make it unlikely that the patient has an acute myocardial infarction (Table 10.1).

In a more recent study, Roghi et al. measured NTBI in 15 patients with ST-segment elevation MI (STEMI) immediately before percutaneous coronary intervention and at 3, 6, 9, 12, and 24 h post-procedure. NTBI was detected in 13/15 patients, with the highest values in 4 patients with evidence of microvascular obstruction and hemorrhage on cardiac magnetic resonance imaging. NTBI levels were significantly related to CK-MB and troponin T values [21].

Table 10.1 Utility of catalytic iron in diagnosis of acute coronary syndrome

Catalytic iron (units)	Sensitivity	Specificity	Positive predictive value	Negative predictive value	Accuracy
0.10	100 (100–100)	44 (39–48	53 (48–58)	100 (100–100)	66 (61–70)
0.20	93 (90–95)	88 (85–91)	77 (73–81)	97 (95–98)	90 (87–93)
0.30	84 (81–88)	95 (93–97)	87 (84–90)	93 (91–96)	92 (89–94)
0.40	75 (71–79)	98 (98–100)	93 (91–96)	90 87–93)	91 (88–94)
0.50	67 (62–71)	99 (98–100)	97 (95–98)	88 (85–91)	89 (87–92)
0.60	61 (57–66)	99 (99–100)	98 (96–99)	86 (83–89)	88 (85–91)

Steen et al. assessed catalytic iron from samples obtained from the Thrombosis in Myocardial Infarction (TIMI) Trial [22]. In this study, they evaluated the association of catalytic iron with clinical outcomes in 1701 patients with unstable angina, non-STEMI, or STEMI [23]. These patients were followed for a median of 10 months. High catalytic iron (median value) was significantly associated with mortality (0.45 μ[mu]mol/L) compared with survivors (0.37μ[mu] mol/L; $P = 0.016$). The highest quartile had an almost fourfold risk compared to baseline (hazard ratio: 3.94, $P = 0.035$), which persisted after adjustment for age, diabetes, prior MI, prior congestive heart failure, ST-segment deviation, creatinine clearance, B-type natriuretic peptide, smoking, and Killip class (adjusted hazard ratio: 3.97, $P = 0.036$) (Fig. 10.1). No association was found between catalytic iron and risk of MI, recurrent ischemia, heart failure, or bleeding. Increased catalytic iron levels were associated with increased all-cause mortality, which suggests the possibility that the therapeutic strategies aimed at reducing catalytic iron may be useful.

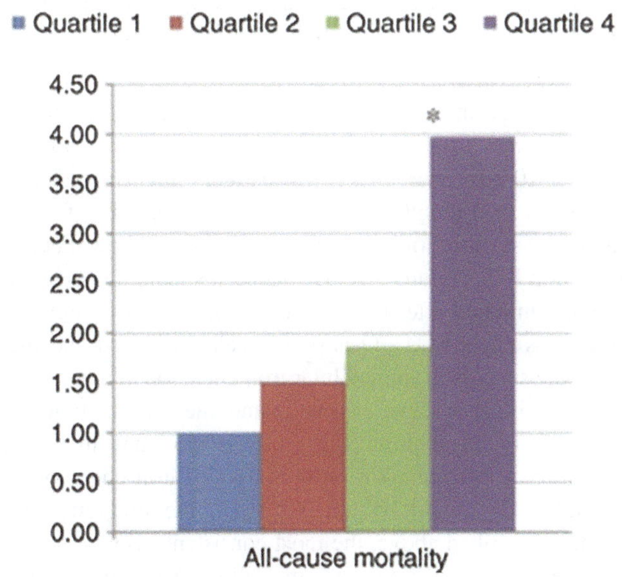

Fig. 10.1 Prognostic evaluation of catalytic iron in patients with acute coronary syndrome. Reprinted with permission from Steen DL et al. Catalytic iron in ACS patients. Clin Cardiol 36, 3, p. 143, 2013, Wiley

Lele et al. measured catalytic iron in patients with acute coronary syndrome undergoing a contrast study [24]. In the study population of 803 patients, the mortality was 1.6% at 30 days. Catalytic iron was significantly higher in patients who died (0.45 μ[mu]mol/L) compared with survivors (0.31 μ[mu]mol/L; $P = 0.004$), with an approximately eightfold increase in patients in the highest quartile compared with the lower three quartiles ($P = 0.001$) after adjustment for age, diabetes, Killip class, ejection fraction, baseline creatinine, hemoglobin level, and troponin (Table 10.2; Fig. 10.2). Interestingly, patients who developed contrast nephropathy had about a one-third increase in median catalytic iron at 48 h compared to virtually no increase in those without contrast nephropathy, and had significantly higher mortality compared with those without contrast nephropathy (9.1 vs. 1.1%, $P = 0.001$) (Fig. 10.3).

Diabetes is associated with a two- to threefold increase in mortality following AMI that cannot be entirely explained by differences in infarct size or recurrent ischemia. Sulieman et al. measured catalytic iron in diabetic and nondiabetic patients who presented to the coronary care unit with acute myocardial infarction [25]. In participants without diabetes ($n = 322$), about 15% showed significant labile plasma iron (LPI) levels. In contrast, about one-third (116 of 329) of the diabetic individuals had significant LPI ($P < 0.0001$). The mean (±SD) LPI level in diabetic subjects was significantly greater than in nondiabetic subjects (0.43 ± 0.7 vs. 0.14 ± 0.23 μ[mu]mol/L, $P < 0.001$). Approximately 10% of the patients died within a 30-day period, with the unadjusted mortality rate 2.5-fold higher in diabetic patients compared to nondiabetic patients (i.e., 13.9 vs. 5.5%, respectively, $P < 0.001$). In diabetic patients but not nondiabetic patients, LPI was associated with an increase in mortality (24.1 vs. 8.5%, odds ratio [OR] 3.4 [95% CI 1.8–6.6], $P < 0.001$ in diabetic patients, as opposed to 4.7 vs. 5.7%, $P = 0.7$ in nondiabetic patients). After adjustment for all covariates found to be significant predictors of 30-day mortality in univariate analysis, elevated LPI was found to be an independent determinant of mortality at 30 days in the

Table 10.2 Adverse cardiac events in the first three quartiles together compared to the fourth quartile of baseline CI (CI levels expressed as medians with interquartile ranges)

Event	Quartile 1 to 3 (n = 605) (0.32, 0.08) (%)	Quartile 4 (n = 201) (0.51, 0.18) (%)	P value
Mortality	4 (0.66)	9 (4.47)	<0.001
Reinfarction	10 (1.65)	6 (2.98)	0.241
Stent thrombosis	0 (0)	2 (0.99)	0.014
Heart failure	33 (5.45)	14 (6.96)	0.428
Stroke	1 (0.16)	1 (0.49)	0.412
Composite	47 (7.76)	26 (12.9)	0.027

Reprinted from American Heart Journal, 165, Suhas S. Lele et al., Impact of catalytic iron on mortality in patients with acute coronary syndrome exposed to iodinated radiocontrast—The Iscom Study, 744–51, Copyright 2013, with permission from Elsevier

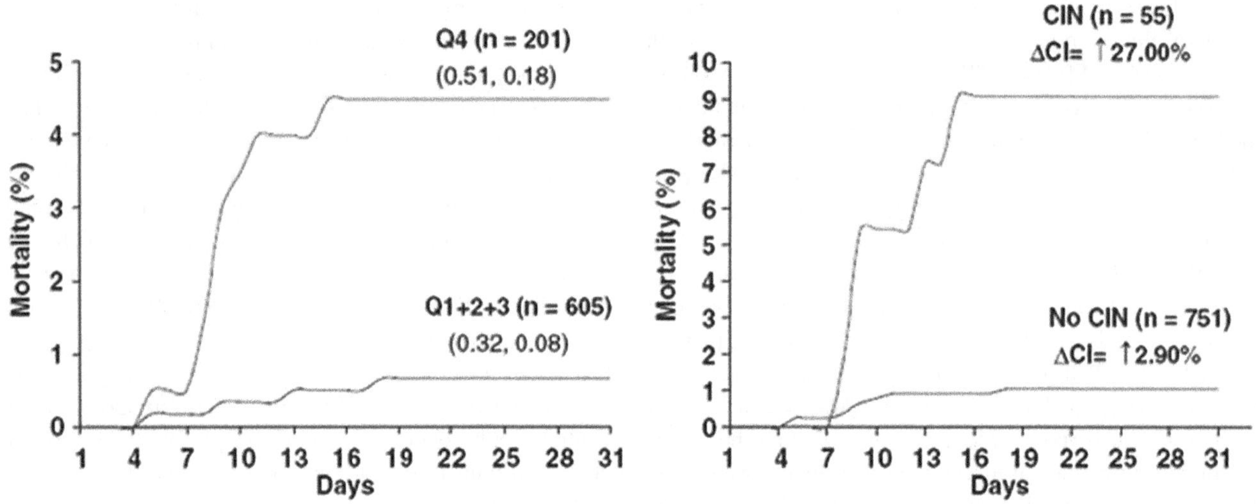

Fig. 10.2 Relationship between baseline CI levels and mortality in the 806 patient with ACS divided into the lower 3 quartiles (Q) + 2n + n3) and the fourth quartile (Q4) and the relationship between mortality and presence or absence of CIN (Δ [delta] CI = change in CI from baseline up to 48 h.) Reprinted from American Heart Journal, 165, Suhas S. Lele et al., Impact of catalytic iron on mortality in patients with acute coronary syndrome exposed to iodinated radiocontrast—The Iscom Study, 744-51, Copyright 2013, with permission from Elsevier

diabetic cohort (2.7 [1.2–6.2], P = 0.02). This study demonstrates that LPI is elevated in over one-third of all diabetic individuals presenting with AMI and that it is an independent and powerful predictor of mortality in diabetic individuals presenting with AMI.

There is very limited information on the therapeutic value of iron chelators in patients with acute MI. Deferoxamine (DFO) has been shown to improve outcomes in humans following coronary artery bypass graft surgery [26]. Chan et al. [27] randomly assigned 60 patients with STEMI to receive an intravenous bolus of DFO (500 mg) immediately before primary percutaneous coronary intervention followed by a 12-hour infusion (50 mg/kg of body weight) (n = 28) or normal saline bolus and infusion (placebo group, n = 32). In DFO-treated patients, there was a significant reduction in plasma F2-isoprostane levels immediately after primary percutaneous coronary intervention (PPCI) (2878 ± 1461 versus 2213 ± 579 pmol/L, P = 0.04). However, there was no difference in contrast-enhanced cardiac MRI-determined infarct size (DFO, 17.4 ± 10.8%, versus placebo, 18.6 ± 10.2%; P = 0.73), myocardial salvage index at 3 days or at 3 months, or the area-under-the-curve for creatine kinase or troponin I. This study does not show that iron chelation limits infarct size. However, it should be noted that therapy initiated after there is clear evidence of infarct may not be as effective. DFO is poorly cell-permeated and may limit the success of intracellular iron chelation and reduction in intracellular reactive oxygen metabolites, production, and cytotoxicity. In addition, this study is too small to have a meaningful interpretation on the effect of iron chelation on mortality. It should be noted that, in the previous large studies described above, the most consistent association was between catalytic iron and mortality. Additionally, two recent studies by Leaf et al. have also shown an association between catalytic iron and death. Of 250 patients undergoing cardiac surgery, patients in the highest quartile of catalytic

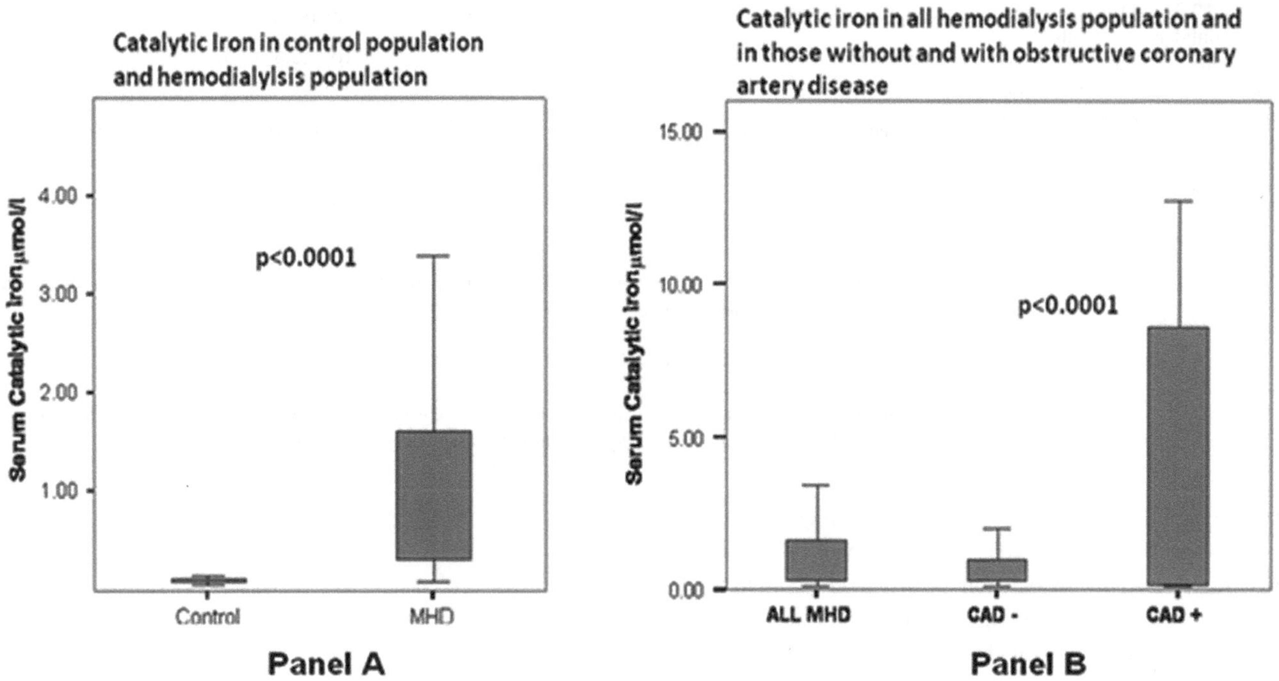

Fig. 10.3 Panel A: Box plots showing catalytic iron (Mean ± SEM) levels in normal control population, $n = 250$ (catalytic iron—0.1 ± 0.06 µ[mu]mol/L) as compared to hemodialysis (maintenance hemodialysis) patients, $n = 59$ (catalytic iron—4.18 ± 1.61 µ[mu] mol/L). Panel B: Box plots showing catalytic iron (mean ± SEM) levels in all he ± 4.12 µ[mu]mol/L). *Boxes* show interquartile ranges and hemodialysis patients (4.18 ± 1.61 µ[mu]mol/L), without coronary artery disease (CAD−) (1.35 ± 0.338 µ[mu]mol/L) and with CAD + (8.92 the bar represents highest and lowest values

iron had greater odds of experiencing hospital mortality, post-operative myocardial injury, and acute kidney injury (AKI) [28]. In a single-center prospective study of 121 critically ill patients admitted to ICU, plasma catalytic iron levels were higher among patients who reached the primary end point of in-hospital mortality or AKI requiring renal replacement therapy [29].

Association of Catalytic Iron with Cardiovascular Diseases

The iron-heart hypothesis was first postulated by Sullivan in the early 1980s [30]. He suggested that the lower incidence of coronary heart disease in premenopausal women when compared with men of the same age is attributable to lower body-iron stores caused by regular blood loss. Several animal studies support a role for iron in atherosclerosis [31, 32]. In contrast, human observational studies evaluating CVD associations with measures of iron stores [33–36], dietary intake [37], and blood donation [38, 39] provide inconsistent results. A study of Finnish men found that serum ferritin of 200 µ[mu]g/L or higher was associated with a 2.2-fold risk of myocardial infarction compared to men with lower levels [40]. de Valk and Marx concluded that there is strong evidence in observational studies that iron is important in atherosclerosis [34]. However, Sempos reported in 2002 that only 3 of 22 observational studies of the association between ferritin and heart disease had statistically significant associations [33]. Data from cross-sectional, case-control, and prospective studies that have used serum ferritin to assess iron stores are also conflicting, with some reporting a positive association with cardiovascular disease [36, 41] and others no association with cardiovascular disease [42]. The discrepancies in findings relating iron stores to cardiovascular disease may be due to the use of varying outcomes [43]. Importantly, ferritin is increased by inflammation, making it difficult to distinguish the effects of iron stores from inflammatory effects. Thus, a potential confounder in studies using ferritin as an indicator of total iron stores is that the majority of the studies did not account for inflammation in their design and analysis [40–42]. Total body iron is not consistently related to the level of biologically active iron [44] and thus it is important to measure catalytic iron rather than total body iron to understand the pathophysiological impact of iron in cardiovascular disease.

Rajapurkar et al. examined the association between catalytic (labile) iron and cardiovascular disease (CVD) in a cross-sectional study of 496 participants [45]. Serum catalytic iron was measured using the bleomycin-detectable iron assay that detects biologically active iron. Eighty-five subjects had CVD. The odds of existing CVD for subjects in

Table 10.3 Odds ratios and 95% confidence intervals indicating association for upper one-third versus lower two-thirds of serum catalytic iron and existing cardiovascular disease

Model (n = 496)	Level of catalytic iron	OR (95% CI)	P value
Unadjusted	Upper 1/3	10.1 (5.8–17.5)	<0.0001
	Lower 2/3	1	
Adjusted for age, gender	Upper 1/3	4.9 (2.6–9.5)	<0.0001
	Lower 2/3	1	
Full model† [45]	Upper 1/3	3.8 (1.4–10.1)	<0.0072
	Lower 2/3	1	

CI confidence interval
* Wald Chi-square test for upper 1/3 versus lower 2/3 for serum catalytic iron from logistic regression models
†Adjusted for age, Framingham 10-year coronary heart disease risk score, estimated glomerular filtration rate, high-density lipoprotein cholesterol, systolic blood pressure, and hypertension

the upper third of catalytic iron were 10 times that of subjects with lower catalytic iron in unadjusted analyses (Table 10.3). This association persisted even after adjustment for age and the Framingham Risk Score (odds ratio 3.8, 95% confidence interval 1.4–10.1). This study provides evidence for a strong detrimental association between high serum catalytic iron and CVD even after adjusting for several co-morbid conditions.

Cardiovascular disease is the leading cause of morbidity and mortality in maintenance hemodialysis (MHD) patients. Rajapurkar et al. evaluated serum catalytic iron (SCI) as a potential biomarker for underlying coronary artery disease (CAD) in patients on maintenance hemodialysis [46]. Fifty-nine asymptomatic stable hemodialysis patients underwent coronary angiography. Significant CAD (defined as >70% narrowing) was detected in 22 (37.3%) patients, with one-vessel disease in 14 (63.63%) and multi-vessel disease in eight (36.36%) patients. Levels of catalytic iron in these patients were compared with a group of healthy controls. The hemodialysis patients had very elevated levels of catalytic iron (4.70 ± 1.79 μ[mu]mol/L) compared with normal controls (0.11 ± 0.01 μ[mu]mol/L) ($P < 0.0001$) (Fig. 10.3). Most importantly, hemodialysis patients with no CAD had SCI levels of 1.36 ± 0.34 μ[mu]mol/L compared with those having significant CAD (8.92 ± 4.12 μ[mu] mol/L) ($P < 0.0001$) (Figs. 10.3 and 10.4). Patients on hemodialysis with diabetes had a stronger correlation between SCI and prevalence of CAD compared with non-diabetics. In multivariate analysis, SCI and diabetes mellitus were independently associated with significant CAD. Elevated catalytic iron levels are associated with presence of significant coronary disease in such patients. Thus, the measurement of catalytic iron may be a useful test to detect coronary artery in otherwise asymptomatic patients. In addition, reducing catalytic iron by using an iron chelator may be an important therapeutic modality to prevent and treat coronary artery disease in hemodialysis patients.

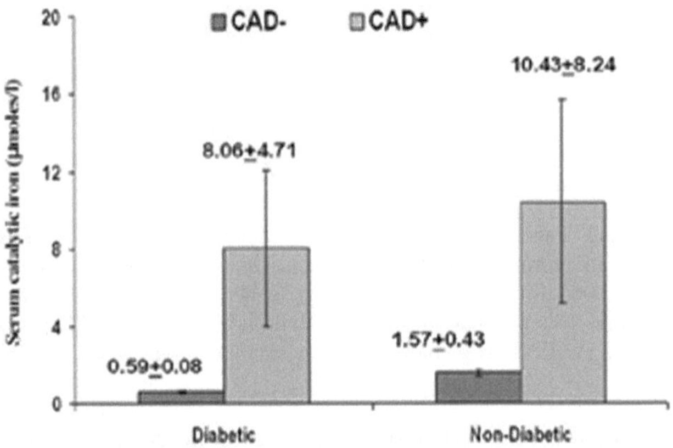

Fig. 10.4 Histogram showing catalytic iron levels in μ[mu]mol/L (Mean ± SEM) in diabetic and nondiabetic patients, with respect to those having coronary artery disease (CAD+) and those without (CAD-)

Lee et al. reported NTBI levels (measured by high-performance liquid chromatography) were increased in 92% of patients with at least 5 years' duration of diabetes and 59% of the patients with newly diagnosed diabetes compared to controls, with mean values of 0.62 ± 0.43 versus 0.24 ± 0.29 versus 0.04 ± 0.13 μ[mu]mol/L Fe, respectively [47].

Providing evidence for the role of catalytic iron in cardiovascular disease requires not only demonstrating an association but, more importantly, demonstrating that removing catalytic iron results in clinical benefit. It should be noted that the first randomized, multicenter Iron and Atherosclerosis trial (FeAST) reported no significant benefit in all-cause mortality or nonfatal myocardial infarction in patients who underwent reduction in iron stores by phlebotomy [38]. Sullivan has argued that, among other reasons, the FeAST trial may have failed because the study design did not achieve full iron depletion. Regardless, in our opinion, the study results were not surprising because iron status does not reflect the iron available to catalyze free radical reactions, as we reported in animal studies a few years ago. In two models of glomerular disease, an iron-deficient diet that was accompanied by a reduction in catalytic iron provided protection [48]. Conversely, an iron-deficient diet was not protective in ischemia-reperfusion injury. In this model, animals that had been fed an iron-deficient diet had identical amounts of catalytic iron in the kidney cortex [44]. Thus, iron status per se may not dictate susceptibility to injury but, rather, iron that is catalytically available to participate in free-radical reactions. Additionally, there is emerging data that measurement of iron in vessel walls and plaques may correlate with atherosclerosis [49, 50].

No clinical trials have examined the effect of an iron chelator on cardiovascular events, either in a normal population or in a population with high levels of catalytic iron such as patients with diabetes or patients on hemodialysis. However, there is some information related to EDTA chelation therapy, which chelates not only calcium but also metals such as iron and copper. The Trial to Assess Chelation Therapy (TACT) was developed in response to a Request for Proposals by the National Center for Complementary and Alternative Medicine and the National Heart Lung and Blood Institute. TACT was a randomized, double-blind placebo-controlled trial that enrolled patients $\geq$ 50 years of age and with a history of prior myocardial infarction. TACT studied the effect of EDTA infusions and high-dose vitamins on cardiovascular outcomes compared to placebo using a 2×2 factorial design. EDTA provided a modest but significant reduction in the primary composite cardiovascular endpoint (HR 0.82, 95% CI 0.69–0.99, $P = 0.035$) [51–53]. Furthermore, a more robust benefit of chelation therapy was apparent among two prespecified subgroups of 'high-risk patients' with diabetes (HR 0.61, 95% CI 0.45–0.83, $P = 0.02$) or anterior MI (HR 0.63, 95% CI 0.47–0.86, $P = 0.03$).

Concluding Remarks

The data presented indicate that high catalytic iron is associated with higher mortality in patients with acute MI, particularly those with diabetes. High catalytic iron is associated with prevalent cardiovascular disease in the general population and particularly in patients with diabetes and patients on hemodialysis. There have been no clinical trials examining the effect of iron chelators in patients with suspected acute myocardial infarction or in patients at high risk for cardiovascular events (e.g., hemodialysis patients and patient with diabetes). Several iron chelators have been approved for use in iron overload states. Desferroxamine (deferoxamine or DFO) is parenteral and therefore less suitable for chronic use. Of the two oral iron chelators currently approved for human use in iron overload states, deferasirox (DFRA) may potentially be beneficial for treating or preventing cardiovascular events, particularly as a short-term therapy such as in patients with suspected acute coronary syndrome, and has an advantage of once-daily administration. However, the recent recognition of side effects must be considered in choosing an appropriate oral iron chelator. Deferiprone (1,2-dimethyl-3-hydroxypyridin-4–1 or L1) has been approved for treatment of iron overload states in Europe, India, and recently in 2011 in North America. In addition to its suitability for long-term treatment (because of oral administration), the high-membrane permeability of deferiprone is well documented, as shown by its capacity to access and deplete intracellular iron pools and ability to remove labile iron from nuclei, endosomes, and mitochondria [9]. The major adverse effect reported so far in several thousand patients receiving deferiprone for periods of up to 14 years is transient agranulocytosis in less than 1% of patients. There is evidence of potentially differential efficacy among available iron chelators. For example, in beta-thalassemia major, well-conducted randomized controlled trials show that cardiovascular function is better preserved with use of deferiprone versus deferoxamine alone, while deferasirox and deferoxamine show equivalence [54]. This suggests that, as a monotherapy, deferiprone is likely the most efficacious iron-chelating agent. Furthermore, in contrast to the other available iron chelators, deferiprone fulfills some of the requirements of being a reversed siderophore which aims to bind labile iron and transfer it to other acceptors or other intra/extracellular compartments [55]. An additional potential beneficial mechanism for these agents may be their ability to reduce oxidative damage caused by other metals such as copper, aluminum, and zinc [56]. Based on the collective evidence to date, randomized, controlled, double-blind trials may be warranted to evaluate the efficacy and safety of iron chelators [57] to prevent or treat cardiovascular disease.

REFERENCES

1. Kruszewski M. The role of labile iron pool in cardiovascular diseases. Acta Biochim Pol. 2004;51(2):471–80.
2. Halliwell B, Gutteridge JM. Role of free radicals and catalytic metal ions in human disease: an overview. Methods Enzymol. 1990;186:1–85.
3. Kakhlon O, Cabantchik ZI. The labile iron pool: characterization, measurement, and participation in celullar processes. Free Rad Biol Med. 2002;33(8):1037–46.
4. Andrews NC. Forging a field: the golden age of iron biology. Blood. 2008;112(2):219–30.

5. Gutteridge JMC, Rowley DA, Halliwell B. Superoxide-dependent formation of hydroxyl radicals in the presence of iron salts. Detection of 'free' iron in biological systems by using bleomycin-dependent degradation of DNA. Biochem J. 1981;199:263–5.
6. Hershko C, Graham G, Bates GW, Rachmilewitz EA. Non-specific serum iron in thalassaemia: an abnormal serum iron fraction of potential toxicity. Br J Haematol. 1978;40:255–63.
7. Brissot P, Ropert M, Le Lan C, Loréal O. Non-transferrin bound iron: a key role in iron overload and iron toxicity. Biochim Biophys Acta. 2012;1820(3):403–10.
8. Esposito BP, Breuer W, Sirankapracha P, Pootrakul P, Hershko C, Cabantchik I. Labile plasma iron in iron overload: redox activity and susceptibility to chelation. Blood. 2003;102(7):2670–7.
9. Sohn YS, Breuer W, Munnich A, Cabantchik ZI. Redistribution of accumulated cell iron: a modality of chelation with therapeutic implications. Blood. 2008;111(3):1690–9.
10. Rajapurkar MM, Baliga R, Shah SV. Catalytic (labile) iron in kidney disease. In: Alpern RJ, Caplan MJ, Moe OW, editors. Seldin and Giebisch's the kidney, physiology & pathophysiology. 5th ed. San Diego: Elsevier, Academic Press; 2012. p. 3003–15.
11. Boddaert N, Le Quan Sang KH, Rötig A, Leroy-Willig A, Gallet S, Brunelle F, et al. Selective iron chelation in Friedreich ataxia: biologic and clinical implications. Blood. 2007;110(1):401–8.
12. Rowley D, Gutteridge JM, Blake D, Farr M, Halliwell B. Lipid peroxidation in rheumatoid arthritis: thiobarbituric acid-reactive material and catalytic iron salts in synovial fluid from rheumatoid patients. Clin Sci (Lond). 1984;66(6):691–5.
13. Kell DB. Iron behaving badly: inappropriate iron chelation as a major contributor to the aetiology of vascular and other progressive inflammatory and degenerative diseases. BMC Med Genomics. 2009;2:2.
14. Chevion M, Jiang Y, Har-El R, Berenshtein E, Uretzky G, Kitrossky N. Copper and iron are mobilized following myocardial ischemia: possible predictive criteria for tissue injury. Proc Natl Acad Sci USA. 1993;90:1102–6.
15. Voogd A, Sluiter W, van Eijk HG, Koster JF. Low molecular weight iron and the oxygen paradox in isolated rat hearts. J Clin Invest. 1992;90:2050–5.
16. Reddy BR, Kloner RA, Przyklenk K. Early treatment with deferoxamine limits myocardial ischemic/reperfusion injury. Free Rad Biol Med. 1989;7:45–52.
17. van der Kraaij AMM, Mostert LJ, van Eijk HG, Koster JF. Iron-load increases the susceptibility of rat hearts to oxygen reperfusion damage. Protection by the antioxidant (+)-cyanidanol-3 and deferoxamine. Circulation. 1988;78:442–9.
18. van der Kraaij AMM, van Eijk HG, Koster JF. Prevention of postischemic cardiac injury by the orally active iron chelator 1,2-dimethyl-3-hydroxy-4-pyridone (L1) and the antioxidant (+)-cyanidanol-3. Circulation. 1989;80:158–64.
19. Nicholson SC, Squier M, Ferguson DJP, Nagy Z, Westaby S, Evans RD. Effect of desferrioxamine cardioplegia on ischemia-reperfusion in isolated rat heart. Ann Thorac Surg. 1997;63:1003–11.
20. Lele S, Shah S, McCullough PA, Rajapurkar M. Serum catalytic iron as a novel biomarker of vascular injury in acute coronary syndromes. EuroIntervention. 2009;5:336–42.
21. Roghi A, Poggiali E, Duca L, Mafrici A, Pedrotti P, Paccagnini S, et al. Role of non-transferrin-bound iron in the pathogenesis of cardiotoxicity in patients with ST-elevation myocardial infarction assessed by cardiac magnetic resonance imaging. Int J Cardiol. 2015;199:326–32.
22. Cannon CP, McCabe CH, Wilcox RG, Langer A, Caspi A, Berink P, et al. Oral glycoprotein IIb/IIIa inhibition with orbofiban in patients with unstable coronary syndromes (OPUS-TIMI 16) trial. Circulation. 2000;102(2):149–56.
23. Steen DL, Cannon CP, Lele SS, Rajapurkar MMM, Mukhopadhyay B, Scirica BM, et al. Prognostic evaluation of catalytic iron in patients with acute coronary syndromes. Clin Invest. 2013;36(3):139–45.
24. Lele SS, Mukhopadhyay BN, Mardkar MM, Patel TA, Vasavada AK, Banker DN, et al. Impact of catalytic iron on mortality in patients with acute coronary syndrome exposed to iodinated radiocontrast—The Iscom Study. Am Heart J. 2013;165:744–51.
25. Sulieman M, Asleh R, Cabantchik ZI, Breuer W, Aronson D, Suleiman A, et al. Serum chelatable redox-active iron is an independent predictor of mortality after myocardial infarction in individuals with diabetes. Diabetes Care. 2004;27(11):2730–2.
26. Paraskevaidis JA, Iliodromitis EK, Vlahakos D, Tsiapras DP, Nikolaidis A, Marathias A, et al. Deferoxamine infusion during coronary artery bypass grafting ameliorates lipid peroxidation and protects the myocardium against reperfusion injury: immediate and long-term significance. Euro Heart J. 2005;26(3):263–70.
27. Chan W, Taylor AJ, Ellims AH, Lefkovits L, Wong C, Kingwell BA, et al. Effect of iron chelation on myocardial infarct size and oxidative stress in ST-elevation-myocardial infarction. Circ Cardiovasc Interv. 2012;5(2):270–8.
28. Leaf DE, Rajapurkar M, Lele SS, Mukhopadhyay B, Rawn JD, Frendl G, et al. Increased plasma catalytic iron in patients may mediate acute kidney injury and death following cardiac surgery. Kidney Int. 2015;87(5):1046–54.
29. Leaf DE, Rajapurkar M, Lele SS, Mukhopadhyay B, Waikar SS. Plasma catalytic iron, AKI, and death among critically ill patients. Clin J Am Soc Nephrol. 2014;9(11):1849–56.
30. Sullivan JL. Iron and the sex difference in heart disease risk. Lancet. 1981;1(8233):1293–4.
31. Zhang W-J, Wei H, Frei B. The iron chelator, desferrioxamine, reduces inflammation and atherosclerotic lesion development in experimental mice. Exp Biol Med. 2010;235:633–41.
32. Day SM, Duquaine D, Mundada LV, Menon RG, Khan BV, Rajagopalan S, et al. Chronic iron administration increases vascular oxidative stress and accelerates arterial thrombosis. Circulation. 2003;107:2601–6.
33. Sempos CT. Do body iron stores increase the risk of developing coronary heart disease? Am J Clin Nutr. 2002;76(3):501–3.
34. de Valk B, Marx JJM. Iron, atherosclerosis, and ischemic heart disease. Arch Intern Med. 1999;159(14):1542–8.
35. van der A DL, Marx JJM, Grobbee DE, Kamphuis MH, Georgiou NA, van Kats-Renaud JH, et al. Non-transferrin-bound iron and risk of coronary heart disease in postmenopausal women. Circulation. 2006;113(6):1942–9.
36. Wolff B, Volzke H, Ludemann J, Robinson D, Vogelgesang D, Staudt A, et al. Association between high serum ferritin levels and carotid atherosclerosis in the Study of Health in Pomerania (SHIP). Stroke. 2004;35:453–7.
37. Derstine JL, Murray-Kolb LE, Yu-Porth S, Hargrove RL, Kris-Etherton PS, Beard JL. Iron status in association with cardiovascular disease risk in 3 controlled feeding studies. Am J Clin Nutr. 2003;77:56–62.
38. Zacharski LR, Chow BK, Howes PS, Shamayeva G, Baron JA, Dalman RL, et al. Reduction of iron stores and cardiovascular outcomes in patients with peripheral arterial disease: a randomized controlled trial. JAMA. 2007;297(6):603–10.
39. Zheng H, Cable R, Spencer B, Votto N, Katz SD. Iron stores and vascular function in voluntary blood donors. Arterioscler Thromb Vasc Biol. 2005;25:1577–83.
40. Salonen JT, Nyyssonen K, Korpela H, Tuomilehto J, Seppanen R, Salonen R. High stored iron levels are associated with excess risk of myocardial infarction in eastern Finnish men. Circulation. 1992;86:803–11.

41. Kiechl S, Willeit J, Egger G, Poewe W, Oberhollenzer F. Group. BS. Body iron stores and the risk of carotid atherosclerosis. Prospective results from the Bruneck study. Circulation. 1997;96:3300–7.
42. Rauramaa R, Vaisanen S, Mercuri M, Rankinen T, Penttila I, Bond MG. Association of risk factors and body iron status to carotid atherosclerosis in middle-aged eastern Finnish men. Eur Heart J. 1994;15:1020–7.
43. Ahluwalia N, Genoux A, Ferrieres J, Perret B, Carayol M, Drouet L, et al. Iron status is associated with carotid atherosclerotic plaques in middle-aged adults. J Nutr. 2010;140(4):812–6.
44. Baliga R, Ueda N, Shah SV. Increase in bleomycin-detectable iron in ischaemia/reperfusion injury to rat kidneys. Biochem J. 1993;291 (3):901–5.
45. Rajapurkar MM, Shah SV, Lele SS, Hegde UN, Lensing SY, Gohel K, et al. Association of catalytic iron with cardiovascular disease. Am J Cardiol. 2012;109(3):438–42.
46. Rajapurkar MM, Lele SS, Malavade TS, Kansara MR, Hegde UN, Gohel KD, et al. Serum catalytic iron: A novel biomarker for coronary artery disease in patients on maintenance hemodialysis. Indian J Nephrol. 2013;3(5):332–7.
47. Lee D-H, Liu DY, Jacobs DR, Shin H-R, Song K, Lee I-K, et al. Common presence of non-transferrin-bound iron among patients with type 2 diabetes. Diabetes Care. 2006;29:1090–5.
48. Baliga R, Ueda N, Shah SV. Kidney iron status in passive Heymann nephritis and the effect of iron deficient diet. J Am Soc Nephrol. 1996;7:1183–8.
49. Raman SV, Sharkey-Toppen TP, Tran T, Liu JX, McCarthy B, He X, et al. Iron, inflammation and atherosclerosis risk in men vs. perimenopausal women. Atherosclerosis. 2015;241(1):249–54.
50. Winner MW, Sharkey-Toppen T, Zhang X, Pennell ML, Simonetti OP, Zweier JL, et al. Iron and noncontrast magnetic resonance T2* as a marker of intraplaque iron in human atherosclerosis. J Vasc Surg. 2015;61(6):1556–64.
51. Ouyang P, Gottlieb SH, Culotta VL, Navas-Acien A. EDTA chelation therapy to reduce cardiovascular events in persons with diabetes. Curr Cardiol Rep. 2015;17(11):96.
52. Lamas GA, Goertz C, Boineau R, Mark DB, Rozema T, Nahin RL, et al. Effect of disodium EDTA chelation regimen on cardiovascular events in patients with previous myocardial infarction: the TACT randomized trial. JAMA. 2013;309(12):1241–50.
53. Escolar E, Lamas GA, Mark DB, Boineau R, Goertz C, Rosenberg Y, et al. The effect of an EDTA-based chelation regimen on patients with diabetes mellitus and prior myocardial infarction in the Trial to Assess Chelation Therapy (TACT). Circ Cardiovasc Qual Outcomes. 2014;7(1):15–24.
54. Pennell DJ, Udelson JE, Arai AE, Bozkurt B, Cohen AR, Galanello R, et al. Cardiovascular function and treatment in β[beta]-thalassemia major: a consensus statement from the American Heart Association. Circulation. 2013;128(3):281–308.
55. Kakhlon O, Breuer W, Munnich A, Cabantchik ZI. Iron redistribution as a therapeutic strategy for treating diseases of localized iron accumulation. Can J Physiol Pharmacol. 2010;88:187–96.
56. Kontoghiorghes GJ. Comparative efficacy and toxicity of desferrioxamine, deferiprone and other iron and aluminum chelating drugs. Toxicol Lett. 1995;80:1–18.
57. Kontoghiorghes GJ. New concepts of iron and aluminium chelation therapy with oral L1 (deferiprone) and other chelators. Analyst. 1995;120:845–51.

11 Erythropoietin and Its Cardiovascular Effects

Nupur Gupta and Jay B. Wish

Introduction

Erythropoietin (EPO) is a cytokine involved in red cell production. EPO was approved for the treatment of anemia in the US in 1989 by the Food and Drug Administration as the first human recombinant biomedicine produced in heterologous mammalian cells [1]. Although it has been known since the 19th century that erythrocyte production is controlled by oxygen tension, it was not until 1948 that the word "erythropoietins" was first used to describe "unidentified plasma factors that [are] produced in anoxic conditions" to stimulate erythrocyte production [2]. In 1906, Carnot and Mademoiselle suggested that hypoxia generates a humoral factor capable of stimulating red blood cell (RBC) production [3]. Erslev demonstrated that injection of a large volume of plasma from donor rats after a bleeding stimulus into normal recipient rats produced a marked reticulocytosis [4]. Eschbach and Adamson demonstrated that daily infusions of EPO-rich plasma into sheep with subtotal nephrectomy corrected the anemia in all subject sheep. The purification of sufficient EPO to sequence using gas phase protein sequencing allowed for the design of effective DNA probes for isolating the EPO gene from a human genome bank. The gene was subsequently cloned and expressed in Chinese hamster ovary cells, resulting in the production of recombinant human EPO (rHuEPO). Publication of phase 3 studies demonstrating the safety and effectiveness rHuEPO in 333 anemic dialysis patients in 9 centers occurred in December 1989, six months after rHuEPO received approval by the FDA for the treatment of anemia in patients with ESKD. Increased blood pressure was noted in 35% of the study participants receiving rHuEPO [5]. The development of rHuEPO was aimed at replacing the insufficient endogenous EPO production related to chronic kidney disease (CKD) progression. It still remains unclear whether the main cause of anemia in CKD is a loss of kidney EPO production capacity or a derangement in oxygen sensing.

N. Gupta · J.B. Wish (✉)
Division of Nephrology, Indiana University School of Medicine, IU Health University Hospital, 550 N. University Blvd., Suite 6100, Indianapolis, IN 46202, USA
e-mail: jwish@iu.edu

N. Gupta
e-mail: nugupta@iu.edu

J. Rangaswami et al. (eds.), *Cardio-Nephrology*,
DOI 10.1007/978-3-319-56042-7_11

Physiology of Erythropoietin

Structure

Human EPO is a glycoprotein characterized by its large carbohydrate chains, which occupy close to 40% of its total mass. Sixty percent of the molecular weight of the recombinant protein is contributed by amino acids. The sugar moieties were thought to be important for the biological activity of EPO, but detailed studies were not performed until the structures were elucidated [1]. EPO exhibits several isoforms that differ in biological activity [6].

Site of Production

Initial studies in mice had shown that the kidney was the site of production of EPO. This awakened more interest in the exact location [7]. In situ hybridization studies demonstrated that the cells containing EPO mRNA are in a peritubular (interstitial or endothelial) location in anemic mouse kidneys [8]. Hepatic production is contributed primarily by hepatocytes but is a much less important source than is the kidney. During fetal life, however, hepatic EPO production is of major importance for RBC production [9].

Receptor

Erythropoietin is secreted as needed; it is not stored. Circulating rHuEPO and presumably native EPO have a half-life of 4–12 h [8]. EPO is degraded once it binds to the EPO receptor (EPOR). EPO binds to an erythroid progenitor cell surface receptor to regulate bone marrow erythroid cell proliferation, differentiation, and survival. EPOR is expressed primarily on erythroid cells between the colony forming unit-erythrocyte (CFU-E) and the pronormoblast stage of erythroid cell development [10]. EPOR is a preformed homodimer that undergoes a structural change upon binding with EPO. The cytoplasmic portion of EPOR contains a positive regulatory domain that interacts with Janus kinase 2 (JAK2) [11]. Immediately after EPO binding, JAK2 cross-phosphorylates the EPOR itself and other proteins that initiate a cascade of erythroid-specific signaling.

Regulation of Erythropoietin Production

The advent of reliable bioassays for EPO led to evidence supporting the concept that oxygen delivery to the tissues regulates circulating levels of EPO. EPO levels were shown to be elevated in patients with acute or chronic anemia and acute or chronic hypoxemia [6]. The main functions of EPO are to maintain hemoglobin and to hasten RBC recovery after hemorrhage. The basal plasma concentration of EPO ranges from 4 to 24 IU/mL. In the basal state, a small number of fibroblasts at the corticomedullary junction of the kidney express EPO mRNA. When stimulated, recruitment spreads outwards, with some evidence that individual cells are recruited in an all-none form.

Hypoxia is the principal regulator of erythropoiesis. Adaptive physiologic responses to hypoxia help to (1) increase O_2 delivery to cells, (2) allow cells to survive under reduced O_2 by activating glycolysis, and (3) reduce the formation of reactive oxygen species. The response to hypoxia is controlled by transcriptional factors termed hypoxia-inducible factors (HIFs) [12]. HIFs are heterodimeric transcription factors composed of a highly-regulated 02-labile α[alpha] subunit and a constitutively expressed β[beta] sub-unit [13]. HIF-2 has been identified as the primary transcription factor inducing EPO expression. The half-life of HIF-1α[alpha] in the cell is minutes under normoxic conditions. The targeting and subsequent polyubiquitination of HIF α[alpha] subunits requires vonHippel Lindau protein (pVHL), iron, O_2, and proline hydroxylase activity, and this complex constitutes the oxygen sensor. When hydroxylated, HIF then couples with the pVHL, and the resultant complex is targeted for proteasomal degradation. Thus, inhibiting prolyl hydroxylase results in stabilization of HIF and consequently transcription of the **EPO** gene. When oxygen delivery decreases, the pVHL complex no longer executes proteolysis of HIF and EPO production is increased.

Non-hematologic Effects of Erythropoietin on the Cardiovascular System

The structure of surface cell receptor that mediates biological effect of EPO and its derivatives in non-hematopoietic tissues remain to be characterized. These receptors are located on various non-hematopoietic organs (Table 11.1).

Angiogenesis

EPO is an angiogenic and vascular-protectant cytokine. EPO signaling modulates the regulation of angiogenesis. It plays an important role in regulation of angiogenesis in embryo, female reproductive organ, and wound healing. EPOR expression in various types of vascular endothelial cells has been associated with the ability of EPO to promote the migration and proliferation of endothelial cells in in vitro models [14]. This property of angiogenesis has been postulated as an etiology of diabetic retinopathy [15]. The neovascularization effect has been associated with a cardioprotective effect of EPO in the setting of myocardial infarction. The mechanism for neovascularization is medicated by migration of bone marrow derived endothelial progenitors cells (EPCs) into circulation [16]. These cells have main role in angiogenesis. Taken together, EPO upregulation and blockade both have effects in vascular repair and tone.

Cardiac Effects of EPO

EPOR expression in the heart and in isolated primary cardiac myocytes is associated with EPO-mediated activation of specific signal transduction pathways [17]. The induction of

Table 11.1 Summary of non-hematological effects of erythropoietin on the cardiovascular system

	Possible mechanism	Clinical implication
Angiogenesis	Migration of bone marrow derived endothelial progenitor cells	Neovascularization may be of benefit in myocardial infarction
Cardiac muscles	Reduction of ischemia induced apoptosis	Recovery of LV function*
Hypertension	Increased endothelin, angiotensin, altered calcium homeostasis	Increased cardiovascular mortality
Thrombosis	Increased blood viscosity	Increased thromboembolic events

*Controvertial as some studies have shown harmful effects on LV remodelling

these pathways leads to reduction of ischemia-induced cardiac myocyte apoptosis and improved recovery of LV function in the ex vivo perfused heart. EPO is cardioprotective when administered at the time of ischemia or even at reperfusion in different experimental models leading to significant reduction in infarct size and attenuation of LV dysfunction [18]. In contrast, the chronic and repeated non-biologic stimulation of cardiac EPO receptors during erythropoiesis stimulating agent (ESA) treatment for anemia could have untoward effects, particularly on remodeling of the myocardium through prevention of apoptosis. Some studies have hypothesized repetitive stimulation and resetting of cardiac growth signals could disorder cardiac modeling, increasing vulnerability to stress [19]. The long-term effects of EPO on the heart remain uncertain but are of critical importance as cardiovascular disease is the most common cause of mortality in patients with CKD.

Hypertension

Initial reports showing the efficacy of rHuEPO found hypertension to be the most common side effect. It was thought initially that higher hemoglobin (Hb) levels were responsible for the hypertension. Administration of rHuEPO has been reported to increase systemic vascular resistance and decrease cardiac output [20], perhaps a result of increased endothelin [21], angiotensin [22], impaired endothelium dependent relaxation [23] and altered calcium homeostasis in vascular smooth muscle cells. Hypertension is established as an independent risk factor for cardiovascular mortality.

Thrombosis

After the introduction of rHuEPO, nephrologists observed an increase in thromboembolic events among dialysis patients. It has been known that EPO increases platelet aggregability and may decrease proteins C and S [24, 25]. The increased platelet aggregation appears to be mediated through tyrosine phosphorylation [24], but can be easily reversed by aspirin [26]. Hemodialysis vascular access thrombosis is not prevented by aspirin, and there are no published studies to examine whether cardiovascular outcomes in patients receiving ESAs are improved with aspirin therapy. The exact mechanism by which rHuEPO increases the risk of vascular access thrombosis is unclear, but it is thought to be secondary to increased blood viscosity as seen in polycythemia.

Target Hemoglobin for Anemia of Chronic Kidney Disease

When rHuEPO was approved by the FDA in 1989 for treatment of anemia in dialysis patients, the goal was to improve quality of life, decrease transfusion requirements, and prevent the iron overload that resulted from multiple transfusions. The initial post-approval Hb target was 9–10 g/dL although pre-approval studies had a Hb goal >11 g/dl [27]. When first NKF-DOQI guidelines were released in 1997, the Hb goal was increased to 11–12 g/dl. This was followed by increased rHuEPO usage and the Centers for Medicare and Medicaid Services instituted a clinical performance quality measure to target 80% of dialysis patients with Hb $\geq$ 11 g/dl [28].

In the 1990s, as experience with rHuPEO grew, questions arose whether complete normalization of the Hb to 14 g/dL or the hematocrit (Hct) to 42% could provide additional clinical benefit. The Normal Hematocrit Cardiovascular Trial (NHCT) enrolled 1233 patients with clinical evidence of congestive heart failure or ischemic heart disease that were undergoing dialysis and receiving maintenance rHuEPO therapy [29]. Patients were randomly assigned to receive increasing doses of epoetin alfa to reach and maintain a "normal" Hct value of 42 $\pm$ 3% or to continue to receive epoetin alfa therapy to maintain a Hct value of 30 $\pm$ 3%. The trial was halted after an interim analysis showing at a median follow-up time of 14 months, 33% of patients in the "normal" Hct group had died or had a nonfatal myocardial infarction, as compared with 27% of those in the low Hct group (risk ratio 1.3; 95% confidence interval [CI] 0.9–1.9). The patients with higher target Hct also had a higher incidence of vascular access thrombosis. After NHCT, there were many smaller randomized control trials in dialysis and CKD patients; these did not show increased mortality with higher target Hb levels. A major ground-breaking change came in 1996 with the publication of two clinical trials: Cardiovascular Risk Reduction by Early Anemia Treatment with Epoetin (CREATE) [30] and Correction of Hemoglobin and Outcomes in Renal Insufficiency (CHOIR) [31].

The CREATE study randomly assigned 603 patients with estimated glomerular filtration rate (GFR) 15–35 ml/min/1.73 m^2 and baseline Hb 11–12.5 g/dL to one of the two groups. Group 1 patients were immediately treated with rHuEPO to target Hb of 13–15 g/dl. Group 2 patients were treated only when Hb fell to <10.5 g/dl with target of 10.5–11.5 g/dl. There was no difference in primary cardiovascular end points between the groups. Although rate of decline of GFR was similar in both groups, a greater percentage of patients required dialysis in group 1 [30].

Table 11.2 Large randomized controlled trails of erythropoiesis-stimulating agents in anemia of chronic kidney disease

	NHCT [29]	CREATE [30]	CHOIR [31]	TREAT [32]
Published	1998	2006	2006	2009
Centers	USA	Europe	USA	International
Agent	Epoetin alfa	Epoetin alfa	Epoetin alfa	Darbepoetin alfa
Dialysis	Yes	No	No	No
CKD	No	yes	Yes	Yes
Number of patients	1223	603	1432	4038
High Hb target (g/dl)	14	13–15	13.5	13
Low Hb target (g/dl)	10	10.5–11.5	11.3	9
CV endpoints	RR +1.3 in high Hct group	No difference	Higher in high Hb group	No difference except stroke in high Hb group

CKD chronic kidney disease, *CV* cardiovascular, *RR* relative risk, *Hb* hemoglobin

The Correction of Hemoglobin and Outcomes in Renal Insufficiency (CHOIR) study included 1432 patients with CKD stages 3–4 and Hb < 11 g/dL [31]. Patients were randomized to target Hb of 11.3 versus 13.5 g/dl. The CHOIR trial was also terminated after an interim analysis. After a median follow-up period of 16 months, the composite end point including death, myocardial infarction, hospitalization for congestive heart failure, or stroke had occurred in 17.5% of patients in the high Hb target group and in 13.5% of patients in the low Hb target group (hazard ratio 1.34; 95% CI 1.03–1.74; P = 0.03) [31].

Based on the results of CHOIR and CREATE, FDA changed package insert for epoetin alfa and darbepoetin alfa adding a warning regarding the risk of death and serious cardiovascular events when an ESA is administered to achieve a target Hb of 13.5–14.5 versus 10–11.3 g/dl. The FDA product information for these agents also recommended individualizing the therapy to achieve and maintain Hb target of 10–12 g/dl.

The Trial to Reduce Cardiovascular Events with Aranesp Therapy (TREAT), published in 2009 [32], enrolled 4038 patients with CKD stages 3–4, type 2 diabetes, and baseline Hb < 11 g/dL; 2012 received darbepoetin alfa, and 2026 received placebo with darbepoetin rescue if Hb fell below 9 g/dL. The median achieved Hb levels were 12.5 g/dL in the darbepoetin alfa group and 10.6 g/dL the placebo group. The median follow-up time was 29 months; there was no evidence of benefit and a trend toward overall harm with darbepoetin alfa. Death or a nonfatal cardiovascular event occurred in 31.4% of patients receiving darbepoetin alfa and 29.7% of patients receiving placebo. There was higher rate of thromboembolic events in the darbepoetin alfa group. Based on the results of TREAT, the FDA changed product information on epoetin and darbepoetin in 2011, eliminating the target Hb range of 10–12 g/dl and adding a black box warning regarding the risk of death, myocardial infarction, stroke, venous thromboembolism, thrombosis of vascular access and tumor progression and recurrence. The findings of the NHCT, CHOIR, CREATE and TREAT studies are summarized in Table 11.2. The timeline of clinical and regulatory changes impacting on ESA use among CKD/ESKD patients in the US is summarized in Table 11.3. The 2013 Kidney Disease Improving Global Outcomes (KDIGO) recommendations regarding ESA use in patients with anemia associated with CKD are summarized in Table 11.4.

Potential Mechanism of Increased Cardiovascular Risk with High Hb Targets in Studies

It is not possible from the data published in the above mentioned studies to determine the relative quantitative importance of increased Hb itself versus the amount of ESA used and/or iron treatment as playing a causative role in the risk of adverse cardiovascular outcomes from higher target Hb levels. Since the intention to treat (ITT) analyses are based on target Hb level, it can be concluded that the association between higher target (not achieved) Hb levels is cause and effect. However, secondary analyses of both NHCT and CHOIR noted that patients randomized to the higher target Hb arms that required the highest ESA doses and failed to achieve the target Hb level had worse cardiovascular outcomes than those patients who succeeded in

Table 11.3 Timeline of clinical and regulatory changes for the use of ESAS in patients with CKD/ESRD in the US

1989	rHuEPO approved by the FDA rHuEPO reimbursed at $40 (USD) per treatment for dialysis patients, irrespective of dose
1991	rHuEPO reimbursed at $11 (USD) per 1000 U for dialysis patients
1997	Original NKF/DOQI anemia guidelines published with target Hct 33–36% for patients receiving rHuPEO Medicare denies payment for rHuEPO if 3 month avg. Hct > 36%
1998	Medicare denies rHuEPO payment if 3 month avg. Hct > 36.5%
2001	Revised NKF/KDOQI anemia guidelines published with target Hb 11–12 g/dL for patients receiving rHuEPO
2006	Newly revised NKF/KDOQI anemia guidelines published with target Hb 11–13 g/dL for patients receiving ESAs Medicare denies ESA payment if Hct > 39% without modifier CHOIR and CREATE studies published Congress holds hearings on ESA use in ESRD
2007	FDA issues "black box" warning on ESAs NKF/KDOQI revises guideline regarding target Hb range to 10–12 g/dL Medicare reduces ESA payment by 50% if Hb > 13 g/dL ×3 month
2008	New clinical performance measures for anemia management in ESRD patents with Hb target of 10–12 g/dL for patients receiving ESAs
2009	TREAT study published
2011	Bundled composite rate payment for dialysis including ESAs Payment for performance for anemia management with penalty for Hb < 10 or >12 g/dL for payment year 2012 for ESRD patients FDA changes ESA warning to decrease or discontinue drug when Hb approaches 11 g/dL and to use lowest dose needed to avoid transfusion Payment for performance for anemia management eliminates penalty for Hb < 10 g/dL for payment year 2013 and beyond for ESRD patients
2013	KDIGO anemia guidelines recommend initiating ESA when Hb 9–10 g/dL and target Hb level no greater than 11.5 g/dL
2015	Payment for performance for anemia management eliminates penalty for Hb > 12 g/dL for payment year 2017 and beyond for ESRD patients

CKD chronic kidney disease, *ESRD* end stage renal disease, *rHuEPO* recombinant human erythropoietin, *FDA* Food and Drug Administration, *NKF* National Kidney Foundation, *DOQI* Dialysis Outcomes Quality Initiative, *KDOQI* Kidney Disease Outcomes Quality Initiative, *Hct* hematocrit, *Hb* hemoglobin, *ESA* erythropoiesis stimulating agent, *CHOIR* Correction of Hemoglobin and Outcomes in Renal Insufficiency, *CREATE* Cardiovascular Risk Reduction by Early Anemia Treatment with Epoetin Beta, *TREAT* Trial to Reduce Cardiovascular Events with Aranesp Therapy, *KDIGO* Kidney Disease Improving Global Outcomes

achieving the higher target Hb levels with the lowest Hb doses. An FDA analysis of NHCT and CHOIR found the ITT association between Hct/Hb target and adverse outcomes to be misleading. There was actually an inverse relationship between achieved Hb level and adverse outcomes in both studies. There was a significant association between outcome and the rate of rise of Hb in both arms of both studies, with the "sweet spot" of fewest adverse events occurring in patients with a Hb rise of 0.25 g/dL per week or around 1 g/dL per month. Patients whose Hb rose or fell >0.5 g/dl per week had the worse outcomes in every group [33]. Szczech et al. revealed in a secondary analysis of CHOIR that when the data are adjusted for EPO dose and patients not achieving the Hb target, the differences in outcomes between the patients in the high and low target Hb arms becomes insignificant. The use of a high dose of ESA becomes the major predictor of adverse events in both groups [34]. These analyses suggest an association (but not cause and effect since they were not part of the ITT analysis) between higher ESA doses and adverse cardiovascular outcomes. The numerous factors which may play a role in increasing cardiovascular risk among patients treated with ESAs are summarized in Fig. 11.1. These factors interact amongst each other, and there is no certainty as to any one single mechanism of increased risk.

Role of Higher Hb Level

Reduction in oxygen-carrying capacity with the development of anemia induces compensatory mechanisms, including systemic vasodilation and increased cardiac output. Both left ventricular mass and end-diastolic volume increase in response to anemia. With the correction of

Table 11.4 Highlights of 2013 KDIGO anemia guidelines with regards to ESA use

• Address all correctable causes of anemia before initiation of ESA therapy
• Balance the potential benefits of reducing blood transfusions and anemia-related symptoms against the risks of harm
– Stroke
– Vascular access loss
– Hypertension
• Use ESAs with great caution in patients with active malignancy when cure is the anticipated outcome
• To avoid having the Hb level fall below 9.0 g/dL, start ESA therapy when the Hb level is 9–10 g/dL
• Individualization of therapy is reasonable as some patients may have improvement in QOL at higher Hb levels and their ESA therapy may be started at Hgb levels above 10 g/dL
• In general, ESAs should not be used to maintain Hb levels of >11.5 g/dL
• Individualization of therapy will be necessary as some patients may have improvements in QOL at Hb levels >11.5 g/dL
• ESAs should not be used to intentionally increase the Hb level to >13 g/dL
• Determine the initial ESA dose based on patient's Hb level, body weight and clinical status
• ESA dose adjustments should be made based on:
– Hb level
– Rate of change of Hb level
– Current ESA dose
– Clinical circumstances
• Decrease ESA dose in preference to withholding dose
• Reevaluate ESA dose if patient has an ESA-related event or has an illness that may cause ESA hyporesponsiveness

KDIGO Kidney Disease Outcomes Quality Initiative, *ESA* erythropoiesis stimulating agent, *ESA* erythropoiesis stimulating agent, *Hb* hemoglobin

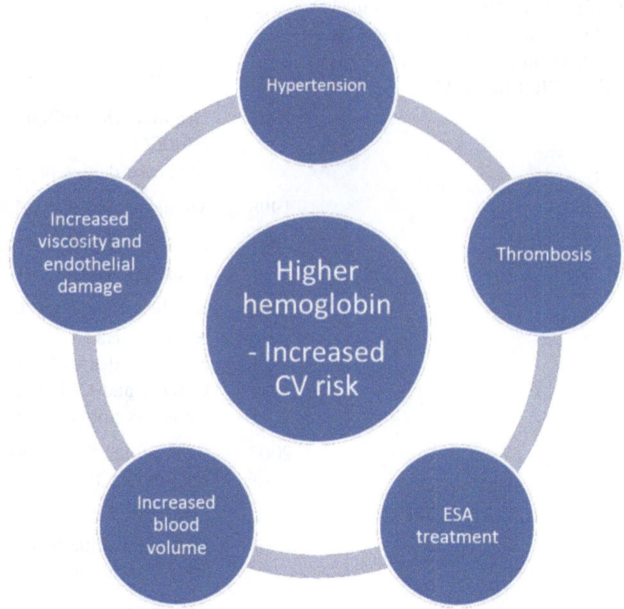

Fig. 11.1 Possible mechanism of increased cardiovascular risk with higher hemoglobin targets. *CV* cardiovascular, *ESA* erythropoiesis stimulating agent

anemia in patients with advanced CKD, there is increased blood volume; this can have negative effect on LVEF and function [35]. For cardiac function to improve with anemia correction, blood volume needs to be managed. Relative hypervolemia may be one of the mechanisms for increased blood pressure (BP) with ESA use.

As anemia is corrected with ESA treatment, the rise in Hb is associated with increased blood viscosity. The relationship between viscosity and Hb level is not linear; viscosity increases slowly until Hct increases to 40–50%, at which point it inflects sharply higher. At very high Hb levels, as seen in states of primary or secondary erythrocytosis, shear stress produces endothelial injury that may result in increased risk for vascular thrombosis [31, 36]. Patients with kidney disease and atherosclerosis may have multiple areas of unstable atherosclerotic plaque and/or ulcerations that are vulnerable to increased viscosity-associated sheer stress.

With correction of anemia, dialysis induced hemoconcentration poses risk for thrombosis. The Hb levels on the non-dialysis day results in a spuriously low measured Hb concentration but the pre-dialysis Hb value is used to adjust ESA dosage. Because Hb targets tend to be the same in patients on hemodialysis (HD) and those with nondialysis CKD, actual time-averaged Hb levels are actually raised to a greater extent in HD patients. Hemoconcentration will be greater in patients with higher Hb resulting in vascular stress on the blood vessels. This is more relevant in patients with increased interdialytic weight gain.

Another effect of increasing Hb and correcting anemia is to improve platelet function and number; this comes with a consequence. Up to 11% of patients experience clotting of dialyzers or blood lines after ESA therapy and, depending on the type of membranes used, the heparin requirements at final target Hb of 10–12.5 g/dL have to be increased by 50% [37]. At higher Hb targets in CKD, the increased platelet function could increase platelet exposure and activation at areas of vascular plaque and injury, thereby increasing risk for thrombosis. It should be noted there is no increase in mortality among HD patients with "natural" Hb levels >12 g/dL not requiring ESA therapy [38].

Role of ESA Dose in Increased Cardiovascular Mortality

A second hypothesis is that some aspect of anemia therapy itself, the amount of ESA used and/or iron treatment, may play a causative role in increased mortality risk. Most of the Hb target studies in HD used epoetin alfa, which is very similar in structure and function to native EPO. EPO is continuously secreted under normal physiological conditions. In the anemic state, EPO levels remain chronically elevated. Treatment with ESA results in serum EPO kinetics that are different from normal physiology. With ESA treatment there is very rapid rise in serum levels after injection, a high peak serum concentration, and rapid decline in level which in some patients is to very low serum concentrations [39]. The potential risks are mediated by protective effects of EPO on non-erythroid receptors, particularly in the central nervous system, spinal cord, retina, vasculature, and heart, where EPO acts in a paracrine manner [40]. As the dose required for this effect is much more than used in treatment of anemia, sufficient levels are not achieved. Using US Renal Data System administrative claims data, a retrospective cohort study of 94,569 prevalent HD patients in 2000 and 2001 showed that epoetin alfa dosage requirement was an independent predictor of total mortality in HD patients after adjustment for Hct and other variables [41]. Patients who were administered higher dosages of epoetin had significantly lower Hct values and greater mortality rates. Bradbury et al. retrospectively examined 22,995 patients in a large dialysis organization and found increased mortality risk of 1.31 per log unit increase in EPO dose in an unadjusted model and 1.21 per long unit increase in EPO dose in case-mix adjusted model, both statistically significant. However, in lagged time-dependent analyses, the increase in mortality risk was no longer statistically significant. The authors caution against drawing any conclusions regarding the relationship between EPO dose, Hb level and mortality in nonexperimental studies [42]. Because of the effect of confounding by indication, namely that patients requiring higher ESA doses could be ESA resistant due to an underling inflammatory state which may in itself increase the risk of cardiovascular disease, it remains uncertain whether the ESA dose has effects on cardiovascular mortality. Indeed, using a marginal structural model which attempts to eliminate time-dependent confounding by indication, Wang and al demonstrated that higher EPO dose is not associated with increased mortality [43].

Using a metaregression analysis, Koulouridis et al. examined 33 trials of ESA treatment of anemia in patients with CKD regardless of dialysis status [44]. Higher total-study-period mean ESA dose was associated with increased rate of hypertension, stroke, and thrombotic events, including dialysis vascular access-related thrombotic events, independent of Hb level. All-cause mortality was associated with higher first 3-month mean ESA dose and higher total-study period mean ESA dose; both remained significant after adjusting for target Hb level.

A natural experiment regarding the relationship between ESA dose and clinical outcomes examined 62,710 HD patients treated with either subcutaneously (SC) or intravenously (IV) administered EPO between 1997 and 2005 per facility protocol [45]. The patients receiving IV EPO required a 25% higher average EPO dose to achieve an equivalent Hb response as the SC group. Relative risk for significant adverse event composite outcomes was 1.11 in the IV group (CI 1.04–1.08), suggesting an association between higher EPO dose and adverse outcomes. These data raise the hypothesis that the adverse cardiovascular effects of ESAs may be related to their pharmacokinetics (e.g. peak plasma concentration, which is higher when the drug is administered IV) as well as to the total dose administered.

Role of Hypertension

One of the modifiable factors for cardiovascular risk reduction is the control of BP. This particularly relevant in CKD patients as they have high prevalence of cardiovascular disease and increased incidence of sudden cardiac death. The reporting of BP from the major trials has been sparse. The initial CHOIR study report did not contain information on BP. However in a secondary analysis of CHOIR participants, higher Hb targets, increases in ESA dose and in achieved Hb levels were associated both with increases in diastolic BP and with higher event rates; however, increasing diastolic BP was not associated with adverse outcomes [46]. The CREATE study demonstrated an approximate 52% increase in risk for increased BP in the 13- to 15-g/dL target group. The initial report of the NHCT did not indicate an increase in BP in the normal Hct target group.

Role of Iron and Thrombocytosis

Streja et al. conducted a logistic regression and survival analysis in a retrospective cohort of long-term HD patients to examine their hypothesis that the induced iron depletion with reactive thrombocytosis may be a possible contributor to the association between high ESA dose-associated Hb level of >13 g/dL and mortality. They found that a prescribed EPO dose of >20,000 U/week was associated with a greater risk of iron depletion (transferrin saturation [TSAT] <20%, case-mix adjusted odds ratio 2.53; 95% CI 2.37–2.69), relative thrombocytosis (platelet count >300,000, case-mix adjusted odds ratio 1.37, 95% CI 1.30–1.42) and increased 3 year mortality (death rate ratio 1.59, 95% CI 1.54–1.65); all $p < 0.001$ [47]. In an accompanying editorial Littlewood [48] pointed out that reports have demonstrated similar findings in anemic patients undergoing cancer chemotherapy receiving ESAs; patients not receiving supplemental iron were more likely to develop thrombocytosis (platelet count >350,000) which was associated with a fourfold increase in thrombotic events. The editorial cited observational data demonstrating a link between low TSAT and decreased survival in patients with CKD, but appropriately noted that this may be a reflection of underling inflammatory illness resulting in impaired iron mobilization. Littlewood's conclusion is that the mechanism for the increased mortality among CKD patients receiving ESAs with target Hb > 13 g/dL remains uncertain, but reactive thrombosis from iron deficiency could be a contributing factor in some patients.

Future of the Anemia Treatment in Patients with Chronic Kidney Disease

Studies have demonstrated that treating anemia related to kidney disease with EPO increases Hb levels, reduces transfusion requirements, and improves the quality of life (QOL) [49]. However, clinical events related to higher Hb targets in some trials have included higher vascular access thrombosis, cerebrovascular events, cardiovascular events, earlier need for renal replacement therapy and higher mortality [30, 31]. As a result of these studies, the FDA recommends in its product information for ESAs that treatment be initiated only when the Hb level is <10 g/dL, the rate of Hb decline indicates the likelihood of the patient requiring a red blood cell (RBC) transfusion, and lowering the risk of alloimmunization and/or RBC transfusion risk is a goal. The FDA further recommends that if the Hb level exceeds 10 g/dL the ESA dose should be reduced or interrupted and the lowest dose used sufficient to reduce the need for RBC transfusions. These recommendations, as well as those by the Kidney Disease Outcomes Quality Initiative (KDOQI) in the United States and the Kidney Disease Improving Global Outcomes (KDIGO) international initiative have significantly curtailed ESA use and led to lower Hb targets among patients with CKD-related anemia since 2011. In its commentary on the 2012 KDIGO clinical practice guideline for anemia in CKD, KDOQI workgroup members found a paucity of evidence that Hb targets between 11 and 11.5 g/dL are associated with a safety risk [50].

Nonetheless, ESA use among anemic patients with non-dialysis CKD has significantly decreased due to safety concerns from the clinical trials and the imposition of lower Hb targets by prescription drug plans; the ESA use among dialysis patients has significantly decreased since 2011 due to safety concerns from the clinical trials, FDA warnings, inclusion of ESAs into a bundled payment system to dialysis facilities and, for payment years 2012–2016, a financial penalty to dialysis providers for having an excessive percentage of patients with Hb > 12 g/dL who are receiving ESAs. Between the onset of a bundled payment system for dialysis in the US in January 2011 and June 2015, mean monthly EPO doses received (90 day average) for dialysis patients decreased from 16,036 to 9618 U and mean Hb levels decreased from 11.48 to 10.82 g/dL. This has been accompanied by a modest increase in SC ESA administration (1.5–4.5%) and a modest decrease in mean monthly (90 day average) IV iron dose (292–247 mg) [51]. In a retrospective analysis of anemia management of ESRD patients in the US before and after the aforementioned regulatory and payment changes, Chertow et al. [49] examined outcomes between patients treated 2005–2010 and 2011–2012. During 2012 observed rates of stroke, venous thromboembolic disease and heart failure were lower than expected (accounting for secular trends and case-mix), but there was no change from expected in the observed rates of all-cause mortality, cardiovascular mortality, and myocardial infarction as the result of efforts taken to mitigate risks associated with ESA use and changes in payment policy.

A novel approach to the treatment of EPO deficiency in anemic patients with CKD is the use of agents which stimulate endogenous EPO production in renal and non-renal tissues. Such a strategy might decrease adverse outcomes by allowing for a more continuous physiologic level of EPO to stimulate RBC production rather than the high intermittent blood levels of ESA that result from pharmacological administration of an exogenous ESA. One such class of agents is those that stabilize hypoxia inducible factor (HIF) by inhibiting the prolyl hydroxylase (PH) enzyme which leads to the rapid degradation of HIF in absence of tissue hypoxia. HIF directly stimulates EPO gene transcription and indirectly decreases hepcidin levels. Hepcidin is thought to be responsible for impaired iron mobilization in the setting of inflammation, so its suppression by HIF-PH inhibitors allows for more effective erythropoiesis. Several versions of HIF-PH inhibitors are currently under investigation. Results of phase 2 studies of these oral agents have demonstrated a dose-dependent increase in Hb levels among CKD patients with anemia, decreased hepcidin levels, and evidence of improved iron mobilization [38, 52]. Mean peak serum EPO levels were 600 mIU/mL in screened patients receiving EPO to achieve target Hb level compared to 100 mIU/mL in patients receiving the HIF-PH inhibitor to the same target Hb level. Phase 3 studies of these agents are expected to last 3 years to ascertain whether there are any safety signals and whether cardiovascular outcomes are improved by the lower peak serum EPO levels.

In conclusion, although ESAs remain a godsend to dialysis patients and very few nephrologists would wish to return to the pre-1989 era of transfusion-dependence, the illusion that these agents would be devoid of adverse effects was naive and ignored the history of all other therapeutic agents. The lesson learned is that every pharmacologic agent, even one that is close to identical to a naturally occurring protein, has a therapeutic window above which untoward events can occur. The 40% decrease in mean ESA dosing between 2011 and 2015 among dialysis patients in the US with only a 0.7 g/dL decrease in mean Hb level is a demonstration that more effective anemia management strategies can be achieved that may put patients at less risk for adverse cardiovascular outcomes. Although a number of mechanisms link ESA doses, higher Hb targets and adverse cardiovascular outcomes based on physiology and the results of clinical trials, the confounding of these factors in clinical practice makes it impossible to be certain how to change practice to improve outcomes. The common denominator in all studies, both prospective and retrospective, is that the patients who are the most ESA resistant (highest ESA doses and lowest achieved Hb levels) are at the greatest risk for adverse outcomes, so it seems prudent to consider less aggressive ESA doses in such patients even if that increases the likelihood of transfusion.

References

1. Takeuchi M, Kobata A. Structures and functional roles of the sugar chains of human erythropoietins. Glycobiology. 1991;1(4):337–46.
2. Bonsdorff E. On the presence of erythropoietins in the plasma from sheep foetuses during the latter half of gestation. Acta Physiol Scand. 1949;18(1):51–62.
3. Fisher JW. Erythropoietin: physiology and pharmacology update. Exp Biol Med (Maywood). 2003;228(1):1–14.
4. Erslev A. Humoral regulation of red cell production. Blood. 1953;8(4):349–57.
5. Adamson JW, Eschbach JW. Management of the anaemia of chronic renal failure with recombinant erythropoietin. Q J Med. 1989;73(272):1093–101.
6. Jelkmann W. Regulation of erythropoietin production. J Physiol. 2011;589(Pt 6):1251–8.
7. Jacobson LO, Goldwasser E, Fried W, Plzak L. Role of the kidney in erythropoiesis. Nature. 1957;179(4560):633–4.
8. Lacombe C, Da Silva JL, Bruneval P, Fournier JG, Wendling F, Casadevall N, et al. Peritubular cells are the site of erythropoietin synthesis in the murine hypoxic kidney. J Clin Invest. 1988;81(2):620–3.
9. Schuster SJ, Koury ST, Bohrer M, Salceda S, Caro J. Cellular sites of extrarenal and renal erythropoietin production in anaemic rats. Br J Haematol. 1992;81(2):153–9.
10. Sawada K, Krantz SB, Dai CH, Koury ST, Horn ST, Glick AD, et al. Purification of human blood burst-forming units-erythroid and demonstration of the evolution of erythropoietin receptors. J Cell Physiol. 1990;142(2):219–30.
11. Constantinescu SN, Keren T, Socolovsky M, Nam H, Henis YI, Lodish HF. Ligand-independent oligomerization of cell-surface erythropoietin receptor is mediated by the transmembrane domain. Proc Natl Acad Sci USA. 2001;98(8):4379–84.
12. Hirota K, Semenza GL. Regulation of angiogenesis by hypoxia-inducible factor 1. Crit Rev Oncol Hematol. 2006;59(1):15–26.
13. Fukuda R, Zhang H, Kim JW, Shimoda L, Dang CV, Semenza GL. HIF-1 regulates cytochrome oxidase subunits to optimize efficiency of respiration in hypoxic cells. Cell. 2007;129(1):111–22.
14. Carlini RG, Gupta A, Liapis H, Rothstein M. Endothelin-1 release by erythropoietin involves calcium signaling in endothelial cells. J Cardiovasc Pharmacol. 1995;26(6):889–92.
15. Grimm C, Wenzel A, Groszer M, Mayser H, Seeliger M, Samardzija M, et al. HIF-1-induced erythropoietin in the hypoxic retina protects against light-induced retinal degeneration. Nat Med. 2002;8(7):718–24.
16. Heeschen C, Aicher A, Lehmann R, Fichtlscherer S, Vasa M, Urbich C, et al. Erythropoietin is a potent physiologic stimulus for endothelial progenitor cell mobilization. Blood. 2003;102(4):1340–6.
17. Cai Z, Manalo DJ, Wei G, Rodriguez ER, Fox-Talbot K, Lu H, et al. Hearts from rodents exposed to intermittent hypoxia or erythropoietin are protected against ischemia–reperfusion injury. Circulation. 2003;108(1):79–85.
18. Lipsic E, van der Meer P, Henning RH, Suurmeijer AJ, Boddeus KM, van Veldhuisen DJ, et al. Timing of erythropoietin treatment for cardioprotection in ischemia/reperfusion. J Cardiovasc Pharmacol. 2004;44(4):473–9.
19. Fishbane S, Besarab A. Mechanism of increased mortality risk with erythropoietin treatment to higher hemoglobin targets. Clin J Am Soc Nephrol. 2007;2(6):1274–82.
20. Pascual J, Teruel JL, Ortuno J. Hypertensive effect of erythropoietin. Ann Intern Med. 1991;114(12):1063.
21. Carlini RG, Dusso AS, Obialo CI, Alvarez UM, Rothstein M. Recombinant human erythropoietin (rHuEPO) increases endothelin-1 release by endothelial cells. Kidney Int. 1993;43(5):1010–4.
22. Kuriyama S, Tomonari H, Tokudome G, Kaguchi Y, Hayashi H, Kobayashi H, et al. Association of angiotensinogen gene polymorphism with erythropoietin-induced hypertension: a preliminary report. Hypertens Res. 2001;24(5):501–5.
23. Wada Y, Matsuoka H, Tamai O, Kohno K, Okuda S, Imaizumi T. Erythropoietin impairs endothelium-dependent vasorelaxation through cyclooxygenase-dependent mechanisms in humans. Am J Hypertens. 1999;12(10 Pt 1):980–7.
24. Diaz-Ricart M, Etebanell E, Cases A, Lopez-Pedret J, Castillo R, Ordinas A, et al. Erythropoietin improves signaling through tyrosine phosphorylation in platelets from uremic patients. Thromb Haemost. 1999;82(4):1312–7.
25. Jaar B, Denis A, Viron B, Verdy E, Chamma F, Siohan P, et al. Effects of long-term treatment with recombinant human erythropoietin on physiologic inhibitors of coagulation. Am J Nephrol. 1997;17(5):399–405.
26. Taylor JE, Henderson IS, Stewart WK, Belch JJ. Erythropoietin and spontaneous platelet aggregation in haemodialysis patients. Lancet. 1991;338(8779):1361–2.
27. Eschbach JW, Downing MR, Egrie JC, Browne JK, Adamson JW. USA multicenter clinical trial with recombinant human erythropoietin (Amgen). Results in hemodialysis patients. Contrib Nephrol. 1989;76:160–5 discussion 212–8.
28. National Kidney Foundation - Dialysis Outcomes Quality Initiative. NKF-DOQI clinical practice guidelines for the treatment of anemia of chronic renal failure. Am J Kidney Dis. 1997;30(4 Suppl 3):S192–240.
29. Besarab A, Bolton WK, Browne JK, Egrie JC, Nissenson AR, Okamoto DM, et al. The effects of normal as compared with low hematocrit values in patients with cardiac disease who are receiving hemodialysis and epoetin. N Engl J Med. 1998;339(9):584–90.
30. Drueke TB, Locatelli F, Clyne N, Eckardt KU, Macdougall IC, Tsakiris D, et al. Normalization of hemoglobin level in patients with chronic kidney disease and anemia. N Engl J Med. 2006;355(20):2071–84.
31. Singh AK, Szczech L, Tang KL, Barnhart H, Sapp S, Wolfson M, et al. Correction of anemia with epoetin alfa in chronic kidney disease. N Engl J Med. 2006;355(20):2085–98.

32. Pfeffer MA, Burdmann EA, Chen CY, Cooper ME, de Zeeuw D, Eckardt KU, et al. A trial of darbepoetin alfa in type 2 diabetes and chronic kidney disease. N Engl J Med. 2009;361(21):2019–32.
33. FDA Advisory Committee Briefing Document Joint meeting of the Cardiovascular and Renal Drugs Advisory Committee and the Drug Safety Risk Management Committee. [cited 2016 Feb 14]. Available from: http://www.fda.gov/ohrms/dockets/ac/07/briefing/2007–4315b1–01-FDA.pdf.
34. Szczech LA, Barnhart HX, Inrig JK, Reddan DN, Sapp S, Califf RM, et al. Secondary analysis of the CHOIR trial epoetin-alpha dose and achieved hemoglobin outcomes. Kidney Int. 2008;74(6):791–8.
35. Anand IS, Chandrashekhar Y, Wander GS, Chawla LS. Endothelium-derived relaxing factor is important in mediating the high output state in chronic severe anemia. J Am Coll Cardiol. 1995;25(6):1402–7.
36. Weiskopf RB, Feiner J, Hopf H, Viele MK, Watson JJ, Lieberman J, et al. Heart rate increases linearly in response to acute isovolemic anemia. Transfusion. 2003;43(2):235–40.
37. Schwartz AB, Prior JE, Mintz GS, Kim KE, Kahn SB. Cardiovascular hemodynamic effects of correction of anemia of chronic renal failure with recombinant-human erythropoietin. Transplant Proc. 1991;23(2):1827–30.
38. Besarab A, Chernyavskaya E, Motylev I, Shutov E, Kumbar LM, Gurevich K, et al. Roxadustat (FG-4592): correction of anemia in incident dialysis patients. J Am Soc Nephrol. 2016;27(4):1225–33.
39. Besarab A, Flaharty KK, Erslev AJ, McCrea JB, Vlasses PH, Medina F, et al. Clinical pharmacology and economics of recombinant human erythropoietin in end-stage renal disease: the case for subcutaneous administration. J Am Soc Nephrol. 1992;2 (9):1405–16.
40. Goodnough LT, Price TH, Parvin CA. The endogenous erythropoietin response and the erythropoietic response to blood loss anemia: the effects of age and gender. J Lab Clin Med. 1995;126(1):57–64.
41. Abraham PA, Opsahl JA, Keshaviah PR, Collins AJ, Whalen JJ, Asinger RW, et al. Body fluid spaces and blood pressure in hemodialysis patients during amelioration of anemia with erythropoietin. Am J Kidney Dis. 1990;16(5):438–46.
42. Bradbury BD, Fissell RB, Albert JM, Anthony MS, Critchlow CW, Pisoni RL, et al. Predictors of early mortality among incident US hemodialysis patients in the Dialysis Outcomes and Practice Patterns Study (DOPPS). Clin J Am Soc Nephrol. 2007;2(1):89–99.
43. Wang O, Kilpatrick RD, Critchlow CW, Ling X, Bradbury BD, Gilbertson DT, et al. Relationship between epoetin alfa dose and mortality: findings from a marginal structural model. Clin J Am Soc Nephrol. 2010;5(2):182–8.
44. Koulouridis I, Alfayez M, Trikalinos TA, Balk EM, Jaber BL. Dose of erythropoiesis-stimulating agents and adverse outcomes in CKD: a metaregression analysis. Am J Kidney Dis. 2013;61(1):44–56.
45. Wright DG, Wright EC, Narva AS, Noguchi CT, Eggers PW. Association of erythropoietin dose and route of administration with clinical outcomes for patients on hemodialysis in the United States. Clin J Am Soc Nephrol. 2015;10(10):1822–30.
46. Inrig JK, Sapp S, Barnhart H, Patel UD, Reddan D, Singh A, et al. Impact of higher hemoglobin targets on blood pressure and clinical outcomes: a secondary analysis of CHOIR. Nephrol Dial Transplant. 2012;27(9):3606–14.
47. Streja E, Kovesdy CP, Greenland S, Kopple JD, McAllister CJ, Nissenson AR, et al. Erythropoietin, iron depletion, and relative thrombocytosis: a possible explanation for hemoglobin-survival paradox in hemodialysis. Am J Kidney Dis. 2008;52(4):727–36.
48. Littlewood TJ. Intravenous or oral iron? Am J Hematol. 2012;87 (2):134–5.
49. Stone WJ, Graber SE, Krantz SB, Dessypris EN, O'Neil VL, Olsen NJ, et al. Treatment of the anemia of predialysis patients with recombinant human erythropoietin: a randomized, placebo-controlled trial. Am J Med Sci. 1988;296(3):171–9.
50. Kliger AS, Foley RN, Goldfarb DS, Goldstein SL, Johansen K, Singh A, et al. KDOQI US commentary on the 2012 KDIGO clinical practice guideline for anemia in CKD. Am J Kidney Dis. 2013;62(5):849–59.
51. Monitor DOaPPSDP. [cited 2016 Feb 14]. Available from: www.dopps.org/dpm.
52. Provenzano R, Besarab A, Wright S, Dua S, Zeig S, Nguyen P, et al. Roxadustat (FG-4592) versus epoetin alfa for anemia in patients receiving maintenance hemodialysis: a phase 2, randomized, 6- to 19-week, open-label, active-comparator, dose-ranging, safety and exploratory efficacy study. Am J Kidney Dis. 2016;67 (6):912–24.

Part III
Cardio-Renal Syndrome

12 Pathophysiology of the Cardiorenal Syndromes Types 1–5: Updates from the Eleventh Consensus Conference of the Acute Dialysis Quality Initiative (ADQI)

Luca Di Lullo, Antonio Bellasi, and Mario Cozzolino

Background

According to the recent definition proposed by the Consensus conference on Acute Dialysis Quality Initiative Group [1], the term cardiorenal syndrome (CRS) has been used to define different clinical conditions in which heart and kidney dysfunction overlap. The aim of this chapter is to provide a detailed outline of the pathophysiology of the subtypes of CRS, to help the cardiologist and nephrologist to be able to identify the clinical phenotypes of CRS, and to initiate appropriate therapy. The classification of CRS proposed in the Consensus Conference by the Acute Dialysis Quality Group essentially divides CRS into two main groups, cardiorenal and renocardiac CRS, on the basis of the primum movens of disease (cardiac or renal). Both cardiorenal and renocardiac CRS are then divided into acute and chronic, according to disease's acuity of onset. Type 5 of CRS integrates simultaneous cardiorenal involvement induced by systemic disease (Table 12.1).

Type 1 Cardiorenal Syndrome

Type 1 CRS occurs in about 25% of patients hospitalized for acute decompensated heart failure (ADHF) [2, 3]. Among these patients, underlying chronic kidney disease (CKD) is quite common and contributes to acute kidney injury (AKI) in 60% of all cases studied. AKI is an independent mortality risk factor in acute decompensated heart failure patients, including those with acute myocardial infarction (AMI) and/or reduced left ventricular ejection fraction [1].

Pathophysiology

Type 1 CRS (acute cardiorenal syndrome) is characterized by acute worsening of cardiac function leading to AKI [4, 5] in the setting of active cardiac disease such as ADHF. Preliminary observations highlight the importance of timing in the development of AKI and its early diagnosis (Fig. 12.1).

Hemodynamic mechanisms play a major role in type 1 CRS in presence of ADHF leading to decreased renal arterial flow and a consequent fall in glomerular filtration rate (GFR). Once hemodynamics have been restored, renal and cardiac parameters come back to normal [6]. Different hemodynamic profiles have been proposed [2]: In "cold" pattern patients, reduction in effective circulation fluid volume (ECFV) represents the main hemodynamic change, while there is a marked increase in central venous pressure (CVP) in "wet" pattern patients.

"Cold" patients also present with decrease in renal blood flow related to the renin–angiotensin–aldosterone system (RAAS) and systemic nervous system activation causing afferent vasoconstriction, decreased renal blood flow, and decreased effective glomerular perfusion pressure. Patients who present with a "wet" hemodynamic profile display increased pulmonary and/or systemic congestion. In these patients, high CVP directly affects renal vein and kidney perfusion pressure [3, 7]; CVP increase also results in increased interstitial pressure with tubular' collapse and progressive decline in GFR [8].

"Warm and wet" patients represent the most frequent profile in acute and chronic advanced heart failure [9, 10]. Mechanisms of increased CVP are quite similar to "cold" profile patients, but renal perfusion pressure is less affected because of higher arterial blood pressures [3].

L. Di Lullo (✉)
Department of Nephrology and Dialysis, L. Parodi-Delfino Hospital, Piazza Aldo Moro, 1, 00046 Colleferro, Rome, Italy
e-mail: dilullo.luca@inwind.it

A. Bellasi
Nephrology and Dialysis, S. Anna Hospital, Via Domea, 4, 22063 Cantù, Como, Italy
e-mail: antoniobellasi@gmail.com

M. Cozzolino
Department of Health Sciences, Hospital of San Paolo, University of Milan, Via Di Rudini, 8, 20142 Milan, Italy
e-mail: mario.cozzolino@unimi.it

J. Rangaswami et al. (eds.), *Cardio-Nephrology*,
DOI 10.1007/978-3-319-56042-7_12

Table 12.1 Classification of cardiorenal syndrome

Type	Denomination	Description	Example
1	Acute cardiorenal	Heart failure leading to AKI	Acute coronary syndrome leading to acute heart and kidney failure
2	Chronic cardiorenal	Chronic heart failure leading to CKD	Chronic heart failure
3	Acute nephrocardiac	AKD leading to acute heart failure	AKI-related uremic
4	Chronic nephrocardiac	CKD leading to heart failure	Left ventricular hypertrophy and diastolic heart failure due to CKD
5	Secondary	Systemic disease leading to heart and kidney failure	Sepsis, vasculitis, diabetes mellitus, amyloidosis

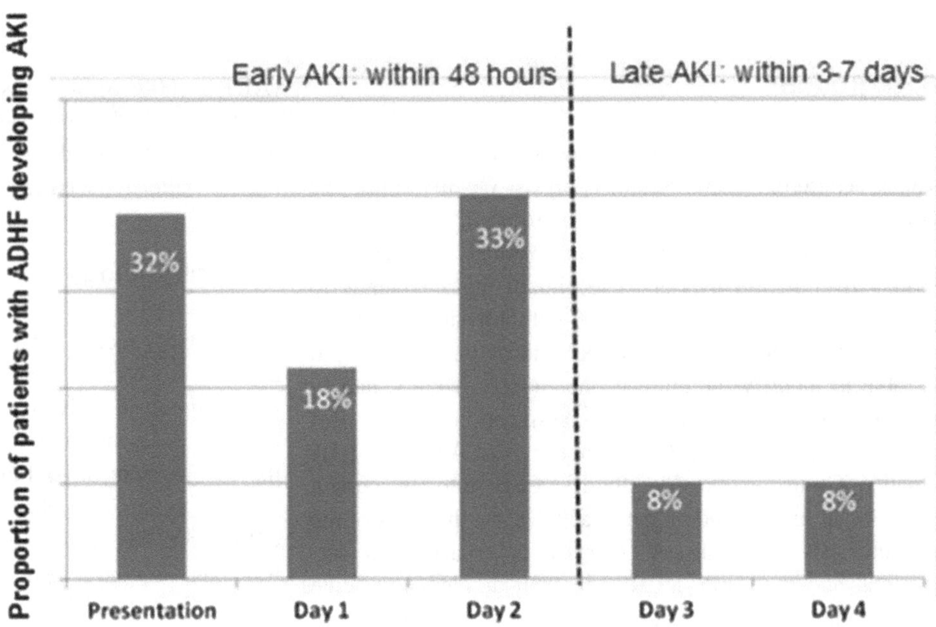

Fig. 12.1 Timing of acute kidney injury in the setting of acute decompensated heart failure

Non-hemodynamic mechanisms were also proposed as involved in type 1 CRS including sympathetic nervous system (SNS) and RAAS activation, chronic inflammation, and imbalance in the proportion of reactive oxygen species (ROS)/nitric oxide (NO) production (Fig. 12.2). Patients with ADHF show more frequently defective regulation of monocyte apoptosis and activation of inflammatory pathways compared with healthy subjects [11, 12].

Several pathophysiological processes contribute to perpetuating AKI, including endothelial and epithelial cell death, and a primary role for apoptotic mechanisms due to renal ischemia, toxic injury, radiation, and tubular obstruction has been suggested in experimental models [13].

Renal tubular epithelium is particularly vulnerable to ischemic injury resulting in cell death by apoptosis and necrosis with consequent loss of r epithelial cell structure and function [14]. Renal tubular cells represent major site of cell damage during AKI with strong associations between intrarenal inflammatory activity and renal cell apoptosis [15].

Sera from type 1 CRS patients' show high levels of proinflammatory cytokines and proapoptotic factors [16]. There are two main intracellular pathways for apoptosis (intrinsic and extrinsic), characterized by activation of different activator caspases [16] and linked by caspase-3 [16]. Cleavage of caspase-3 and its activation causes DNA fragmentation, demolition of cellular cytoskeletal, and nuclear proteins and consequent formation of apoptotic bodies [16, 17]. Fragmentation of renal tubular cells genomic DNA represents a biochemical hallmark of apoptosis, an irreversible process leading to cell's death [17]. The final pathway of apoptotic process is characterized by phagocytosis of apoptotic bodies [17].

Oxidative stress is a hallmark of type 1 CRS, as evidenced by a significant increase in circulating reactive oxygen species (ROS) and reactive nitrogen species (RNS), coupled with increased expression of interleukin-6 (IL-6). Increased levels of NADPH oxidase and myeloperoxidase (MPO), with upregulation of proinflammatory mediators via

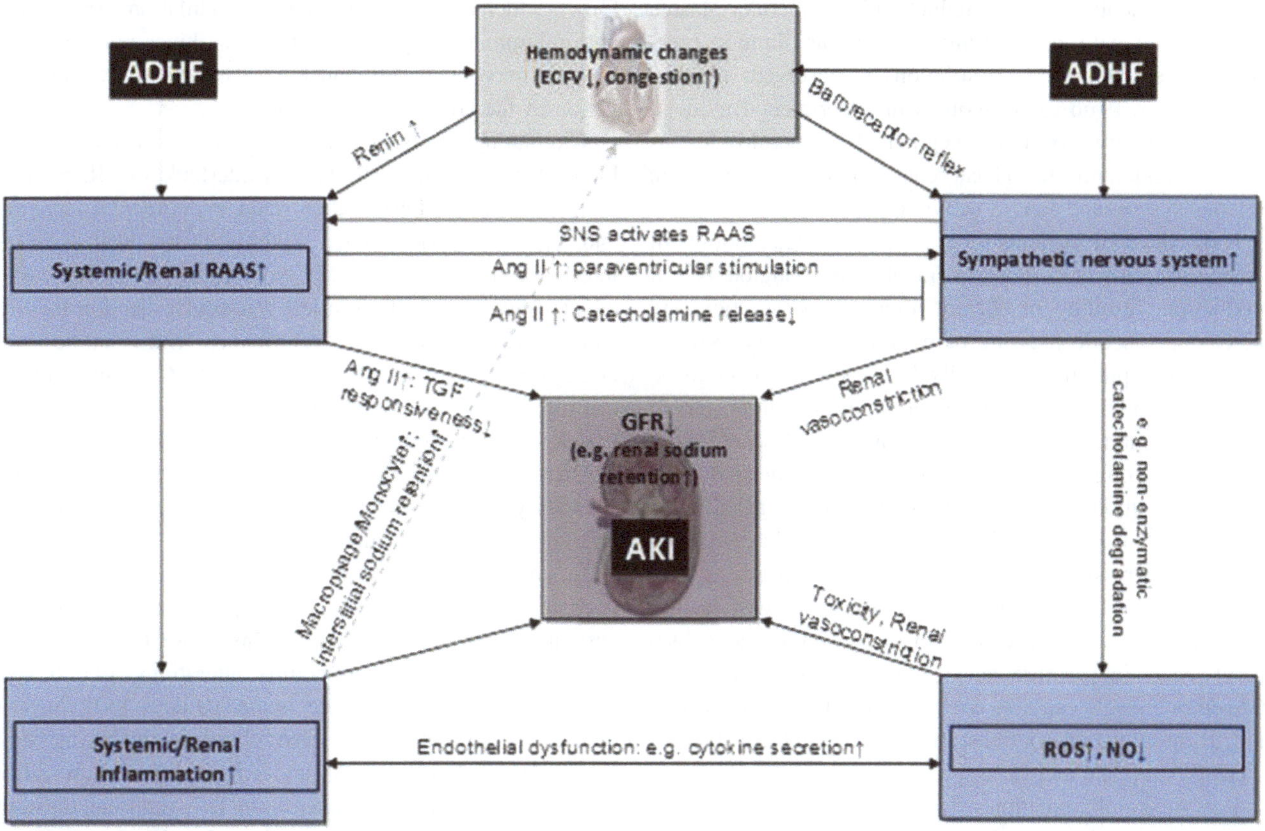

Fig. 12.2 Non-hemodynamic network of pathophysiological interactions in CRS type 1. Note the emerging potential role of macrophages/monocytes as mediator of sodium and fluid retention. Reproduced with permission from ADQI

powerful oxidants such as peroxynitrite, have also been recently demonstrated [18].

MPO acts as primary enzyme in ROS generation by promoting hydrogen peroxide (H_2O_2) conversion into nitrogen dioxide (NO_2) and other species involved in oxidative damage of several critical compounds (lipids, lipoproteins) implicated in the pathogenesis of atherosclerosis, cancer, diabetic vasculopathy, and CKD [18, 19]. Gut under-perfusion and endotoxin release in patients with ADHF have also been proposed as pathophysiologic mechanisms accelerating progression of HF and CRS [20].

Type 2 Cardiorenal Syndrome

Type 2 cardiorenal syndrome is characterized by chronic abnormalities in cardiac function leading to kidney injury or dysfunction. Chronic heart and kidney disease often coexist, but large cohort studies assessing the onset of one disease (e.g., chronic heart failure [HF]) subsequently describe the prevalence of the other (chronic kidney disease [CKD]) [21, 22]. CKD has been observed in 45–63% of CHF patients [21–23], but it is unclear how to classify these patients often including those ones shifting from a clinical condition of Type 1 CRS to distinguish these patients from Type 4 CRS (chronic renocardiac syndrome) [24].

Pathophysiology

Intrinsic to its definition, type 2 CRS is characterized by the development of CKD in HF patients, but two fundamental features are proposed: CHF and CKD are to be simultaneously present and CHF causally underlies CKD occurrence or progression [25]. Examples of type 2 CRS can be provided by "cyanotic nephropathy" occurring in patients with congenital heart disease, when heart disease clearly precedes kidney involvement or acute coronary syndrome leading to left ventricular dysfunction and onset/progression of co-existing CKD. Neuro-hormonal activation, renal hypoperfusion and venous congestion, inflammation, atherosclerosis, and oxidative stress represent most important pathophysiological mechanisms of type 2 CRS. These mechanisms are operative in recurrent episodes of acute heart and/or kidney decompensation, which are associated with HF and CKD progression [26].

In experimental studies, a reduction in glomerular plasma flow together with elevated intra-glomerular filtration pressure (efferent arteriolar constriction) is observed; if these changes persist (up to six months in experimental models) podocytes injury, focal and segmental glomerulosclerosis can occur, often related to local renal increase in sympathetic nervous system and RAAS activation [27].

Kidneys of HF patients seem to release large amounts of circulating renin with consequent abnormal angiotensin II production, resulting in efferent arteriolar constriction and increase in oncotic pressure of peritubular capillaries [28]. High venous pressure is described as a key factor in worsening GFR in HF patients, especially in those with preserved ejection fraction. Patients with decompensated heart failure and venous congestion often have t with significant RAAS activation without decreased circulating volume as stimulus [29]. Persistent RAAS and SNS activation could contribute to CKD progression in type 2 cardiorenal syndrome.

Angiotensin II production and aldosterone release lead to distal nephron-augmented sodium reabsorption and subsequent systemic pressure and volume overload. Increased aldosterone levels can also contribute to glomerular fibrosis due to upregulation of transforming growth factor-β[beta] (TGF-β[beta]) and increased secretion of fibronectin [30, 31].

Persistent inflammation triggered by ongoing cardiac decompensation is also responsible for CKD progression in ADHF [32].

Type 3 Cardiorenal Syndrome

Type 3 cardiorenal syndrome, also defined as acute renocardiac syndrome, occurs when acute kidney injury (AKI) contributes and/or precipitates development of acute cardiac injury. AKI may directly or indirectly produce an acute cardiac event; triggered by the inflammatory surge, oxidative stress, and secretion of neurohormones following AKI [33, 34]. Other triggers for cardiac injury and dysfunction include AKI-related volume overload, metabolic acidosis, and electrolytes disorders such as hyperkalemia and hypocalcemia. Acute, left ventricular dysfunction, and accelerated fibrosis have been also described in patients with AKI [35]. Finally, AKI can affect cardiac function contributing to alterations in drug pharmacokinetics and dynamics (such as excretion of digoxin).

Pathophysiology

Direct Effects of AKI on Cardiac Function

Pathophysiological interactions between the kidney and heart in AKI have been referred to "cardiorenal connectors" [36], which include immune modulation (pro- and anti-inflammatory cytokines and chemokines release), sympathetic nervous system and RAAS hyperactivity, and activation of the coagulation cascade.

Circulating levels of tumor necrosis factor-alpha (TNFα [alpha]), interleukin-1 (IL-1), and interleukin-6 (IL-6) seem to increase immediately after renal experimental ischemia and, together with other cytokines as well as and interferon-alfa (IFN-α[alpha]), have direct cardio-depressant effects, such as reduction in left ventricular ejection fraction and elevation of left ventricular end-diastolic and end-systolic volumes and areas [37, 38]. Cytokines release can affect myocardial cells directly on their contractility or by close interactions with extracellular matrix leading to negative inotropic effects. Cellular mechanisms involve secondary mediators such as sphingolipids, arachidonic acid. and intracellular Ca^{2+} alterations [30].

In animal models, infusion of TNF-α[alpha] results in decrease of left ventricular diastolic pressure with secondary coronary vasoconstriction. Infusions cause time-dependent dysfunction (regional contractility alterations) of left ventricle and its dilation lasting up to 10 days [30]. Several diastolic abnormalities are also observed, including slow relaxation of left ventricle and raised left atrium filling pressure to indicate an increase in left ventricle diastolic stiffness [39]. In the presence of renal ischemia, rat hearts show increased expression of adhesion molecules such as ICAM-1 together with myocardial apoptosis (this is not true in case of bilateral nephrectomy) to prove that systemic inflammation, and not AKI, plays an immediate role in myocardial damage and dysfunction [40]. In animal experiments, it has been shown that left ventricular dilation, increased left ventricular end-diastolic and end-systolic diameters, increased relaxation time, and decreased fractional shortening can occur 48 h after renal injury [37].

Hyperactivity of the SNS with abnormal secretion of norepinephrine impairs myocardial activity in several ways: direct norepinephrine effect, impairment in Ca^{2+} metabolism, increase in myocardial oxygen demand with potential evolution to myocardial ischemia, myocardial cells β[beta] 1-adrenergic-mediated apoptosis, stimulation of α[alpha]1 receptors, and, finally, activation of RAAS. Abnormal and uncontrolled RAAS activation leads to angiotensin II release with consequent systemic vasoconstriction and elevation of vascular resistance. In addition, angiotensin II itself directly promotes cellular hypertrophy and apoptosis [41]. Increased RAAS activity could be accountable for diminished coronary response to adenosine, bradykinin, and L-arginine [42]. Other animal models exemplify how the inflammatory cascade of AKI can contribute to altered permeability of lung vessels, with resultant interstitial edema and micro-hemorrhage mediated by inflammatory mediators and altered expression of epithelial sodium channel and aquaporin-5 [43].

Myocardial cells apoptosis and neutrophil activation greatly contribute to the pathophysiologic pathways of cardiac injury following AKI, leading to lethal major cardiac events as can be seen in rat transgenic models [44]. Cardiac myocyte apoptosis and neutrophil infiltration represent two of the most important contributors to the pathophysiology of myocardial infarction during AKI [38]. The cardiorenal link between AKI and cardiac fibrosis is shown with the upregulation of beta-galactoside-binding lectin galectin-3, mRNA expression renal ischemia. It is also implicated in the development of myocardial fibrosis and heart failure in AKI, and its inhibition can delay progression of myocardial fibrosis [45].

Indirect Effects of AKI on Heart Function

As renal function declines, it can result in significant pathophysiological derangement, leading to cardiac injury. Oliguria can lead to sodium and water retention with consequent fluid overload and development of volume overload, hypertension, pulmonary edema, and myocardial injury. Electrolytes imbalances (primarily hyperkalemia) can contribute to raised risk of fatal arrhythmias and sudden death. Acidemia also can worsen pulmonary vasoconstriction, increased right ventricular afterload, and contribute to a negative cardiac inotropic effect. Finally, uremia itself can directly affect myocardial cells contractility through myocardial depressant factors and promote pericardial effusions and pericarditis [46, 47].

In response to systemic and renal hemodynamic changes, baroceptor and intrarenal chemoreceptors lead to SNS and RAAS activation. As described previously, SNS activation directly affects intrarenal hemodynamics and stimulates renin incretion, and also causes cardiomyocyte apoptosis. Neuropeptide Y, a vascular growth factor accountable for neointimal formation and following vasoconstriction, is also stimulated by RAAS activation [48, 49].

Electrophysiological Effects

Classical ECG changes in hyperkalemic patients are represented by tenting of T wave due to rapid and consistent elevation in extracellular potassium levels, leading to increased activity of potassium channel (and inactivation of sodium channel) with faster repolarization and predisposition to arrhythmias [50]. Hyperkalemia reduces resting membrane potentials (both atrial and ventricular) and induces ST-T segment abnormalities (i.e., elevations in V1 and V2) simulating an ischemic pattern. In some patients, hyperkalemia can simulate a Brugada-like pattern, characterized by right bundle branch block and persistent ST-T segment elevation [50].

Type 4 Cardiorenal Syndrome

Type 4 CRS, also defined as chronic renocardiac disease, is characterized by cardiovascular involvement in patients affected by chronic kidney disease at any stage according to National Kidney Foundation (NKF) classification. It is well established that renal dysfunction is an independent risk factor for cardiovascular disease with higher mortality risk for myocardial infection and sudden death in CKD [51].

Pathophysiology

Figures 12.3 and 12.4 show close interactions between chronic kidney disease (CKD) and cardiovascular involvement. Chronic kidney disease independently accelerates ischemic heart disease and contributes to pressure and volume overload, leading to left ventricular hypertrophy [52].

Left ventricular hypertrophy (LVH) is highly prevalent in patients starting hemodialysis. Pressure overload leading to LVH results from hypertension and calcific valvular disease as early as CKD-2, but is particularly prevalent in hemodialysis and pre-dialysis patients [53, 54]. Hyperphosphatemia and secondary hyperparathyroidism can produce ossification of cardiac vessels and valves because of "osteoblastic" transformation of vascular smooth muscle cells [55]. Congestive heart failure is exacerbated by volume overload central to CKD with underlying anemia of chronic disease and the presence of hemodialysis arteriovenous fistulae being common contributing factors [56, 57].

Chronic inflammation, insulin resistance, hyperhomocysteinemia, and malnutrition–inflammation-associated dyslipidemia can also contribute to accelerated cardiovascular disease in CKD. As GFR declines, gradual accumulation of a spectrum of toxins (β[beta]2 microglobulin, guanidines, phenols, indoles, aliphatic amines, furans, polyols, nucleosides, leptin, serum amyloid A protein, asymmetric dimethylarginine, parathyroid hormone, and erythropoiesis inhibitors) can occur [58–60], which contribute to the inflammatory milieu of progressive CKD. B-type natriuretic peptide (BNP) and related N-terminal proBNP (NT-proBNP) are both elevated in CKD patients compared to age- and sex-matched cohorts with preserved renal function, reflecting myocardial cells injury due to hypertension, volume overload, LVH, cardiac remodeling, and fibrosis [61, 62].

Congestive Heart Failure and Left Ventricular Hypertrophy

Echocardiographic abnormalities (impairment of ejection fraction, increased end-systolic, and end-diastolic left

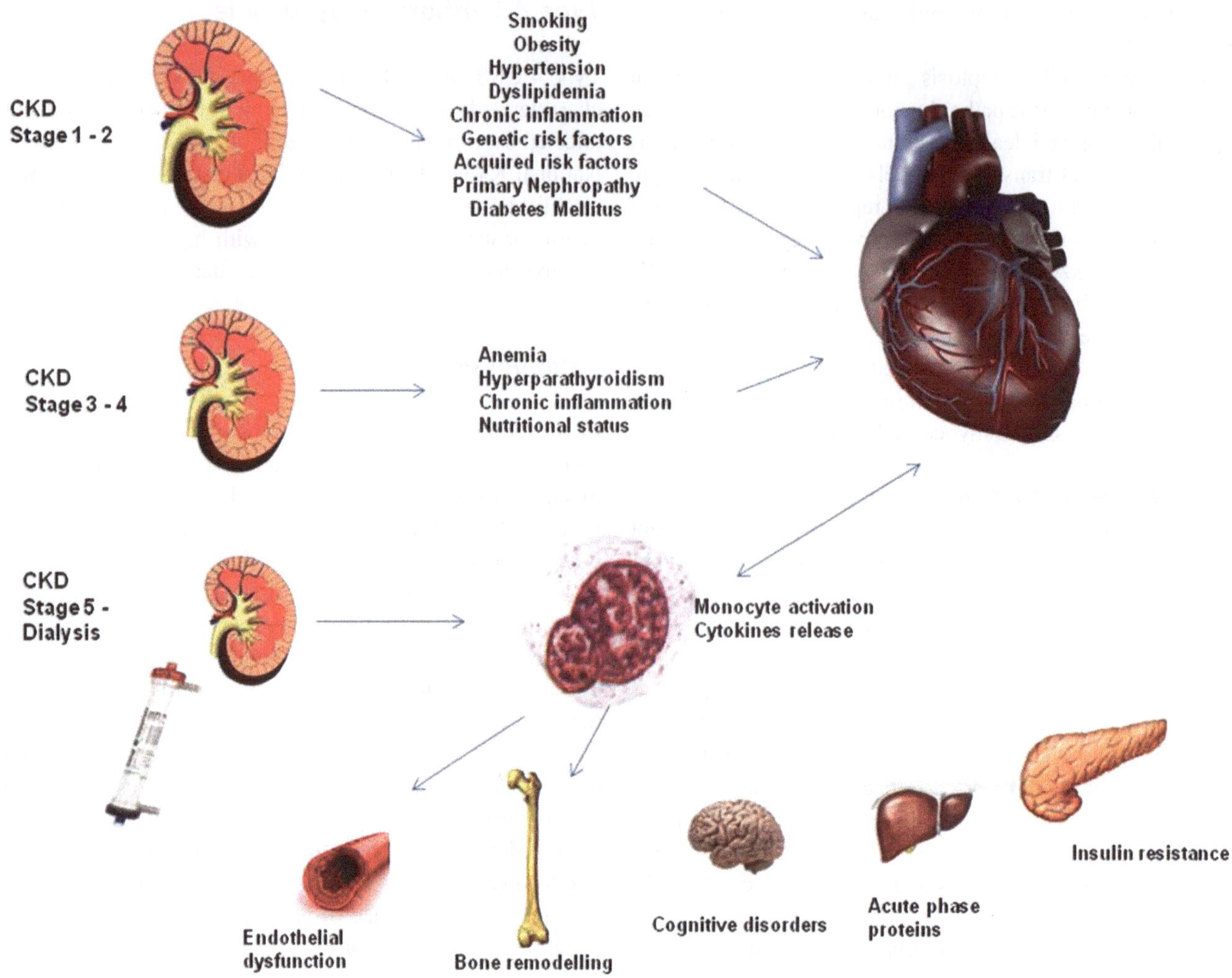

Fig. 12.3 Pathophysiological pathways of type 4 cardiorenal syndrome

ventricular diameter and volume) are frequently reported since early stages of CKD to ESKD. Incident dialysis patients show higher rates of systolic dysfunction (15%), LVH (74%), and left ventricular dilation (36%) [63, 64]. Pathophysiological mechanisms proposed include pressure and volume overload in parallel with progressive GFR decline. Pressure overload is also exacerbated by co-existing hypertension, valvular heart disease (accelerated by secondary hyperparathyroidism), and impaired vascular compliance. Consequent increase in cardiac workload leads to compensatory hypertrophy and excessive myocardial cells stress relative to increased oxygen demand resulting in myocyte fibrosis and death, cardiac chamber dilation, and systolic dysfunction [64].

Fibroblast growth factor-23 (FGF-23), a member of fibroblast growth factor family (implicated in regulation, growth, and differentiation of cardiac myocytes), has paracrine functions in kidneys because of its phosphaturic properties blocking vitamin D3 synthesis [65]. During CKD progression, accumulation of phosphate leads to increase in FGF-23 secretion that promotes LVH and cardiac remodeling. Echocardiographic assays demonstrated a 5% LVMI (left ventricular mass index) rise for every log increase in plasma FGF-23 levels [66].

Cardiac Arrhythmias and Sudden Cardiac Death

CKD patients, especially those on hemodialysis, are more prone to develop arrhythmias, especially atrial fibrillation and ventricular tachyarrhythmias. Significant shifts of electrolytes and blood pressures/volumes levels are common in intra- and inter-dialytic periods leading to myocardial cells mechanical (regional wall motion abnormalities) and arrhythmogenic potential [67]. Almost half of cardiovascular deaths in the end-stage kidney disease population are related to cardiac arrhythmia or sudden death [67]. Increased risk for sudden death seems to be particularly related to longer inter-dialytic intervals in subjects undergoing thrice weekly hemodialysis treatment, because of extreme shifts of

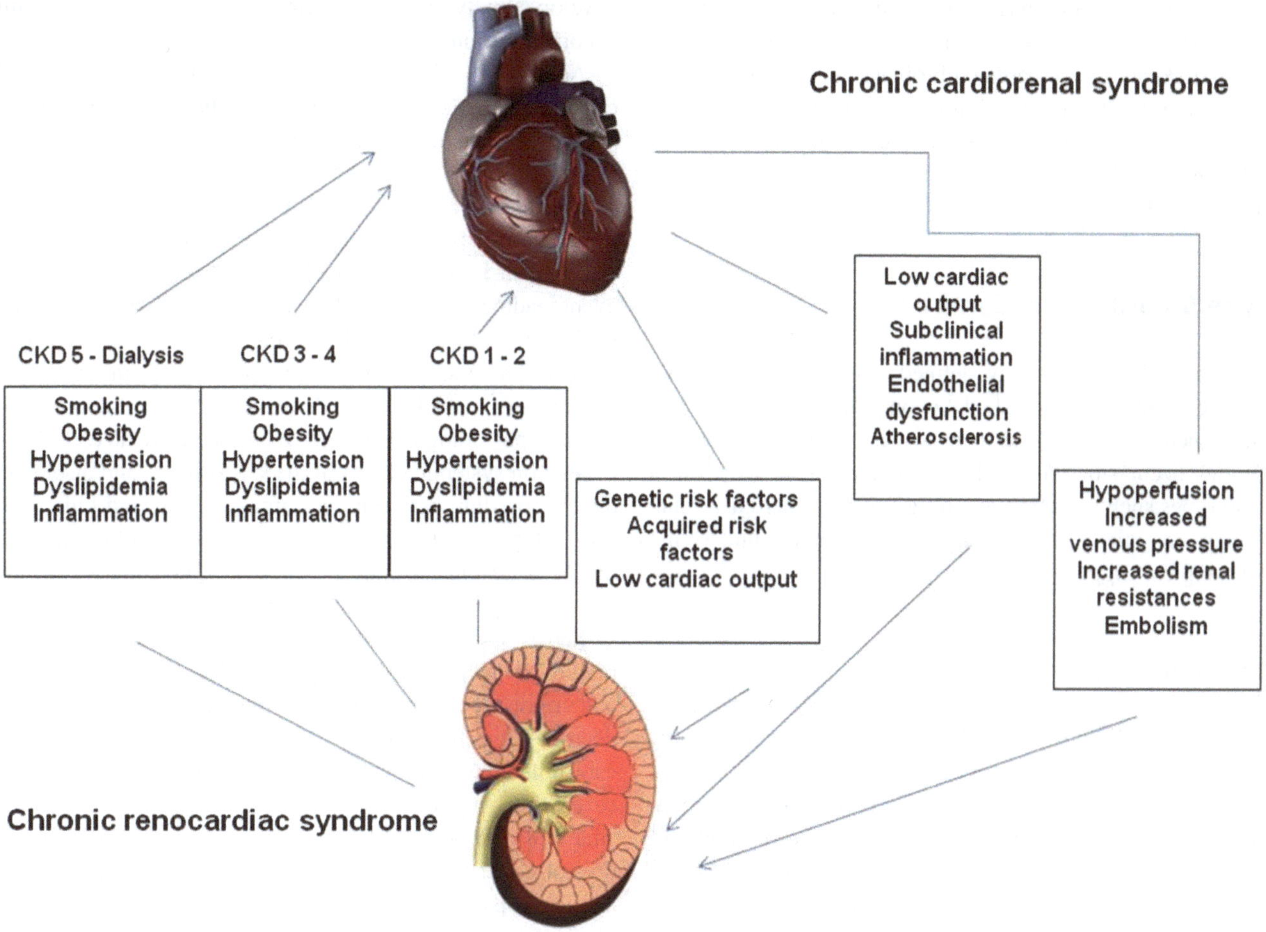

Fig. 12.4 Clinical correlation between kidney and heart disease

electrolytes and fluids [68]. In the non-dialysis CKD population, a 1.11 hazard ratio for sudden cardiac death exists for every 10 ml/min/1.73 m2 fall in GFR [69].

Atrial fibrillation is a common arrhythmia in the CKD/ESKD population. In the Chronic Renal Insufficiency Cohort (CRIC) study, an 18% prevalence of atrial fibrillation was found [70]. The incidence of atrial fibrillation (ECG-detected) correlates with the degree of CKD with a 4–5% prevalence in stage 4–5 CKD patients. After multivariate analysis, the odds ratios for ECG-defined atrial fibrillation were 2.20 in CKD stage 1–2 patients, 1.51 in CKD 3, and 2.86 in CKD 4–5 patients, respectively, compared to control subjects with normal renal function [70]. The burden of atrial fibrillation is complicated by the increased hemorrhagic risk in this population from anticoagulation [70].

Coronary Atherosclerotic Heart Disease

CKD patients present higher prevalence of coronary artery disease at angiographic evaluation with multivessel disease and ECG evidence of previous ischemia [71].

Conchol et al. assessed CAD prevalence in early stages of CKD with coronary catheterization procedures in 261 patients with GFR between 30 and 90 ml/min. More than half the patients with GFR < 90 mls/min/1.73 m^2 had a 70% stenosis in at least one coronary artery, and more than 84% patients with GFR < 30 ml/min/1.73 m^2 showed significant CAD mainly involving the left coronary arterial territory [72].

Uremia and Cardiac Fibrosis

End-stage CKD patients develop cardiac fibrosis similar to hypertensive and chronic ischemic heart disease patients in which endocardial and epicardial fibrosis predominate [73]. Uremic toxins such as indoxyl sulfate and p-cresol can contribute to cardiac fibrosis in CKD patients. Indoxyl sulfate concentrations are 300-fold higher than control population and it directly contributes to cardiac fibrosis by synthesis of TGF-β[beta], tissue inhibitor of metalloproteinase-1 (TIMP-1), and alpha-1 collagen [74, 75].

Recent evidence shows upregulation of galectin-3, a member of the β[beta]-galactoside-binding lectin family synthesized by macrophages, which interacts with extracellular matrix protein like laminin, synexin, and integrins. Galectin-3 can bind to cardiac fibroblasts increasing collagen production in the myocardium. Lok et al. [75] enrolled 232-stage 3–4 CKD patients and demonstrated that galectin-3 levels were independent predictors of cardiovascular mortality.

Type 5 Cardiorenal Syndrome

Type 5 CRS is a recently defined clinical syndrome and complete epidemiological data on this entity are still incomplete. Type 5 CRS occurs when cardiac and renal injuries occur simultaneously, encompassing many clinical syndromes such as sepsis, and drug toxicity where heart and kidney are involved secondary to a common underlying pathological trigger [1].

Pathophysiology

The pathophysiology of CRS-5 depends on the underlying disease. Acute CRS-5 results from systemic processes, e.g., sepsis, infections, drugs, toxins, and connective tissue disorders such as lupus, Wegener's granulomatosis, and sarcoidosis. The temporal course of the development of CRS 5 is variable. For example, in sepsis-induced acute CRS-5, there is a fulminant disease process with an acute impact on both the kidney and the heart, with obvious clinical manifestations. On the other hand in cirrhosis, CRS-5 has a more insidious onset and the kidney and cardiac dysfunction may develop slowly, until a crucial point is reached and full decompensation occurs.

Acute CRS-5 develops into four following steps and it can be hyper-acute (0–72 h after diagnosis), acute (3–7 days), sub-acute (7–30 days), and chronic (over 30 days) (Table 12.2).

Chronic CRS-5 (i.e., CRS in cirrhotic patients) presents time sequence quite variable because in most cases of CRS-5 there is an underlying condition and related precipitating event leading to attention. For instance, cirrhotic patients are subject to infections and an acute CRS-5 can overlap a chronic process. The mechanisms invoked in acute and chronic forms of CRS-5 are described in Figs. 12.5 and 12.6.

Pathophysiological changes in sepsis-related CRS 5 depend on systemic effects of the sepsis itself, and also, from direct cross-talk between the damaged heart and kidney. In early stages of sepsis, microcirculation is often initially involved despite normal systemic hemodynamics [38, 44] and strongly correlates with morbidity and mortality rates.

Sepsis-associated cardiomyopathy represents one of main predictors of mortality in septic patients [76]. Both the left and right ventricles can be injured with dilation and decreased ejection fraction, often unresponsive to fluid and catecholamine therapy [77]. Septic cardiomyopathy, when severe, can mimic cardiogenic shock but it is usually reversible [78]. Myocardial blood flow and oxygen consumption do not seem to be involved in pathophysiology of septic cardiomyopathy [79]. Proinflammatory mediators and complement factors have been proposed as crucial actors in the development of cardiac involvement during sepsis [80, 81].

In sepsis-associated AKI, there are clear changes in intra-parenchymal blood flow independent of systemic

Table 12.2 Temporal considerations in pathophysiology of CRS-5

Attribute	CRS5 acute (sepsis) (Fig. 12.1)	CRS5 chronic (cirrhosis) (Fig. 12.2)
Time for organ dysfunction	Short: hours to days	Long: weeks to months
Underlying organ function	May be superimposed on underlying cardiac and kidney disease	Heart and kidney have adaptive responses that fail over time
Sequence of organ involvement	Generally simultaneous or in close proximity to each other	One organ precedes the other, e.g., cardiac dysfunction precedes renal in cirrhosis
Underlying disease	Systemic event contributes to CRS5	Precipitating events can transition to an acute deterioration in CRS5, e.g., GI bleed can precipitate hepatorenal syndrome
Pathophysiology	Direct effects on organs	Failure of adaptive responses over time
Mechanisms	Determined by underlying disease	Determined by adaptive changes
Reversibility	Possible with control of sepsis and organ support	Limited unless there is replacement of diseased organ, e.g., liver transplant

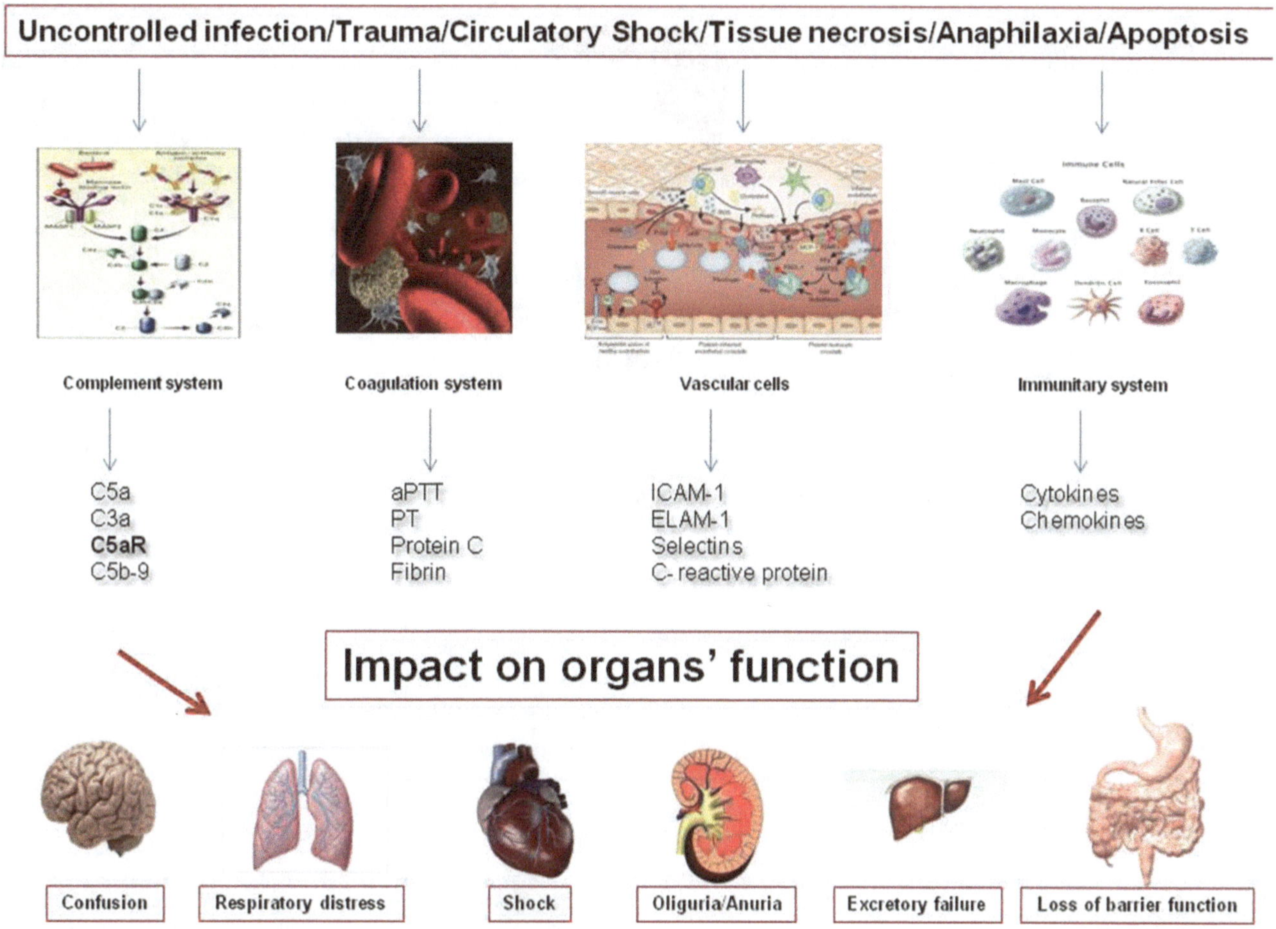

Fig. 12.5 Pathophysiology of sepsis-induced organ dysfunction

hemodynamic changes linked to the septic process [82, 83]. Recent experimental data have compared two different sepsis models in pigs in which, irrespective of systemic hemodynamics, only pigs developing septic AKI demonstrated increased renal vascular resistance and early rises in proinflammatory cytokines (IL-6) and oxidative stress markers [83].

Sepsis is able to affect the autonomic nervous system (ANS), RAAS, and hypothalamus–pituitary gland–adrenal gland axis (HPA) independently which can impact, in several and distinctive steps, cardiac and/or renal function. Severity of ANS dysfunction correlates with morbidity and mortality [84, 85]; autonomic dysfunction can be assessed by observing decreased heart rate variability (HRV), often associated with release of inflammatory biomarkers such as IL-6, IL-10, and C-reactive protein (CRP) [68]. It is clear that during combined heart and kidney dysfunction, as in sepsis, several cellular and molecular changes occur in both tissues. Activation and induction of cytokines (TNF-α[alpha] and IL-6) and leukocytes (macrophages, neutrophils, and lymphocytes) is well documented both in heart and kidney during [86, 87]. Myocardial contractility is significantly affected and muscle protein expression (actin and myosin) is abnormal in sepsis as well as membrane-associated proteins, as dystrophin, normally regulating cell shape, mechanical strength, and myocardial cells contractility. Mean amount of dystrophin and other similar glycoproteins are reduced in septic myocardium [88]. Sepsis induces tubular damage in kidneys affected by increased secretion of lipopolysaccharide that alters HC03 transport leading to abnormalities in urine acidification [89]. Lipopolysaccharide also modifies megalin, a glomerular protein involved in increasing albuminuria, and consequently intrarenal inflammation [90].

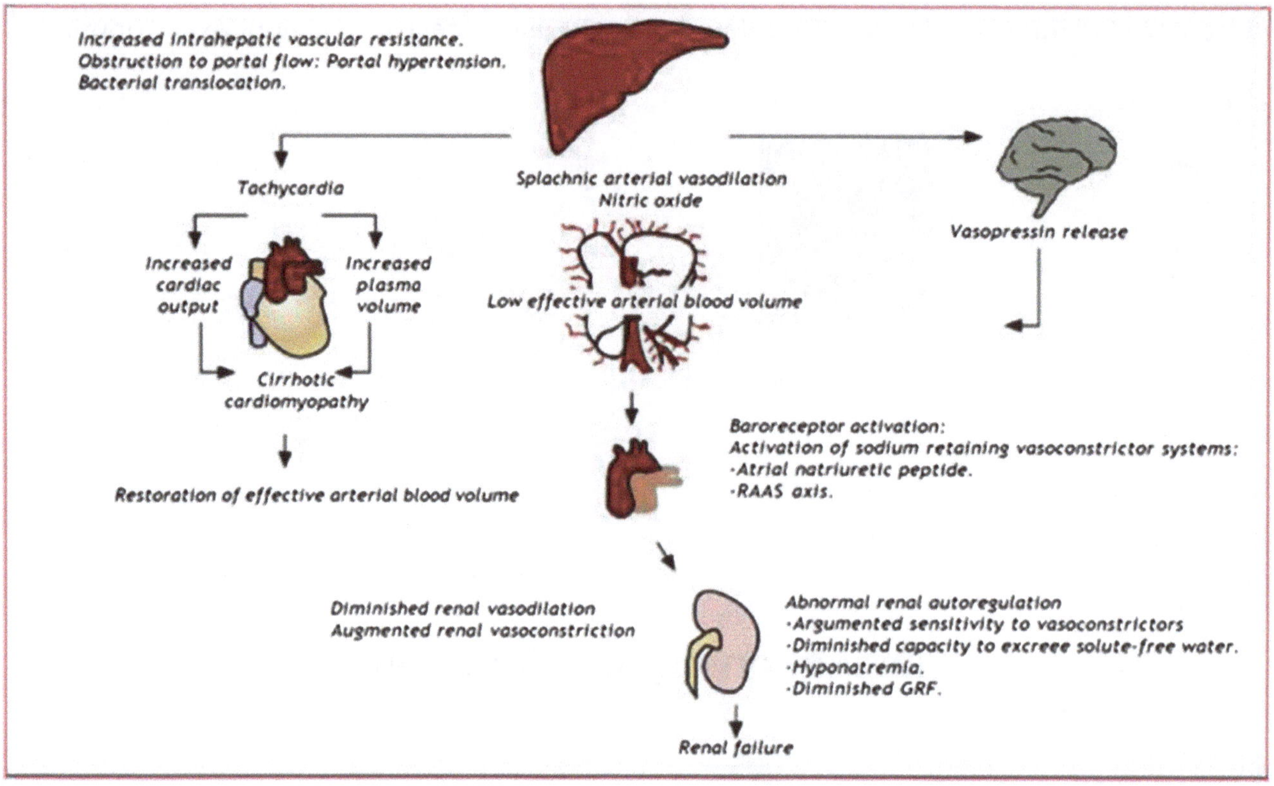

Fig. 12.6 Pathophysiology of cirrhosis-induced CRS-5

Summary

The pathophysiology and clinical impact of the various subtypes of cardiorenal syndrome exemplify the intricate cross-talk between the heart and the kidney. Given the huge morbidity and mortality of the dual burden of these organ system afflictions, early recognition of the clinical phenotype of cardiorenal syndrome and interventions to slow down end-organ damage is crucial in positively influencing the burden of this pathological symbiosis.

References

1. Ronco C. The cardiorenal syndrome: basis and common ground for a multidisciplinary patient-oriented therapy. Cardiorenal Med. 2011;1:3–4.
2. Ronco C. Cardiorenal syndromes: definition and classification. Contrib Nephrol. 2010;164:33–8.
3. Eren Z, Ozveren O, Buvukoner E, Kaspar E, Degertekin M, Kantarci G. A Single-centre study of acute cardiorenal syndrome: incidence, risk factors and consequences. Cardiorenal Med. 2012;2:168–76.
4. Bargshaw SM, Cruz DM, Aspromonte N, for the Acute Dialysis Quality Initiative (ADQI) Consensus Group, et al. Epidemiology of cardio-renal syndromes: workgroup statements from the 7th ADQI consensus conference. Nephrol Dial Transplant. 2010;25:1406–16.
5. Damman K, Navis G, Voors AA, et al. Worsening renal function and prognosis in heart failure: systematic review and meta-analysis. J Card Fail. 2007;13:599–608.
6. McCullough PA. Cardiorenal syndromes: pathophysiology to prevention. Int J Nephrol. 2010;2010:762590.
7. Hanada S, Takewa Y, Mizuno T, Tsukiyan T, Taenaka Y, Tatsumi E. Effect of the technique for assisting renal blood circulation on ischemic kidney in acute cardiorenal syndrome. J Artif Organs. 2012;15:140–5.
8. Stevenson LW, Perloff JK. The limited reliability of physical signs for estimating hemodynamics in chronic heart failure. JAMA. 1989;261:884–8.
9. Mullens W, Abrahams Z, Francis GS, Sokos G, Taylor DO, Starling RC, Young JB, Tang WH. Importance of venous congestion for worsening of renal function in advanced decompensated heart failure. J Am Coll Cardiol. 2009;53:589–96.
10. Uthoff H, Breidthardt T, Klima T, Aschwanden M, Arenja N, Socrates T, Heinisch C, Noveanu M, Frischknecht B, Baumann U, Jaeger KA, Mueller C. Central venous pressure and impaired renal function in patients with acute heart failure. Eur J Heart Fail. 2011;13:432–9.
11. Braam B, Cupples WA, Joles JA, Gaillard C. Systemic arterial and venous determinants of renal hemodynamics in congestive heart failure. Heart Fail Rev. 2012;17:161–75.
12. De Silva R, Loh H, Rigby AS, Nikitin NP, Witte KK, Goode K, Bhandari S, Nicholson A, Clark AL, Cleland JG. Epidemiology, associated factors, and prognostic outcomes of renal artery stenosis in chronic heart failure assessed by magnetic resonance angiography. Am J Cardiol. 2007;100:273–9.
13. Nohria A, Tsang SW, Fang JC, Lewis EF, Jarcho JA, Mudge GH, Stevenson LW. Clinical assessment identifies hemodynamic

profiles that predict outcomes in patients admitted with heart failure. J Am Coll Cardiol. 2003;41:1797–804.
14. Machnik A, Neuhofer W, Jantsch J, Dahlmann A, Tammela T, Machura K, Park JK, Beck FX, Müller DN, Derer W, Goss J, Ziomber A, Dietsch P, Wagner H, van Rooijen N, Kurtz A, Hilgers KF, Alitalo K, Eckardt KU, Luft FC, Kerjaschki D, Titze J. Macrophages regulate salt-dependent volume and blood pressure by a vascular endothelial growth factor-C-dependent buffering mechanism. Nat Med. 2009;15:545–52.
15. Virzì GM, Torregrossa R, Cruz DN, Chionh CY, de Cal M, Soni SS, Dominici M, Vescovo G, Rosner MH, Ronco C. Cardiorenal syndrome type 1 may be immunologically mediated: a pilot evaluation of monocyte apoptosis. Cardiorenal Med. 2012;2:33–42.
16. Havasi A, Borkan SC. Apoptosis and acute kidney injury. Kidney Int. 2011;80:29–40.
17. Bonventre JV. Dedifferentiation and proliferation of surviving epithelial cells in acute renal failure. J Am Soc Nephrol. 2003;14 (suppl 1):S55–61.
18. Akcay A, Nguyen Q, Edelstein CL. Mediators of inflammation in acute kidney injury. Mediators Inflamm. 2009;2009:137072.
19. Elmore S. Apoptosis: a review of programmed cell death. Toxicol Pathol. 2007;35:495–516.
20. Pastori S, Virzì GM, Brocca A, De Cal M, Cantaluppi V, Castellani C, Fedrigo M, Thiene G, Valente ML, Angelini A, Vescovo G, Ronco C. Cardiorenal syndrome type-1: activation of dual apoptotic pathways. Cardiorenal Med. 2015;5:306–15.
21. Virzì GM, Clementi A, De Cal M, Brocca A, Day S, Pastori S, Bolin C, Vescovo G, Ronco C. Oxydative stress: dual pathway induction in cardiorenal syndrome type 1 pathogenesis. Oxid Med Cell Longev. 2015;Article ID 391790.
22. Maruyama Y, Lindholm B, Stenvinkel P. Inflammation and oxidative stress in ESRD—the role of myeloperoxydase. J Nephrolgy. 2004;17(Suppl 8):S72–6.
23. Kraut EJ, Chen S, Hubbard NE, Erickson KI, Wisner DH. Tumor necrosis factor depresses myocardial contractility in endotoxemic swine. J Trauma. 1999;46:900–6.
24. Heywood JT, Fonarow GC, Costanzo MR, Mathur VS, Wigneswaran JR, Wynne J. High prevalence of renal dysfunction and its impact on outcome in 118,465 patients hospitalized with acute decompensated heart failure: a report from the ADHERE database. J Card Fail. 2007;13(6):422–30.
25. Hebert K, Dias A, Delgado MC, Franco E, Tamariz L, Steen D, Trahan P, Major B, Arcement LM. Epidemiology and survival of the five stages of chronic kidney disease in a systolic heart failure population. Eur J Heart Fail. 2010;12(8):861–5.
26. Cruz DN, Bagshaw SM. Heart-kidney interaction: epidemiology of cardiorenal syndromes. Int J Nephrol. 2010;2011:351291.
27. Bagshaw SM, Cruz DN, Aspromonte N, Daliento L, Ronco F, Sheinfeld G, Anker SD, Anand I, Bellomo R, Berl T, et al. Epidemiology of cardiorenal syndromes: workgroup statements from the 7th ADQI Consensus Conference. Nephrol Dial Transplant. 2010;25(5):1406–16.
28. Cruz DN, Schmidt-Ott KM, Vescovo G, House AA, Kellum JA, Ronco C, McCullough PA. Pathophysiology of cardiorenal syndrome type 2 in stable chronic heart failure: workgroup statements from the eleventh consensus conference of the Acute Dialysis Quality Initiative (ADQI). Contrib Nephrol. 2013;182:117–36.
29. Setoguchi S, Stevenson LW, Schneeweiss S. Repeated hospitalizations predict mortality in the community population with heart failure. Am Heart J. 2007;154(2):260–6.
30. Bongartz LG, Cramer MJ, Doevendans PA, Joles JA, Braam B. The severe cardiorenal syndrome: 'Guyton revisited'. Eur Heart J. 2005;26(1):11–7.
31. Merrill AJ, Morrison JL, Branno ES. Concentration of renin in renal venous blood in patients with chronic heart failure. Am J Med. 1946;1(5):468.
32. Kishimoto T, Maekawa M, Abe Y, Yamamoto K. Intrarenal distribution of blood flow and renin release during renal venous pressure elevation. Kidney Int. 1973;4(4):259–66.
33. Remuzzi G, Cattaneo D, Perico N. The aggravating mechanisms of aldosterone on kidney fibrosis. J Am Soc Nephrol. 2008;19 (8):1459–62.
34. Onozato ML, Tojo A, Kobayashi N, Goto A, Matsuoka H, Fujita T. Dual blockade of aldosterone and angiotensin II additively suppresses TGF-beta and NADPH. Nephrol Dial Transplant. 2007 May;22(5):1314–22.
35. Colombo PC, Ganda A, Lin J, Onat D, Harxhi A, Iyasere JE, Uriel N, Cotter G. Inflammatory activation: cardiac, renal, and cardio-renal interactions in patients with the cardiorenal syndrome. Heart Fail Rev. 2012;17(2):177–90.
36. Yap SC, Lee HT. Acute kidney injury and extrarenal organ dysfunction: new concepts and experimental evidence. Anesthesiology. 2012;116(5):1139–48.
37. Prabhu SD. Cytokine-induced modulation of cardiac function. Circ Res. 2004;95(12):1140–53.
38. Kingma JG Jr, Vincent C, Rouleau JR, Kingma I. Influence of acute renal failure on coronary vasoregulation in dogs. J Am Soc Nephrol. 2006;17(5):1316–24.
39. Ma XL, Lefer DJ, Lefer AM, Rothlein R. Coronary endothelial and cardiac protective effects of a monoclonal antibody to intercellular adhesion molecule-1 in myocardial ischemia and reperfusion. Circulation. 1992;86(3):937–46.
40. Blake P, Hasegawa Y, Khosla MC, Fouad-Tarazi F, Sakura N, Paganini EP. Isolation of "myocardial depressant factor(s)" from the ultrafiltrate of heart failure patients with acute renal failure. ASAIO J. 1996;42(5):M911–5.
41. Edmunds NJ, Lal H, Woodward B. Effects of tumour necrosis factor-alpha on left ventricular function in the rat isolated perfused heart: possible mechanisms for a decline in cardiac function. Br J Pharmacol. 1999;126(1):189–96.
42. Rauchhaus M, Doehner W, Francis DP, et al. Plasma cytokine parameters and mortality in patients with chronic heart failure. Circulation. 2000;102(25):3060–7.
43. Chuasuwan A, Kellum JA. Cardio-renal syndrome type 3: epidemiology, pathophysiology, and treatment. Semin Nephrol. 2012;32(1):31–9.
44. Kajstura J, Cigola E, Malhotra A, et al. Angiotensin II induces apoptosis of adult ventricular myocytes in vitro. J Mol Cell Cardiol. 1997;29(3):859–70.
45. Nath KA, Grande JP, Croatt AJ, et al. Transgenic sickle mice are markedly sensitive to renal ischemia-reperfusion injury. Am J Pathol. 2005;166(4):963–72.
46. Kelly KJ. Distant effects of experimental renal ischemia/reperfusion injury. J Am Soc Nephrol. 2003;14 (6):1549–58.
47. Bryant D, Becker L, Richardson J, et al. Cardiac failure in transgenic mice with myocardial expression of tumor necrosis factor-alpha. Circulation. 1998;97:1375–81.
48. Liu YH, D'Ambrosio M, Liao TD, et al. *N*-acetyl-seryl-aspartyl-lysyl-proline prevents cardiac remodeling and dysfunction induced by galectin-3, a mammalian

adhesion/growth-regulatory lectin. Am J Physiol Heart Circ Physiol. 2009;296(2):H404–12.
49. De Deyn PP, Vanholder R, D'Hooge R. Nitric oxide in uremia: effects of several potentially toxic guanidino compounds. Kidney Int. 2003;84(Suppl):S25–8.
50. Scheuer J, Stezoski W. The effects of uremic compounds on cardiac function and metabolism. J Mol Cell Cardiol. 1973;5:287–300.
51. Jackson G, Gibbs CR, Davies MK, Lip GY. ABC of heart failure. Pathophysiology. Br Med J. 2000;320:167–70.
52. Li L, Lee EW, Ji H, Zukowska Z. Neuropeptide Y-induced acceleration of postangioplasty occlusion of rat carotid artery. Arterioscler Thromb Vasc Biol. 2003;23:1204–10.
53. Karnik JA, Young BS, Lew NL, Herget M, Dubinsky C, Lazarus JM, Chertow GM. Cardiac arrest and sudden cardiac death in dialysis units. Kidney Int. 2001;60:350–7.
54. Redón J, Cea-Calvob L, Lozanoc JV, Fernández-Pérez C, Navarroe J, Bonete A, Gonzalo-Esteban J. Kidney function and cardiovascular disease in the hypertensive population: the ERIC-HTA study. Journal of Hypertension. 2006;24:663–9.
55. Levin A, Singer J, Thompson CR, Ross H, Lewis M. Prevalent left ventricular hypertrophy in the predialysis population: Identifying opportunities for intervention. Am J Kidney Dis. 1996;27(3):347–54.
56. Lezaic V, Tirmenstajn-Jankovic B, Bukvic D, Vujisic B, Perovic M, Novakovic N, Dopsaj V, Maric I, Djukanovic L. Efficacy of hyperphosphatemia control in the progression of chronic renal failure and the prevalence of cardiovascular calcification. Clin Nephrol. 2009;71(1):21–9.
57. Di Lullo L, Floccari F, Santoboni A, Barbera V, Rivera RF, Granata A, Morrone L, Russo D. Progression of cardiac valve calcification and decline of renal function in CKD patients. J Nephrol. 2013;26(4):739–44.
58. Olgaard K, Lewin E, Silver J. Calcimimetics, vitamin D and ADVANCE in the management of CKD-MBD. Nephrol Dial Transplant. 2011 Apr;26(4):1117–9.
59. MacRae JM, Pandeya S, Humen DP, Krivitski N, Lindsay RM. Arteriovenous fistula-associated high-output cardiac failure: a review of mechanisms. Am J Kidney Dis. 2004;43(5):e17–22.
60. Di Lullo L, Floccari F, Polito P. Right ventricular diastolic function in dialysis patients could be affected by vascular access. Nephron Clin Pract. 2011;118:c258–62.
61. Fort J. Chronic renal failure: a cardiovascular risk factor. Kidney Int. 2005;99(Suppl):S25–9.
62. Schiffrin EL, Lipman ML, Mann JF. Chronic kidney disease: effects on the cardiovascular system. Circulation. 2007;116(1):85–97.
63. Bologa RM, Levine DM, Parker TS, et al. Interleukin-6 predicts hypoalbuminemia, hypocholesterolemia, and mortality in hemodialysis patients. Am J Kidney Dis. 1998;32(1):107–14.
64. Maisel AS, Katz N, Hillege HL, et al. Biomarkers in kidney and heart disease. Nephrol Dial Transplant. 2011;26(1):62–74.
65. Foley RN, Parfrey PS, Sarnak MJ. Clinical epidemiology of cardiovascular disease in chronic renal disease. Am J Kidney Dis. 1998;32(5 Suppl 3):S112–9.
66. Harnett JD, Foley RN, Kent GM, et al. Congestive heart failure in dialysis patients: prevalence, incidence, prognosis and risk factors. Kidney Int. 1995;47(3):884–90.
67. Foley RN, Parfrey PS, Harnett JD, et al. The prognostic importance of left ventricular geometry in uremic cardiomyopathy. J Am Soc Nephrol. 1995;5(12):2024–31.
68. Bougle A, Duranteau J. Pathophysiology of sepsis-induced acute kidney injury: the role of global renal blood flow and renal vascular resistance. Contrib Nephrol. 2011;174:89–97.
69. Jovanovich A, Ix JH, Gottdiener J, McFann K, Katz R, Kestenbaum B, de Boer IH, Sarnak M, Shlipak MG, Mukamal KJ, Siscovick D, Chonchol M. Fibroblast growth factor 23, left ventricular mass, and left ventricular hypertrophy in community-dwelling older adults. Atherosclerosis. 2013;231(1):114–9.
70. Shamseddin MK, Parfrey PS. Medscape: sudden cardiac death in chronic kidney disease: epidemiology and prevention. Nat Rev Nephrol. 2011.
71. Chan CT, Levin NW, Chertow GM, et al. Determinants of cardiac autonomic dysfunction in ESRD. Clin J Am Soc Nephrol. 2010;5(10):1821–7.
72. Winkelmayer WC, Patrick AR, Liu J, et al. The increasing prevalence of atrial fibrillation among hemodialysis patients. J Am Soc Nephrol. 2011;22(2):349–57.
73. Boerrigter G, Costello-Boerrigter LC, Abraham WT, Sutton MG, Heublein DM, Kruger KM, Hill MR, McCullough PA, Burnett JC Jr. Cardiac resynchronization therapy improves renal function in human heart failure with reduced glomerular filtration rate. J Card Fail. 2008;14(7):539–46.
74. Cai Q, Mukku VK, Ahmad M. Coronary artery disease in patients with chronic kidney disease: a clinical update. Curr Cardiol Rev. 2013;9(4):331–9.
75. Chonchol M, Whittle J, Desbien A, Orner MB, Petersen LA, Kressin NR. Chronic kidney disease is associated with angiographic coronary artery disease. Am J Nephrol. 2008;28(2):354–60.
76. Lok DJ, Lok SI, Bruggink-André de la Porte PW, Badings E, Lipsic E, van Wijngaarden J, de Boer RA, van Veldhuisen DJ, van der Meer P. Galectin-3 is an independent marker for ventricular remodeling and mortality in patients with chronic heart failure. Clin Res Cardiol. 2013;102(2):103–10.
77. Lundy DJ, Trzeciak S. Microcirculatory dysfunction in sepsis. Crit Care Clin. 2009;25(4):721–31.
78. Trzeciak S, et al. Early microcirculatory perfusion derangements in patients with severe sepsis and septic shock: relationship to hemodynamics, oxygen transport, and survival. Ann Emerg Med. 2007;49(1):88–98, 98e1–2.
79. Jardin F, et al. Sepsis-related cardiogenic shock. Crit Care Med. 1990;18(10):1055–60.
80. Lambermont B, et al. Effects of endotoxic shock on right ventricular systolic function and mechanical efficiency. Cardiovasc Res. 2003;59(2):412–8.
81. Parker MM, et al. Profound but reversible myocardial depression in patients with septic shock. Ann Intern Med. 1984;100(4):483–90.
82. Dhainaut JF, et al. Coronary hemodynamics and myocardial metabolism of lactate, free fatty acids, glucose, and ketones in patients with septic shock. Circulation. 1987;75(3):533–41.
83. Kumar A, et al. Tumor necrosis factor alpha and interleukin 1beta are responsible for in vitro myocardial cell depression induced by human septic shock serum. J Exp Med. 1996;183(3):949–58.
84. Torre-Amione G, et al. Proinflammatory cytokine levels in patients with depressed left ventricular ejection fraction: a report from the Studies of Left Ventricular Dysfunction (SOLVD). J Am Coll Cardiol. 1996;27(5):1201–6.
85. Benes J, et al. Searching for mechanisms that matter in early septic acute kidney injury: an experimental study. Crit Care. 2011;15(5):R256.

86. Schmidt H, et al. Autonomic dysfunction predicts both 1- and 2-month mortality in middle-aged patients with multiple organ dysfunction syndrome. Crit Care Med. 2008;36(3):967–70.
87. Tateishi Y, et al. Depressed heart rate variability is associated with high IL-6 blood level and decline in the blood pressure in septic patients. Shock. 2007;28(5):549–53.
88. Mortensen EM, et al. Impact of previous statin and angiotensin II receptor blocker use on mortality in patients hospitalized with sepsis. Pharmacotherapy. 2007;27(12):1619–26.
89. Chopra M, et al. Modulation of myocardial mitochondrial mechanisms during severe polymicrobial sepsis in the rat. PLoS ONE. 2011;6(6):e21285.
90. Liu M, et al. Transcription factor Nrf2 is protective during ischemic and nephrotoxic acute kidney injury in mice. Kidney Int. 2009;76(3):277–85.

13 Hemodynamic Cross-Talk in Cardiorenal Syndrome: Era of Biomarkers

Faeq Husain-Syed, Salvador Lopez-Giacoman, and Horst-Walter Birk

The Quest for Biomarkers in Cardiorenal Syndrome—On the Right Track

The sequence of cardiorenal involvement can vary depending on the acuteness of disease onset, nature of the underlying disorder, and organ reserve [1]. Cardiorenal syndrome may represent a lifelong course that begins with the evolution of risk factors contributing to the development of subclinical disease, or it may arise due to a major event (e.g., myocardial infarction), and culminate in overt cardiac and/or renal failure. The onset of the involvement of either organ portends a poor outcome with a greater risk of incomplete recovery, recurrent events, morbidity, and mortality. For example, cardiac remodeling with increased apoptosis and fibrosis occurs in response to both cardiac and renal stimuli. With an improved understanding of the complex interactions in disease states, it is increasingly clear that complementary tools are needed to aid clinical assessment and enhance clinicians' ability to identify the "vulnerable" patient at risk for acute injury or progression to chronic disease.

Biomarkers are by definition objective, quantifiable characteristics of biological processes at the cellular or molecular level—even in the absence of clinical symptoms—and can serve as indicators of disease trait (risk marker), disease state (subclinical or clinical), or disease rate (progression) [2]. The measurement of biomarkers must be applied in relation to the clinical context and must never be used in isolation, as expertise is required for a meaningful interpretation. Regardless of the purpose for its use, a biomarker will be of clinical value if it is accurate, is reproducibly obtained in a standardized fashion, and has high sensitivity and high specificity. To alter patient care, a cardiac/renal biomarker (for example, in heart failure [HF]) should either aid in the timely diagnosis of the underlying disease (HF) and/or injury of the organ not directly involved in the primary disease (the kidney in the case of HF) or provide additional information not obtainable by conventional methods. In the cardiovascular field, biomarker research has greatly improved clinicians' decision-making ability in the last decade and enabled the detection of myocardial stretch (b-type natriuretic peptide) and injury (troponin). In the field of nephrology, however, early diagnostic biomarkers for acute kidney injury (AKI) remain research tools, but it is expected that further validation will define their clinical role.

According to the current definition of AKI, an acute deterioration of renal function is linked to increased creatinine and/or reduced urinary output, while chronic kidney disease (CKD) is defined using the estimated glomerular filtration rate (GFR) and albuminuria. Due to creatinine kinetics, however, AKI is diagnosed 24–48 h after it has occurred, and factors such as hydration, nutrition, and lean tissue status further confound the diagnosis. Importantly, renal dysfunction is not a single disease entity, and consists of more than impaired glomerular filtration alone, including for instance, tubulointerstitial damage, proteinuria, sodium and water retention, and dysregulation of calcium and phosphate metabolism—all of which are altered in HF [3, 4]. Thus, new markers are needed to diagnose AKI at a much earlier stage, even in patients who do not fulfill the current consensus criteria but are still expected to have poor renal, cardiac, or overall outcomes (biomarker-positive, creatinine-negative—the so-called "subclinical"—AKI) [5]. It should be noted that patients undergo all types of different

F. Husain-Syed (✉) · H.-W. Birk
Division of Nephrology, Pulmonology and Critical Care Medicine, Department of Internal Medicine II, University Clinic Giessen and Marburg (UKGM) – Campus Giessen, Klinikstr. 33, Giessen, Hessen 35392, Germany
e-mail: faeqhusain@yahoo.de

H.-W. Birk
e-mail: Horst-Walter.Birk@innere.med.uni-giessen.de

S. Lopez-Giacoman
Hospital General Isssste Zacatecas, Blvd. Adolfo López Mateos, Zacatecas Centro, 98000 Zacatecas, Zacatecas, Mexico
e-mail: shava32@hotmail.com

J. Rangaswami et al. (eds.), *Cardio-Nephrology*,
DOI 10.1007/978-3-319-56042-7_13

exposures during their hospital stay, which differ in terms of pathophysiology and timelines; for example, a patient may be exposed to a nephrotoxic drug, and then 6 h later, undergo an examination with intravenous contrast media, and 12 h later, develop cardiogenic shock. No biomarker can forecast these developments, and thus biomarkers may only be useful within a definable time window.

Given the different time frames and the heterogeneous nature of cardiorenal syndrome, it is unlikely that a single-marker strategy can meet all criteria. Instead, a combination of selected biomarkers is required to detect disease, assist therapy, and predict recovery or progression to chronic disease (Table 13.1). The use of biomarkers as a panel is a relatively new development, but may soon become available to clinicians. It should be noted that limited data are available on the performance of biomarkers in predicting recovery or progression to chronic disease, in particular, in concomitant cardiac and renal failure. Below, we review a selected group of currently established and promising future biomarkers, and the evidence linking them to cardiorenal syndrome. We also discuss our current pathobiological understanding of the biomarkers beyond being a diagnostic tool.

Biomarkers in Heart Disease

High-Sensitivity Cardiac Troponin

Cardiac troponins are components of the contraction apparatus of cardiac myocytes, and are established diagnostic and prognostic tools for acute myocardial infarction (Fig. 13.1). High-sensitivity cardiac troponin (cTn) I and T assays that measure cTn in the single-digit range of nanograms per liter have been introduced in clinical practice. With these assays, acute myocardial infarction can be detected at a much earlier stage, and a diagnosis can often be made based on laboratory results alone within 1–3 h of a patient's arrival in the emergency department [6]. However, the cTn level may be above the 99th percentile in a number of clinical conditions, and elevated levels can persist until 10 (cTn I) to 14 days (cTn T) after the onset of myocardial injury. Thus, the interpretation of cTn assays depends on serial testing and the clinical context. Chronic conditions causing sustained cTn elevation include non-coronary conditions (hypoxemia, global hyperperfusion) and coronary conditions resulting from ischemic imbalance (e.g., increased demand in the setting of known and putatively stable coronary artery disease lesions), classified as type II myocardial infarction. Furthermore, a significant overlap can be seen with kidney disease, where levels of cTn are frequently elevated in the absence of acute coronary syndrome, and the prevalence of elevated cTn increases with the severity of CKD [7]. To diagnose acute myocardial infarction in these patients, a dynamic change in cTn is useful. There is compelling evidence that in asymptomatic patients, a sustained cTn increase indicates kidney disease-related microvascular heart disease rather than a reduced clearance rate, and this may help to stratify CKD patients at high risk for structural heart damage and subsequent all-cause mortality. The Kidney Disease Outcomes Quality Initiative recommends the use of cardiac troponins for prognostication. In hemodialysis patients, measurements should be obtained before dialysis, as the modality alters the serum concentration of troponins.

B-Type Natriuretic Peptide and N-Terminal Pro-B-Type Natriuretic Peptide

B-type natriuretic peptide (BNP) and its inactive cleavage protein N-terminal pro-B-type natriuretic peptide (NT-proBNP) are markers of cardiac stretch from increased wall tension, and are established diagnostic, prognostic, and management tools for acutely decompensated HF, chronic HF, and acute coronary syndrome [8]. The two markers significantly differ in their half-life (BNP: 20 min, NT-proBNP: 120 min). BNP levels correlate with ventricular filling pressures and increase in proportion to the severity of systolic and diastolic dysfunction. As a vasoactive protein, BNP counterbalances the neurohormonal activation that is a fundamental aspect of the pathophysiology of HF and regulates blood pressure and volume through direct effects on the kidney and systemic vasculature. However, there is a lack of robust evidence that recombinant BNP can be used to improve cardiac, renal, and overall outcomes. As AKI is a heterogeneous disease, the utilization of BNP in addition to other renal biomarkers may further distinguish cardiorenal syndrome from other forms of AKI in HF. Elevations in BNP in the setting of acute HF and ACS are associated with an increased risk of AKI [8, 9]. Patients with CKD have higher levels of BNP than age- and gender-matched patients with normal renal function, probably because of increased cardiac production of BNP due to subclinical pressure overload, volume overload, and uremic cardiomyopathy as well as decreased renal clearance, which is more notable with NT-proBNP than BNP.

Soluble Suppressor of Tumorigenicity 2

Suppressor of tumorigenicity 2 (ST2), which exists both as a transmembrane ligand and in a soluble form (sST2), is a member of the interleukin (IL)-1 receptor family and has been identified as a marker integrating inflammation, myocyte hypertrophy, and tissue fibrosis. The circulating isoform sST2 is of particular interest, as it abrogates the anti-fibrotic effects of IL-33/ST2L signaling. Since sST2 lacks organ

Table 13.1 Current utility of biomarkers in diagnosis, targeted treatment, and prognosis of cardiorenal syndromes

Biomarkers	Diagnosis	Targeted treatment	Prognosis
Markers in heart disease			
High-sensitivity cTn	+++ (myocardial ischemia)	+	+
BNP	++	++	+++
sST2	None	None	+
Galectin-3	None	None	+
Markers in renal disease			
Biomarkers of glomerular integrity			
Serum creatinine	+	+	+++
Cystatin C	+++ (CKD)	None	+++
Albuminuria	+	+	+++
Biomarkers of renal tubular injury			
Urine sediment	++ (AKI)	(+)	++(+) (Renal recovery)
α[Alpha] 1-Microglobulin	+(+) (AKI)	(+)	(+)
TIMP-2*IGFBP7	++(+) (AKI)	None	++(+) (Renal recovery)
Serum NGAL	+	None	+
Urinary NGAL	+	None	+
L-FABP	+	None	+
H-FABP	+(+)	None	+
KIM-1	++	+	None
IL-18	+	None	+
Urinary angiotensinogen	++	None	++

The pluses indicate the level of the evidence available; +++: strong, ++: moderate, +: weak, (+): expected future evidence or absence of characteristics. None: no evidence

AKI acute kidney injury, *BNP* b-type natriuretic peptide, *CKD* chronic kidney disease, *H-LABP* heart-type fatty acid-binding protein, *cTn* cardiac troponin, *IGFBP7* insulin-like growth factor-binding protein 7, *IL* interleukin, *KIM-1* kidney injury molecule-1, *L-FABP* liver-type fatty acid-binding protein, *NGAL* neutrophil gelatinase-associated lipocalin, *sST2* soluble suppressor of tumorigenicity 2, *TIMP-2* tissue inhibitor of metalloproteinase-2

specificity, it cannot serve as a diagnostic tool. However, the 2013 American College of Cardiology Foundation (ACCF)/ American Heart Association (AHA) guidelines included sST2 for additive risk stratification of acute and chronic HF, as its concentration gives relevant information beyond that which can be obtained using other prognosticators, such as cTn and BNP [10]. sST2 is not adversely influenced by age and impaired renal function, and current data suggest that its level correlates with CKD severity [11]. Its prognostic value in cardiorenal syndrome has not been tested.

Galectin-3 and Urinary Angiotensinogen

Galectin-3 is a non-organ-specific β[beta]-galactoside-binding lectin with putative roles in immunomodulation, cell transformation, and fibrogenesis. Galectin-3 has garnered much attention in the fields of heart and kidney research, as it is implicated in the shared common pathogenesis of aldosterone-induced fibrosis via the transforming growth factor-β[beta]/Smad3-mediated activation of fibroblasts. Galectin-3 levels are influenced by age and renal function in progressive fashion, and it remains a matter of debate if an increase in galectin-3 is associated with cardiac functional and structural abnormalities in the absence of renal impairment [12]. Galectin-3 has been included in the 2013 ACCF/AHA guidelines for additive risk stratification of acute and chronic HF, and has additional prognostic value over cTn and BNP. In patients with kidney disease, galectin-3 is associated with a rapid decline in GFR, with incident CKD, as well as with adverse cardiovascular events and all-cause mortality [13].

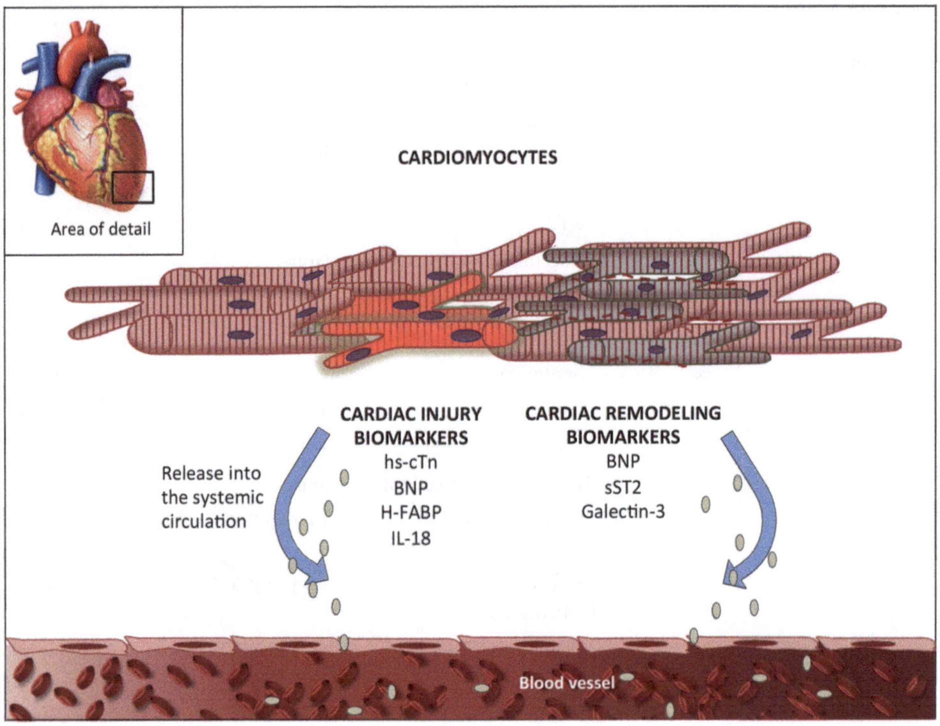

Fig. 13.1 Biomarkers in heart disease. Strategically selected biomarkers can be useful to identify the sequence of acute injury and risk of progression to chronic disease. Figure illustrates established and promising future biomarkers in heart disease. BNP, b-type natriuretic peptide; H-LABP, heart-type fatty acid-binding protein; hs-cTn, high-sensitivity cardiac troponin; IL, interleukin; sST2, soluble suppressor of tumorigenicity 2

Urinary angiotensinogen reflects intrarenal renin–angiotensin system activation and is currently being investigated as a biomarker of renal hemodynamic alterations as well as hypertension and CKD progression. In type 1 cardiorenal syndrome, urinary angiotensinogen level peaks on the first day (on admission) and appears to be a strong prognosticator for AKI (area under the curve [AUC], 0.84), hospital readmission, and 1-year mortality [14]. Complementary prospective studies are needed to assess the value of galectin-3- and urinary angiotensinogen-guided therapy with anti-renin–angiotensin–aldosterone agents in terms of cardiac/renal remodeling and fibrosis.

Biomarkers in Renal Disease

Markers of Glomerular Integrity

Albuminuria

Albuminuria is recognized as the best biomarker of glomerular dysfunction, but can also develop after proximal tubular damage (Fig. 13.2). At the time microalbuminuria becomes manifest, the phase of glomerular hyperfiltration is shifting to that of progressive renal function loss. Therefore, albuminuria is generally used as a biomarker for monitoring AKI progression to CKD and hypertension in non-HF patients. It is an established and inexpensive tool to screen and classify individuals in all CKD stages, and the National Kidney Foundation and AHA include microalbuminuria (30–300 mg/day albumin or 30–300 mg albumin/g creatinine) as a puissant risk factor for renal and cardiovascular diseases.

However, data on the performance of albuminuria in AKI are limited. After cardiac surgery [15], albuminuria predicts AKI with an AUC of 0.81 and correlates with future renal development. Current data support that its combination with tubular damage biomarkers can improve AKI prediction models. Microalbuminuria is present in one-third of acute [16] and chronic HF patients [17], and has been linked to endothelial dysfunction, venous congestion, and fluid overload. The reduction of albuminuria in acute HF correlates with improvement in BNP level and in the clinical symptoms of congestion, regardless of changes in renal function. In chronic HF, albuminuria has independent prognostic value in addition to that of GFR, but no evidence exists that it can be used to indicate therapeutic efficacy.

Markers of Renal Tubular Injury

Urine Sediment

Urine sediment is the oldest established diagnostic and prognostic biomarker for the evaluation of kidney disease. It is inexpensive and indicates the site of nephron injury—either glomerular or tubulointerstitial. Unfortunately, its use is hampered as urine microscopy is time-consuming and requires experience and clinical correlation. Urine sediment scores based on composites of granular casts and renal

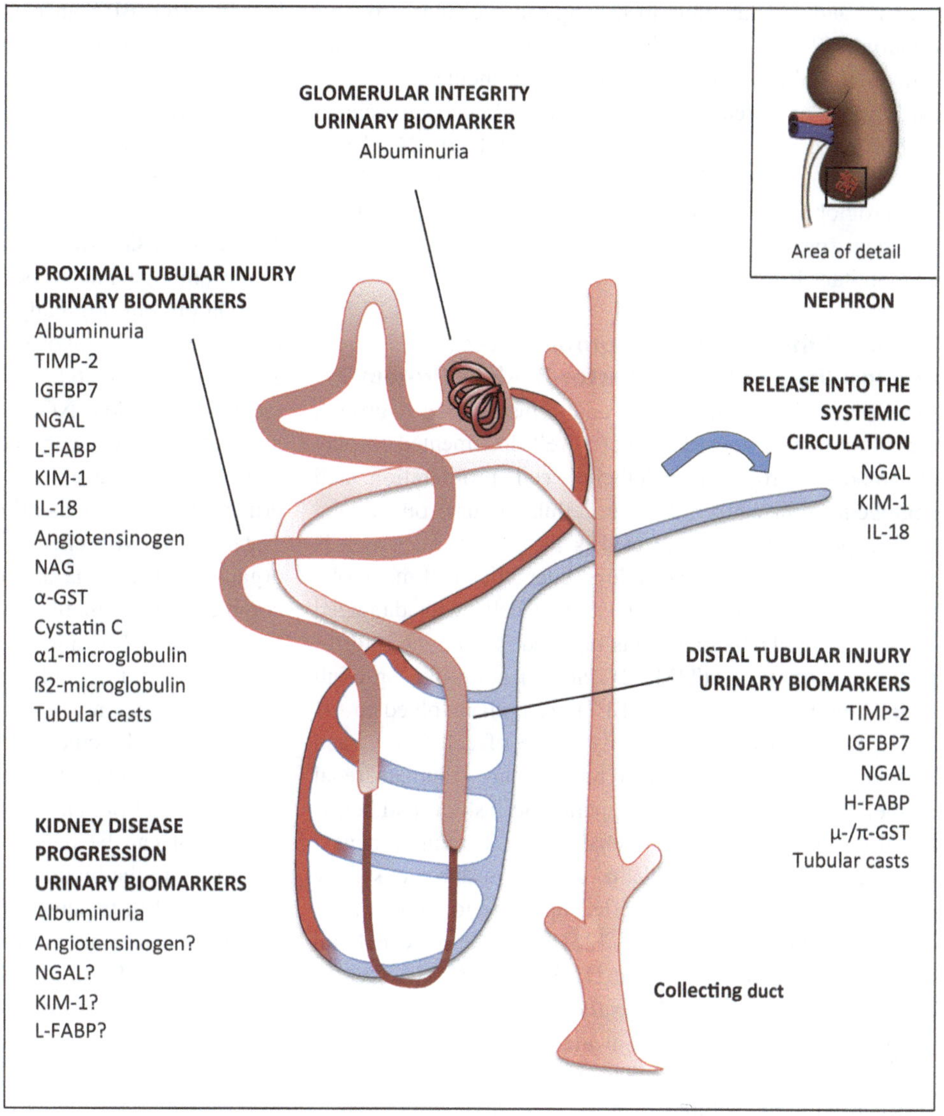

Fig. 13.2 Biomarkers in renal disease. Strategically selected biomarkers can be useful to identify the sequence of acute injury and risk of progression to chronic failure. Figure illustrates established and promising future biomarkers in renal disease, categorized by specific regions of the nephron. CKD, chronic kidney disease; GST, glutathione S-transferase; IGFBP7, insulin-like growth factor-binding protein 7; IL, interleukin; KIM-1, kidney injury molecule-1; L-/H-FABP, liver-type/heart-type fatty acid-binding protein; NAG, *N*-acetyl-β[beta]-D-glucosaminidase; NGAL, neutrophil gelatinase-associated lipocalin; TIMP-2, tissue inhibitor of metalloproteinase-2

tubular epithelial cells have been evaluated in the acute setting, and show a strong association with AKI stage, with an AUC for worsening AKI of 0.66–0.85 [18]. Although highly specific in discriminating AKI from non-AKI, it lacks sensitivity, which might be improved by the use of novel tubular damage biomarkers. Beyond providing valuable information about the course of AKI, urine sediment scores can predict non-renal recovery with an AUC of 0.79 [19]. Urine sediment microscopy has not been described in cardiorenal syndrome.

α[Alpha]1-Microglobulin

α[Alpha]1-Microglobulin is a low-molecular-weight protein (33 kDa) synthesized in the liver, and its unbound form is freely filtered through the glomerular capillaries and reabsorbed by the proximal tubular cells via endocytotic uptake. Therefore, its increased urinary excretion (indicating tubular proteinuria) can serve as a sensitive marker for proximal tubular damage. In clinical practice, α[alpha]1-microglobulin is generally used as an inexpensive biomarker for screening and monitoring acquired tubular disorders (e.g., those caused by nephrotoxins) and inherited tubulopathies (e.g., Fanconi syndrome). Its role in AKI and concomitant heart disease is, however, not well explored and remains inconclusive.

In a heterogeneous population of patients with non-oliguric AKI, α[alpha]1-microglobulin was found to be an early indicator of the requirement for renal replacement therapy (AUC: 0.86) [20], albeit its performance in predicting early AKI (AUC: 0.62) [21] and renal recovery (AUC: 0.69) [22] was moderate. However, its lack of sensitivity can be improved using it in combination with novel tubular damage biomarkers. In the chronic setting, the assessment of urinary α[alpha]1-microglobulin may allow an early diagnosis of hypertensive nephropathy in non-HF patients and is analogous to the appearance of microalbuminuria [23]. It should be noted that α[alpha] 1-microglobulin is not associated with incident HF and cardiovascular disease-related mortality but is associated with other causes of death (e.g., due to CKD) [24]. Liver dysfunction can alter serum levels of α[alpha] 1-microglobulin, and therefore, this marker may not have sufficient specificity and sensitivity for AKI in patients with concomitant liver disease.

Tissue Inhibitor of Metalloproteinase-2 and Insulin-Like Growth Factor-Binding Protein 7

Matrix metalloproteinases and insulin-like growth factor-binding proteins have been well documented to play an important role in endothelial cell proliferation and angiogenesis in cancer. During cellular injury, one of the earliest processes to be affected is the cell cycle, which is downregulated to preserve cellular energetics and metabolic functions, and prevent the division of cells with damaged DNA until the DNA damage is repaired. Tissue inhibitor of metalloproteinase-2 (TIMP-2) and insulin-like growth factor-binding protein 7 (IGFBP7) are both involved in G1 cell cycle arrest during the early phase of cell injury, and current data suggest that their release may stimulate renal epithelium in an autocrine and paracrine fashion and sensitize it for upcoming insults ("renal alert"). Through repeated episodes of self-limited sublethal cellular insults, the kidney may precondition and increase its capability to recover after alterations in cellular processes [25]. Both the proximal and distal renal tubular cells release TIMP-2 and IGFBP7, which can be detected in urine. Recently, commercialized in-vitro diagnostic tests have become available for both markers.

The performance of TIMP-2 and IGFBP7 has been validated in different settings of AKI, and seems to be consistent. In critically ill patients (with evidence of respiratory or cardiovascular failure) [26], and cardiac [27] and non-cardiac [28] surgery patients, each cell cycle arrest marker showed an AUC value of more than 0.76 to predict the development of AKI (Acute Kidney Injury Network stage 2 or 3) within 4–12 h, while the combination of the two markers [TIMP-2*IGFBP7] resulted in an AUC above 0.8. This result was significantly superior to those of other available biomarkers (urine: KIM-1, NGAL, L-FABP, IL-18, pi-GST; serum: NGAL, cystatin C), which might be due in part to the varying kinetics of the two markers. When added to clinical scoring systems, [TIMP-2*IGFBP7] significantly improved risk prediction of AKI. To ensure high sensitivity/high negative predictive value and high specificity/high positive predictive value, cutoffs of 0.3 and 2.0 (ng/ml)2/1000, respectively, have been validated [26]. Additionally, current data indicate that the decline in [TIMP-2*IGFBP7] urinary concentrations in the first 24 h after cardiac surgery can predict renal recovery (defined by serum creatinine value at hospital discharge < the baseline value) with an AUC of 0.79 [27]. The relationship of cell cycle arrest markers in cardiorenal syndrome has not yet been described.

Neutrophil Gelatinase-Associated Lipocalin

Neutrophil gelatinase-associated lipocalin (NGAL) is a 25-kDa protein originally found in neutrophil granules, and is secreted by the myocardium, renal tubules (loop of Henle and collecting ducts), activated immune cells, lung, hepatocytes, and colon. NGAL is freely filtered in the glomerulus, but is nearly completely reabsorbed in the proximal convoluted tubule unless tubular damage exists. Therefore, urinary NGAL reflects primarily intrarenal damage, whereas systemic NGAL reflects injury to the kidneys and other organs. Both plasma and urine NGAL can be tested using commercially available assays. Among the new biomarkers for cardiorenal syndrome detection, NGAL is the most extensively and carefully studied, with a focus on its ability to serve as a diagnostic tool for AKI and its prognostic value in patients with acute and chronic HF.

NGAL is activated and released after myocardial ischemia and inflammation, and seems to be an early marker of renal injury that can be detected with high sensitivity and high specificity in the blood and urine, increasing 24–48 h before creatinine [29]. In acute HF, serum NGAL level >140 ng/ml on hospital admission or on the third day after admission has been associated with a 7.4-fold increase in AKI (86% sensitivity and 54% specificity) [30]. Recently, a meta-analysis demonstrated the very early utility of urinary NGAL (intraoperative measurement) and plasma NGAL (postoperative measurement) to predict cardiac surgery-associated AKI to be moderate (AUC < 0.7) [31]. Serial measurements of serum NGAL in acute HF appear to strengthen its ability to predict AKI; the degree of change in NGAL from the baseline to its peak produced an AUC for AKI of 0.91 compared to an AUC of only 0.69 for NGAL at admission [32]. However, the results reported to date are not entirely conclusive, possibly because of the lack of cutoff values for cardiorenal syndrome and the variations in NGAL level due to disease activity and several clinical factors (e.g., age, gender, sepsis). Breidthardt et al. showed that creatinine outperforms plasma NGAL, and is a more independent predictor of AKI in acute HF [33]. Plasma but not urinary NGAL increases markedly with GFR reduction, and can possibly generate a high number of false-positive diagnoses of AKI in stable CKD patients. Thus, acute rather than chronic cardiorenal syndromes may be a more suitable setting for the clinical implementation of NGAL (GISSI-HF study) [34].

L-Type Fatty Acid-Binding Protein and H-Type Fatty Acid-Binding Protein

Liver-type fatty acid-binding protein (L-FABP) binds unsaturated fatty acids and lipid peroxidation products in hypoxic tissue, and thus plays a putative antioxidant and renoprotective role predominantly in the renal proximal tubular cells, which use fatty acids as their major source of energy. The heart-type fatty acid-binding protein (H-FABP) can be found in cardiomyocytes and distal tubules. Both biomarkers are diagnostic and prognostic tools for AKI, HF, and myocardial ischemia.

The 14-kDa heavy cytosolic L-FABP has been shown to be an early urinary marker of AKI, and a commercialized test is available for this molecule. In the setting of cardiac surgery, urinary L-FABP peaks after 6 h and shows an overall AUC of 0.72 in predicting AKI; its utility can be increased within a biomarker panel [31]. Serum H-FABP has been tested as a diagnostic marker of HF, where it might improve the diagnostic accuracy of NT-proBNP and predict HF-related rehospitalization. It also predicts the occurrence of AKI with an AUC of 0.79, outperforming L-FABP, and urinary NGAL [35]. In the setting of acute myocardial ischemia without elevated high-sensitivity cTn, H-FABP might identify patients at high risk for adverse cardiac events [36].

Kidney Injury Molecule-1

Kidney injury molecule-1 (KIM-1) is a 38.7-kDa transmembrane tubular protein solely expressed in response to ischemic or nephrotoxic insults in the proximal renal tubular cells. In the setting of AKI, KIM-1 is upregulated and sheds its ectodomain, which can be measured as a diagnostic marker in urine. Experimental studies and the late timing of its peak changes (>48 h) indicate that KIM-1 may also be involved in the repair response to injury, as well as the transition from AKI to CKD; therefore, KIM-1 might serve as a prognostic tool as well [4]. KIM-1 levels are associated with ejection fraction, functional status, and incident HF risk [37]. KIM-1 levels also predict an increased risk of AKI in chronic HF [35] and show an overall AUC of 0.72 to develop AKI after cardiac surgery [31].

Interleukin-18

The 22-kD cytokine IL-18 mediates inflammation and acute injury through the nuclear factor-κ[kappa]B pathway, and induces the upregulation of other proinflammatory markers, such as tumor necrosis factor- α[alpha], inducible nitric oxide synthase, and chemokines, which lead to cell infiltration in multiple organs. In the kidney, IL-18 is of particular interest given its possible role in promoting and exacerbating ischemic renal injury. IL-18 is released from the proximal convoluted tubules and can be measured in urine within the first 6 h of renal injury and peaks after 12–18 h. In post-cardiac surgery patients, IL-18 shows a moderate overall predictive AUC value of 0.68 for AKI [31]. In addition, there is evidence that IL-18 is upregulated in HF [38], and may translocate into the systemic circulation and cause end-organ dysfunction, including renal dysfunction. IL-18 may be important as a long-term prognostic marker of persistent renal impairment after acute HF, implicating the ongoing inflammatory process in the kidney [39].

Time-Dependent Release of Biomarkers and Their Clinical Implications

Cardiorenal biomarkers give valuable information regarding the pathobiology and timeline of molecular events implicated in the initiation and progression of this complex heterogeneous disease [4]. For instance, myocardial infarction is accompanied by progressive mechanical obstruction, plaque inflammation and rupture, reduced coronary vasoreactivity, and superimposed thrombosis. Myocardial ischemia and necrosis are the consequences, followed by cardiac remodeling. Thus, the activation of selected markers during different phases of the process can be detected. Plaque inflammation is associated with release of IL-18. The development of myocardial necrosis is accompanied by the time-dependent release of troponin, myoglobin, and creatine kinase-MB. The hemodynamic consequences of myocardial infarction are reflected by an increase in BNP. Galectin-3 and sST2 are implicated in the pathogenesis of myocardial fibrosis.

Analogous to myocardial infarction, different phases can be drawn throughout the continuum of AKI, though these may not necessarily be applicable to all forms of AKI [4, 40]. Several studies have investigated blood and urinary biomarker kinetics in cardiac surgery-associated AKI simply because the timing of injury is known and the dominant mechanism of AKI is thought to be intraoperative ischemia–reperfusion injury [41]. The initial insult causes alterations in vasoreactivity and renal perfusion, which is followed by vascular obstruction/coagulation and epithelial inflammation. Apoptosis and necrosis of tubular epithelial cells are the sequelae, and current data suggest that the early release of IL-18 exacerbates renal injury during the extension phase of AKI. Contrarily, NGAL and L-FABP are implicated in re-epithelialization and antioxidant mechanisms, and thus mitigate renal injury. The protective role of TIMP-2 and IGFBP7 was mentioned before, and current data suggest that an upregulation of TIMP-2 and IGFBP7 might "alert" surrounding renal tubular cells to potential renal insults. This fits into the patchy nature of AKI, which can lead to profound dysfunction even though only few cells seem to be significantly affected. Renal repair occurs 2–3 days after renal injury, and is characterized by the stabilization of glomerular function and proliferation/migration of tubular epithelial cells to the damaged epithelium. Persistent elevation of NGAL, KIM-1, and L-FABP suggests that these markers have a potential role in these phases and beyond. Finally, activation of the renin–angiotensin system, best reflected by the sustained elevation of urinary angiotensinogen, may play an important role in ongoing kidney injury and progression to CKD.

Use of Biomarkers in Combination

We have summarized the current biomarker-integrated concept of cardiorenal syndrome, including their possible role in the pathobiology of injury, followed by recovery or progression to chronic disease. Biomarkers cannot replace clinical evaluation, and expertise is required for their meaningful interpretation. Both conventional (cTn, BNP, creatinine, albuminuria, urine sediment, α[alpha]1-microglobulin) as well as new biomarkers (e.g., galectin-3, urinary angiotensinogen, TIMP-2*IGFBP7, NGAL, KIM-1) provide mechanistic insights, permit monitoring, and lead to a better understanding of the various disease states in cardiorenal syndrome. Furthermore, they can provide insights into disease biology and help to better classify at-risk individuals in the absence of overt clinical disease. The combination of strategically selected biomarkers may distinguish cardiorenal syndrome from other forms of AKI in heart disease. It is expected that in the future, a panel of biomarkers will provide sufficient risk prediction and early diagnosis to allow for the prevention and treatment of cardiorenal syndrome and the determination of prognosis.

Funding No funding to declare

Conflict of interest The authors do not have any relationship that may be perceived as an actual or possible conflict of interest with the content of the manuscript.

References

1. Husain-Syed F, McCullough PA, Birk HW, Renker M, Brocca A, Seeger W, Ronco C. Cardio-pulmonary–renal interactions: a multidisciplinary approach. J Am Coll Cardiol. 2015;65 (22):2433–48.
2. Biomarkers Definitions Working Group. Biomarkers and surrogate endpoints: preferred definitions and conceptual framework. Clin Pharmacol Ther. 2001;69(3):89–95.
3. Damman K, Testani JM. The kidney in heart failure: an update. Eur Heart J. 2015;36(23):1437–44.
4. Alge JL, Arthur JM. Biomarkers of AKI: a review of mechanistic relevance and potential therapeutic implications. Clin J Am Soc Nephrol. 2015;10(1):147–55.
5. Haase M, Kellum JA, Ronco C. Subclinical AKI—an emerging syndrome with important consequences. Nat Rev Nephrol. 2012;8 (12):735–9.
6. de Lemos JA, Drazner MH, Omland T, Ayers CR, Khera A, Rohatgi A, Hashim I, Berry JD, Das SR, Morrow DA, McGuire DK. Association of troponin T detected with a highly sensitive assay and cardiac structure and mortality risk in the general population. JAMA. 2010;304(22):2503–12.
7. Wang AY, Lai KN. Use of cardiac biomarkers in end-stage renal disease. J Am Soc Nephrol. 2008;19(9):1643–52.
8. Oremus M, McKelvie R, Don-Wauchope A, Santaguida PL, Ali U, Balion C, Hill S, Booth R, Brown JA, Bustamam A, Sohel N, Raina P. A systematic review of BNP and NT-proBNP in the management of heart failure: overview and methods. Heart Fail Rev. 2014;19(4):413–9.
9. Ronco C, McCullough P, Anker SD, Anand I, Aspromonte N, Bagshaw SM, Bellomo R, Berl T, Bobek I, Cruz DN, Daliento L, Davenport A, Haapio M, Hillege H, House AA, Katz N, Maisel A, Mankad S, Zanco P, Mebazaa A, Palazzuoli A, Ronco F, Shaw A, Sheinfeld G, Soni S, Vescovo G, Zamperetti N, Ponikowski P, Acute Dialysis Quality Initiative (ADQI) consensus group. Cardio-renal syndromes: report from the consensus conference of the acute dialysis quality initiative. Eur Heart J. 2010;31(6):703–11.
10. Gandhi PU, Testani JM, Ahmad T. The current and potential clinical relevance of heart failure biomarkers. Curr Heart Fail Rep. 2015;12(5):318–27.
11. Bao YS, Na SP, Zhang P, Jia XB, Liu RC, Yu CY, Mu SH, Xie RJ. Characterization of interleukin-33 and soluble ST2 in serum and their association with disease severity in patients with chronic kidney disease. J Clin Immunol. 2012;32(3):587–94.
12. deFilippi CR, Christenson RH. Evolving role of galectin-3 as a cardiac biomarker: heart failure with preserved ejection fraction and renal function, important pieces of the puzzle. JACC Heart Fail. 2015;3(3):253–6.
13. Drechsler C, Delgado G, Wanner C, Blouin K, Pilz S, Tomaschitz A, Kleber ME, Dressel A, Willmes C, Krane V, Krämer BK, März W, Ritz E, van Glist WH, van der Harst P, de Boer RA. Galectin-3, renal function, and clinical outcomes: results from the LURIC and 4D studies. J Am Soc Nephrol. 2015;26(9):2213–21.
14. Yang X, Chen C, Tian J, Zha Y, Xiong Y, Sun Z, Chen P, Li J, Yang T, Ma C, Liu H, Wang X, Hou FF. Urinary angiotensinogen level predicts AKI in acute decompensated heart failure: a prospective, two-stage study. J Am Soc Nephrol. 2015;26 (8):2032–41.
15. Molnar AO, Parikh CR, Sint K, Coca SG, Koyner J, Patel UD, Butrymowicz I, Shlipak M, Garg AX. Association of postoperative proteinuria with AKI after cardiac surgery among patients at high risk. Clin J Am Soc Nephrol. 2012;7(11):1749–60.
16. Koyama S, Sato Y, Tanada Y, Fujiwara H, Takatsu Y. Early evolution and correlates of urine albumin excretion in patients presenting with acutely decompensated heart failure. Circ Heart Fail. 2013;6(2):227–32.
17. van de Wal RM, Asselbergs FW, Plokker HW, Smilde TD, Lok D, van Veldhuisen DJ, van Gilst WH, Voors AA. High prevalence of microalbuminuria in chronic heart failure patients. J Card Fail. 2005;11(8):602–6.
18. Perazella MA. The urine sediment as a biomarker of kidney disease. Am J Kidney Dis. 2015;66(5):748–55.
19. Chawla LS, Dommu A, Berger A, Shih S, Patel SS. Urinary sediment cast scoring index for acute kidney injury: a pilot study. Nephron Clin Pract. 2008;110(3):c145–50.
20. Herget-Rosenthal S, Poppen D, Hüsing J, Marggraf G, Pietruck F, Jakob HG, Philipp T, Kribben A. Prognostic value of tubular

proteinuria and enzymuria in nonoliguric acute tubular necrosis. Clin Chem. 2004;50(3):552–8.
21. Liangos O, Tighiaouart H, Perianayagam MC, Kolyada A, Han WK, Wald R, Bonventre JV, Jaber BL. Comparative analysis of urinary biomarkers for early detection of acute kidney injury following cardiopulmonary bypass. Biomarkers. 2009;14(6):423–31.
22. Aregger F, Uehlinger DE, Witowski J, Brunisholz RA, Hunziker P, Frey FJ, Jörres A. Identification of IGFBP-7 by urinary proteomics as a novel prognostic marker in early acute kidney injury. Kidney Int. 2014;85(4):909–19.
23. Aznaouridis K, Vlachopoulos C, Masoura K, Pietri P, Vyssolis G, Ioakeimidis N, Stefanadis C, Tousoulis D. Office blood pressure is a predictor of aortic elastic properties and urinary protein excretion in subjects with white coat hypertension. Int J Cardiol. 2015;21 (203):98–103.
24. O'Seaghdha CM, Hwang SJ, Larson MG, Meigs JB, Vasan RS, Fox CS. Analysis of a urinary biomarker panel for incident kidney disease and clinical outcomes. J Am Soc Nephrol. 2013;24 (11):1880–8.
25. Zarbock A, Schmidt C, Van Aken H, Wempe C, Martens S, Zahn PK, Wolf B, Goebel U, Schwer CI, Rosenberger P, Haeberle H, Görlich D, Kellum JA, Meersch M. RenalRIPC Investigators. Effect of remote ischemic preconditioning on kidney injury among high-risk patients undergoing cardiac surgery: a randomized clinical trial. JAMA. 2015;313(21):2133–41.
26. Kashani K, Al-Khafaji A, Ardiles T, Artigas A, Bagshaw SM, Bell M, Bihorac A, Birkhahn R, Cely CM, Chawla LS, Davison DL, Feldkamp T, Forni LG, Gong MN, Gunnerson KJ, Haase M, Hackett J, Honore PM, Hoste EA, Jiannes-Boyau O, Joannidis M, Kim P, Koyner JL, Laskowitz DT, Lissauer ME, Marx G, McCullough PA, Mullaney S, Ostermann M, Rimmele T, Shapiro NI, Shaw AD, Shi J, Sprague AM, Vincent JL, Vinsonneau C, Wagner L, Walker MG, Wilkerson RG, Zacharowski K, Kellum JA. Discovery and validation of cell cycle arrest biomarkers in human acute kidney injury. Crit Care. 2013;17(1): R25.
27. Meersch M, Schmidt C, Van Aken H, Martens S, Rossaint J, Singbartl K, Görlich D, Kellum JA, Zarbrock A. Urinary TIMP-2 and IGFBP7 as early biomarkers of acute kidney injury and renal recovery following cardiac surgery. PLoS ONE. 2014;9(3): e93460.
28. Gocze I, Koch M, Renner P, Zeman F, Graf BM, Dahlke MH, Nerlich M, Schlitt HJ, Kellum JA, Bein T. Urinary biomarkers TIMP-2 and IGFBP7 early predict acute kidney injury after major surgery. PLoS ONE. 2015;10(3):e0120863.
29. Mishra J, Dent C, Tarabishi R, Mitsnefes MM, Ma Q, Kelly C, Ruff SM, Zahedi K, Shao M, Bean J, Mori K, Barasch J, Devarajan P. Neutrophil gelatinase-associated lipocalin (NGAL) as a biomarker for acute renal injury after cardiac surgery. Lancet. 2005;365(9466):1231–8.
30. Aghel A, Shrestha K, Mullens W, Borowski A, Tang WH. Serum neutrophil gelatinase-associated lipocalin (NGAL) in predicting worsening renal function in acute decompensated heart failure. J Card Fail. 2010;16(1):49–54.
31. Ho J, Tangri N, Komenda P, Kaushal A, Sood M, Brar R, Gill K, Walker S, MacDonald K, Hiebert BM, Arora RC, Rigatto C. Urinary, plasma, and serum biomarkers' utility for predicting acute kidney injury associated with cardiac surgery in adults: a meta-analysis. Am J Kidney Dis. 2015;66(6):993–1005.
32. Mortara A, Bonadies M, Mazzetti S, Fracchioni I, Delfino P, Chioffi M, Bersano C, Specchia G. Neutrophil gelatinase-associated lipocalin predicts worsening of renal function in acute heart failure: methodological and clinical issues. J Cardiovasc Med. 2013;14(9):629–34.
33. Breidthardt T, Socrates T, Drexler B, Noveanu M, Heinisch C, Arenja N, Klima T, Züsli C, Reichlin T, Potocki M, Twerenbold R, Steiger J, Mueller C. Plasma neutrophil gelatinase-associated lipocalin for the prediction of acute kidney injury in acute heart failure. Crit Care. 2012;16(1):R2.
34. Damman K, Masson S, Hillege HL, Voors AA, van Veldhuisen DJ, Rossignol P, Proietti G, Barbuzzi S, Nicolosi GL, Tavazzi L, Maggioni AP, Latini R. Tubular damage and worsening renal function in chronic heart failure. JACC Heart Fail. 2013;1(5):417–24.
35. Shirakabe A, Hata N, Kobayashi N, Okazaki H, Shinada T, Tomita K, Yamamoto M, Tsurumi M, Matsushita M, Yamamoto Y, Yokoyama S, Asai K, Shimizu W. Serum heart-type fatty acid-binding protein level can be used to detect acute kidney injury on admission and predict an adverse outcome in patients with acute heart failure. Circ J. 2015;79(1):119–28.
36. Viswanathan K, Kilcullen N, Morrell C, Thistlethwaite SJ, Sivananthan MU, Hassan TB, Barth JH, Hall AS. Heart-type fatty acid-binding protein predicts long-term mortality and re-infarction in consecutive patients with suspected acute coronary syndrome who are troponin-negative. J Am Coll Cardiol. 2010;55(23):2590–8.
37. Driver TH, Katz R, Ix JH, Magnani JW, Peralta CA, Parikh CR, Fried L, Newman AB, Kritchevsky SB, Sarnak MJ, Shlipak MG, Health ABC. Study. Urinary kidney injury molecule 1 (KIM-1) and interleukin 18 (IL-18) as risk markers for heart failure in older adults: the Health, Aging, and Body Composition (Health ABC) Study. Am J Kidney Dis. 2014;64(1):49–56.
38. Mallat Z, Heymes C, Corbaz A, Logeart D, Alouani S, Cohen-Solal A, Seidler T, Hasenfuss G, Chvatchko AM, Tedgui A. Evidence for altered interleukin 18 (IL)-18 pathway in human heart failure. FASEB J. 2004;18(14):1752–4.
39. Verbrugge FH, Dupont M, Shao Z, Shrestha K, Singh D, Finucan M, Mullens W, Tang WH. Novel urinary biomarkers in detecting acute kidney injury, persistent renal impairment, and all-cause mortality following decongestive therapy in acute decompensated heart failure. J Card Fail. 2013;19(9):621–8.
40. Sutton TA, Fisher CJ, Molitoris BA. Microvascular endothelial injury and dysfunction during ischemic acute renal failure. Kidney Int. 2002;62(5):1539–49.
41. Parikh CR, Thiessen-Philbrook H, Garg AX, Kadiyala D, Shlipak MG, Koyner JL, Edelstein CL, Devarajan P, Patel UD, Zappitelli M, Krawczeski CD, Passik CS. Coca SG; TRIBE-AKI Consortium. Performance of kidney injury molecule-1 and liver fatty acid-binding protein and combined biomarkers of AKI after cardiac surgery. Clin J Am Soc Nephrol. 2013;8(7):1079–88.

Kidney Attack: Is NGAL Set to Take the Stage with Troponins?

14

Prasad Devarajan

Concept of Kidney Attack

The symptoms, consequences, and urgency for intervention in subjects with heart attack (myocardial infarction), brain attack (stroke), or lung attack (exacerbation of COPD) are widely acknowledged. Dramatic advances in the early diagnosis and management of these conditions have been made possible by objective measurement of structural injury biomarkers. Examples include troponins that are released from damaged cardiomyocytes in acute myocardial injury, and sensitive imaging biomarkers that detect structural brain injury in strokes. In striking contrast, the syndrome of kidney attack, now widely referred to as acute kidney injury (AKI), is less well recognized by clinicians and is almost unknown to the lay public [1]. The overall incidence of AKI is similar to that of heart attacks and higher than that of brain attacks. However, AKI is largely asymptomatic and often occurs in the wake of other underlying conditions such as cardiac surgical procedures, sepsis, critical illness, and nephrotoxin use. Establishing the diagnosis in the estimated 5% of all hospitalized patients and a third of intensive care patients who suffer from AKI and its devastating consequences currently hinges on serial measurements of functional biomarkers such as serum creatinine. This approach is flawed due to several reasons [2]. First, several non-renal factors such as age, gender, diet, muscle mass, and medications can influence serum creatinine concentration independent of changes in kidney structure or function. Second, a previously healthy kidney is endowed with significant functional reserve, such that over 50% of kidney function can be lost due to an acute damaging insult without any change in serum creatinine. Third, a rise in serum creatinine concentration accompanies any condition that leads to transient renal hypoperfusion; these episodes of "prerenal azotemia" are usually fully reversible without consequences, and must be differentiated from the more ominous forms of "intrinsic AKI" with accompanying structural damage. Fourth, there is typically a lag period of hours to days after an acute injurious event before serum creatinine rises, reflective of the time elapsed before a new equilibrium between steady-state production and decreased excretion of creatinine is established. During this time, structural damage is known to occur to the kidney tubules, and experimental evidence accumulated over the last four decades clearly demonstrates the efficacy of several interventions that can prevent and/or treat AKI during this "subclinical" phase, before the serum creatinine rises. The paucity of a troponin-like early biomarker of structural AKI has crippled our ability to translate these promising interventions to human AKI in a timely manner.

P. Devarajan (✉)
Department of Nephrology and Hypertension, Cincinnati Children's Hospital Medical Center, University of Cincinnati School of Medicine, 3333 Burnet Avenue, MLC 7022, Cincinnati, OH 45229-3039, USA
e-mail: prasad.devarajan@cchmc.org

Desirable Characteristics of a Troponin-like Biomarker of Kidney Attack

Like troponins, AKI biomarkers should be rapidly measurable using standardized clinical laboratory platforms and easily accessible samples such as urine or blood. They should be sensitive to facilitate early detection, with a wide dynamic range and cutoff values that establish or predict the diagnosis with confidence. They should exhibit strong predictive performance by area under the receiver-operating characteristic curve (AUC) analysis.

Given the myriad complexities of kidney function and pathophysiology, AKI biomarkers should ideally display several additional characteristics [3]. First and foremost, they should be specific for structural damage and differentiate intrinsic AKI from other conditions that also cause the serum creatinine to rise (such as functional prerenal azotemia and chronic kidney disease). Indeed, the ideal AKI biomarker should be able to predict "subclinical" structural AKI and its

J. Rangaswami et al. (eds.), *Cardio-Nephrology*,
DOI 10.1007/978-3-319-56042-7_14

consequences independent of the bronze standard functional marker, serum creatinine. Second, they should allow for risk stratification (duration and severity of AKI) and prognostication (need for dialysis, length of hospital stay, mortality). Third, they should represent real-time indicators of disease and recovery, so that the response to AKI interventions can be monitored in clinical trials and in clinical practice.

The search for biomarkers for the early diagnosis of AKI and its outcomes is an area of intense contemporary research that has yielded several promising candidates. Neutrophil gelatinase-associated lipocalin (NGAL) is the most widely studied and validated AKI biomarker that is clinically available at the present time, and is the focus of this chapter.

NGAL as a Biologically Plausible Kidney Attack Biomarker

Unbiased transcriptome profiling studies reported in over 150 distinct studies performed in AKI models from several species ranging from mouse to man have consistently revealed NGAL to be one of the most dramatically upregulated genes in the kidney soon after an ischemic or nephrotoxic insult [4, 5]. The 25 kDa NGAL protein is also highly induced in regenerating and recovering kidney tubule cells [6]. NGAL binds siderophores, which in turn bind iron. Chelation of toxic iron from the extracellular environment is an important mechanism that protects the kidney from worsening injury in the early phases of AKI. In addition, the NGAL-mediated delivery of iron to intracellular sites promotes regeneration and proliferation of tubule cells in the repair phase of AKI. Thus, the biologic role of NGAL in AKI is one of the marked preservations of function, and an enhanced tubule cell proliferative response [7]. The serendipitous findings that the induced NGAL protein is rapidly secreted both into the urine as well as plasma in animal models of AKI have launched a decade of translational studies evaluating NGAL as a noninvasive biomarker of human AKI. These studies have now established a definitive role for NGAL as a biomarker to predict AKI and its adverse outcomes independent of serum creatinine, for the differential diagnosis of intrinsic structural AKI from a prerenal state, and for facilitating AKI clinical trials. The bulk of these studies have been conducted in clinical situations that are highly pertinent to cardio-nephrology, including cardiac surgery, contrast nephropathy, and critical illness, and are reviewed below.

NGAL for the Early Prediction of Kidney Attack

Cardiac surgery-associated acute kidney injury (CS-AKI) is the second most common cause of AKI in critically ill adults and children, with a reported incidence of 20–60% [8]. However, the diagnosis is typically delayed, with an increase in serum creatinine occurring only 1–3 days after cardiopulmonary bypass [2, 3]. As first highlighted by Mishra et al. [9], a dramatic increase in both urine and plasma NGAL is easily detected within 2–6 h of cardiopulmonary bypass in patients destined for AKI, with a predictive AUC of over 0.9. These findings have now been confirmed in more than 30 publications of good methodological quality, involving well over 7500 patients, and have now been the subject of three meta-analyses and systematic reviews [10–12]. Collectively, the published data have confirmed the high diagnostic accuracy of NGAL in the early detection of CS-AKI, with measurements obtained within 4–6 h after initiation of cardiopulmonary bypass yielding an overall predictive pooled AUC of 0.86, surpassing the performance of all other biomarkers tested to date. The overall pooled sensitivity of NGAL for the diagnosis of AKI was 0.68 and overall specificity was 0.79 (Table 14.1). The predictive performance for CS-AKI was similar for both urine and plasma NGAL. Subgroup analyses revealed that NGAL displays the highest predictive accuracy for CS-AKI in children (AUC 0.89 vs. 0.83 in adults) and in subjects without pre-existing renal insufficiency (AUC 0.87 vs. 0.81 with pre-existing renal insufficiency) [12].

Critical illness, including sepsis, is the most common cause of AKI worldwide, with a reported incidence of 30–50%. The utility of serum creatinine in this clinical scenario

Table 14.1 NGAL for the early prediction of kidney attack in various clinical settings

Clinical setting	Number of studies	Number of patients	Urine or plasma	Pooled sensitivity	Pooled specificity	Pooled AUC	Reference
AKI in cardiac surgery	24	4066	Both	0.68	0.79	0.86	[12]
AKI in sepsis	6	433	Plasma	0.83	0.57	0.86	[13]
AKI in sepsis	12	1263	Urine	0.80	0.80	0.90	[13]
AKI after contrast	14	1520	Both	0.84	0.89	0.93	[15]

As reported in recent meta-analyses [12, 13, 15]. AUC, area under the receiver-operating characteristic curve is limited by several factors, including the delay in rise, the confounding influence of a prerenal state, the varying degrees of established AKI prior to initial presentation, and the diminished endogenous production of creatinine in sepsis. The ability of NGAL to predict AKI in this heterogeneous population has been examined in over 8500 critically ill patients [11]. Collectively, the data from 25 publications have confirmed the high diagnostic accuracy of NGAL in the early detection of AKI in critical illness, with measurements obtained within 6 h of clinical presentation yielding an overall predictive AUC of 0.8 [11]. A recent meta-analysis [13] has specifically examined the value of NGAL for the prediction of AKI in patients with sepsis, in whom NGAL concentrations can potentially be elevated even in the absence of kidney damage due to release from activated neutrophils. As would be expected, the specificity of plasma NGAL for predicting AKI was inferior to that of urine NGAL in sepsis, although the sensitivities and pooled AUCs were similar and promisingly high (Table 14.1).

Contrast-induced acute kidney injury (CI-AKI) is a common cause of AKI after cardiac catheterization. In general, advances in diagnostic and interventional imaging techniques have resulted in an ever-increasing number of patients exposed to iodinated contrast media. CI-AKI is the third most common cause of hospital-acquired AKI, accounting for more than 10% of cases. However, the diagnosis is once again typically delayed, with an increase in serum creatinine occurring only 1–3 days after contrast administration. As first described by Hirsch et al. [14], both urine and plasma NGAL concentrations increase within 2–6 h of contrast administration, with a predictive AUC of over 0.9. A recent meta-analysis [15] of 14 publications and a total of 1520 patients has confirmed the high diagnostic accuracy of NGAL in the early detection of CI-AKI, with measurements obtained 2–24 h after contrast administration yielding a pooled AUC of 0.93, pooled sensitivity of 84%, and pooled specificity 89% (Table 14.1). The performance of both urine and plasma NGAL was similar for predicting CI-AKI. Subgroup analyses revealed that NGAL levels obtained within 4 h of exposure to contrast yielded an improved predictive performance (pooled AUC 0.96) when compared to NGAL measurements made beyond 4 h (pooled AUC 0.89).

NGAL for the Differential Diagnosis of Kidney Attack

Serum creatinine measurements cannot distinguish true structural (intrinsic) AKI from functional volume-responsive prerenal azotemia or from chronic kidney disease. It is critical to make these distinctions in the acute setting, since the medical management of each is dramatically different and mismanagement is deleterious [16]. Nickolas et al. [17] first demonstrated the ability of a single measurement of urinary NGAL at the time of initial patient encounter to accurately differentiate those who subsequently developed intrinsic AKI from those who would follow a more benign course of prerenal azotemia, with an AUC of 0.95, sensitivity of 0.99, and specificity approaching unity. These findings have now been confirmed in three additional publications involving over 2000 patients [18–20] (Table 14.2). Collectively, the published data have confirmed the diagnostic accuracy of NGAL in the early prediction of intrinsic AKI, with AUCs in the 0.81–0.87 range, surpassing the performance of all other biomarkers tested to date.

NGAL for the Prediction of Adverse Outcomes After Kidney Attack

Kidney attack due to structural nephron damage portends a number of adverse outcomes, including worsening severity, need for dialysis, prolonged length of hospital stay, mortality, and development of chronic kidney disease. A prognostic biomarker that could predict the consequences of AKI would be invaluable for risk stratification and for planning resource utilization. Initial single-center studies of cardiac surgical patients by Bennett et al. [21] and Dent et al. [22] identified the correlation of early NGAL measurements in the urine and plasma, respectively, with severity and duration of AKI, length of stay, dialysis requirement, and death. An initial meta-analysis of 10 studies involving about 2000 patients with predominantly cardiorenal syndrome [10] identified early NGAL measurements as a predictor of dialysis and death with a pooled AUC of 0.78 and 0.75, respectively. In a more recent meta-analysis of six large studies that included

Table 14.2 NGAL for the differentiation between intrinsic structural AKI and a functional (prerenal) state in the emergency department setting

Number of patients	Urine or plasma	Sensitivity	Specificity	AUC for intrinsic AKI	Reference
635	Urine	0.99	1.0	0.95	[17]
1635	Urine	0.68	0.81	0.81	[18]
161	Urine	0.75	0.88	0.87	[19]
616	Plasma	0.54	0.89	0.82	[20]

AUC, area under the receiver-operating characteristic curve

about 2000 heterogeneous intensive care patients [23], the pooled AUC for prediction of renal replacement therapy was 0.82 and the pooled AUC for mortality prediction was 0.67.

Remarkably, NGAL signals structural kidney injury and poor outcomes even in the absence of an increase in serum creatinine. In a multicenter pooled analysis of 10 prospective studies involving over 2300 patients with predominantly cardiorenal syndrome, approximately 20% displayed NGAL concentrations above the optimal cutoff value as defined by each study, but no increase in serum creatinine [24]. This previously undetectable condition (termed "subclinical AKI") was associated with an almost threefold increased risk of mortality or dialysis requirement and a doubling of median length of hospital stay. Notably, even in patients with significant loss of renal function, NGAL measurements still added prognostic information, since patients with increased concentrations of both NGAL and serum creatinine displayed by far the worst prognosis. This "added value" of NGAL measurements for the prediction of AKI and its adverse consequences over and above clinical and functional scores has now been repeatedly demonstrated in several large studies involving cardiac surgical patients, using advanced statistical techniques such as net reclassification improvement and integrated discrimination improvement [25–27].

The Economic Implications of NGAL Use in Kidney Attack

The economic impact and cost-effectiveness of NGAL after cardiac surgery have been examined using a decision analysis model comparing the ability to diagnose AKI with versus without NGAL [28]. Even though the analysis assumed the lowest possible diagnostic performance (AUC 0.60–0.69) and highest possible cost (£25) for the NGAL test, the cost per quality-adjusted life year for a strategy of early NGAL measurements for predicting AKI was approximately 30% less compared to one without NGAL. The use of NGAL in this theoretical decision analysis model was an economically advantageous strategy because it lowered overall expected costs as a result of earlier AKI diagnosis. The cost-effectiveness increased further when the likelihood of clinical benefit from therapy triggered by elevated NGAL was considered.

Clinical Platforms for NGAL Measurement in Kidney Attack

NGAL is protease resistant and remarkably stable in urine and blood. Short-term storage of samples at 4 °C for up to 24 h and long-term storage at −80 °C for up to 5 years result in no clinically significant loss in NGAL signal [29]. These findings are reassuring for the deployment of NGAL assays in standard clinical platforms as well as in prospective clinical studies that require long-term sample storage.

There are currently three clinical analytic platforms for NGAL measurement in patient samples, with results available within 15–30 min. These include a point-of-care immunoassay for plasma NGAL (Alere Triage® NGAL Test), a urine immunoassay developed for an exclusive platform (ARCHITECT, Abbott Diagnostics), and a particle-enhanced turbidimetric immunoassay for urine and plasma NGAL that can be run on a large variety of standard automated clinical chemistry analyzers (NGAL TestTM, BioPorto Diagnostics). Thus, the NGAL TestTM gives any hospital or clinical laboratory immediate access to NGAL measurements both in the urine and blood. All of these three tests are CE-marked and launched for clinical diagnostic use worldwide, but are currently pending FDA approval for diagnostic use in the USA.

The Clinical Use of NGAL in Kidney Attack: A Proposed Framework

In the clinical setting, the two most likely applications of the NGAL test remain (a) for the prediction of AKI and its adverse outcomes, and (b) to differentiate intrinsic structural AKI from a prerenal state. In both these settings, NGAL performs well independent of the serum creatinine and results in substantial added value to serum creatinine measurements. However, specific cutoff values for NGAL need to be determined, and these cutoffs may vary depending on the assay used, regulatory intended use guidelines, as well as the specific clinical setting. Based on the available data included in the eight meta-analyses published to date [10–13, 15, 23–25], the following approximate conclusions can be derived regarding urine and plasma NGAL concentrations measured on a standardized clinical laboratory platform:

- NGAL cutoff of <50 ng/ml effectively rules out intrinsic structural AKI
- NGAL cutoff of >150 ng/ml strongly predicts intrinsic structural AKI
- NGAL cutoff of >300 ng/ml strongly predicts severe AKI and adverse outcomes.

As is true for most biomarkers in clinical medicine, there appears to be a "gray zone" for NGAL (approximately 50–150 ng/ml), in which predictions are somewhat indeterminate. Under these circumstances, it is likely that careful assessment of clinical risk factors as well as repeated serial NGAL measurements will clarify the situation [20]. A proposed guideline for the use of NGAL in the clinical setting is illustrated in Table 14.3.

These proposed guidelines are closely aligned with recent expert opinion [30] focused on cardiac surgery-associated

Table 14.3 Proposed guideline for the use of NGAL in the clinical setting

• Measure NGAL only if AKI is clinically suspected
– False positives may include urinary tract infections and sepsis without AKI
• <50 ng/ml
– Low risk of AKI, repeat measures only if clinically indicated
• 50–150 ng/ml
– Gray zone, repeat measures
• 150–300 ng/ml
– High risk for structural tubular injury, obtain daily NGAL measurements, monitor ins and outs, monitor electrolytes and kidney function, avoid nephrotoxins, avoid hypotension, consider Nephrology consult
• >300 ng/ml
– High risk for severe structural tubular injury, obtain daily NGAL measurements, keep in ICU setting, closely monitor ins and outs, closely monitor electrolytes and kidney function, avoid nephrotoxins, avoid hypotension, low threshold for pressor use, obtain Nephrology consult, strongly consider early interventions

AKI, proposing the derivation of a cardiac surgery-associated NGAL (CSA-NGAL) score based on both the absolute NGAL concentration as well as the increase in NGAL concentration on serial measurements. The authors propose a CSA-NGAL score of 0–3, with a score of 0 (urine NGAL <50 and plasma NGAL <100 ng/ml) indicating that tubular damage is unlikely, score of 1 (urine NGAL 50–150 and plasma NGAL 100–200 ng/ml) suggesting that tubular damage is possible, score of 2 (urine NGAL 150–999 and plasma NGAL 200–999 ng/ml) signaling definite tubular damage, and score of 3 (urine or plasma NGAL >1000 ng/ml) indicating severe tubular damage. The authors have also provided a clinical decision algorithm based on the CSA-NGAL score that mirrors what is proposed in Table 14.3.

The Use of NGAL in Clinical Trials for Kidney Attack

A structural kidney injury biomarker such as NGAL can be employed in many strategies to facilitate clinical trials. Extrapolating from guidelines provided by the US Food and Drug Administration (FDA) in the context of biomarker use for drug development [31], biomarkers can be used in the following settings:

- Before structural AKI develops. NGAL can be used as a diagnostic biomarker to preferentially enroll patients destined for structural intrinsic AKI
- At the time structural AKI develops. NGAL can be used as a prognostic biomarker to identify patients destined for severe AKI
- After structural AKI develops. NGAL can be used as a pharmacodynamic biomarker to monitor response to therapy

Parikh et al. [32] have recently reported on simulated clinical trials of AKI using data from a multicenter prospective cohort study of patients undergoing cardiac surgery, to illustrate the added utility of structural injury biomarkers. First, the addition of NGAL and interleukin-18 to clinical risk factors as eligibility criteria for enrollment in an AKI trial (diagnostic biomarker) increases the proportion of patients who will experience true AKI progression and will reduce trial cost. Second, in a trial of an effective therapy at the time of structural AKI development, use of NGAL (prognostic biomarker) instead of serum creatinine increases the proportion of true intrinsic AKI cases enrolled, thereby increasing the statistical power and decreasing the sample size needed. Third, the use of NGAL as an outcome measure (pharmacodynamic biomarker) to monitor response to therapy, the sample size to detect a reduction in AKI is lower than if serum creatinine was used instead. The proposed use of NGAL in a hypothetical future clinical trial is illustrated in Fig. 14.1.

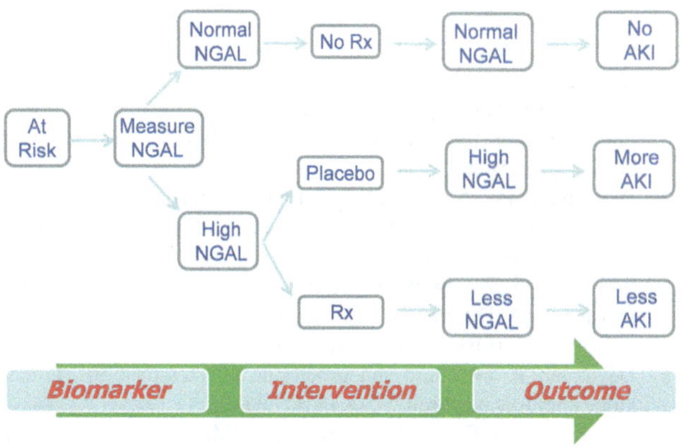

Fig. 14.1 The proposed use of NGAL in a hypothetical future clinical trial. Patients at clinical risk for AKI and with high NGAL (diagnostic biomarker) would be enrolled and randomized to placebo versus a specific therapy. The highest NGAL levels will be encountered in placebo-treated patients who would develop the most severe AKI (prognostic biomarker). Serial NGAL measurements can be used as an outcome measure (pharmacodynamic biomarker) to monitor response to intervention

Summary: NGAL is Set for Center Stage in Kidney Attack

The biologic plausibility of NGAL as an early predictive biomarker of structural AKI is irrefutable. Unbiased preclinical transcriptomic interrogations reported in AKI models from several species ranging from mouse to man have consistently revealed NGAL to be one of the most dramatically upregulated genes in the kidney soon after an ischemic or nephrotoxic insult. The 25 kDa NGAL protein is also highly induced in kidney tubule cells, where its iron-chelating properties result in an enhanced tubule cell proliferative response and a robust nephron protection. The induced NGAL protein is rapidly secreted into the urine and plasma in animal and human models of AKI. Over a decade of intense translational studies that have now established NGAL as a noninvasive biomarker of human AKI. These studies have now defined a role for NGAL as a cost-effective biomarker to predict AKI and its adverse outcomes independent of serum creatinine, for the differentiation of structural intrinsic AKI from a functional prerenal state, and for facilitating AKI clinical trials by increasing statistical power, decreasing sample size, and reducing cost. Standardized clinical platforms for the rapid and accurate measurement of NGAL have been launched globally and can be made available in every clinical setting. Expert opinion is consistent with the notion that NGAL is poised for center stage in kidney attack, as a troponin-like diagnostic, prognostic, and pharmacodynamic biomarker.

References

1. Kellum JA, Bellomo R, Ronco C. Kidney attack. JAMA. 2012;307(21):2265–6.
2. Devarajan P. Neutrophil gelatinase-associated lipocalin: a promising biomarker for human acute kidney injury. Biomark Med. 2010;4(2):265–80.
3. Devarajan P. Neutrophil gelatinase-associated lipocalin: a troponin-like biomarker for human acute kidney injury. Nephrology (Carlton). 2010;15(4):419–28.
4. Supavekin S, Zhang W, Kucherlapati R, Kaskel FJ, Moore LC, Devarajan P. Differential gene expression following early renal ischemia/reperfusion. Kidney Int. 2003;63(5):1714–24.
5. Devarajan P. Genomic and proteomic characterization of acute kidney injury. Nephron. 2015;131(2):85–91.
6. Mishra J, Ma Q, Prada A, Mitsnefes M, Zahedi K, Yang J, Barasch J, Devarajan P. Identification of neutrophil gelatinase-associated lipocalin as a novel early urinary biomarker for ischemic renal injury. J Am Soc Nephrol. 2003;14(10):2534–43.
7. Mishra J, Mori K, Ma Q, Kelly C, Yang J, Mitsnefes M, Barasch J, Devarajan P. Amelioration of ischemic acute renal injury by neutrophil gelatinase-associated lipocalin. J Am Soc Nephrol. 2004;15(12):3073–82.
8. Jefferies JL, Devarajan P. Early detection of acute kidney injury after pediatric cardiac surgery. Prog Pediatr Cardiol. 2016. doi:10.1016/j.ppedcard.2016.011.
9. Mishra J, Dent C, Tarabishi R, Mitsnefes MM, Ma Q, Kelly C, Ruff SM, Zahedi K, Shao M, Bean J, Mori K, Barasch J, Devarajan P. Neutrophil gelatinase-associated lipocalin (NGAL) as a biomarker for acute renal injury after cardiac surgery. Lancet. 2005;365(9466):1231–8.
10. Haase M, Bellomo R, Devarajan P, Schlattmann P, Haase-Fielitz A, NGAL Meta-analysis Investigator Group. Accuracy of neutrophil gelatinase-associated lipocalin (NGAL) in diagnosis and prognosis in acute kidney injury: a systematic review and meta-analysis. Am J Kidney Dis. 2009;54(6):1012–24.
11. Haase-Fielitz A, Haase M, Devarajan P. Neutrophil gelatinase-associated lipocalin as a biomarker of acute kidney injury: a critical evaluation of current status. Ann Clin Biochem. 2014;51(Pt 3):335–51.
12. Zhou F, Luo Q, Wang L, Han L. Diagnostic value of neutrophil gelatinase-associated lipocalin for early diagnosis of cardiac surgery-associated acute kidney injury: a meta-analysis. Eur J Cardiothorac Surg. 2016;49(3):746–55.
13. Zhang A, Cai Y, Wang P-F, Qu J-N, Luo Z-C, Chen X-D, Huang B, Liu Y, Huang W-Q, Wu J, Yin Y-H. Diagnosis and prognosis of neutrophil gelatinase-associated lipocalin for acute kidney injury with sepsis: a systematic review and meta-analysis. Crit Care. 2016;20:41.
14. Hirsch R, Dent C, Pfriem H, Allen J, Beekman RH 3rd, Ma Q, Dastrala S, Bennett M, Mitsnefes M, Devarajan P. NGAL is an early predictive biomarker of contrast-induced nephropathy in children. Pediatr Nephrol. 2007;22(12):2089–95.
15. Wang K, Duan CY, Wu J, Liu Y, Bei WJ, Chen JY, He PC, Liu YH, Tan N. Predictive value of neutrophil gelatinase-associated lipocalin for contrast-induced acute kidney injury after cardiac catheterization: a meta-analysis. Can J Cardiol. 2016 Aug;32(8):1033.e19–29.
16. Devarajan P. NGAL for the detection of acute kidney injury in the emergency room. Biomark Med. 2010;8(2):1–3.
17. Nickolas TL, O'Rourke MJ, Yang J, Sise ME, Canetta PA, Barasch N, Buchen C, Khan F, Mori K, Giglio J, Devarajan P, Barasch J. Sensitivity and specificity of a single emergency department measurement of urinary neutrophil gelatinase-associated lipocalin for diagnosing acute kidney injury. Ann Intern Med. 2008;148(11):810–9.
18. Nickolas TL, Schmidt-Ott KM, Canetta P, Forster C, Singer E, Sise M, Elger A, Maarouf O, Sola-Del Valle DA, O'Rourke M, Sherman E, Lee P, Geara A, Imus P, Guddati A, Polland A, Rahman W, Elitok S, Malik N, Giglio J, El-Sayegh S, Devarajan P, Hebbar S, Saggi SJ, Hahn B, Kettritz R, Luft FC, Barasch J. Diagnostic and prognostic stratification in the emergency department using urinary biomarkers of nephron damage: a multicenter prospective cohort study. J Am Coll Cardiol. 2012;59(3):246–55.
19. Singer E, Elger A, Elitok S, Kettritz R, Nickolas TL, Barasch J, Luft FC, Schmidt-Ott KM. Urinary neutrophil gelatinase-associated lipocalin distinguishes pre-renal from intrinsic renal failure and predicts outcomes. Kidney Int. 2011;80(4):405–14.
20. Soto K, Papoila AL, Coelho S, Bennett M, Ma Q, Rodrigues B, Fidalgo P, Frade F, Devarajan P. Plasma NGAL for the diagnosis of AKI in patients admitted from the emergency department setting. Clin J Am Soc Nephrol. 2013;8(12):2053–63.
21. Bennett M, Dent CL, Ma Q, Dastrala S, Grenier F, Workman R, Syed H, Ali S, Barasch J, Devarajan P. Urine NGAL predicts severity of acute kidney injury after cardiac surgery: a prospective study. Clin J Am Soc Nephrol. 2008;3(3):665–73.
22. Dent CL, Ma Q, Dastrala S, Bennett M, Mitsnefes MM, Barasch J, Devarajan P. Plasma neutrophil gelatinase-associated lipocalin

predicts acute kidney injury, morbidity and mortality after pediatric cardiac surgery: a prospective uncontrolled cohort study. Crit Care. 2007;11(6):R127.

23. Hjortrup PB, Haase N, Wetterslev M, Perner A. Clinical review: predictive value of neutrophil gelatinase-associated lipocalin for acute kidney injury in intensive care patients. Crit Care. 2013;17(2):211.
24. Haase M, Devarajan P, Haase-Fielitz A, Bellomo R, Cruz DN, Wagener G, Krawczeski CD, Koyner JL, Murray P, Zappitelli M, Goldstein SL, Makris K, Ronco C, Martensson J, Martling CR, Venge P, Siew E, Ware LB, Ikizler TA, Mertens PR. The outcome of neutrophil gelatinase-associated lipocalin-positive subclinical acute kidney injury: a multicenter pooled analysis of prospective studies. J Am Coll Cardiol. 2011;57(17):1752–61.
25. Krawczeski CD, Goldstein SL, Woo JG, Wang Y, Piyaphanee N, Ma Q, Bennett M, Devarajan P. Temporal relationship and predictive value of urinary acute kidney injury biomarkers after pediatric cardiopulmonary bypass. J Am Coll Cardiol. 2011;58(22):2301–9.
26. Parikh CR, Devarajan P, Zappitelli M, Sint K, Thiessen-Philbrook H, Li S, Kim RW, Koyner JL, Coca SG, Edelstein CL, Shlipak MG, Garg AX, Krawczeski CD, TRIBE-AKI Consortium. Postoperative biomarkers predict acute kidney injury and poor outcomes after pediatric cardiac surgery. J Am Soc Nephrol. 2011;22(9):1737–47.
27. Parikh CR, Coca SG, Thiessen-Philbrook H, Shlipak MG, Koyner JL, Wang Z, Edelstein CL, Devarajan P, Patel UD, Zappitelli M, Krawczeski CD, Passik CS, Swaminathan M, Garg AX, TRIBE-AKI Consortium. Postoperative biomarkers predict acute kidney injury and poor outcomes after adult cardiac surgery. J Am Soc Nephrol. 2011;22(9):1748–57.
28. Shaw AD, Chalfin DB, Kleintjens J. The economic impact and cost-effectiveness of urinary neutrophil gelatinase-associated lipocalin after cardiac surgery. Clin Ther. 2011;33(11):1713–25.
29. Schuh MP, Nehus E, Ma Q, Haffner C, Bennett M, Krawczeski CD, Devarajan P. Long-term stability of urinary biomarkers of acute kidney injury in children. Am J Kidney Dis. 2016;67(1):56–61.
30. de Geus HR, Ronco C, Haase M, Jacob L, Lewington A, Vincent JL. The cardiac surgery-associated neutrophil gelatinase-associated lipocalin (CSA-NGAL) score: a potential tool to monitor acute tubular damage. J Thorac Cardiovasc Surg. 2016;151(6):1476–81.
31. Guidance for Industry and FDA Staff: Qualification Process for Drug Development Tools. Center for Drug Evaluation and Research, US Food and Drug Administration, Department of Health and human Services; 2014.
32. Parikh CR, Moledina DG, Coca SG, Thiessen-Philbrook HR, Garg AX. Application of new acute kidney injury biomarkers in human randomized controlled trials. Kidney Int. 2016;89(6): 1372–9.

15 Ultrafiltration Therapy in Decompensated Heart Failure

Dan Negoianu

Introduction

Volume overload is a cardinal feature of decompensated heart failure. Decongestion with diuretics is the standard of care for treatment of patients with either acute or chronic volume overload. However, decongestion can also be achieved through mechanical means. Ultrafiltration (UF) results when hydrostatic or osmotic forces drive fluid across a semipermeable membrane. Mechanical UF is typically achieved by passing blood through hollow fibers made of semipermeable material while applying negative pressure to the space surrounding the fibers. A pressure gradient across the membrane (i.e., the transmembrane pressure) causes isotonic fluid to be removed from the blood (see Fig. 15.1).

While the mechanism of removal of fluid via UF is clear, its role in the management of heart failure remains uncertain. While significant physiologic differences between decongestion via UF compared to decongestion by diuretics have been demonstrated, the clinical impact of these differences remain unclear.

Physiological Differences Between Decongestion with Ultrafiltration Versus Loop Diuretics

Composition of the Removed Fluid

The electrolyte composition of fluid that is removed by UF is typically very different from the urine produced in response to diuretics [1]. For substances small enough to easily pass through the semipermeable membrane, ultrafiltrate will have approximately the same composition as plasma. Because sodium is the major cation in the extracellular fluid, it is also the major cation in ultrafiltrate. Since extracellular fluid volume is proportional to total body sodium content, sodium removal is critical for decongestion in heart failure.

On average, urine produced by loop diuretics has a lower sodium content and a much higher potassium content than ultrafiltrate [1]. Since sodium is a largely extracellular ion and potassium is a largely intracellular ion, it is reasonable to suspect that removal of one liter of sodium-rich ultrafiltrate will have a greater impact upon extracellular fluid volume than the loss of one liter of urine containing less sodium and more potassium. However, this hypothesis has not been proven by directly measuring extracellular fluid volume in randomized trials of ultrafiltration compared to diuretics.

It is important to draw a distinction between extracellular fluid volume and extracellular sodium concentration. Serum sodium concentration reflects the ratio of total body electrolytes to total body water. Because of this, losses of potassium have a similar effect upon serum sodium concentration as do losses of sodium [2]. However, sodium concentration does not reflect the volume of extracellular fluid (which is the key derangement in volume overload).

Diuretic Holiday

UF allows the removal of fluid without the need for loop diuretics. Withdrawal of loop diuretics may be beneficial by avoiding potassium wasting. Patients with congestive heart failure tend to be chronically potassium depleted [3]. In addition to the well-known risk of arrhythmias with hypokalemia, potassium depletion has also been shown to directly lead to vasoconstriction in hypertensive patients [4, 5]. Such vasoconstriction could be detrimental patients with heart failure, though it remains to be well demonstrated in this patient population.

Withdrawal of loop diuretics may also decrease renin release. In animal models, loop diuretics directly enhance

D. Negoianu (✉)
Renal Electrolyte and Hypertension Division, Hospital of the University of Pennsylvania, 3400 Spruce St, 1 Founders Pavilion, Philadelphia, PA 19104, USA
e-mail: dan.negoianu@uphs.upenn.edu

J. Rangaswami et al. (eds.), *Cardio-Nephrology*,
DOI 10.1007/978-3-319-56042-7_15

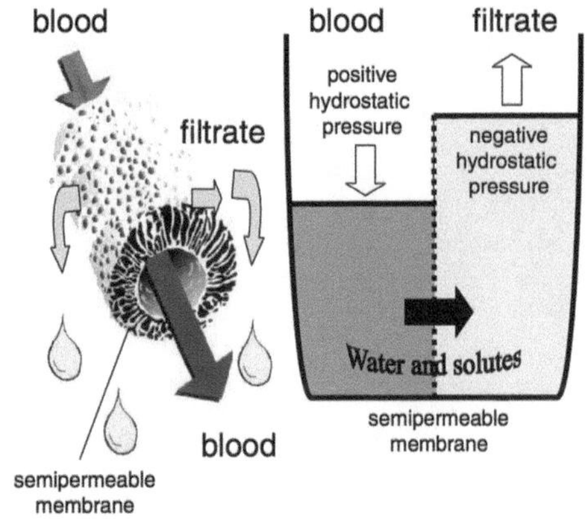

Fig. 15.1 Ultrafiltration resulting from a hydrostatic pressure gradient across a semipermeable membrane. Solutes small enough to pass through the membrane pores are removed as well. The rate of fluid removal is controlled by changing the pressure on the ultrafiltrate side of the membrane rather than the blood side. Reproduced with permission from John S, Eckardt KU. Renal replacement strategies in the ICU. Chest. 2007;132(4):1379–88

renin secretion by blocking chloride from entering cells of the macula densa [6]. This physiology may help explain the fact that in a small trial of 16 patients with chronic HF randomized to either UF or diuretic therapy, the UF group had significantly less elevation in renin and aldosterone levels [7]. Another RCT of 30 subjects with acute decompensated HF (ADHF) showed decreased aldosterone levels in the UF group, but not in the diuretic group [8]. Renin was not measured in this study, so it is impossible to be certain if decreased aldosterone levels in the UF group were, in fact, due to decreased renin activity. Of course, there are multiple factors impacting the renin–angiotensin system in HF, and it is impossible to be certain if decreased stimulation of the macula densa played a role in these observations in human trials.

Avoidance of Hypertrophy of Distal Nephron

Treatment with loop diuretic leads to decreased diuretic response over time even if volume depletion is prevented [9]. This may be partly due to the fact that chronic exposure to loop diuretics leads to hypertrophy of the distal nephron in experimental animals [10]. UF allows decongestion to continue while without exposing the distal nephron to high loads of sodium, thereby potentially minimizing diuretic resistance in these patients on maintenance loop diuretics.

Reduction of Renal Vein Congestion

Elevated renal venous pressures may lower glomerular filtration rate and sodium excretion in experimental animals [11, 12]. Renal congestion may contribute to diuretic resistance in some patients, leading to a vicious cycle that causes further volume overload. UF may therefore provide the ability to break this cycle in selected patients.

Risks of Hypovolemia with Ultrafiltration

The major risk of any form of decongestion is excessive intravascular volume depletion. From this perspective, the decreased effectiveness of loop diuretics in the setting of intravascular volume depletion may actually be protective. A UF machine, however, will keep removing fluid regardless of the patient's volume status. Furthermore, as UF continues, plasma refill rate declines [13] (see Fig. 15.2). Therefore, patients treated with UF must be closely monitored for evidence of worsening intravascular volume depletion. In particular, UF rates will generally need to be

Fig. 15.2 Plasma refilling rate (PRR) during extracorporeal UF. *$P < 0.01$ versus PRR after 1 l fluid removed. Reproduced with permission from Marenzi et al. [13]

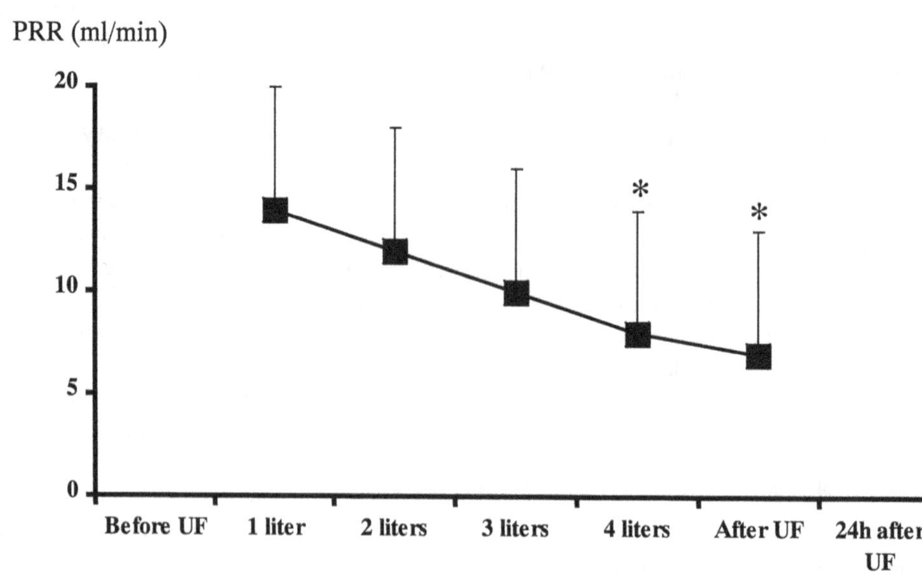

lowered over the course of UF treatment in order to mirror the changes in plasma refill rate.

Summary

The ability of UF to remove isotonic, sodium-rich fluid without stimulating the macula densa or the distal nephron suggests that decongestion via UF is physiologically different from decongestion with diuretics. However, "different" does not necessarily mean "better" (especially given that UF is a more invasive therapy). The hypotheses generated by the above differences in physiology require confirmation by trials that measure clinically relevant outcomes.

Clinical Trials of UF Versus Diuretics

There have only been seven clinical trials of UF versus diuretics in ADHF [14]. Even the largest clinical trial is relatively small (224 subjects). With this degree of limited statistical power, the ability to study clinically meaningful endpoints is limited. The two smallest studies focused on physiologic parameters obtained by right heart catheterization. We will therefore focus on the remaining five studies, which examined clinical endpoints. There are significant differences among these trials in selection criteria, management of the treatment arms, and the outcomes measured. Discussing these trials in the order that they were published gives insight not only into their differences, but also into the changes in the field of UF over the past decade. The results of the four largest trials are summarized in Table 15.1.

The Relief for Acutely Fluid-Overloaded Patients with Decompensated Congestive Heart Failure (Rapid-CHF, 2005)

This was the first randomized trial of UF for patients hospitalized with ADHF [15]. This investigator-initiated trial-randomized 40 patients to either usual care plus a single 8-hour UF session versus usual care alone. There was no statistically significant difference in the primary outcome of weight loss at 24 h after enrolment. However, there was a non-significant trend toward greater weight loss in the UF group, which lead the authors to conclude that a larger study was needed.

Ultrafiltration Versus Intravenous Diuretics for Patients Hospitalized for Acute Decompensated Heart Failure (UNLOAD, 2007)

This industry-sponsored trial-randomized 200 patients within 24 h of hospitalization for ADHF to either IV loop diuretic or UF [16].

Patients were required to have evidence of volume overload as defined by at least 2 of the following:

- Peripheral edema of 2+ or greater,
- Jugular venous distension of 7 cm or greater,
- Radiographic pulmonary edema or pleural effusion,
- Enlarged liver or ascites,
- Pulmonary rales, paroxysmal nocturnal dyspnea, or orthopnea.

For the IV diuretic group, the minimum daily dose was twice the outpatient dose of oral diuretic. Average intravenous furosemide-equivalent diuretic dose during the 48 h after randomization was 181 ± 121 mg/day. Diuretic therapy could be given either as bolus therapy or as a continuous drip (at the discretion of the treating physician). For the UF group, duration and rate of UF was left up to the treating physician. The average UF rate was 241 ml/h for 12.3 ± 12 h.

The study had two primary "efficacy" outcomes measured at 48 h: weight loss and dyspnea score. Weight loss was significantly greater in the UF group (5.0 ± 0.68 vs. 3.1 ± 0.75 kg, $P = 0.001$). Dyspnea score was not significantly different between the two groups. While the authors reported that there was no statistically significant difference in creatinine at any time point between the two groups, there was a trend toward higher creatinine in the UF group during hospitalization (which did not persist at 30 days after discharge). Importantly, the secondary outcome of 90-day rehospitalization rates showed significantly greater freedom from rehospitalization for the UF group (Fig. 15.3).

While the reduction in rehospitalization rates was an exciting finding, there are number of important limitations to this study. First of all, the most clinically relevant finding of the trial—reduction in rehospitalization—was a secondary outcome. Second, it was unclear if the diuretic group could have also achieved a similar readmission rate had they received an even more aggressive escalation in diuretic dose. Finally, the inclusion criteria for this trial are very broad. Given that UF is a more invasive therapy than IV diuretic therapy, it is unlikely that it would ever be first-line therapy for patients that do not have some evidence of functional diuretic resistance over and above the typical patient with ADHF.

Table 15.1 The largest trials of ultrafiltration in heart failure

Variables	UNLOAD Trial, 2007	CARRESS-HF Trial, 2012	CUORE Trial, 2014	AVOID-HF Trial, 2016
Number of patients	200 (100 UF, 100 PT)	188 (94 UF, 94 PT)	56 (27 UF, 29 PT)	224 (110 UF, 114 PT)
Study design and protocol	Multicenter; single-session early UF therapy for ADHF (within 24 h)	Multicenter; rescue therapy for patients with both ADHF and WRF	Two centers; one or two early UF treatments for ADHF (within 24 h)	Multicenter; single-session early UF therapy for ADHF (within 24 h)
Primary end point	Weight loss and dyspnea at 48 h (efficacy); changes in renal function and hypotension (safety)	Changes in Scr and weight at 96 h (bivariate)	Rehospitalization rate for HF at 1 year	Time to first HF event within 90 days after discharge
UF regimen	Duration and rate of UF flexible; maximum UF rate, 500 ml/h; average UF rate, 241 ml/h for 12.3 ± 12 h	Fixed initial UF rate, 200 ml/h; median duration of UF, 40 h; median duration of 40 h	Duration and rate of UF flexible; maximum UF rate, 500 ml/h; average duration of 19 ± 10 h	Duration and rate of UF flexible; maximum UF rate, 500 ml/h; average UF rate, 138 ml/h for 80 ± 53 h
Medical therapy	Conventional PT (no preplanned algorithm)	Stepped PT (algorithm based)	Conventional PT (no preplanned algorithm)	Adjustable IV loop diuretics (algorithm based)
Baseline renal function	Scr 1.5 mg/dl; UF, 1.5 mg/dl; PT (Scr > 3 mg/dl excluded)	Scr 1.9 mg/dl; UF, 2.09 mg/dl; PT (Scr > 3.5 mg/dl excluded)	Scr 1.7 mg/dl; UF, 1.9 mg/dl; PT (Scr > 3 mg/dl excluded)	Scr 1.5 mg/dl; UF, 1.6 mg/dl; PT (Scr ≥ 3 mg/dl excluded)
Effect on renal function	No significant difference in renal function between UF and PT	Significant increase in Scr level with UF; no change in Scr for PT	Higher Scr and BUN in the PT group at 6 mo; no difference in eGFR, Scr, and BUN between UF and PT at 1 year	No significant difference in eGFR, Scr, BUN, and BUN/Scr ratio during treatment and ≤90 days between UF and PT
Effect on congestion	Greater weight loss with UF; greater net fluid loss with UF	Weight loss and total amount of fluid removal similar for both groups	Weight loss similar for both groups at discharge; lower bodyweight for UF at 1 year	Higher total amount of fluid removed with UF; no difference in weight loss between UF and PT
Other findings	Fewer patients in the UF group rehospitalized at 90 days, with fewer hospitalization days and unscheduled visits; a trend for WRF for UF at 24 and 48 h and discharge (statistically not significant)	Higher rate of serious adverse events in the UF group; enrollment ended prematurely because of a lack of benefit and an excess of adverse events with UF; similar mortality rates for both groups at 60 days	No difference in mortality between UF and PT at 1 year; UF group had a lower HF readmission and mortality rate (combined) at 1 year	UF group had fewer patients admitted for HF within 30 days post-discharge and fewer days in the hospital for HF; higher rate of adverse events in the UF group; no difference in mortality at 90 days; trial ended prematurely because of slow recruitment

UNLOAD ultrafiltration versus intravenous diuretics for patients hospitalized for acute decompensated heart failure, *CARRESS-HF* cardiorenal rescue study in acute decompensated heart failure, *CUORE* continuous ultrafiltration for congestive heart failure, *AVOID-HF* aquapheresis versus intravenous diuretics and hospitalization for heart failure, *UF* ultrafiltration, *PT* pharmacologic therapy, *ADHF* acute decompensated heart failure, *WRF* worsening renal function, *Scr* serum creatinine, *HF* heart failure

Reproduced with permission from Kazory A. Ultrafiltration Therapy for Heart Failure: Balancing Likely Benefits against Possible Risks. Clin J Am Soc Nephrol. 2016;11(8):1463–71

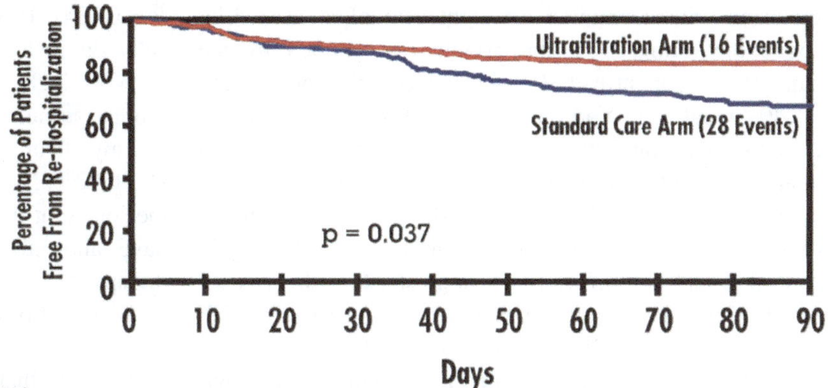

No. Patients at Risk

Ultrafiltration Arm	88	85	80	77	75	72	70	66	64	45
Standard Care Arm	86	83	77	74	66	63	59	58	52	41

Fig. 15.3 Kaplan–Meier estimate of freedom from rehospitalization for heart failure within 90 days after discharge in the UF (*red line*) and standard care (*blue line*) groups from the UNLOAD trial. Reproduced with permission from Costanzo et al. [16]

Cardiorenal Rescue Study in Acute Decompensated Heart Failure (CARRESS-HF, 2012)

This landmark trial enrolled 188 patients admitted for ADHF and worsening renal function (WRF) [17]. Criteria for volume overload were similar to UNLOAD, while WRF was defined as an increase in creatinine of at least 0.3 mg/dl within 12 weeks before admission or 10 days afterward. Almost all of the study participants (95%) sustained WRF after admission rather than before. The average time from admission to qualifying creatinine was 34 h, and the median increase in creatinine was 0.45 mg/dl.

Therapy in the control arm differed from the prior studies as well. A detailed algorithm guided escalation of diuretic therapy [18]. This sought to eliminate the critique of prior trials that the diuretic arm was not sufficiently aggressive.

Guidance for the UF arm was not nearly as detailed. UF was to be initiated at 200 cc/h in all patients and continued until clinical decongestion was achieved. There was a general recommendation that UF be decreased to 100 cc/h or discontinued in the setting of significant intravascular volume depletion, but no specific criteria for this were given [19].

The primary endpoint was a bivariate change in weight and creatinine 96 h after randomization. There was no significant difference in weight loss between the pharmacologic therapy and UF groups (5.5 ± 5.1 and 5.7 ± 3.9 kg, respectively; $P = 0.58$). However, the UF group had an increase in creatinine of 0.23 mg/dl versus a decrease of 0.04 ± 0.53 mg/dl in the pharmacologic therapy group ($P = 0.003$). Furthermore, there was no benefit seen for UF in any secondary endpoints, including 60-day readmission. On the contrary, patients in the UF group had a significantly higher percentage of serious adverse events (72 vs. 57%, $P = 0.03$).

Why were the results from this study so different from the prior UNLOAD Trial? First, the inclusion criteria of the two trials differed significantly. Rather than randomizing patients immediately upon admission for ADHF, patients in CARRESS-HF had to first demonstrate worsening renal function in the context of standard management. These patients may therefore have been more tenuous than those studied in UNLOAD [20]. Furthermore, the initiation of UF at a fixed rate of 200 cc/h may have been too aggressive in this population. There were clearly challenges in delivering the UF therapy. Patients in the UF arm received therapy for an average of only 40/96 h prior to the primary endpoint (as opposed to 92/96 h for the pharmacologic therapy arm). In addition, 30% of patients in the UF arm received IV diuretics during the 96 h prior to the primary endpoint. This suggests UF needed to be abandoned well before maximum fluid removal could be achieved in many patients.

Regardless of these issues, CARRESS-HF provides a strong argument against the use of UF as a therapy to "rescue" patients with rising creatinine in the setting of attempted decongestion for ADHF. This conclusion is supported by the poor outcomes reported in case series of patients where UF is attempted as "rescue" in the setting of severe diuretic resistance [21, 22].

While the trial does provide a strong argument against the use of UF in the population it studied, these results may not be generalizable to other sub-populations of patients with HF [20].

Continuous Ultrafiltration for Congestive Heart Failure (CUORE, 2012)

This trial sought to study a population of patients hospitalized for ADHF who had larger amounts of fluid retention than those enrolled in the previously discussed trials [23].

Inclusion criteria required a weight gain of at least 4 kg above the estimated normal weight (as reported by the patient). All patient had HF with reduced ejection fraction ($\leq$40%) and New York Heart Association Class III or IV. Patients were randomized within 24 h of admission to treatment with UF versus IV loop diuretics. Both groups had similar amounts of weight reduction at discharge (7.5 ± 5.6 kg in ultrafiltration group vs. 7.9 ± 9.0 kg in control group; P = 0.75). This was greater than the average weight reduction in the UF groups of CARRESS-HF (5.7 kg) and AVOID-HF (5.0 kg). This difference suggests CUORE may indeed have studied a different patient population than these previously published trials. Interestingly, loop diuretics were continued in the UF group during UF treatments. This was not the case in the other trials.

In spite of similar weight reduction between the two arms, the primary outcome of rate of HF readmission was significantly better in the UF group (hazard ratio 0.14, 95%, confidence interval 0.04–0.48; P = 0.002). This study therefore suggested that UF may be of benefit in patients who not only have substantial volume overload, but also have sufficient functional reserve to tolerate a large volume of fluid removal. However, this was a very small study performed at only two centers. The authors appropriately state that a larger study would be needed to lend credence to these results.

Aquapheresis Versus Intravenous Diuretics Hospitalizations for Heart Failure (AVOID-HF, 2016)

This industry-sponsored trial sought to randomize 810 patients to UF versus diuretic therapy [24]. Inclusion criteria were similar to UNLOAD. In the wake of the publication of CARRESS-HF, a detailed pharmacologic algorithm, modeled on the CARRESS-HF algorithm, was added to the protocol. A detailed UF algorithm was added simultaneously. The study sponsor, Baxter International, chose to terminate the trial prior to completion, citing slower than projected enrolment. At this point, 224 patients had been enrolled. Pre-specified follow-up procedures were completed for all enrolled patients.

The UF group showed a trend toward decreased hospital readmission, but this did not achieve statistical significance (hazard ratio of 0.663 with 95% confidence interval: 0.402 to 1.092). It is obviously impossible to know if statistical significance would have been reached had the trial recruited the planned 810 patients. A number of pre-specified secondary outcomes were significantly different at 30 days post-discharge. For example, the patients in the UF arm had significantly fewer HF rehospitalisations within 30 days compared to the diuretic group (9.5 vs. 20.4%, respectively, P = 0.034). However, these trends were no longer statistically significant at 90 days.

Worryingly, a greater percentage of patients in the UF groups sustained serious adverse events related to study therapy than did the diuretic group (14.6 vs. 5.4%; P = 0.026). No single sub-class of adverse event was clearly the source of this difference, and a larger study would likely have allowed better understanding of the risks of UF therapy.

Given all of the above, the authors felt that this negative trial was nevertheless hypothesis-generating, and that further trials of UF therapy were therefore warranted.

Practical Aspects and Future Directions

While current data are insufficient to conclusively answer the question of who or which subset of patients should be considered for UF, they nevertheless do provide some guidance.

Patient Selection

Given the results of CARRESS-HF, UF should not be considered a treatment for cardiorenal syndrome. Patients such as those in CARRESS-HF may simply be "too sick" to easily tolerate UF.

Going further along the "too sick" spectrum, data from case series argue against the use of UF as "rescue" late in the management of patients who are completely refractory to IV diuretics. In one such series of 63 patients, 59% required conversion to continuous dialysis during their hospitalization, 30% died during hospitalization, 6% were discharged to hospice, and 14% were dialysis-dependent at discharge [22].

On the other extreme of the spectrum, the use of UF as first-line therapy for the general population of patients with ADHF is inappropriate given the increased invasiveness of this therapy compared to diuretics.

One potentially promising group of patients is those readmitted for ADHF within 30 days of discharge. Readmission may be a surrogate for functional diuretic resistance, and this patient population is of obvious interest to both healthcare providers and payers.

Another population of interest are patients who require above-average amounts of fluid removal to achieve decongestion—such as the CUORE trial sought to study. These patients will likely require high doses and long durations of IV diuretic therapy. If there are clinically meaningful advantages of UF over diuretics, then they may be more prominent in such patients.

Management of Patients with UF: Avoidance of Hypovolemia

As stated previously, one of the major risks of UF is excessive fluid removal. While diuretics also carry this risk, there is some protection afforded by diuretics' decrease in potency as patients become progressively more volume depleted. With UF, however, it is up to the clinician to anticipate, recognize, and respond to volume depletion. The UF guideline developed for AVOID-HF attempted to codify this [25].

The guideline recommends that vital signs and UOP be assessed every 6 h and that serum chemistries be obtained every 12 h. UF rates are to be dropped if there are alterations in heart rate, blood pressure, or urine output. As an aside, the ability to use a fall in urine output as a surrogate for renal hypo-perfusion is one of the rationales for holding diuretics during UF therapy.

While the guideline itself is opinion-based [25], the overall philosophy is more important that the details of the algorithm. This approach consists of four sequential steps:

- Choice of initial UF rate based on vital signs and clinical history
- Systematic monitoring so that UF rate can be decreased to match the inevitable decline in plasma refill rate
- Recognition of either clinical decongestion or intolerance of further fluid removal
- Re-institution of diuretic therapy with a goal of preventing recurrence of volume overload.

A potential adjunct to algorithms such as this would be real-time monitoring of hematocrit as a surrogate for hemoconcentration. This strategy was used in the CUORE trial, although the authors did not state if specific cutoffs were used to guide alterations in UF rate [23]. In a previous study by the same group, UF was terminated when hematocrit increased 10% above baseline [13].

While the optimal method for monitoring patients and adjusting their treatment to prevent hypovolemia remains unknown, some systematic way to achieve this goal is likely required for clinical UF programs and for any future trials of HF for ADHF.

Outcomes for Future Clinical Trials

The hypothesis-generating trends within the AVOID-HF trial further support the need for adequately powered clinical trials. While it will be impossible to power studies for all-cause mortality, HF readmission is a both clinically meaningful and achievable endpoint. Given that such studies are necessarily open-label, care must be taken to isolate decisions about readmission from authors of the study.

Conclusion

Current data for the use of UF in the treatment of ADHF are inconclusive. Further study is required to define what, if any, sub-population of patients may benefit from UF therapy, and what the optimal manner is to prescribe it.

References

1. Ali SS, Olinger CC, Sobotka PA, Dahle TG, Bunte MC, Blake D, et al. Loop diuretics can cause clinical natriuretic failure: a prescription for volume expansion. Congest Heart Fail. 2009;15 (1):1–4.
2. Edelman IS, Leibman J, O'Meara MP, Birkenfeld LW. Interrelations between serum sodium concentration, serum osmolarity and total exchangeable sodium, total exchangeable potassium and total body water. J Clin Invest. 1958;37(9):1236–56.
3. Cleland JG, Dargie HJ, Robertson I, Robertson JI, East BW. Total body electrolyte composition in patients with heart failure: a comparison with normal subjects and patients with untreated hypertension. Br Heart J. 1987;58(3):230–8.
4. Adrogue HJ, Madias NE. Sodium and potassium in the pathogenesis of hypertension. N Engl J Med. 2007;356(19):1966–78.
5. Krishna GG, Kapoor SC. Potassium depletion exacerbates essential hypertension. Ann Intern Med. 1991;115(2):77–83.
6. Lorenz JN, Weihprecht H, Schnermann J, Skott O, Briggs JP. Renin release from isolated juxtaglomerular apparatus depends on macula densa chloride transport. Am J Physiol. 1991;260(4 Pt 2):F486–93.
7. Agostoni P, Marenzi G, Lauri G, Perego G, Schianni M, Sganzerla P, et al. Sustained improvement in functional capacity after removal of body fluid with isolated ultrafiltration in chronic cardiac insufficiency: failure of furosemide to provide the same result. Am J Med. 1994;96(3):191–9.
8. Giglioli C, Landi D, Cecchi E, Chiostri M, Gensini GF, Valente S, et al. Effects of ULTRAfiltration vs. DIureticS on clinical, biohumoral and haemodynamic variables in patients with deCOmpensated heart failure: the ULTRADISCO study. Eur J Heart Fail. 2011;13(3):337–46.
9. Loon NR, Wilcox CS, Unwin RJ. Mechanism of impaired natriuretic response to furosemide during prolonged therapy. Kidney Int. 1989;36(4):682–9.
10. Kaissling B, Bachmann S, Kriz W. Structural adaptation of the distal convoluted tubule to prolonged furosemide treatment. Am J Physiol. 1985;248(3 Pt 2):F374–81.
11. Burnett JC Jr, Knox FG. Renal interstitial pressure and sodium excretion during renal vein constriction. Am J Physiol. 1980;238 (4):F279–82.
12. Firth JD, Raine AE, Ledingham JG. Raised venous pressure: a direct cause of renal sodium retention in oedema? Lancet. 1988;1 (8593):1033–5.
13. Marenzi G, Lauri G, Grazi M, Assanelli E, Campodonico J, Agostoni P. Circulatory response to fluid overload removal by extracorporeal ultrafiltration in refractory congestive heart failure. J Am Coll Cardiol. 2001;38(4):963–8.
14. Jain A, Agrawal N, Kazory A. Defining the role of ultrafiltration therapy in acute heart failure: a systematic review and meta-analysis. Heart Fail Rev. 2016;21(5):611–9.
15. Bart BA, Boyle A, Bank AJ, Anand I, Olivari MT, Kraemer M, et al. Ultrafiltration versus usual care for hospitalized patients with heart failure: the Relief for Acutely Fluid-Overloaded Patients

With Decompensated Congestive Heart Failure (RAPID-CHF) trial. J Am Coll Cardiol. 2005;46(11):2043–6.
16. Costanzo MR, Guglin ME, Saltzberg MT, Jessup ML, Bart BA, Teerlink JR, et al. Ultrafiltration versus intravenous diuretics for patients hospitalized for acute decompensated heart failure. J Am Coll Cardiol. 2007;49(6):675–83.
17. Bart BA, Goldsmith SR, Lee KL, Givertz MM, O'Connor CM, Bull DA, et al. Ultrafiltration in decompensated heart failure with cardiorenal syndrome. N Engl J Med. 2012;367(24):2296–304.
18. Bart BA, Goldsmith SR, Lee KL, Redfield MM, Felker GM, O'Connor CM, et al. Cardiorenal rescue study in acute decompensated heart failure: rationale and design of CARRESS-HF, for the Heart Failure Clinical Research Network. J Card Fail. 2012;18(3):176–82.
19. Bart BA. Protocol: CARRESS-HF. N Engl J Med. 2012.
20. Tang WH. Reconsidering ultrafiltration in the acute cardiorenal syndrome. N Engl J Med. 2012;367(24):2351–2.
21. Liang KV, Hiniker AR, Williams AW, Karon BL, Greene EL, Redfield MM. Use of a novel ultrafiltration device as a treatment strategy for diuretic resistant, refractory heart failure: initial clinical experience in a single center. J Card Fail. 2006;12(9):707–14.
22. Patarroyo M, Wehbe E, Hanna M, Taylor DO, Starling RC, Demirjian S, et al. Cardiorenal outcomes after slow continuous ultrafiltration therapy in refractory patients with advanced decompensated heart failure. J Am Coll Cardiol. 2012;60(19):1906–12.
23. Marenzi G, Muratori M, Cosentino ER, Rinaldi ER, Donghi V, Milazzo V, et al. Continuous ultrafiltration for congestive heart failure: the CUORE trial. J Card Fail. 2014;20(1):9–17.
24. Costanzo MR, Negoianu D, Jaski BE, Bart BA, Heywood JT, Anand IS, et al. Aquapheresis versus intravenous diuretics and hospitalizations for heart failure. JACC Heart Fail. 2016;4(2):95–105.
25. Costanzo MR, Negoianu D, Fonarow GC, Jaski BE, Bart BA, Heywood JT, et al. Rationale and design of the aquapheresis versus intravenous diuretics and hospitalization for heart failure (AVOID-HF) trial. Am Heart J. 2015;170(3):471–82.

Bioimpedance Vectorial Analyses in Cardiorenal Syndrome

16

Nadia Aspromonte, Francesco Monitillo, Roberto Valle, and Massimo Iacoviello

Introduction

Water constitutes approximately 60% of body weight. Total body water (TBW) content is distributed between two main compartments, separated by cell membranes. The intracellular fluid compartment (ICF) contains about two-third of TBW, while the remaining part is the extracellular compartment (ECF). The latter is further divided into the interstitial fluid compartment and plasma, or intravascular space. Water homeostasis results from the balance between total water intake and the combined water loss. The kidney is responsible for the regulation of water excretion and, in most conditions, is the main way to remove water from the body. Renal excretion of water is tightly regulated in order to maintain water balance [1]. Other sources of water loss include evaporation from the cells of the skin and of respiratory tract, sweat, and feces. Many clinical conditions can contribute to the alteration of this fine balanced mechanism, including cardiovascular disease (especially heart failure) and kidney disease. The accurate assessment of volume status is crucial both in steady state as well as in conditions such as end-stage kidney disease (ESKD) and acute decompensated heart failure (ADHF).

In clinical practice, many methods have been proposed, including physical examination, chest X-ray, laboratory parameters and biomarkers (serum creatinine, electrolytes, urinary, and plasma osmolarity, hematocrit, natriuretic peptides), bedside ultrasound, and monitoring of central venous pressure [2, 3]. The simple evaluation of edema and other clinical signs as expression of fluid overload can be inaccurate, requiring an increase of 4–5 l in body fluid volume before detection [4, 5]. Indeed, significant changes in total body water can develop subclinically and can pose challenges in the correct assessment of fluid status and volume responsiveness to therapies. In this context, bioelectrical impedance techniques, providing a reliable assessment of volume status, are being used in the management of patients with ESKD and ADHF.

Principles of Bioelectrical Impedance Techniques

Bioimpedance analysis (BIA) and bioimpedance vector analysis (BIVA) have shown promise as noninvasive, safe, rapid, and reproducible bedside measures of body composition. BIA measures the electric impedance (*Z*) which is the opposition of body tissues to the flow of a sinusoidal alternating current. In practice, a constant alternating current at a fixed 50-kHz frequency is applied across the thorax and two electrodes are placed at the pisiform prominence of the wrist and between the medial and lateral malleoli of the ankle, which measure the voltage drop between the two ends of the circuit. From Ohm's law, when electrical current is passed through human tissue, the voltage difference between two points on the body is proportional to the impedance. Considering that the voltage drop is proportional to changes in the impedance to current flow and that impedance is tightly related to volume, changes in impedance can be assumed as expression of changes in volume [6, 7]. BIVA is an integrated part of BIA measurements and allows to optimize the assessment of volume status and of TBW as a percentage of fat-free body mass.

N. Aspromonte (✉)
Division of Cardiology, San Filippo Neri Hospital, Via Giovanni Martinotti 20, 00135 Rome, Italy
e-mail: naspromonte@yahoo.it

F. Monitillo
Cardiology Unit, Veris Delli Ponti Hospital, Via Giuseppina Delli Ponti, 73020 Scorrano, LE, Italy
e-mail: fmonitillo@libero.it

R. Valle
Department of Cardiology, Ospedale Civile, Chioggia, VE, Italy
e-mail: robertovalle@libero.it

M. Iacoviello
Cardiothoracic Department, Policlinic Hospital of Bari, Bari, Italy
e-mail: massimo.iacoviello@gmail.com

J. Rangaswami et al. (eds.), *Cardio-Nephrology*,
DOI 10.1007/978-3-319-56042-7_16

The electrical impedance (*Z*) is a function of two components, the resistance (*R*) to the applied current and the reactance (X_c). Resistance is a measure of opposition to flow of current through intra- and extracellular fluid volume, and reactance is a function of dielectric material of tissue interfaces and cell membranes, and reflects the capacitance of cells to store energy. R is inversely proportional to the amount of TBW, while X_c is related to the structure, function, and integrity of cell membranes. The measured *R* and X_c are standardized by sex and height (*H*), and BIVA results are graphically displayed by integrating *R*/*H* (Ω/m) on the *x* axis versus *X*/*H* (X_c/H9 on the *y* axis, and generating an output that reflects fluid status and alterations of cellular integrity. The obtained information used to construct a vector in a nomogram which is the expression of the relative hydration status. Shorter vectors are associated with volume overload and longer vectors with lower degrees of TBW. BIVA data are compared with measurements made in healthy reference population that are plotted as tolerance ellipses corresponding to the 50th, 75th, and 90th percentile. Values outside the 95th percentile are considered abnormal. BIVA results can be also graphically presented in the visual scale where they are classified into three classes: normally hydrated, over hydrated, or dehydrated. The vector migration within the nomogram reflects in a variation within the visual numeric scale of the hydration status (Fig. 16.1).

Another parameter resulting from bioimpedance is the "phase angle" (PA), which is the angle of the vector measured from the *x* axis, and represents the phase difference between voltage and current. It corresponds to the portion of the electrical current which is stored and then released in a different phase. This parameter depends on the ability of cells to function as capacitors, which is related to cell membrane permeability and integrity, cellular health, and soft tissue hydration [8]. BIVA has shown high correlation with TBW in comparison with deuterium dilution studies, which is the gold standard for TBW assessment [9]. Despite its limitations including body and limbs position, correct placement of the electrodes on the skin, the presence of sweat and/or skin wounds, consumption of food and beverages, skin temperature, ambient temperature, and ethnic and race variation, BIVA has been employed in various physiological and pathological conditions [3, 7, 10, 11].

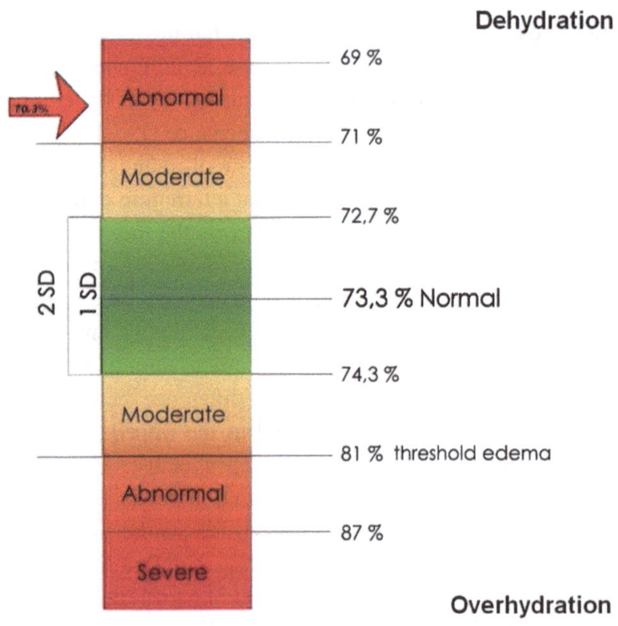

Fig. 16.1 Graphic representation of the hydration state in the visual scale for BIVA

BIVA in Acute Heart Failure

Acute heart failure syndromes (AHFS) are defined as the rapid development of HF signs and symptoms requiring urgent therapy and hospitalization. Fluid overload leading to pulmonary and systemic congestion is the most frequent presentation of AHFS [12, 13].

Currently, the mainstay of therapy for ADHF is represented by diuretics aiming to reduce congestion in order to improve renal perfusion. While this approach often results in substantial improvement of signs and symptoms during hospitalization, patients are frequently discharged with subclinical congestion and with minimal or no weight loss, or even weight gain [12, 14, 15]. The post-discharge period is burdened by high rates of readmissions and the persistent venous congestion has potential unfavorable effects on the kidneys and is associated with acute and chronic cardiorenal syndrome [16]. Moreover, diuretic therapy which often reduces congestion and relieves signs and symptoms can reduce renal perfusion, glomerular filtration rate, responsiveness to natriuretic peptides, and lead to acute kidney injury (AKI) especially during the initial phase of treatment for ADHF, with negative impact on patient's outcome [17, 18].

The detrimental impact of subclinical congestion is often underestimated, and thus an accurate quantification of the volume status of the patient is utmost importance in optimizing these patients. Currently, pre-discharge clinical assessment of congestion is empiric, and established and validated methods and guidelines to assess the degree of congestion are still lacking. Despite several proposed elements in the measurement of congestion, including bedside assessment, laboratory analysis, and dynamic maneuvres, a systematic approach in the assessment of congestion is not prevalent [2]. In this setting, BIVA can be helpful in estimating volume status of the patient before discharge, and in identifying high-risk patients with fluid overload who are more prone to experience recurrent heart failure exacerbations and poor outcomes. BIVA has been demonstrated to correlate with NYHA class [19] and has shown a high diagnostic accuracy in the differential diagnosis of dyspnea related to ADHF. In 292 patients presenting with acute dyspnea to the emergency department (ED), segmental and whole BIA were performed in addition to the conventional diagnostic strategies and BNP measurement. Dyspnea was judged as related to ADHF or to other causes according to an expert team consensus. Patients with ADHF showed significantly lower whole and segmental BIA and resistance in addition to higher BNP values. Moreover, the analyzed BIA parameters correlated significantly with BNP levels, suggesting the usefulness of this technique in the early diagnosis of dyspnea from ADHF, alone or in combination with BNP [20].

Similarly, BIVA has shown high accuracy in discriminating between cardiogenic and non-cardiogenic dyspnea in 315 patients referring to the ED for shortness of breath (69% sensitivity, 79% specificity, and 80% area under the receiver operating characteristic curve). Dyspnea was classified as cardiogenic based on physical examination, electrocardiogram, chest X-ray, NT-proBNP, and presence of Kerley B-lines on ultrasound. Peripheral congestion correlated with vector position, confirming that the combination of BIVA with lung ultrasound is a reliable method to determine the cause of dyspnea in the ED [21].

The role of natriuretic peptides (NP) in the diagnosis and management of patients with AHFs is well established [13, 22]. BNP changes during hospitalization seem to be tightly related to the relief of congestion and high BNP levels at discharge usually reflect persistent congestion predicting medium-term prognosis [23, 24]. Based on these evidences, the combined role of NP measurement and BIVA in ADHF has been the object of attention for researchers, and the accuracy of this approach for volume assessment and its utility in planning proper therapeutic interventions has been evaluated. The assessment of BNP levels together with volume status during BNP-guided treatment may allow the identification of true euvolemia in optimizing therapy and timing of patient discharge. However, BNP levels can remain high because of myocardial stretching even with euvolemia (dry BNP). The incorrect interpretation of these high BNP levels can lead to overtreatment of a euvolemic patient, especially with related kidney impairment [24].

The usefulness of a combined BNP and BIVA-guided therapy approach has been demonstrated in a retrospective study including 186 patients admitted with ADHF. This study demonstrated that the assessment of volume status with BIVA during BNP-guided therapy can improve the timing of patient discharge and predict the occurrence of cardiovascular events at 6 months [23]. Paterna et al. investigated the effect of the combination of high-dose furosemide and small-volume hypertonic saline solution (HSS) on BNP plasma levels and volume status in patients admitted for refractory congestive HF. The study population was divided into two groups depending on the administration of intravenous furosemide plus HSS or intravenous bolus of furosemide alone. BNP levels and volume status assessment by BIA were performed at admission and after discharge. Patients in HSS group displayed lower BNP levels and more optimal volume status than the non-HSS group together with a reduction in hospitalization time and readmission rate [25].

Valle et al. evaluated the role of a BNP/BIVA-guided therapy in reducing congestion and optimizing discharge timing of 300 patients hospitalized for ADHF. Therapy was titrated to reach a BNP value of less than 250 pg/ml. Authors stratified the patients into three groups (early responders, late responders, and non-responders) according to BNP changes in response to therapy. The addition of BIVA to BNP levels measurement allowed the determination of the "true volume status" differentiating high BNP levels reflecting myocardial dysfunction with normal volume status ("dry BNP") from high BNP levels due to volume overload. This approach has proved effective in achieving adequate fluid balance status and avoiding unnecessary aggressive diuretic and prolonged therapy to achieve BNP reduction and preventing AKI [26].

Recently, Di Somma et al. verified the diagnostic and 30-day prognostic value of body fluid assessment at admission by BIVA in 381 patients referring to the Emergency Department for symptoms (dyspnea), signs (edema, jugular venous distension), and other trigger factors for volume status perturbations (gastrointestinal disorders, fever, sepsis). Based on medical records, two cardiologists, blinded for BIVA results, classified the diagnosis of ADHF and these patients underwent standard dosage of drugs according to ESC guidelines. BIVA demonstrated diagnostic utility in assessing congestion in those patients with BNP levels ranging from 100 to 400 pg/ml which are not diagnostic of ADHF. Moreover, the study confirmed the prognostic role of volume status assessed at admission in a follow-up period of 30 days [27].

These results confirmed previous data obtained by the same group in a small population of ADHF patients. The combined use of BIVA and BNP improved the therapeutic management of these patients, preventing excessive volume depletion due to diuretics. In addition, BIVA was able to identify patients with a persistent volume overload and a higher risk of death and rehospitalization [28].

Alves et al. have evaluated the role of BIVA and phase angle in 57 patients during hospitalization for ADHF and after clinical stabilization. Authors have demonstrated that the combination of these methods can allow the detection of significant changes in volume status during ADHF. Moreover, the assessment of congestion by BIVA at admission identified those patients more prone to experience weight loss and improvement of dyspnea during compensation [29].

BIVA in Chronic Kidney Disease and Chronic Heart Failure

It is well known that patients with chronic kidney disease (CKD), especially those receiving renal replacement therapy, are at very high cardiovascular risk with a high risk of death due to cardiovascular causes. Similarly, chronic heart failure (CHF) causes a progressive decline in kidney function resulting in a high prevalence of CKD in these patients [30]. In patients with end-stage kidney disease (ESKD), the hemodialysis (HD) prescription is targeted to fluid removal to achieve optimized fluid balance. The main objective of the treatment is to achieve the "dry weight" defined as the lowest weight a patient can tolerate without the development of intradialytic hypotension, with optimal pre- and post-dialysis blood pressures, in the absence of overt fluid overload [31, 32].

The accurate assessment of the balance between ultrafiltration rates and plasma refilling is of main importance in order to prevent both myocardial stunning due to intradialytic hypotension or persistent chronic volume overload, e.g., suboptimal volume management in ESKD patients has been linked to increase morbidity and long-term cardiovascular complications. Inadequate fluid removal during hemodialysis and chronic subclinical volume overload are associated with hypertension, left ventricular hypertrophy and heart failure, increased arterial stiffness, and stroke, which are among the leading causes of death in dialysis patients. In contrast, excessive fluid removal can lead to hypotension, arrhythmias, muscle cramping, nausea, vomiting, and other adverse effects [23, 33]. Isolated clinical assessment of volume status may be unreliable because the absence of visible edema cannot exclude a significant extracellular volume expansion, and this approach does not account for changes in lean body mass, fat mass, or inflammatory or nutritional status over time. In the absence of overt clinical signs of dehydration or overhydration, changes in body weight or blood pressure cannot be considered as a sensitive index of correct hydration. Therefore, an accurate evaluation of volume changes during HD is required for defining the goal for fluid removal and to develop strategies for safer dialysis treatments.

Several methods to monitor fluid status have been proposed including biochemical markers, vena cava diameter, blood volume monitoring, and bioimpedance analysis [32, 33].

In this setting, BIA and BIVA techniques may represent intriguing and useful tools to monitor and optimize the effectiveness of performed therapies. These methods have proved to be comparable to direct estimation methods of TBW, intracellular fluid volume (ICV), and extracellular fluid volume (ECV) [34].

Considering that at a given phase angle, the bioimpedance vector length reflects the degree of tissue hydration, the relative risk of death associated with different bioimpedance vector lengths has been evaluated in a large population of hemodialysis patients. A significant association between volume status expressed by vector length by BIA and mortality has been demonstrated, confirming the importance of maintaining a dry weight in these patients [33].

In a small population of patients on chronic hemodialysis, it has been demonstrated that changes in BIA variables in the immediate post-dialysis period (dry weight state) seem constant and reproducible, allowing a reliable estimation of total body weight [35].

Kouw et al. using multiple frequencies compared pre- and post-dialysis values of ECV and ICV to normal values obtained in healthy volunteers in order to identify post-dialysis over- and underhydration. The authors observed that ECV of patients in "dry weight" after dialysis was comparable to that of control subjects and was a reliable marker of post-dialysis volume status [36].

In a large population of HD patients, the backward–forward impedance vector displacements on the R-X_c plane accurately reflected the wet–dry weight cycling of HD patients. Indeed, vectors of patients prone to hemodynamic instability were more often out of the reference of the 75% tolerance ellipse, compared to stable patients. Data obtained by BIVA were reliable in guiding dry weight prescription in this study [37].

In 200 patients on continuous ambulatory peritoneal dialysis (CAPD), BIVA was validated based on direct measurements of resistance (R) and reactance (X_c), without knowledge of body weight. Vector distribution was compared with that obtained in healthy volunteers and subjects on hemodialysis and nephrotic subjects. Vector lengths were reduced in patients with edema and demonstrated the sensitivity of BIVA in assessing fluid status [38].

Basile et al. [39] developed and validated a bioimpedance prediction model for the accurate assessment of volume status and especially of "dry weight" in HD patients with good predictive value.

Piccoli et al. verified the role of the combined evaluation of nutrition and volume status in 130 patients undergoing chronic hemodialysis three times a week. Each subject was classified as having normal nutritional status, moderate or severe malnutrition according to subjective global assessment (SGA), whereas volume status was evaluated with BIVA. The study demonstrated the useful role of BIVA in identifying changes in hydration status during fluid removal with hemodialysis in each SGA category [40].

In a study of 131 HD patients, BIA-guided dry weight prescription was more effective than clinical judgment alone in obtaining strict volume fluid control. The primary outcome was all-cause mortality over 2.5 years (the duration of the intervention). The BIA-guided approach was associated with reduction in all-cause deaths with a greater decline in arterial stiffness, relative fluid overload, and systolic BP in comparison to the clinical-methods group [41].

Chen et al. have investigated the combined use of NT-proBNP measurements with BIVA as a marker of fluid status in patients undergoing continuous renal replacement therapy (CRRT). Indeed, BIVA is a measure of static tissue hydration and this data can be supplemented by serum N-terminal pro-B-type natriuretic peptide (NT-proBNP) which reflects the cardiac reaction to volume load, and acts as a biomarker for diagnosis of heart failure. Therefore, the combined use of BIVA and NT-proBNP allows to identify shifts in volume status and the optimal net ultrafiltration rate during CRRT [42]. These results were consistent with data from another study on 92 patients in peritoneal dialysis, where serial measurements of NT-proBNP correlated with changes in volume assessments made by multifrequency bioimpedance [43].

The importance of the assessment of body composition and fat-free mass as marker of disease severity and progression in chronic heart failure (CHF) patients is well established [44]. Uszko-Lencer et al. compared BIA and dual-energy X-ray absorptiometry (DXA) with deuterium dilution (DEU) as a reference method to assess fat-free mass (FFM) in patients with cardiomyopathy. Authors observe that DXA and deuterium dilution are strongly related and interchangeable laboratory methods for assessment of FFM. Moreover, BIA proved to be a reliable tool to estimate FFM in stable outpatients with systolic dysfunction [45].

The prognostic value of the bioelectrical phase angle has been retrospective evaluated and compared with other well-established indicators of outcome in a population of 389 patients. Bioimpedance phase angle was observed to be a significant and independent predictor of all-cause mortality and was associated with malnutrition markers [8]. The bioimpedance phase angle has been also reported to be a good indicator of functional class in 243 patients with HF with significantly shorter and downsloping impedance vector in the NYHA III–IV group compared with the NYHA I–II group [19]. BIVA has been investigated as a tool to assess cardiac cachexia in 519 outpatients with CHF in NYHA classes I–IV. Authors found a significant difference of vector migration between survivors and non-survivors despite average weight loss not being significantly different in cachectic patients when compared with the non-cachectic group [46].

Conclusion

The estimation of body fluid content has proven to be crucial for both diagnosis and prognosis assessment in patients with heart failure and kidney diseases. In the acute and chronic setting the bioelectrical vector analysis (BIVA) associated with laboratory biomarkers might achieve much results in management of AHF or end-stage kidney disease, especially for monitoring, risk stratification, and therapeutic decision-making.

References

1. Berne RM, Levy MN, Koeppen BM, Stanton BA. Physiology. 5th ed. New York: Elsevier; 2004.
2. Gheorghiade M, Follath F, Ponikowski P, Barsuk JH, et al. Assessing and grading congestion in acute heart failure: a scientific statement from the acute heart failure committee of the heart failure association of the European Society of Cardiology and endorsed by the European Society of Intensive Care Medicine. Eur J Heart Fail. 2010;12(5):423–33.
3. Kalantari K, Chang JN, Ronco C, Rosner MH. Assessment of intravascular volume status and volume responsiveness in critically ill patients. Kidney Int. 2013;83:1017–28.
4. Jones SL, Tanaka A, Eastwood GM, Young H, et al. Bioelectrical impedance vector analysis in critically ill patients: a prospective, clinician-blinded investigation. Crit Care. 2015;19:290.
5. Stevenson LW, Perloff JK. The limited availability of physical signs for estimating hemodynamics in chronic heart failure. JAMA. 1989;261:884–8.
6. Peacock WF IV. Use of bioimpedance vector analysis in critically ill and cardiorenal patients. Contrib Nephrol. 2010;165:226–35.
7. Walter-Kroker A, Kroker A, Mattiucci-Guehlke M, Glaab T. A practical guide to bioelectrical impedance analysis using the example of chronic obstructive pulmonary disease. Nutr J. 2011; 21(10):35.
8. Colín-Ramírez E, Castillo-Martínez L, Orea-Tejeda A, Vázquez--Durán M, et al. Bioelectrical impedance phase angle as a prognostic marker in chronic heart failure. Nutrition. 2012;28 (9):901–5.
9. Kushner RF, Schoeller DA. Estimation of total body water by bioelectrical impedance analysis. Am J Clin Nutr. 1986;44(3): 417–24.
10. Tang WH, Tong W. Measuring impedance in congestive heart failure: current options and clinical applications. Am Heart J. 2009;157(3):402–11.
11. Bioelectrical impedance analysis in body composition measurement: national institutes of health technology assessment conference statement. Am J Clin Nutr. 1996;64(3 Suppl):524S–32S **(review)**.
12. Gheorghiade M, Pang PS. Acute heart failure syndromes. J Am Coll Cardiol. 2009;53(7):557–73.
13. McMurray JJ, Adamopoulos S, Anker SD, Auricchio A, et al. ESC guidelines for the diagnosis and treatment of acute and chronic heart failure 2012: the Task Force for the Diagnosis and Treatment of Acute and Chronic Heart Failure 2012 of the European Society of Cardiology. Developed in collaboration with the Heart Failure Association (HFA) of the ESC. Eur J Heart Fail. 2012;14:803–69.
14. Adams KF Jr, Fonarow GC, Emerman CL, LeJemtel TH, Costanzo MR, Abraham WT, Berkowitz RL, Galvao M, Horton DP, ADHERE Scientific Advisory Committee and Investigators. Characteristics and outcomes of patients hospitalized for heart failure in the United States: rationale, design, and preliminary observations from the first 100,000 cases in the Acute Decompensated Heart Failure National Registry (ADHERE). Am Heart J. 2005;149:209–16.
15. Gheorghiade M, Zannad F, Sopko G, Klein L, et al. Acute heart failure syndromes: current state and framework for future research. Circulation. 2005;112(25):3958–68.

16. Mullens W, Abrahams Z, Francis GS, Sokos G, Taylor DO, Starling RC, Young JB, Tang WH. Importance of venous congestion for worsening of renal function in advanced decompensated heart failure. J Am Coll Cardiol. 2009;53:589–96.
17. Freda BJ, Slawsky M, Mallidi J, Braden GL. Decongestive treatment of acute decompensated heart failure: cardiorenal implications of ultrafiltration and diuretics. Am J Kidney Dis. 2011;58(6):1005–17.
18. Aspromonte N, Cruz DN, Ronco C, Valle R. Role of bioimpedance vectorial analysis in cardio-renal syndromes. Semin Nephrol. 2012;32(1):93–9.
19. Castillo Martínez L, Colín Ramírez E, Orea Tejeda A, Asensio Lafuente E. Bioelectrical impedance and strength measurements in patients with heart failure: comparison with functional class. Nutrition. 2007;23(5):412–8.
20. Parrinello G, Paterna S, Di Pasquale P, Torres D, et al. The usefulness of bioelectrical impedance analysis in differentiating dyspnea due to decompensated heart failure. J Card Fail. 2008;14 (8):676–86.
21. Piccoli A, Codognotto M, Cianci V, Vettore G, et al. Differentiation of cardiac and noncardiac dyspnea using bioelectrical impedance vector analysis (BIVA). J Card Fail. 2012;18(3): 226–32.
22. Roberts E, Ludman AJ, Dworzynski K, Al-Mohammad A, et al. The diagnostic accuracy of the natriuretic peptides in heart failure: systematic review and diagnostic meta-analysis in the acute care setting. BMJ. 2015;4(350):h910.
23. Valle R, Aspromonte N, Giovinazzo P, Carbonieri E, et al. B-type natriuretic peptide-guided treatment for predicting outcome in patients hospitalized in sub-intensive care unit with acute heart failure. J Card Fail. 2008;14(3):219–24.
24. Valle R, Aspromonte N. Use of brain natriuretic peptide and bioimpedance to guide therapy in heart failure patients. Contrib Nephrol. 2010;164:209–16.
25. Paterna S, Di Pasquale P, Parrinello G, Fornaciari E, et al. Changes in brain natriuretic peptide levels and bioelectrical impedance measurements after treatment with high-dose furosemide and hypertonic saline solution versus high-dose furosemide alone in refractory congestive heart failure: a double-blind study. J Am Coll Cardiol. 2005;45(12):1997–2003.
26. Valle R, Aspromonte N, Milani L, Peacock FW, et al. Optimizing fluid management in patients with acute decompensated heart failure (ADHF): the emerging role of combined measurement of body hydration status and brain natriuretic peptide (BNP) levels. Heart Fail Rev. 2011;16(6):519–29.
27. Di Somma S, Lalle I, Magrini L, Russo V, et al. Additive diagnostic and prognostic value of bioelectrical impedance vector analysis (BIVA) to brain natriuretic peptide 'grey-zone' in patients with acute heart failure in the emergency department. Eur Heart J Acute Cardiovasc Care. 2014;3(2):167–75.
28. Di Somma S, De Berardinis B, Bongiovanni C, Marino R, et al. Use of BNP and bioimpedance to drive therapy in heart failure patients. Congest Heart Fail. 2010;16(Suppl 1):S56–61.
29. Alves FD, Souza GC, Aliti GB, Rabelo-Silva ER, et al. Dynamic changes in bioelectrical impedance vector analysis and phase angle in acute decompensated heart failure. Nutrition. 2015;31(1):84–9.
30. Ronco C, McCullough PA, Anker SD, Anand I, Aspromonte N, Bagshaw SM, Bellomo R, Berl T, Bobek I, Cruz DN, Daliento L, Davenport A, Haapio M, Hillege H, House A, Katz NM, Maisel A, Mankad S, Zanco P, Mebazaa A, Palazzuoli A, Ronco F, Shaw A, Sheinfeld G, Soni S, Vescovo G, Zamperetti N, Ponikowski P, Acute Dialysis Quality Initiative (ADQI) Consensus Group. Cardiorenal syndromes: an executive summary from the consensus conference of the acute dialysis quality initiative (ADQI). Contrib Nephrol. 2010;165:54–67.
31. Henderson LW. Symtomatic hypotension during hemodyalisis. Kidney Int. 1980;17:571–6.
32. Jaeger JQ, Mehta RL. Assessment of dry weight in hemodialysis: an overview. J Am Soc Nephrol. 1999;10(2):392–403.
33. Pillon L, Piccoli A, Lowrie EG, Lazarus JM, et al. Vector length as a proxy for the adequacy of ultrafiltration in hemodialysis. Kidney Int. 2004;66(3):1266–71.
34. Raimann JG, Zhu F, Wang J, Thijssen S, et al. Comparison of fluid volume estimates in chronic hemodialysis patients by bioimpedance, direct isotopic, and dilution methods. Kidney Int. 2014;85 (4):898–908.
35. Di Iorio BR, Scalfi L, Terracciano V, Bellizzi V, et al. A systematic evaluation of bioelectrical impedance measurement after hemodialysis session. Kidney Int. 2004;65(6):2435–40.
36. Kouw PM, Olthof CG, ter Wee PM, Oe LP, et al. Assessment of post-dialysis dry weight: an application of the conductivity measurement method. Kidney Int. 1992;41(2):440–4.
37. Piccoli A. Identification of operational clues to dry weight prescription in hemodialysis using bioimpedance vector analysis. The Italian Hemodialysis-Bioelectrical Impedance Analysis (HD-BIA) Study Group. Kidney Int. 1998;53(4):1036–43.
38. Piccoli A, Italian CAPD-BIA Study Group. Bioelectric impedance vector distribution in peritoneal dialysis patients with different hydration status. Kidney Int. 2004;65(3):1050–63.
39. Basile C, Vernaglione L, Di Iorio B, Bellizzi V, et al. Development and validation of bioimpedance analysis prediction equations for dry weight in hemodialysis patients. Clin J Am Soc Nephrol. 2007;2(4):675–80.
40. Piccoli A, Codognotto M, Piasentin P, Naso A. Combined evaluation of nutrition and hydration in dialysis patients with bioelectrical impedance vector analysis (BIVA). Clin Nutr. 2014;33(4):673–7.
41. Onofriescu M, Hogas S, Voroneanu L, Apetrii M, et al. Bioimpedance-guided fluid management in maintenance hemodialysis: a pilot randomized controlled trial. Am J Kidney Dis. 2014;64(1):111–8.
42. Chen H, Wu B, Gong D, Liu Z. Fluid overload at start of continuous renal replacement therapy is associated with poorer clinical condition and outcome: a prospective observational study on the combined use of bioimpedance vector analysis and serum N-terminal pro-B-type natriuretic peptide measurement. Crit Care. 2015;2(19):135.
43. Davenport A. Changes in N-terminal pro-brain natriuretic peptide correlate with fluid volume changes assessed by bioimpedance in peritoneal dialysis patients. Am J Nephrol. 2012;36(4):371–6.
44. Conraads VM, Bosmans JM, Vrints CJ. Chronic heart failure: an example of a systemic chronic inflammatory disease resulting in cachexia. Int J Cardiol. 2002;85(1):33–49.
45. Uszko-Lencer NH, Bothmer F, van Pol PE, Schols AM. Measuring body composition in chronic heart failure: a comparison of methods. Eur J Heart Fail. 2006;8(2):208–14.
46. Castillo-Martínez L, Colín-Ramírez E, Orea-Tejeda A, González Islas DG, et al. Cachexia assessed by bioimpedance vector analysis as a prognostic indicator in chronic stable heart failure patients. Nutrition. 2012;28(9):886–91.

17 Novel Therapies for Acute Decompensated Heart Failure

Bryan A. Smith and John E.A. Blair

Introduction

Acute decompensated heart failure (ADHF), defined as new onset, gradually or rapidly worsening heart failure (HF) requiring urgent therapy, continues to be a clinical challenge [1]. Hospitalizations for ADHF typically are caused by an increase in left ventricular (LV) filling pressure leading to symptomatic congestion. The prognosis of outpatients with chronic HF has improved significantly in the past 20 years as a result of advancements in medical therapies, implantable cardioverter defibrillators and cardiac resynchronization therapy devices. However, patients hospitalized with HF continue to have a mortality rate of 15% and a readmission rate of 30% within 30–60 days of discharge [2]. Repeated hospitalizations for HF result in a 6-month mortality rate of 10–20% and a 1-year mortality rate of 30–50% after the first hospitalization [3, 4]. Previous trials for ADHF have failed to discover any therapies that significantly improve clinical outcomes. There have also been concerns about the safety of drugs that have been approved because of an increased risk of ventricular arrhythmias and sudden death. As a result, therapies for ADHF have remained relatively unchanged for the past 20 years. This review will discuss a number of novel therapies that have been studied or are currently in development for the management of ADHF.

B.A. Smith · J.E.A. Blair (✉)
Department of Medicine, Section of Cardiology, University of Chicago Pritzker School of Medicine, 5841 S Maryland Avenue, MC 5076, 60637 Chicago, IL, USA
e-mail: jblair2@bsd.uchicago.edu

B.A. Smith
e-mail: bryan.smith2@uchospitals.edu

J. Rangaswami et al. (eds.), *Cardio-Nephrology*,
DOI 10.1007/978-3-319-56042-7_17

Fluid Removal Strategies

Diuretics

Presently, intravenous non-potassium-sparing loop diuretics remain the cornerstone of therapy for relief from congestion in acute decompensated heart failure [5]. The Diuretic Optimization Strategies Evaluation trial (DOSE-AHF) was a prospective, double-blind trial that randomized 308 patients hospitalized with worsening chronic HF regardless of left ventricular ejection fraction (LVEF) in a 2-by-2 factorial design into either high-dose (2.5 times total daily furosemide equivalents) or low-dose (same total daily furosemide equivalent) furosemide, administered in either continuous or bolus intravenous preparations [6]. The primary endpoint of global assessment of symptoms over 72 h demonstrated a favorable trend in the high-dose strategy ($P = 0.06$), but no difference in infusion strategies (Fig. 17.1). The primary safety endpoint of mean change in serum creatinine (sCr) level was not significantly different between groups, and the prespecified secondary endpoints of dyspnea score, weight change, and net fluid loss over 72 h were significantly better in the high-dose versus low-dose strategies, at a cost of more patients with an increase in sCr > 0.3 mg/dL within 72 h (23 vs. 14%, $P = 0.04$), but with no difference in composite death, rehospitalizations, or emergency department visits. A follow-up analysis of this study found that greater that one-third of patients in the DOSE-AHF and Cardiorenal Rescue Study in Acute Decompensated Heart Failure (CARRESS-HF) trials continued to have persistent congestion at discharge, highlighting the limitations of loop diuretic therapy for management of congestion [7].

Although effective, loop diuretics have some detrimental effects, both in their acute and chronic use, by causing electrolyte disturbances and neurohormonal stimulation [8–11]. Retrospective studies in both acute and chronic HF have demonstrated that higher doses of diuretics were associated with increased mortality and worsening renal function, even after correcting for baseline clinical

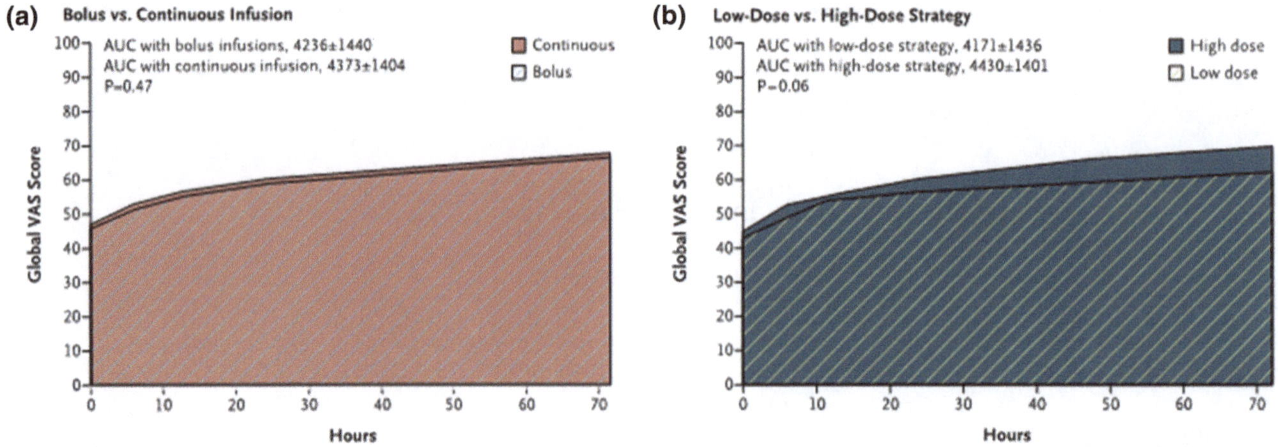

Fig. 17.1 Primary endpoint of the DOSE study: global symptom assessment of symptoms over 72 h in different furosemide dosing strategies for patients hospitalized with worsening chronic heart failure regardless of ejection fraction. Reprinted with permission from Felker et al. [6]

characteristics [12, 13]. Other potential diuretic regimens to relieve congestion include dual blockage of nephrons with thiazide diuretics. This may assist in increasing volume removal, but can cause additional electrolyte disturbances and arrhythmias [14]. The addition of mineralocorticoid receptor antagonists to a loop diuretic regimen can also provide some symptomatic relief, but this has not been studied in a prospective, randomized trial. Given the lack of evidence, as well as the potential untoward drug effects of loop diuretics, additional pharmacologic agents have been developed to remove fluid and relieve the signs and symptoms of congestion, without worsening cardiac or renal function.

Tolvaptan

Arginine vasopressin (AVP) is a nonapeptide hormone that plays an important role in maintaining serum osmolarity and central volume. AVP, also known as antidiuretic hormone (ADH), is synthesized in the hypothalamus and transported in secretory granules to the posterior pituitary, where it is stored until release after appropriate stimulation [13]. The most potent stimulus for AVP secretion is elevated serum osmolarity, through stimulation of osmoreceptors located in the hypothalamus [15]. Nonosmotic factors that stimulate AVP release include reduced cardiac index (CI), hypovolemia, or hemorrhage, which act through baroreceptors located in the carotid sinus, aortic arch, and left atrium [16]. AVP release leads to free water retention. In states of hypovolemia or hemorrhage, AVP is important in maintaining adequate cardiac preload through stimulation of V1a and V2 receptors, and afterload through stimulation of V1a receptors, maintaining circulating volume. In ADHF, however, these effects are maladaptive, resulting in worsening HF and adverse LV remodeling. Vasopressin antagonists have been developed to remove fluid in patients with HF, while modulating the deleterious effects of vasopressin on LV function and correcting hyponatremia [15].

After initial studies showed some short-term efficacy of tolvaptan in mild chronic HF, the Acute and Chronic Therapeutic Impact of a Vasopressin Antagonist in Congestive Heart Failure (ACTIV in CHF) trial was designed to evaluate the clinical effects of tolvaptan in patients hospitalized for HF [17]. This was a randomized, multicenter, double-blind, placebo-controlled phase 2 trial of 319 patients hospitalized with worsening HF, LVEF < 40%, and signs of systemic congestion after initial in-hospital therapy. Eligible patients were randomized in a 1:1:1:1 manner to either placebo or 1 of 3 doses of tolvaptan (30, 60, or 90 mg daily) in addition to standard HF therapy, including diuretics, and followed for 60 days both during the in-hospital and outpatient periods. The primary end points were changed in body weight at 24 h after drug administration, and worsening HF at 60 days after randomization, defined as hospitalization or unscheduled visit for ADHF, escalation of existing therapy or new therapy for ADHF, or death. The primary endpoint of median body weight loss at 24 h ranged from 1.8 to 2.1 kg in the tolvaptan group and did not appear to be dose-dependent, compared to a weight loss of 0.6 kg in the placebo arm, while the other primary endpoint of worsening HF at 60 days was not significantly different between groups (26.7% in patients in the tolvaptan vs. 27.5% in the placebo groups). Body weight was significantly lower at discharge in the groups receiving 30 and 60 mg of tolvaptan compared to placebo, but this difference disappeared at 1-week post-discharge and on the last clinic visit. Urine volume was significantly higher, serum sodium increased and often normalized, and was sustained in patients with hyponatremia, and there appeared to be no differences in potassium or vital signs in the tolvaptan groups compared to placebo [17]. Post hoc analysis revealed a trend toward reduced mortality in patients with severe congestion or elevated blood urea nitrogen treated with tolvaptan compared to placebo [17].

While phase 3 clinical trials were planned or underway, the Effect of Tolvaptan on Hemodynamic Parameters in Subjects with Heart Failure (ECLIPSE) study was designed to evaluate the hemodynamic effects of tolvaptan in severe chronic HF [18]. This study was a randomized, multicenter, double-blind, placebo-controlled trial of 181 patients with at least 3 months of severe HF symptoms and LVEF $\leq$ 40%, on standard HF therapy. Patients were randomized in a 1:1:1:1 manner to either placebo or tolvaptan (15, 30, or 60 mg) given as a single dose, if the pulmonary capillary wedge pressure (PCWP) was >18 mmHg on two consecutive recordings at least 10 min apart after a 2- to 20-h stabilization period. The primary endpoint of PCWP peak change from baseline at 3–8 h was significantly greater with tolvaptan (5.7–6.4 mmHg in the tolvaptan groups compared with 4.2 mmHg with the placebo group). Peak right atrial pressure and pulmonary arterial pressure reductions were significantly greater in the tolvaptan versus placebo groups, with no significant differences in CI, blood pressure, or systemic or pulmonary vascular resistances [18].

The phase 3 Efficacy of Vasopressin Antagonist in Heart Failure Outcome Study with Tolvaptan (EVEREST) trials were designed to determine the short-term and long-term efficacy of tolvaptan when administered to patients hospitalized with HF and LVEF $\leq$ 40% and continued post-discharge [19, 20]. Total enrollment for the EVEREST trials was 4133 patients followed for a median of 9.9 months. The short-term trials demonstrated that tolvaptan resulted in significantly were two identical trials designed to assess improvement in clinical symptoms, and demonstrated that tolvaptan resulted in significantly greater improvement in the composite primary end point of patient-assessed global status and weight loss at day 7 or discharge, driven entirely by reduction in body weight (3.56 vs. 2.76 kg, $P < 0.001$). There was a significantly greater improvement in dyspnea with tolvaptan versus placebo, and significantly greater improvement in edema only in one of the two short-term trials. Adverse event frequencies were similar in both the tolvaptan and placebo groups. For the long-term trial, the dual primary end points did not significantly differ between groups: death at 9.9 months occurred in 25.9% in the tolvaptan group and 26.3% in the placebo group, and composite cardiovascular death or heart failure hospitalization occurred in 42.0% in the tolvaptan group and 40.2% in the placebo group (Fig. 17.2). There was no subgroup, including severe HF, severely depressed LVEF, or hyponatremia, that appeared to benefit from tolvaptan over placebo. Although the EVEREST trials did not show any significant benefit in long-term clinical outcomes, there was a potentially important benefit in volume status and symptoms.

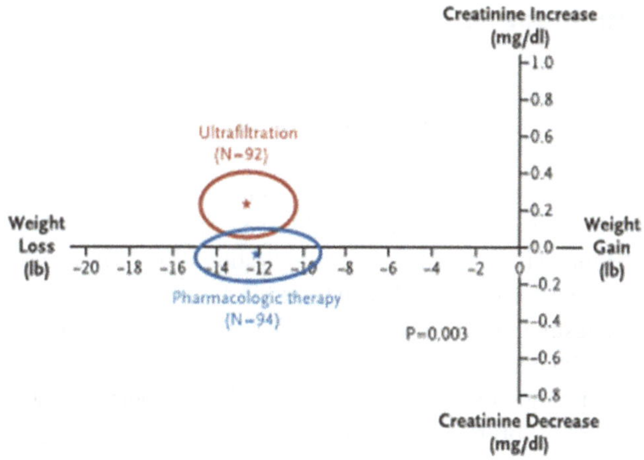

Fig. 17.2 Primary outcome of CARRESS-HF: changes in serum creatinine and weight at 96 h in patients hospitalized with heart failure and worsening renal function. Reprinted with permission from Bart et al. [24]

Two additional clinical trials are currently underway which are further evaluating the effects of tolvaptan on decongestion in ADHF [21]. The Targeting Acute Congestion With Tolvaptan in Congestive Heart Failure Study (TACTICS) compares the effects of oral tolvaptan to placebo in addition to a fixed dose of intravenous furosemide in 250 patients hospitalized with ADHF, with a primary endpoint of dyspnea without need for rescue therapy or death (NCT01644331). This study has completed enrollment and is awaiting publication of the results. The study to Evaluate Challenging Responses to Therapy in Congestive Heart Failure (SECRET of CHF) study is assessing the additive effect on tolvaptan to a short-term diuretic regimen in 250 patients with ADHF who are have one of the following: renal insufficiency, hyponatremia, or inadequate initial response to diuretic therapy, with the primary endpoint of self-assessed 7-point dyspnea score at 8 and 16 h (NCT 01584557). The study is currently enrolling and scheduled to be completed in October 2016.

Despite the promising improvement in symptoms with tolvaptan, studies to date have not demonstrated its role in reduction of mortality in ADHF. Nevertheless, tolvaptan has been approved by the United States Food and Drug Administration (FDA) in May 2009 for the treatment of euvolemic and hypervolemic hyponatremia, to include patients with HF, and has a favorable safety profile and result in normalization of serum sodium, reduction in body weight, and symptomatic improvement, especially in high-risk groups [22]. With further study, vasopressin antagonists still hold promise in the treatment of ADHF.

Ultrafiltration

When pharmacological approaches prove to be ineffective in patients with ADHF, ultrafiltration may be a possible solution. Ultrafiltration is a therapy in which plasma water is moved across a semipermeable membrane due to a transmembrane pressure gradient [7]. The effectiveness of this method was assessed in the Ultrafiltration versus Intravenous Diuretics for Patients Hospitalized for Acute Decompensated Congestive Heart Failure trial (UNLOAD), which randomized 200 patients hospitalized for HF regardless of LVEF, to ultrafiltration or loop diuretics within 24 h of hospitalization [23]. The primary endpoint of weight loss and dyspnea assessment at 48 h was met for ultrafiltration for weight loss (5.0 ± 3.1 vs. 3.1 ± 3.5 kg, $P = 0.001$), but not for dyspnea scores. There was a trend toward larger sCr increases during hospitalization in the ultrafiltration arm, but a decrease in rehospitalization for ADHF at 90 days compared with diuretic therapy (16 vs. 28 events) [23]. This study led to the Cardiorenal Rescue Study in Acute Decompensated Heart Failure (CARRESS-HF), a randomized trial of ultrafiltration versus pharmacological therapy in 188 patients hospitalized for HF regardless of LVEF, with worsened renal function (increase in sCr ≥ 0.3 mg/dL within 12 weeks before or 10 days after admission) [24]. The primary endpoint, a bivariate response in change in sCr level and weight at 96 h, was significantly different between groups, due to the increases in SCr in the ultrafiltration arm (0.23 ± 0.70 mg/dL increase vs. 0.04 ± 0.53 mg/dL, $P = 0.003$) and similar weight reduction in both arms (5.5–5.7 kg in both groups) (Fig. 17.2). There was no significant difference in natriuretic peptide levels, death, rehospitalizations, or emergency room visits, and the ultrafiltration group had a higher percentage of serious adverse events. The FDA approved the Aquadex FlexFlow System [CHF Solutions, Brooklyn Park, MN (now known as Gambro, Lakewood, CO)] in June 2002 for the ultrafiltration of patients with fluid overload who have failed diuretic therapy [25]. Based on available data, ultrafiltration should be used sparingly in select patients who are refractory to intensified diuretic regimens.

Novel Vasodilators

Nesiritide

Patients with heart failure have elevated levels of vasoconstrictors and high systemic vascular resistance. Though they typically have elevated B-type natriuretic peptide (BNP) levels, the level of bioactive BNP may be low. Nesiritide is a recombinant B-type natriuretic peptide that has specific venous, arterial, and coronary vasodilatory properties which increase cardiac output (CO) and reduce afterload without any inotropic effects. Also, it increases the glomerular filtration rate and filtration fraction, causes natriuresis in patients with ADHF, and suppresses the renin–angiotensin–aldosterone axis [26]. It has been extensively studied as a therapy to increase urine output in acute HF, but initial studies showed conflicting data. In the Nesiritide Study Group and Vasodilation in the Management of Acute CHF (VMAC) trial, 432 patients hospitalized for ADHF were enrolled in either a nesiritide efficacy trial or a comparative trial in which nesiritide was compared with nitroglycerine. The primary endpoint was changed from baseline of the PCWP 6 h after the initiation of therapy. Treatment with nesiritide resulted in significant reduction in PCWP, pulmonary artery pressure, systemic vascular resistance, and an increase in CI compared to nitroglycerin and placebo [26].

Based on the success of the VMAC study, the Acute Study of Clinical Effectiveness of Nesiritide and Decompensated Heart Failure (ASCEND-HF) was created. In this study, 7141 patients hospitalized with HF and at least one objective measure (pulmonary edema on chest radiograph, elevated natriuretic peptide, PCWP > 20 mmHg, or LVEF < 40% in previous 12 months) were randomized to either nesiritide or placebo in addition to standard medical therapy [27]. Although the coprimary endpoint of improvement in dyspnea at 6 and 24 h was observed when nesiritide was added to standard therapy, this finding did not meet prespecified criteria for statistical significance, and the other primary endpoint of death or rehospitalization was the same in the nesiritide and placebo groups (Fig. 17.3). There was more hypotension in the nesiritide group (26.6 vs. 15.3%, $P < 0.01$) and there was also no difference in the secondary end point of patients with a >25% decrease in estimated glomerular filtration rate (eGFR) from baseline. Overall, nesiritide had minimal effects on mortality, hospitalizations, and symptoms. A follow-up analysis of this study sought to determine if nesiritide had a significant effect on diuresis in patients with ADHF. The 24-h urine output was 2280 mL for patients who received nesiritide and 2200 mL for patients who received placebo (P = NS). Though nesiritide did cause a slight increase in urine output in patients with worsened renal function, this was not the case after independent predictors of urine output were controlled for [27]. Previous studies that demonstrated a significant effect on urine output with nesiritide enrolled patients without ADHF [28]. Based on ASCEND-HF and similar trials, nesiritide has no effect on urine output in patients with ADHF. Suggested reasons for this effect may be that neurohormonal activation limits the effect of natriuretic peptides in patients with HF. Also, there may be differing vascular effects of BNP in patients with and without HF [29, 30]. Although the FDA approved nesiritide in

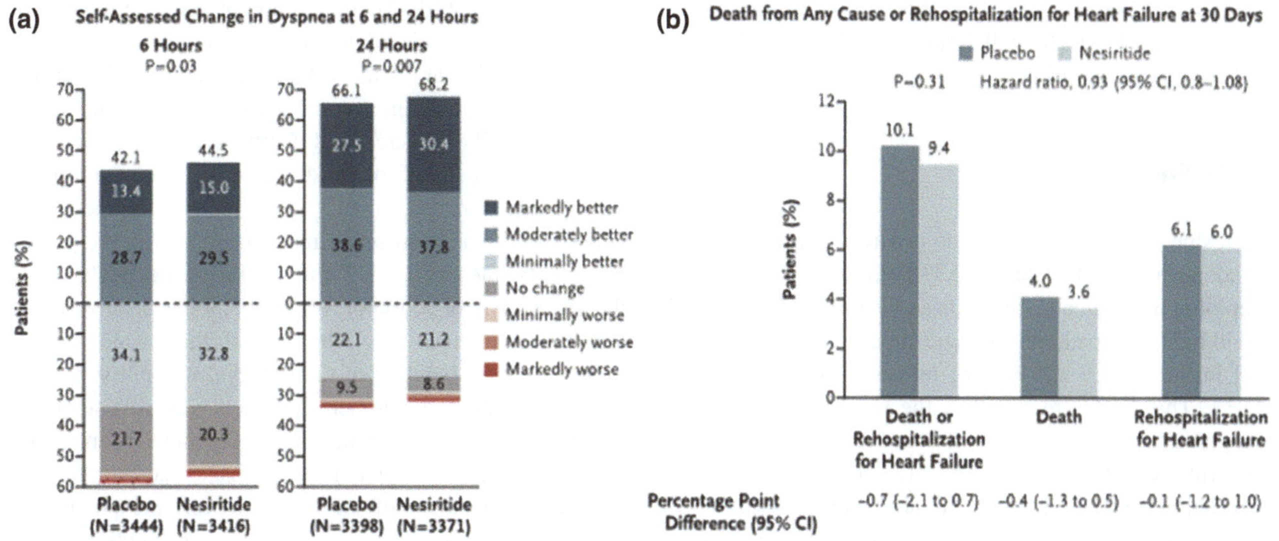

Fig. 17.3 The ASCEND-HF failed to meet coprimary endpoints of self-assessed dyspnea score and death or heart failure rehospitalization when nesiritide was compared to placebo in patients hospitalized with heart failure. Reprinted with permission from O'Connor et al. [27]

August 2001, post-marketing data led to further scrutiny of the medication's efficacy and safety, ultimately leading to the ASCEND-HF trial. In July 2012, the FDA released safety labeling changes reflecting the higher incidence of symptomatic hypotension and worsening renal function with nesiritide. Based on the totality of data available, there is little evidence supporting the use of nesiritide in patients with ADHF.

Relaxin

Relaxin is an endogenous hormone that regulates normal physiological response to pregnancy [31]. In addition, it has numerous effects that may be beneficial to the management of ADHF. Early studies demonstrated that it increases vasodilation and CO, promotes renal blood flow, and increases vascular endothelial growth factor and angiogenesis [32]. It has also been shown to prevent ischemia and reperfusion injury, decrease cardiac fibrosis in hypertension, and reduce cell death and contractile dysfunction in myocardial infarction [33]. Serelaxin, or recombinant relaxin-2, was studied in the Preliminary Study of Relaxin in Acute Heart Failure (Pre-RELAX-AHF) trial, which was a phase II placebo-controlled study of 234 patients hospitalized with HF, mild- to moderate-renal dysfunction, and a systolic blood pressure (SBP) greater than 125 mmHg. This study showed that patients treated with serelaxin had significant improvements in dyspnea score, although hypotension and worsening renal function occurred at higher doses. This small pilot study showed that serelaxin is a safe and well-tolerated therapy with potentially positive clinical outcomes [34]. The RELAX-AHF study enrolled 1161 patients hospitalized with HF within 16 h of presentation who had dyspnea, congestion, mild–moderate-renal insufficiency, a BNP > 350 ng/L or an NT-proBNP > 1400 ng/L, and SBP greater than 125 mmHg. Patients were randomized in a 1:1 fashion to receive either an infusion of serelaxin (30 mcg/kg per day) or placebo for up to 48 h [31]. The primary endpoints were improved in dyspnea from baseline until day 5 as measured by the visual analog scale (VAS) and improvement in dyspnea over 24 h as measured by a 7 point Likert scale. When compared to placebo, serelaxin improved the dyspnea VAS primary end point ($P = 0.007$) but it did not have any significant effect on the shorter term endpoint of self-reported dyspnea improvement at 6, 12, and 24 h. Serelaxin did not have a significant effect on days alive out of the hospital or the combined endpoint of death or HF readmission at 60 days. The serelaxin group had more hypotensive events requiring reduction in dose by 50% ($P < 0.001$) but the placebo group had more renal impairment ($P = 0.03$). In this study, serelaxin did result in reducing cardiovascular death ($P = 0.028$) and all-cause mortality ($P = 0.20$) at 180 days [31].

The FDA voted unanimously to recommend against approval of serelaxin in March 2013, due to the lack of multiple efficacy trials. Therefore, RELAX-AHF-2 (NCT01870778), a 6800 patient trial designed to assess 180-day mortality and worsening HF at 5 days in patients hospitalized with HF, has started enrollment in October 2013 and is expected to conclude enrollment in January 2017. In addition, RELAX-AHF ASIA (NCT02007720) is enrolling 1520 patients to assess improvement of signs and symptoms of inpatients hospitalized with HF, and is expected to conclude in March 2017. The role for serelaxin in the management of ADHF will largely be determined by the results of these two trials.

Rolofylline

Adenosine is a purine nucleoside produced from hydrolysis of adenosine triphosphate (ATP) [35]. The adenosine receptor is found in all body cells and is involved in multiple physiologic and pathophysiologic processes. However, the A1R in the kidney has been of interest in the treatment of ADHF. The A1Rs are found in the renal afferent arteriole and proximal tubules. Their stimulation leads to reduced glomerular filtration rate (GFR) via afferent arteriolar vasoconstriction and increased proximal sodium absorption via stimulation of proximal sodium/bicarbonate transporters, along with suppression of renin release [36, 37]. As adenosine has adverse effects on GFR, the A1R has emerged as a potential target for treating acute HF syndrome in an attempt to preserve GFR.

Phase 1 studies testing different intravenous doses (1–60 mg) of rolofylline in a double-blind, randomized, placebo-controlled trial of 36 patients with ADHF demonstrated a dose-dependent natriuresis with a peak effect at the 30-mg dose, occurring 3 h after drug administration [38]. Promising results from phase 1 and 2 studies led to the design of the phase 3 multicenter, randomized, double-blind, placebo-controlled PROTECT studies. The PROTECT pilot study randomized 301 patients hospitalized with heart failure, irrespective of LVEF, CrCl 20–80 mL/min, and BNP > 250 pg/mL or NT-proBNP > 1000 pg/mL to 1 of 3 intravenous doses of rolofylline (10, 20, or 30 mg) or placebo for 3 days or until discharge, with telephone follow-up at 60 days [39]. Patients treated with rolofylline were more likely to achieve treatment success (53 vs. 37%), defined as improvement in patient-reported dyspnea, and less likely to experience failure (16 vs. 28%), defined as death early heart failure readmission or persistent renal impairment, compared to placebo, though this study was not powered to achieve a statistically significant end point. Other findings included a trend toward reduction in body weight and initial improvement in dyspnea, and a significantly lesser increase in sCr in patients treated with rolofylline compared to placebo, which appeared to be dose-related. There was a nonsignificant trend toward reduced 60-day mortality (5 vs. 10%), and combined mortality, cardiovascular readmission, or renal readmission (16 vs. 29%) at 60 days in the rolofylline versus placebo groups [39].

The favorable trends from the PROTECT pilot led to continuation with the main PROTECT study, which randomized 2033 patients hospitalized with HF regardless of LVEF in a 2:1 ratio to either 30 mg rolofylline or placebo for up to 3 days [40]. There was no difference in the primary tricotomous endpoint of treatment success, unchanged, or failure was similar in the rolofylline and placebo groups, even after stratification according to baseline renal function (Fig. 17.4). There were no differences between rolofylline and placebo in any of the prespecified secondary end points. Importantly, only a small percentage of the population experienced persistent renal impairment in both the placebo and rolofylline arms, 13.7 and 15.0%, respectively. Given the mechanism of action of rolofylline, it has been suggested that the hypothesis for which rolofylline was intended, protection or prevention of the kidneys, was not sufficiently tested given the low number of patients with persistent renal impairment. The results of PROTECT have been a large setback in the development of adenosine receptor blockers for the management of ADHF; however, the potential to augment diuresis while preserving renal function in this population is attractive and would benefit from further investigation.

Novel Inotropes

Omecamtiv Mecarbil

Existing inotropic agents work by increasing the velocity and force of contraction, but they do not prolong the length of systole. Previous trials of inotropic therapies either fail to demonstrate significant efficacy or have shown that there are significant safety concerns with hypotension, myocardial ischemia, and increased mortality [41]. Cardiac myosin activators are a class of medication that increase myocardial contractility and the length of systole, resulting in an improvement in stroke volume and CO [42, 43]. Omecamtiv mecarbil (OM) is the first selective cardiac myosin activator to be studied in humans. It binds to the catalytic domain of cardiac myosin ATPase and increases the transition rate of myosin into the actin-bound state that generates force. As a result, it extends the duration of systole and it increases the force of contraction without increasing myocardial oxygen consumption [43]. In healthy volunteers, it has been shown to increase systolic ejection time, fractional shortening, and LVEF [44]. In a phase II, double-blind placebo-controlled trial, 45 patients on a stable HF regimen and LVEF of <40%, received OM for 2, 24, or 72 h in a dose-escalating fashion to ensure tolerability of the infusion. Over the course of the study, the 45 patients received 151 infusions of the medication. Doses higher than 100 ng/mL were associated with a significant increase in the duration of left ventricular systole, stroke volume, and fractional shortening. This trend continued in a dose-dependent manner that plateaued above 400 ng/mL. There were very few adverse events, with chest pain, tachycardia, and myocardial ischemia observed at high

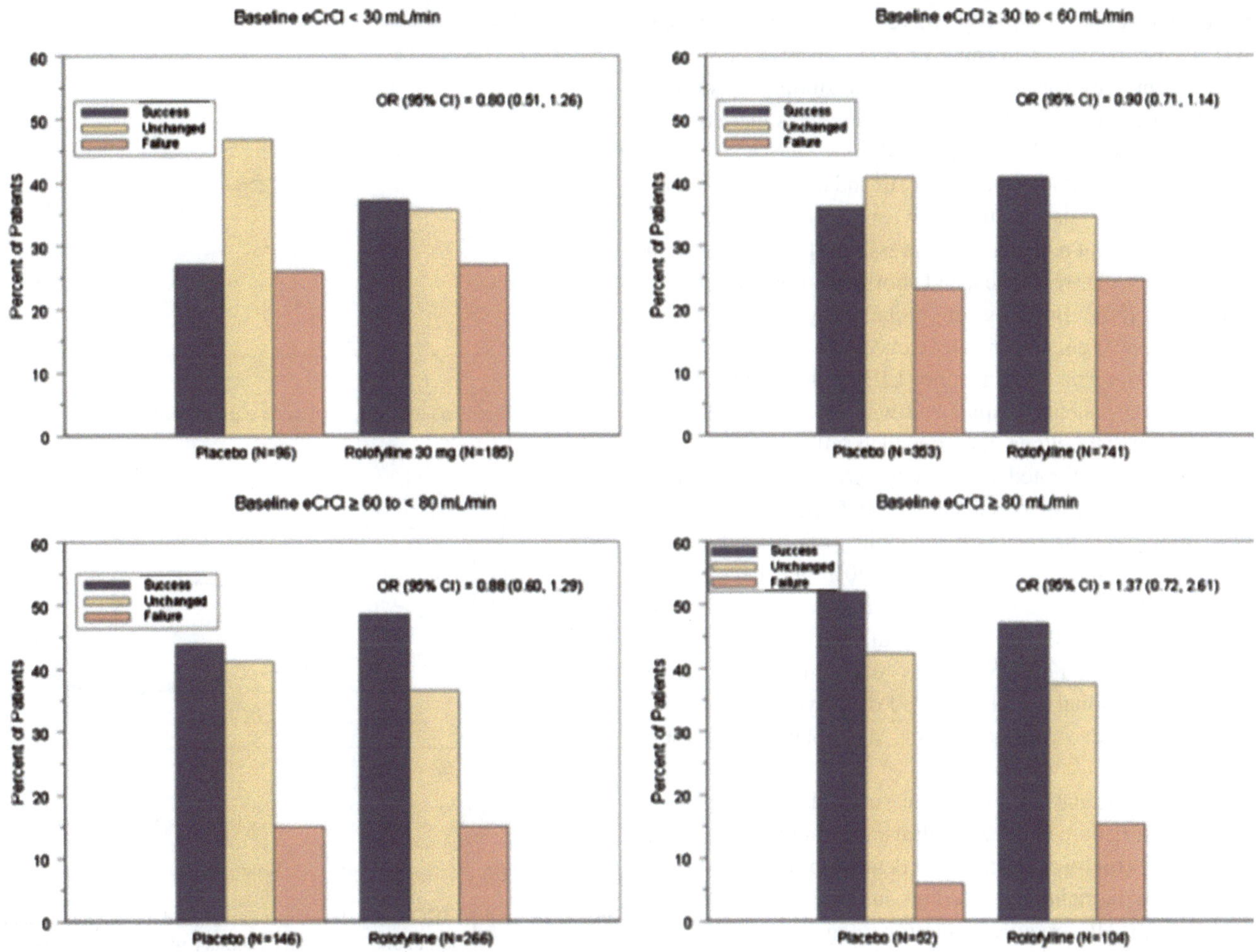

Fig. 17.4 Primary endpoint of the PROTECT study was not different between patients hospitalized with heart failure randomized to rolofylline or placebo. Reprinted with permission from Voors et al. [40]

plasma concentrations. Overall, this study found that omecamtiv mecarbil is a safe, well-tolerated medication with positive effects on CO [45]. This was followed up with the Acute Treatment With Omecamtiv Mecarbil to Increase Contractility in Acute Heart Failure (ATOMIC-AHF) study, which compared OM with placebo in 606 patients with symptoms of HF, with LVEF < 40%, dyspnea, and elevated plasma concentrations of natriuretic peptides [46]. They were randomized 1:1 to either a 48-h infusion of placebo or OM where target mean plasma concentrations of OM at 48 h were 114, 230, and 310 ng/mL using three escalating dose regimens. When compared to placebo, OM did not improve the primary endpoint of dyspnea relief or any secondary endpoints ($P = 0.331$). In a prespecified analysis of the high-dose cohort, OM did result in greater dyspnea relief at 48 h ($P = 0.034$) and at 5 days ($P = 0.038$), along with increases in LV systolic ejection time ($P < 0.0001$) and decreases in LV end-systolic dimension ($P < 0.05$). There were no significant differences in adverse events including ventricular arrhythmias or supraventricular tachyarrhythmias; however, there was a mild increase in troponin in the high-dose OM group, not temporally related to the drug exposure. Though OM did not meet its primary endpoint in this study, it was well tolerated and did have significant physiological effects on systolic ejection time. Also, the study was underpowered to determine if there was any effect on clinical outcomes [46]. The clinical effectiveness of OM is currently being evaluated as an oral regimen in the Chronic Oral Study of Myosin Activation to Increase Contractility in Heart failure (COSMIC-HF) study (NCT01786512).

Levosimendan

Levosimendan is both a calcium sensitizing agent and a potassium channel modulator. It binds to cardiac troponin C in a calcium-dependent manner resulting in increased myocyte calcium sensitivity, thereby increasing inotropy [47]. It also facilitates opening of ATP-sensitive potassium channels in vascular smooth muscle resulting in smooth muscle relaxation [48]. These combined effects increase LV contractility while reducing afterload.

Early clinical studies with levosimendan demonstrated a dose–response relationship between levosimendan and increased CO and reduced filling pressures, [49] reduction in systemic vascular resistance, and short-term improvement in symptoms [50]. Building on these early hemodynamic studies, more promising results came from the Levosimendan Infusion versus Dobutamine (LIDO) study, which randomized 203 patients hospitalized with low-output HF and LVEF < 35% to either levosimendan infusion started at 0.1 mcg/kg/min, titrated to 0.2 mcg/kg/min if CI failed to increase by 30%, or to dobutamine at 5 mcg/kg/min [51]. This trial met its primary endpoint of hemodynamic improvement (increase in CO by $\geq$30% and decrease in $\geq$25% in PCWP) at 24 h: 28% of the levosimendan-group patients versus 15% of the dobutamine-group patients ($P = 0.029$) (Fig. 17.5). Secondary endpoint of days alive out of the hospital at 31 and 180 days was significantly lower in the levosimendan versus the dobutamine group [51].

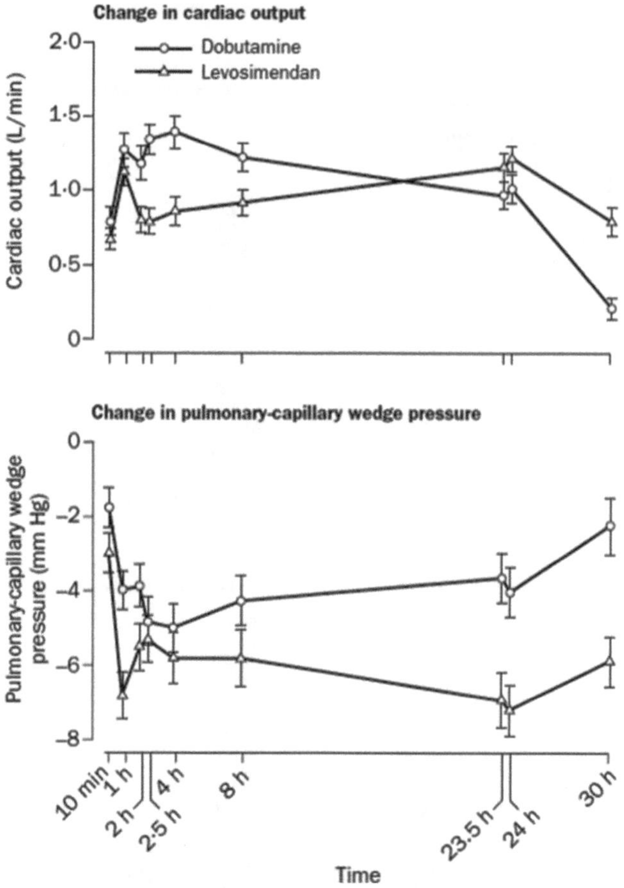

Fig. 17.5 In the LIDO study, levosimendan caused a more significant change in cardiac output and pulmonary capillary wedge pressure when compared to dobutamine. Reprinted with permission from Follath et al. [51]

Based on the above findings, the Survival of Patients with Acute Heart Failure in need of Intravenous Inotropic Support (SURVIVE) trial was designed to detect a primary endpoint of all-cause mortality at 180 days in 1327 patients hospitalized with HF, requiring inotropic agents, and LVEF 30% when comparing 24-h infusions of levosimendan (0.1 mcg/kg/min titrating to 0.2 mcg/kg/min tolerated) to dobutamine (5 mcg/kg/min). Despite a significant initial reduction in plasma BNP level in the levosimendan group compared to the dobutamine group, there was no significant difference in all-cause mortality between groups at 31 and 180 days, and none of the other secondary clinical endpoints were met [52]. In order to determine the performance of levosimendan against placebo, the Randomized Evaluation of Intravenous Levosimendan Efficacy (REVIVE-II) trial randomized a total of 600 patients with LVEF $\leq$ 35% hospitalized for HF to either levosimendan titrated to a target dose of at a target dose of 0.2 mcg/kg/min versus placebo for 24 h, in addition to standard therapy [53]. In this trial, the administration of levosimendan was associated with a slight, but significant ($P = 0.015$) improvement in overall clinical course over 5 days compared to placebo, the trial's primary endpoint. The secondary endpoints of BNP levels at 24 h and global symptom assessment over 5 days were improved with levosimendan versus placebo; however, NYHA functional class at day 5 and mortality at 14, 31, and 90 days after enrollment were not different between groups. Patients randomized to levosimendan had lower blood pressure during infusion, reversible at 12 h, and higher heart rates, persistent at 5 days, compared to placebo. Adverse events were seen in both groups, but the five that were more frequent in the levosimendan group were hypotension (50 vs. 36%), headache (30 vs. 15%), ventricular tachycardia (25 vs. 17%), atrial fibrillation (9 vs. 2%), and ventricular extrasystoles (8 vs. 2%).

Since levosimendan provides positive inotropy and afterload reduction without involving adrenergic receptors, there is a theoretical advantage of this patient in patients receiving beta-blocking agents. Prespecified subanalysis of the LIDO study demonstrated that patients on beta-receptor antagonists had greater increases in CO and decreases in PCWP while on levosimendan compared to those not on beta-receptor antagonists, whereas the opposite was true for patients on beta-receptor antagonists receiving dobutamine [51]. Subgroup analysis of SURVIVE demonstrated a statistically significant reduction in 5-day mortality with levosimendan in patients on beta-receptor antagonists versus dobutamine (1.5 vs. 5.1%, $P = 0.01$), an effect that diminished by 31 days [52]. Levosimendan is not approved for use in the United States; however, these series of trials suggest that this agent has potential in patients hospitalized with ADHF, reduced LVEF, not hypotensive, and on a good chronic HF regimen.

Istaroxime

Istaroxime is a novel agent that has both inotropic and lusitropic properties. The inotropic effects of istaroxime are due to inhibition of sodium–potassium adenosine triphosphate (Na–K ATPase) at the sarcolemma, leading to an increase in cytosolic calcium and thus improved contractility. The lusitropic effects are related to stimulation of the sarcoplasmic reticulum calcium ATPase isoform 2 (SERCA2), leading to rapid sequestration of cytosolic calcium into the sarcoplasmic reticulum during diastole and thereby promoting myocardial relaxation [54].

The phase I–II trial was a multicenter, randomized, double-blind, placebo-controlled, dose-escalation study conducted at centers within the United States. The initial clinical trial with istaroxime was a randomized dose-escalation study designed to evaluate its safety and tolerability. Patients with chronic HF and LVEF $\leq$ 40% randomized to one of three groups receiving istaroxime or placebo, each with escalating doses over 3 h within each low-, medium-, and high-dose cohort [55]. Cohort 1 (low dose) received infusions of 0.005, 0.0167, and 0.05 μ(mu) g/kg/min of istaroxime, cohort 2 (medium dose) received doses of 0.167, 0.5, and 1.0 μ(mu)g/kg/min infusions, and cohort 3 (high dose) received 1.67,3.33, and 5 μ(mu) g/kg/min infusions. Hemodynamics, ECG, and pharmacokinetics were measured for 9 h, as were short-term adverse effects. Istaroxime had no effect on hemodynamic parameters in cohorts 1 and 2. In cohort 3, there was a dose-dependent increase in CI, acceleration index, and velocity index. SBP did not decrease, but there was an increase in pulse pressure. There was no significant change in mean HR, supraventricular ectopy, or ventricular ectopy between istaroxime and placebo. There was a trend toward QTc shortening during the infusion period. There were no significant changes in routine clinical data or BNP. The hemodynamic effects appeared to disappear rapidly within 6 h after termination of the infusion.

HORIZON-HF was a randomized, double-blind, placebo-controlled, dose-escalation study that was conducted in three European countries. The study population included 120 patients hospitalized with HF who had LVEF $\leq$ 35, SBP < 150 and > 90 mmHg, HR < 110 and > 60 and on standard medical therapy for HF. The main exclusion criteria were use of intravenous inotropes, serum digoxin concentration >0.5 ng/mL, recent acute coronary syndromes or coronary revascularization, atrial fibrillation, left bundle branch block, implanted electrical devices, sCr > 3.0 mg/dL, and severe liver enzyme abnormalities [56].

Patients were monitored using a continuous CO pulmonary artery catheter within 48 h of admission and then randomized to receive istaroxime or placebo at a ratio of 3:1 within 3 sequential cohorts of 40 patients each. Cohort 1 (low dose) received 0.5 μ(mu)g/kg/min or placebo, cohort 2 (medium dose) received 1.0 μ(mu)g/kg/min or placebo, and cohort 3 (high dose) received 1.5 μ(mu)g/kg/min or placebo. In this study, PCWP was significantly reduced with all three doses of istaroxime during the entire length of the infusion, blood pressure increased, and HR trended downward in a dose-dependent manner (Fig. 17.6). CI increased in the high-dose cohort versus placebo. Echocardiography showed a dose-dependent decrease in LV end-diastolic volume that reached a statistically significant difference in the high-dose cohort (1.5 μ(mu)g/kg/min) versus placebo. There was no significant change in LVEF, laboratory data, or BNP. Pharmacokinetic analysis shows that istaroxime has a short half-life (<1 h), is not significantly eliminated by the kidneys, but rather is metabolized into less-active species. No deaths occurred during the infusion period in any of the cohorts, but two patients from the medium-dose cohort died within 30 days of randomization—one due to sudden cardiac death and one from worsened HF. Premature discontinuation of the infusion occurred in one patient in the high-dose group due to initiation of a treatment not allowed in the study protocol, and one patient in the placebo group due to clinical worsening. Dominant side effects were gastrointestinal and infusion site-related.

Istaroxime has not undergone further testing to date, but has potential in patients hospitalized with HF and reduced LVEF, in whom inotropy and lusitropy are desired without potential side effects of hypotension and tachycardia.

Neutral Endopeptidase Inhibitors

Neutral endopeptidase (NEP) is a metallopeptidase that is upregulated in HF patients and is responsible for metabolism of peptides such as bradykinin, substance p, endothelin-1, and atrial natriuretic peptides [57, 58]. These endogenous peptides cause vasodilation, reduce sodium retention, and slow down ventricular hypertrophy and remodeling [58]. Enhancing the effects of neutral endopeptidase may reverse some of the adverse pathophysiology associated with HF. The combination of angiotensin converting enzyme (ACE) and NEP inhibition has been shown to decrease the breakdown of bradykinin, reduce blood pressure, and result in symptomatic and hemodynamic improvements in HF more effectively than either enzyme alone [59, 60]. In the OVERTURE trial (The Omipatrilat Versus Enalapril

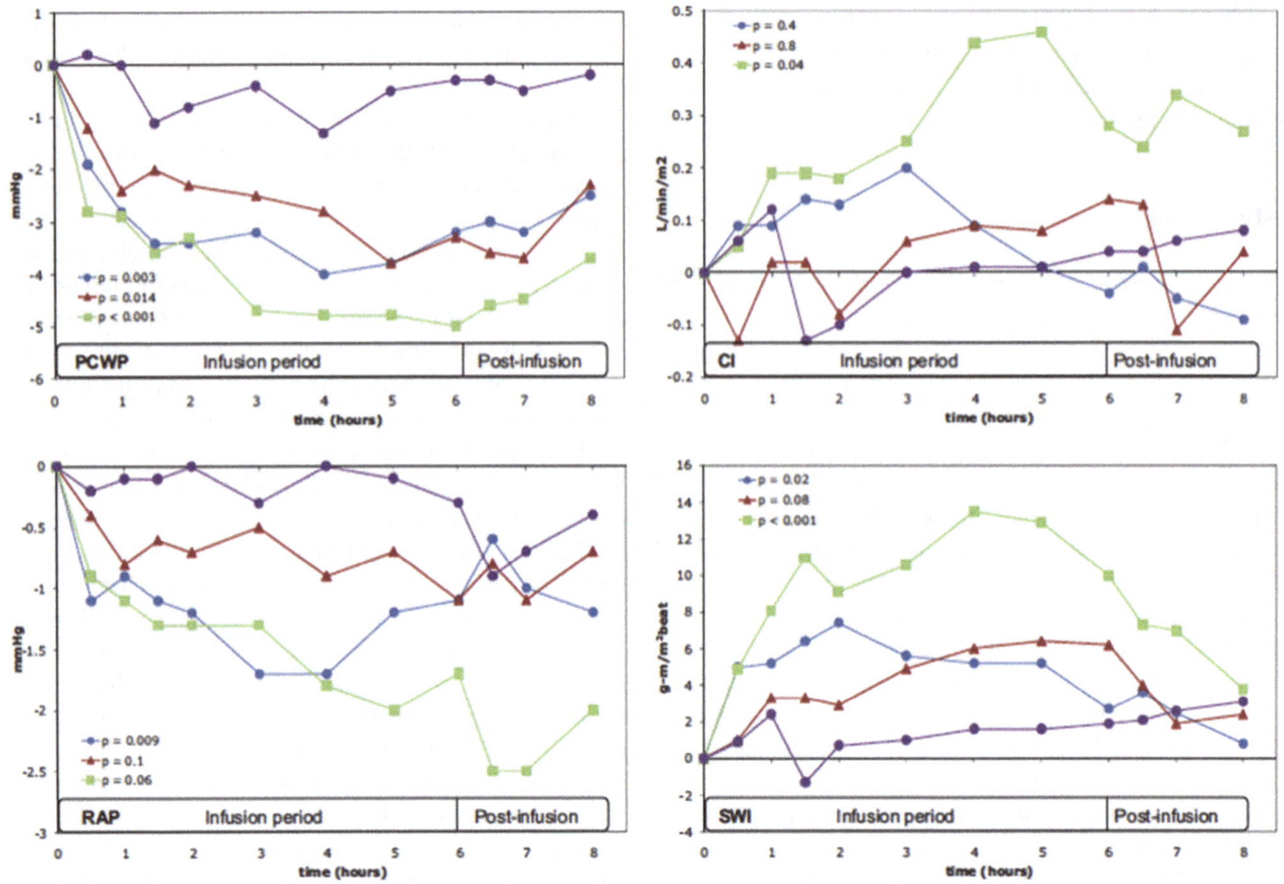

Fig. 17.6 The HORIZON-HF study showed that when compared to placebo, istaroxime resulted in an improvement in both invasive and noninvasive hemodynamics in a dose-dependent manner. Hemodynamics are plotted over the time course of treatment with placebo (*purple*), or istaroxime 0.5 μg/kg/min (*blue*), 1.0 μg/kg/min (*red*), 1.5 μg/kg/min (*green*). Reprinted with permission from Gheorghiade et al. [56]

Randomized Trial of Utility in Reducing Events), the combined ACE and NEP inhibitor omapatrilat was compared with enalapril in symptomatic patients with chronic HF. There were 5770 patients with NYHA class II to IV HF and reduced ejection fraction randomized 1:1 to enalapril at 10 mg twice a day or omipatrilat at 40 mg once daily for an average of 14.5 months. The primary endpoint was the combined risk of death or hospitalization for HF requiring intravenous therapy. Omapatrilat was found to be noninferior to enalapril as the primary endpoint was reached in 973 patients in the enalapril group and 914 patients in the omapatrilat group [hazard ratio (HR) 0.94; 95% confidence interval (CI) 0.86–1.03, $P = 0.187$] [61]. In addition, there was a significant incidence of angioedema in patients treated with omapatrilat thought to be caused by the inhibition of three enzymes that break down bradykinin. Also, in subsequent clinical trials, the combination of ACE and NEP inhibition resulted in an increased risk of angioedema [62].

Neprilysin is an NEP that breaks down numerous endogenous vasoactive peptides such as natriuretic peptides, bradykinin, and adrenomedullin [58, 63]. LCZ696 is a novel combination therapy comprised the angiotensin receptor blocker (ARB) valsartan and the neprilysin inhibitor sacubitril. Unlike omapatrilat, LCZ696 does not inhibit ACE or aminopeptidase P, reducing the risk of angioedema [64, 65]. In one study, 1328 patients with hypertension were randomized to receive treatment for 8 weeks with escalating doses of valsartan or LCZ696. The average reduction in sitting diastolic blood pressure was greater with LCZ696 when compared with similar doses of valsartan (mean reduction: −2.17 mmHg, 95% CI −3.28 to −1.06; $P < 0.0001$). There were very few side effects and no episodes of angioedema associated with the medication [66]. In another phase 2 study, the prospective comparison of ARNI with ARB on management of heart failure with preserved ejection fraction (PARAMOUNT) trial randomized 301 patients with heart failure with preserved LVEF and NT-proBNP greater than 400 pg/mL to either LCZ696 titrated to 200 mg, or valsartan at 160 mg twice a day. The trial met its primary endpoint of higher reduction in

NT-proBNP in the LCZ696 arm compared to valsartan alone, and was found to be well-tolerated with few side effects [67].

These studies supported the safety and efficacy of LCZ696 and led to the development of PARADIGM-HF. In this double blind trial, 8442 patients with chronic NYHA class II–IV HF and LVEF $\leq$ 40% were randomized 1:1 to either LCZ696 at a dose of 200 mg twice daily or enalapril at a dose of 10 mg twice daily in addition to guideline-based therapy. Those who met inclusion criteria were switched from the ACE inhibitor or ARB to enalapril for a period of 2 weeks. Next, they were treated with LCZ696 for 4–6 weeks to ensure that there were no adverse side effects. At the end of this period they were randomly assigned in a 1:1 ratio to treatment with either enalapril at 10 mg twice a day or LCZ696 at 200 mg twice a day. The primary outcome was a composite of death from cardiovascular causes or a first hospitalization for HF. The trial was stopped early after median follow up of 27 months because of the robust clinical benefit seen with LCZ696. Death from cardiovascular causes or hospitalization for HF occurred in 914 patients (21.8%) in the LCZ696 group and 1117 patients (26.5%) in the enalapril group (HR 0.80; 95% CI 0.73–0.87; $P < 0.01$) [65]. All-cause mortality was also reduced in the LCZ696 group compared to valsartan, an effect seen across all prespecified subgroups. Also, from baseline to 8 months, the KCCQ clinical summary score decreased 2.99 points in the LCZ696 group and decreased 4.63 points in the enalapril group, with higher scores indicting fewer symptoms and physical limitations associated with heart failure (95% CI 0.63–2.65; $P = 0.001$). This study also showed LCZ696 to be safe overall as fewer patients in the LCZ696 group stopped their medication because of an adverse event (10.7 vs. 12.3%, $P = 0.03$) or because of renal dysfunction (0.7 vs. 1.4%, $P = 0.002$).

The PARADIGM study has demonstrated remarkable efficacy in reducing both mortality and rehospitalization in patients with symptomatic chronic HF; however, its potential in AHFS has not been prospectively studied. However, retrospective analysis of PARADIGM has demonstrated that once hospitalized for HF, those randomized to LCZ696 (675 patients hospitalized at least once) had lower rates of all-cause and HF rehospitalization at 30- and 60-days compared to those randomized to valsartan (775 patients hospitalized at least once) [68]. Although these data are promising, further investigation into whether initiation of LCZ696 during an index ADHF hospitalization is an efficacious strategy in preventing morbidity and mortality is warranted.

Conclusion

Though there are many therapies for ADHF that are effective in the acute management period, few have proven to have any long-term clinical benefit. Despite the initial promise of a number of different pharmacotherapies, the management of these patients continues to be a challenging moving target. Diuresis and fluid removal strategies remain an integral component of acute management, but have not resulted in an improvement in mortality outcomes. Vasopressin antagonists have modest clinical effects and may be useful in patients with ADHF and symptomatic hyponatremia. Similarly, though studies do not support its use, nesiritide may be beneficial as an adjunct to improve urine output in ADHF on a case-by-case basis. Relaxin and rolofylline are not approved by the FDA for use in ADHF; however, their novel mechanisms of action may be future targets for ongoing study. Adenosine antagonists need further long-term efficacy and safety data to justify their use, given the unfavorable short-term effects on the central nervous system. Promising therapies for ADHF seem to be novel inotropes such as omecamtiv mecarbil, levosimendan, and istaroxime. Currently, additional studies are ongoing to determine their safety and clinical effectiveness, but they may prove to have significant efficacy compared to standard inotropic therapy. Finally, the dramatic reduction in morbidity and mortality of combination angiotensin receptor and neprilysin blockade in patients with chronic HF and reduced LVEF warrants the study of these types of agents the acute phase.

Acknowledgements This research is supported by the American Heart Association 14SDG20380354.

References

1. Gheorghiade M, et al. Congestion in acute heart failure syndromes: an essential target of evaluation and treatment. Am J Med. 2006;119(12 Suppl 1):S3–10.
2. Gheorghiade M, Pang PS. Acute heart failure syndromes. J Am Coll Cardiol. 2009;53(7):557–73.
3. Jong P, et al. Prognosis and determinants of survival in patients newly hospitalized for heart failure: a population-based study. Arch Intern Med. 2002;162(15):1689–94.
4. Solomon SD, et al. Influence of nonfatal hospitalization for heart failure on subsequent mortality in patients with chronic heart failure. Circulation. 2007;116(13):1482–7.
5. Dickstein K, et al. ESC Guidelines for the diagnosis and treatment of acute and chronic heart failure 2008: the Task Force for the Diagnosis and Treatment of Acute and Chronic Heart Failure 2008 of the European Society of Cardiology. Developed in collaboration with the Heart Failure Association of the ESC (HFA) and endorsed

by the European Society of Intensive Care Medicine (ESICM). Eur Heart J. 2008;29(19):2388–442.
6. Felker GM, et al. Diuretic strategies in patients with acute decompensated heart failure. N Engl J Med. 2011;364(9): 797–805.
7. Felker GM, Mentz RJ. Diuretics and ultrafiltration in acute decompensated heart failure. J Am Coll Cardiol. 2012;59 (24):2145–53.
8. Weber KT. Furosemide in the long-term management of heart failure: the good, the bad, and the uncertain. J Am Coll Cardiol. 2004;44(6):1308–10.
9. Hasselblad V, et al. Relation between dose of loop diuretics and outcomes in a heart failure population: results of the ESCAPE trial. Eur J Heart Fail. 2007;9(10):1064–9.
10. Francis GS, et al. Acute vasoconstrictor response to intravenous furosemide in patients with chronic congestive heart failure. Activation of the neurohumoral axis. Ann Intern Med. 1985;103 (1):1–6.
11. McCurley JM, et al. Furosemide and the progression of left ventricular dysfunction in experimental heart failure. J Am Coll Cardiol. 2004;44(6):1301–7.
12. Domanski M, et al. Diuretic use, progressive heart failure, and death in patients in the Studies Of Left Ventricular Dysfunction (SOLVD). J Am Coll Cardiol. 2003;42(4):705–8.
13. Manning M, Sawyer WH. Discovery, development, and some uses of vasopressin and oxytocin antagonists. J Lab Clin Med. 1989;114(6):617–32.
14. Jentzer JC, DeWald TA, Hernandez AF. Combination of loop diuretics with thiazide-type diuretics in heart failure. J Am Coll Cardiol. 2010;56(19):1527–34.
15. Goldsmith SR, Gheorghiade M. Vasopressin antagonism in heart failure. J Am Coll Cardiol. 2005;46(10):1785–91.
16. Oghlakian G, Klapholz M. Vasopressin and vasopressin receptor antagonists in heart failure. Cardiol Rev. 2009;17(1):10–5.
17. Gheorghiade M, et al. Effects of tolvaptan, a vasopressin antagonist, in patients hospitalized with worsening heart failure: a randomized controlled trial. JAMA. 2004;291(16): 1963–71.
18. Udelson JE, et al. Acute hemodynamic effects of tolvaptan, a vasopressin V2 receptor blocker, in patients with symptomatic heart failure and systolic dysfunction: an international, multicenter, randomized, placebo-controlled trial. J Am Coll Cardiol. 2008;52 (19):1540–5.
19. Gheorghiade M, et al. Short-term clinical effects of tolvaptan, an oral vasopressin antagonist, in patients hospitalized for heart failure: the EVEREST Clinical Status Trials. JAMA. 2007;297(12): 1332–43.
20. Konstam MA, et al. Effects of oral tolvaptan in patients hospitalized for worsening heart failure: the EVEREST Outcome Trial. JAMA. 2007;297(12):1319–31.
21. Felker GM, et al. Tolvaptan in patients hospitalized with acute heart failure: rationale and design of the TACTICS and the SECRET of CHF trials. Circ Heart Fail. 2015;8(5):997–1005.
22. Ghali JK, et al. Tolvaptan. Nat Rev Drug Discov. 2009;8(8): 611–2.
23. Costanzo MR, et al. Ultrafiltration versus intravenous diuretics for patients hospitalized for acute decompensated heart failure. J Am Coll Cardiol. 2007;49(6):675–83.
24. Bart BA, et al. Ultrafiltration in decompensated heart failure with cardiorenal syndrome. N Engl J Med. 2012;367(24):2296–304.
25. Dahle TG, Sobotka PA, Boyle AJ. A practical guide for ultrafiltration in acute decompensated heart failure. Congest Heart Fail. 2008;14(2):83–8.
26. Publication Committee for the, V.I. Intravenous nesiritide vs nitroglycerin for treatment of decompensated congestive heart failure: a randomized controlled trial. JAMA. 2002;287(12): 1531–40.
27. O'Connor CM, et al. Effect of nesiritide in patients with acute decompensated heart failure. N Engl J Med. 2011;365(1):32–43.
28. Holmes SJ, et al. Renal, endocrine, and hemodynamic effects of human brain natriuretic peptide in normal man. J Clin Endocrinol Metab. 1993;76(1):91–6.
29. Jensen KT, Carstens J, Pedersen EB. Effect of BNP on renal hemodynamics, tubular function and vasoactive hormones in humans. Am J Physiol. 1998;274(1 Pt 2):F63–72.
30. Bie P, et al. Enhanced atrial peptide natriuresis during angiotensin and aldosterone blockade in dogs. Am J Physiol. 1990;258(5 Pt 2): R1101–7.
31. Teerlink JR, et al. Serelaxin, recombinant human relaxin-2, for treatment of acute heart failure (RELAX-AHF): a randomised, placebo-controlled trial. Lancet. 2013;381(9860):29–39.
32. Teichman SL, et al. Relaxin: review of biology and potential role in treating heart failure. Curr Heart Fail Rep. 2010;7(2):75–82.
33. Du XJ, et al. Cardiovascular effects of relaxin: from basic science to clinical therapy. Nat Rev Cardiol. 2010;7(1):48–58.
34. Teerlink JR, et al. Relaxin for the treatment of patients with acute heart failure (Pre-RELAX-AHF): a multicentre, randomised, placebo-controlled, parallel-group, dose-finding phase IIb study. Lancet. 2009;373(9673):1429–39.
35. Shah RH, Frishman WH. Adenosine1 receptor antagonism: a new therapeutic approach for the treatment of decompensated heart failure. Cardiol Rev. 2009;17(3):125–31.
36. Modlinger PS, Welch WJ. Adenosine A1 receptor antagonists and the kidney. Curr Opin Nephrol Hypertens. 2003;12(5):497–502.
37. Takeda M, Yoshitomi K, Imai M. Regulation of Na(+)-3HC03-cotransport in rabbit proximal convoluted tubule via adenosine A1 receptor. Am J Physiol. 1993;265(4 Pt 2):F511–9.
38. Chaparro S, Dittrich HC, Tang WW. Rolofylline (KW-3902): a new adenosine A1-receptor antagonist for acute congestive heart failure. Future Cardiol. 2008;4(2):117–23.
39. Cotter G, et al. The PROTECT pilot study: a randomized, placebo-controlled, dose-finding study of the adenosine A1 receptor antagonist rolofylline in patients with acute heart failure and renal impairment. J Card Fail. 2008;14(8):631–40.
40. Voors AA, et al. Effects of the adenosine A1 receptor antagonist rolofylline on renal function in patients with acute heart failure and renal dysfunction: results from PROTECT (Placebo-Controlled Randomized Study of the Selective Adenosine A1 Receptor Antagonist Rolofylline for Patients Hospitalized with Acute Decompensated Heart Failure and Volume Overload to Assess Treatment Effect on Congestion and Renal Function). J Am Coll Cardiol. 2011;57(19):1899–907.
41. Hasenfuss G, Teerlink JR. Cardiac inotropes: current agents and future directions. Eur Heart J. 2011;32(15):1838–45.
42. Shen YT, et al. Improvement of cardiac function by a cardiac Myosin activator in conscious dogs with systolic heart failure. Circ Heart Fail. 2010;3(4):522–7.
43. Malik FI, et al. Cardiac myosin activation: a potential therapeutic approach for systolic heart failure. Science. 2011;331(6023): 1439–43.
44. Teerlink JR, et al. Dose-dependent augmentation of cardiac systolic function with the selective cardiac myosin activator, omecamtiv mecarbil: a first-in-man study. Lancet. 2011;378 (9792):667–75.
45. Cleland JG, et al. The effects of the cardiac myosin activator, omecamtiv mecarbil, on cardiac function in systolic heart failure: a

double-blind, placebo-controlled, crossover, dose-ranging phase 2 trial. Lancet. 2011;378(9792):676–83.
46. Teerlink JR, et al. Acute treatment with omecamtiv mecarbil to increase contractility in acute heart failure: the ATOMIC-AHF study. J Am Coll Cardiol. 2016;67(12):1444–55.
47. Pollesello P, et al. Binding of a new $Ca2^+$ sensitizer, levosimendan, to recombinant human cardiac troponin C. A molecular modelling, fluorescence probe, and proton nuclear magnetic resonance study. J Biol Chem. 1994;269(46):28584–90.
48. Yokoshiki H, et al. Levosimendan, a novel $Ca2^+$ sensitizer, activates the glibenclamide-sensitive K^+ channel in rat arterial myocytes. Eur J Pharmacol. 1997;333(2–3):249–59.
49. Nieminen MS, et al. Hemodynamic and neurohumoral effects of continuous infusion of levosimendan in patients with congestive heart failure. J Am Coll Cardiol. 2000;36(6):1903–12.
50. Slawsky MT, et al. Acute hemodynamic and clinical effects of levosimendan in patients with severe heart failure. Study Investigators. Circulation. 2000;102(18):2222–7.
51. Follath F, et al. Efficacy and safety of intravenous levosimendan compared with dobutamine in severe low-output heart failure (the LIDO study): a randomised double-blind trial. Lancet. 2002;360 (9328):196–202.
52. Mebazaa A, et al. Levosimendan vs dobutamine for patients with acute decompensated heart failure: the SURVIVE Randomized Trial. JAMA. 2007;297(17):1883–91.
53. Packer M, et al. Effect of levosimendan on the short-term clinical course of patients with acutely decompensated heart failure. JACC Heart Fail. 2013;1(2):103–11.
54. Mattera GG, et al. Istaroxime: a new luso-inotropic agent for heart failure. Am J Cardiol. 2007;99(2A):33A–40A.
55. Ghali JK, et al. A phase 1–2 dose-escalating study evaluating the safety and tolerability of istaroxime and specific effects on electrocardiographic and hemodynamic parameters in patients with chronic heart failure with reduced systolic function. Am J Cardiol. 2007;99(2A):47A–56A.
56. Gheorghiade M, et al. Hemodynamic, echocardiographic, and neurohormonal effects of istaroxime, a novel intravenous inotropic and lusitropic agent: a randomized controlled trial in patients hospitalized with heart failure. J Am Coll Cardiol. 2008;51 (23):2276–85.
57. Roques BP, et al. Neutral endopeptidase 24.11: structure, inhibition, and experimental and clinical pharmacology. Pharmacol Rev. 1993;45(1):87–146.
58. Cruden NL, et al. Neutral endopeptidase inhibition augments vascular actions of bradykinin in patients treated with angiotensin-onverting enzyme inhibition. Hypertension. 2004;44(6):913–8.
59. Favrat B, et al. Neutral endopeptidase versus angiotensin converting enzyme inhibition in essential hypertension. J Hypertens. 1995;13(7):797–804.
60. Trippodo NC, et al. Vasopeptidase inhibition with omapatrilat improves cardiac geometry and survival in cardiomyopathic hamsters more than does ACE inhibition with captopril. J Cardiovasc Pharmacol. 1999;34(6):782–90.
61. Packer M, et al. Comparison of omapatrilat and enalapril in patients with chronic heart failure: the Omapatrilat Versus Enalapril Randomized Trial of Utility in Reducing Events (OVERTURE). Circulation. 2002;106(8):920–6.
62. Kostis JB, et al. Omapatrilat and enalapril in patients with hypertension: the Omapatrilat Cardiovascular Treatment vs. Enalapril (OCTAVE) trial. Am J Hypertens. 2004;17(2):103–11.
63. Rademaker MT, et al. Neutral endopeptidase inhibition: augmented atrial and brain natriuretic peptide, haemodynamic and natriuretic responses in ovine heart failure. Clin Sci (Lond). 1996;91(3):283–91.
64. Fryer RM, et al. Effect of bradykinin metabolism inhibitors on evoked hypotension in rats: rank efficacy of enzymes associated with bradykinin-mediated angioedema. Br J Pharmacol. 2008;153 (5):947–55.
65. McMurray JJ, et al. Angiotensin–neprilysin inhibition versus enalapril in heart failure. N Engl J Med. 2014;371(11):993–1004.
66. Ruilope LM, et al. Blood-pressure reduction with LCZ696, a novel dual-acting inhibitor of the angiotensin II receptor and neprilysin: a randomised, double-blind, placebo-controlled, active comparator study. Lancet. 2010;375(9722):1255–66.
67. Solomon SD, et al. The angiotensin receptor neprilysin inhibitor LCZ696 in heart failure with preserved ejection fraction: a phase 2 double-blind randomised controlled trial. Lancet. 2012;380 (9851):1387–95.
68. Desai AS, et al. Influence of Sacubitril/Valsartan (LCZ696) on 30-day readmission after heart failure hospitalization. J Am Coll Cardiol. 2016;68(3):241–8.

Kidney Injury in Patients with Ventricular Assist Devices

18

Ami M. Patel, Karan Kapoor, and Michael R. Rudnick

Overview of LVADs

Mechanical circulatory support (MCS) with LVADs is a rapidly evolving field and a potentially life-saving therapy for patients with decompensating advanced HF who fail to improve or stabilize with optimal medical management (OMM). This evolution has been mandated by the growing discrepancy between the number of patients qualified for cardiac transplantation and the number of available donor organs [1]. Over the past two decades, the implantable LVAD has transformed the treatment of advanced late-stage systolic HF. The REMATCH study was a landmark trial that demonstrated the increased survival with LVAD implantation over OMM in patients with class IV HF who were ineligible for cardiac transplantation [2]. The clinical approach to the management of end-stage HF with LVADs has been streamlined into three distinct pathways:

- Bridge to transplantation (BTT), in patients with deteriorating clinical status who are candidates for heart transplantation but are too unstable to wait any longer without circulatory support
- Destination therapy (DT), in patients who are considered ineligible for transplantation and for whom long-term use of an LVAD serves as an alternative; and
- Bridge to recovery (BTR), in patients for whom there is reason to believe will have eventual recovery of myocardial function allowing for eventual device removal.

A.M. Patel (✉)
Division of Nephrology, Department of Medicine, University of Maryland Medical Center, 22 S. Greene St. N3W143, Baltimore, MD 21201, USA
e-mail: apatel1@som.umaryland.edu

K. Kapoor
Department of Internal Medicine, University of Maryland Medical Center, 22 South Greene Street, Baltimore, MD 21201, USA
e-mail: kkapoor@umm.edu

M.R. Rudnick
Department of Medicine, University of Pennsylvania, 3400 Spruce Street, Philadelphia, PA 19104, USA
e-mail: rudnickm@uphs.upenn.edu

Although LVADs have evolved with differences in design and indications for use, they have in common a number of basic components. All LVAD systems consist of an inflow cannula that drains blood from the heart to a pump and an outflow cannula that carries blood back to the arterial system. LVADs are surgically implanted in a preperitoneal position relative to the left hemidiaphragm or in the pericardial sac. The power supply for the LVAD is delivered through a percutaneous lead that connects to an external power system. Another external component is a small portable computer (called a controller) that controls device speed and monitors device function (Fig. 18.1).

An important distinction between first generation and newer generation devices is the transition from pulsatile to continuous-flow rotary pumps. The pulsatile flow system utilized by first generation devices was based upon a volume displacement design with pulsatile flow that mimicked the phasic contractions of a normal cardiac cycle. First generation LVADs include the HeartMate I, Novacor, and Thoratec Paracorporeal Ventricular Assist Device. Due to a variety of limitations, including limited durability, need for extensive surgical dissection at time of implant and presence of a large external lead (more vulnerable to infection), pulsatile devices are now rarely (if ever) used [1]. Newer generation devices (HeartMate II, Jarvik 2000, Berlin Heart INCOR, HeartMate III, and HeartWare) differ significantly from first generation devices in their utilization of continuous-flow pumps instead of pulsatile pumps and clinically have replaced pulsatile devices. This paradigm shift to continuous-flow devices has been driven by a variety of technical and mechanistic advantages, including smaller size and fewer moving parts, resulting in greater durability and reliability. An important point of clarification is that blood

J. Rangaswami et al. (eds.), *Cardio-Nephrology*,
DOI 10.1007/978-3-319-56042-7_18

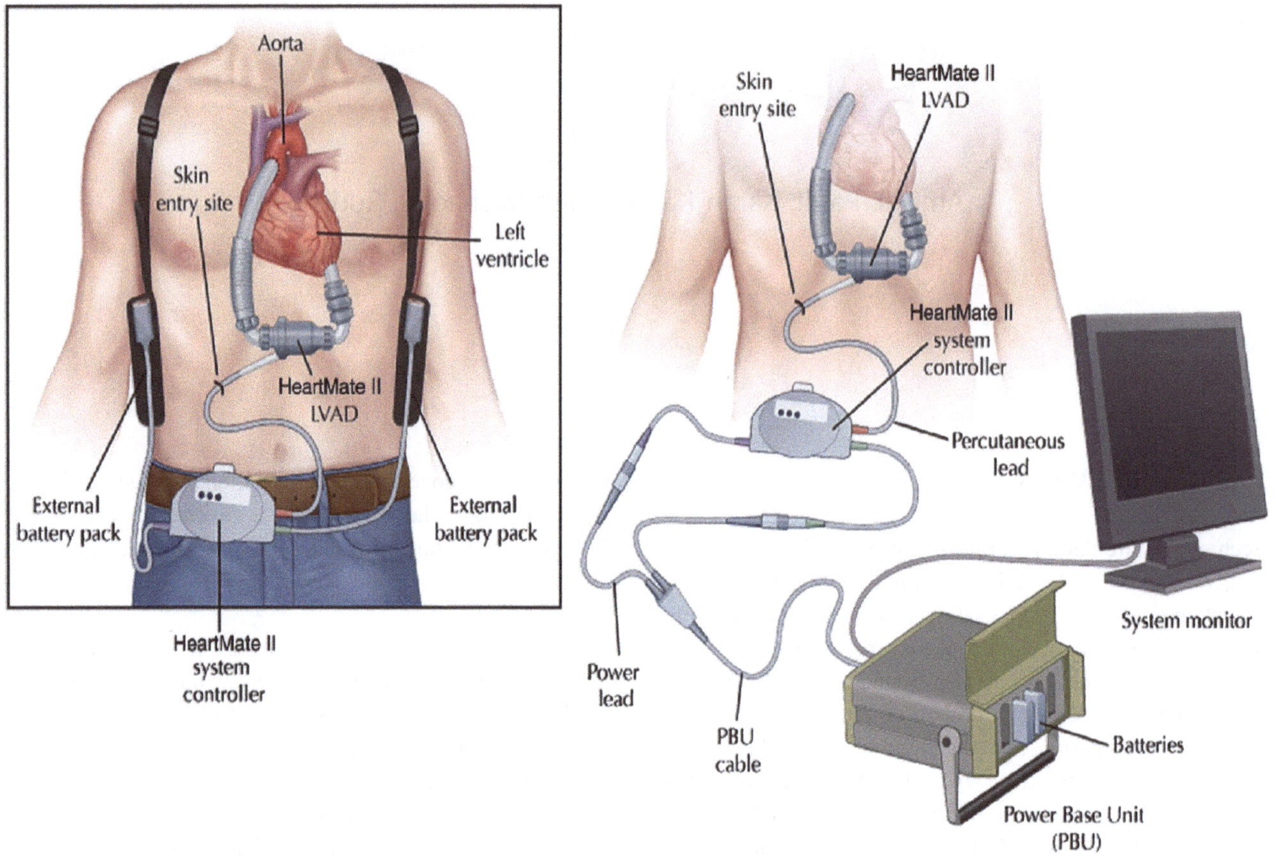

Fig. 18.1 Components of HeartMate II Apparatus. The HeartMate II LVAD consists of a blood pump, percutaneous lead, external power source, and system controller. The system controller can be connected to a monitor, which can display key parameters such as pump speed, pulsatility index, and pump power. Power may be delivered either through a power base unit or battery packs, which allow for increased mobility. *LVAD* left ventricular assist device. Reprinted with permission from Wilson SR, Givertz MM, Stewart GB, Mudge GH. Ventricular assist devices the challenges of outpatient management. J Am Coll Cardiol 2009; 54: 1648

flow in continuous-flow LVAD recipients has some pulsatility, albeit low, from residual native left ventricular function.

Presently, the HeartMate II is one of the most commonly used long-term continuous-flow LVADs, gaining FDA approval as a BTT in 2008 and for DT in 2010 [2]. To date, data on over 10,000 patients receiving durable MCS therapy have been reported to the national Interagency Registry for Mechanically Assisted Circulatory Support (INTERMACS), which is the largest available data repository for the study of durable MCS outcomes. The overall survival rate for all patients undergoing primary implantation of a durable MCS device is approximately 80% at 1 year and 70% at 2 years [1].

Impact of Baseline Renal Function on Outcome After LVAD

Nearly two-thirds of the hospitalized patients with HF have CKD with 44% having stage 3 CKD, 14% with stage 4 CKD, and 7% with stage 5 CKD [3]. Coexistent cardiac and renal dysfunction, the form of CRS, increases the risk of death, both with advanced HF and after LVAD implantation. Type I CRS describes AKI resulting from acute HF, which is potentially reversible following LVAD implantation. However, in type II CRS, chronic HF causes progressive CKD, which is irreversible post-LVAD. In the LVAD literature, the term *renal dysfunction* is commonly used and is defined as an estimated glomerular filtration rate (eGFR) of less than 60 ml/min/1.73 m^2. This term along with the term *kidney impairment* (KI, which is used in this chapter) are non-specific, since it is unclear if these terms refer to patients with CKD, AKI (including CRS), or AKI superimposed on CKD. Therefore, it is not surprising that the literature is conflicting when describing the outcomes in patients with KI. Of the 4917 LVAD recipients in the INTERMACS registry, 64% had no or mild KI [defined as eGFR $\geq$ 60 ml/min using the Cockcroft–Gault formula and Blood urea nitrogen (BUN) < 60 mg/dl], 30% had moderate KI (defined as eGFR = 30 to 59 ml/min or BUN > 60 mg/dl), and 6% had severe KI (defined as dialysis and/or eGFR < 30 ml/min) [4]. Impaired renal function in HF patients is likely related to a combination of factors including intrinsic disease from long-standing comorbidities such as diabetes and hypertension, and acute or chronic ischemia from hemodynamic changes causing poor renal perfusion and venous congestion.

Early studies of LVAD implantation have shown that baseline KI prior to LVAD insertion negatively impacts LVAD morbidity and mortality. In one study by Sandner et al. [5] the 6 month survival was 73% for LVAD recipients with baseline eGFR > 60 ml/min/1.73 m^2 versus 48% in recipients with baseline eGFR < 60 ml/min per 1.73 m^2. In addition, recipients with baseline eGFR > 60 ml/min/ 1.73 m^2 had a higher rate of cardiac transplantation (63 vs. 40%) and decreased requirement of continuous renal replacement therapy (CRRT) post-implantation (28 vs. 42%) in comparison to those recipients with baseline eGFR < 60 ml/min/1.73 m^2. In another study, the cumulative survival rates following LVAD implantation at 30, 90 days, and 1 year were 96, 88, and 77%, respectively, in patients with a serum creatinine < 1.96 mg/dl (n = 26) versus 60, 47, and 31% in patients with serum creatinine ≥ 1.96 mg/dl (n = 15) [6]. Progressive degrees of KI constitute incremental risk with a 20% reduction in 2-year survival going from pre-implant eGFR ≥ 60 ml/min to eGFR < 30 ml/min. The requirement for dialysis pre-implantation carried a mortality of >30% within the first 3 months and was particularly lethal if the patient was in critical cardiogenic shock, with 3 month mortality approaching 50%. In patients with eGFR < 30 ml/min and other major comorbidities, initial support with a temporary device while awaiting organ recovery should be considered before implanting a more durable pump [4]. A more recent INTERMACS report from 2014 suggests that percentage of patients receiving LVAD implantation in critical cardiogenic shock has declined from 29% before 2010 to 15% [1].

Other studies have shown that it is the post-implantation kidney function rather than the pre-implant that is a critical determinant of survival. Recovering renal function to eGFR > 60 ml/min/1.73 m^2 after LVAD insertion was associated with improved survival equivalent to those with normal renal function pre-LVAD insertion [5]. Iwashima et al. [7] demonstrated that VAD recipients with an eGFR ≥ 82 ml/min at 2 weeks postimplantation had greater survival compared with recipients whose eGFR was <82 ml/min/1.73 m^2. This study concluded that the 2-week postimplantation eGFR was a stronger predictor of survival than baseline eGFR. Even those patients with severe KI prior to VAD implantation who had subsequent renal recovery experienced enhanced outcomes. Khot et al. [8] reported that those recipients with serum creatinine ≥ 3.0 (4.0 ± 0.7) mg/dl preimplantation but recovered renal function post implantation had comparable outcomes to patient with serum creatinine < 3.0 mg/dl with similar 30 day (83 vs. 83%, p = 0.999) and 6-month survival (72 vs. 67%, p = 0.651) after VAD placement, survival to transplantation (61 vs. 68%, p = 0.549), and survival 1 year post transplantation (82 vs. 88%, p = 0.628). Additionally, more than half of the patients who required CRRT were able to survive to transplantation. These studies demonstrate that patients with even severe baseline KI requiring CRRT, may have a significant component of AKI that recovers after LVAD implantation and have decreased mortality (Fig. 18.2) [4, 8].

Furthermore, the renal outcome following LVAD implantation is predictive of renal function after cardiac transplantation. Singh et al. [9] demonstrated that patients with creatinine clearance (CrCl) > 60 ml/min following LVAD implantation and before cardiac transplantation experienced similar 1 year post-transplant CrCl regardless of baseline renal function prior to LVAD support. However, the ability to attain this level of renal function post-LVAD was less likely in those LVAD recipients with worst baseline renal function prior to LVAD. These studies suggest that survival after LVAD support and renal outcome after cardiac transplant is more dependent on the level of renal function achieved with LVAD rather than the baseline renal function. Kidney impairment is considered the most common modifiable contraindication to cardiac transplant. Thus, LVAD support prior to cardiac transplant may help differentiate between reversible and nonreversible KI [10].

In summary, given worse post-LVAD outcomes of patients with baseline KI at the time of LVAD implantation, it becomes imperative to determine whether the KI is due to poor renal perfusion which may be reversible and associated with better outcomes, or irreversible and could contribute to higher mortality. Future studies are needed to help identify patient characteristics that predict those with KI who will recover. Separating out the subgroups with different causes of KI will be useful in this regard. It is important to consider LVAD implantation without delay for patients with end-stage HF before advanced (irreversible) CRS occurs [4]. Generally individuals with CKD with serum creatinine above 2.5–3 mg/dl or with long-term dialysis are considered high risk and may not be suitable candidates for LVAD implantation [10, 11]. A brief trial of inotropic therapy and/or intra-aortic balloon pump may help determine reversibility of KI and aid in the assessment of LVAD candidacy [11, 12].

Impact of Continuous Blood Flow on Renal Outcome

Theoretical concerns about the impact of continuous blood flow on end-organ function including kidneys, brain, and gut have been the subject of considerable study and debate. The observation that short-term continuous cardiopulmonary

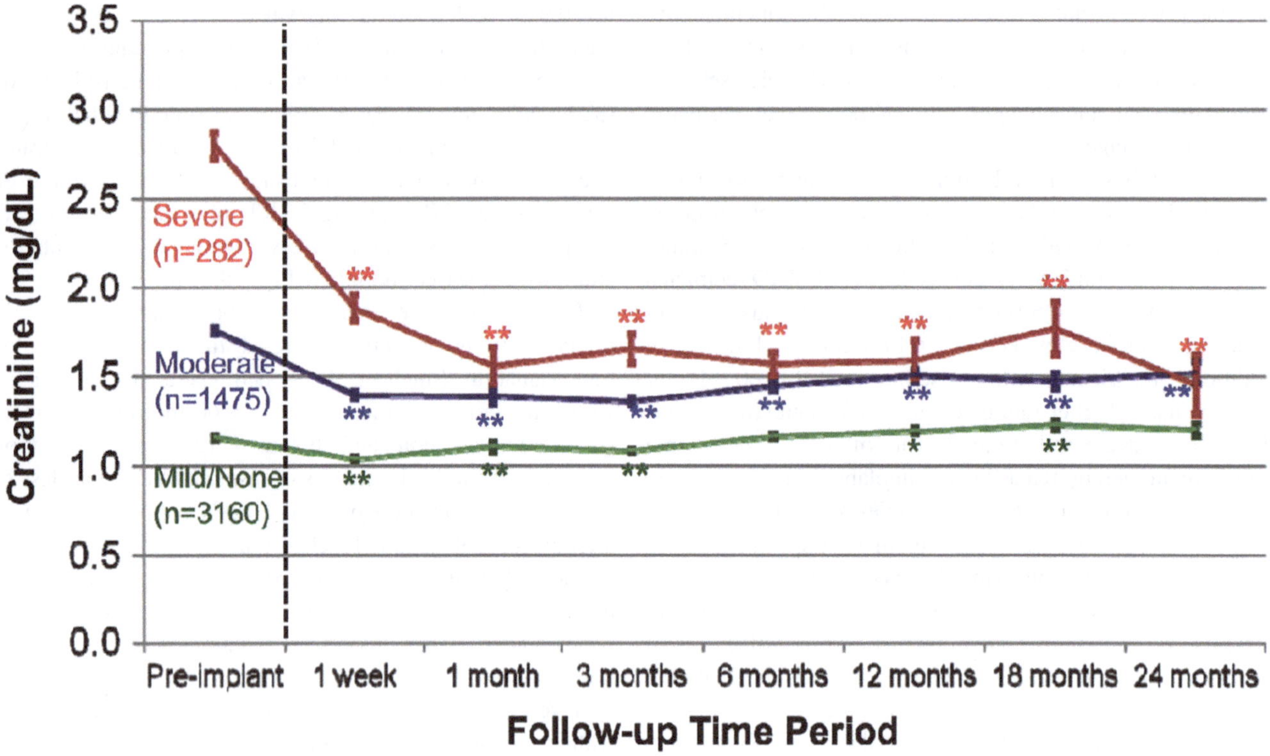

Fig. 18.2 Time course of serum creatinine according to pre-implant kidney impairment. Time course of average serum creatinine among surviving patients (n = 4917) with continuous-flow LVAD and BIVAD implants in the INTERMACS registry from June 2006 to March 2012, including for DT and BTT. Follow-up points of serum creatinine are stratified by severity of pre-implant kidney impairment. Severe was defined as requiring dialysis and/or eGFR < 30 ml/min; moderate if eGFR was 30–59 ml/min or BUN was >60 mg/dl; and mild or no kidney impairment if eGFR was $\geq$60 ml/min and BUN was <60 mg/dl. The *error bars* indicate $\pm$1 standard error. *BIVAD* biventricular assist device, *BTT* bridge to transplant, *DT* destination therapy, *LVAD* left ventricular assist device, *eGFR* estimated glomerular filtration rate, *BUN* blood urea nitrogen. Reprinted with permission from Kirklin JK, Naftel DC, Kormos RL, Pagani FD, Myers SL, Stevenson LW, Givertz MM, Young JB. Quantifying the effect of cardiorenal syndrome on mortality after left ventricular assist device implant. J Heart Lung Transplant 2013; 32: 1211

bypass surgeries, in use since the 1950s, are not associated with long-term clinical sequelae provided the initial evidence that continuous flow may be sufficient for end-organ function. Animal studies have shown preserved renal function with continuous-flow LVAD for prolonged periods as long as 340 days postimplantation [13].

However, in a model of cardiogenic shock in pigs, pulsatile VAD was more effective in restoring renal microcirculation than continuous VAD [14]. Alterations in renal morphology associated with continuous perfusion have been detected, including smooth muscle cell hypertrophy of renal cortical arteries, periarteritis, and interstitial nephritis [15–17]. In another study, increased upregulation of angiotensin II receptor and angiotensin-converting enzyme was observed in the mononuclear inflammatory cells in the kidney. Reduced pulsatile circulation can activate local renin–angiotensin system which may promote inflammatory reaction and vascular proliferation resulting in severe periarteritis, which is not seen in animals supported by pulsatile devices [16, 17]. Such changes have been implicated to cause decreased peripheral vascular reactivity, and it has been suggested that continuous flow can lead to vascular stiffness [18]. Interestingly, Welp et al. [19] compared levels of renin and aldosterone with pulsatile and continuous-flow LVADs. After implantation, there was a greater decrease in levels of renin and aldosterone in the pulsatile group compared to continuous flow. It is unclear whether this disparity in levels has any long-term clinical effects. The applicability of these findings to patients with LVADs is unclear since animal subjects with LVADs have different flow characteristics with intact left ventricular function while patients who underwent continuous LVAD have advanced bi-ventricular HF. Surprisingly, a recent study using calves by Cooper et al. observed morphologically identical systemic arteritis involving the kidney following intravenous administration of cephalosporin antibiotics, potentially *confounding* the findings of these medical device studies in calves as possible idiosyncratic drug reaction [18, 20]. Nevertheless, findings in other animal studies remain intriguing. Ohnishi et al. [16] observed smooth muscle cell proliferation of renal afferent arterioles in goats with continuous VAD. Ootaki et al. [17] detected periarteritis in the kidney only in the calves with continuous LVAD implantation which were not found in the group with RVAD or total heart. In contrast to the animal studies, Tromp et al. [18] investigated renal samples in 10 human LVAD recipients who underwent autopsy and they found no evidence of periarterial inflammation or medial wall thickening in the renal arcuate arteries. It is important to note that the absence of structural lesions in this small study does not rule out for potential adverse effect of LVAD on renal function.

In patients, many studies have demonstrated improved or stable renal function after continuous LVAD implantation for periods up to 3.7 years similar to pulsatile LVAD [5, 21–23]. In contrast, two studies have noted a slow progressive decline in renal function following an initial improvement in kidney function after continuous-flow device implantation raising the concern for possible adverse renal effect from long-term continuous flow [24, 25]. However, a recent analysis of the INTERMACS data revealed that the gradual late decline in renal function was observed in both continuous and pulsatile flow LVADs, suggesting that the decline in renal function cannot solely be attributed to reduced pulsatility [26].

Presently, there is scant data in humans on the cumulative effects of chronic continuous flow on the renal microcirculation. With the growing number of patients undergoing DT and that LVAD support are being used significantly longer, additional studies on renal function and histology are necessary to further confirm the long-term renal safety of continuous-flow LVADs.

Post-Implant Acute Kidney Injury

Post-implant AKI is a serious adverse event that manifests early after device implantation and is associated with poor outcomes. The incidence of post-implant AKI has been reported within a wide range, from 4 to 56%, in part attributable to heterogeneity in the definition of AKI between studies [27]. Despite this heterogeneity, more recent studies report an incidence of 7–14%, a reduction likely driven by increased surgical experience and widespread trend to implant LVADs primarily in more hemodynamically stable patients [28] (see Table 18.1). Interestingly, the incidence of post-implant AKI does not appear to differ among patients receiving continuous-flow versus pulsatile devices, although randomized trials to confirm this have not been performed [36]. An important subset of patients experiencing post-implant AKI are those whose renal injury is severe enough to require RRT, generally in the form of CRRT. The need for post-implant RRT has been reported in 11 to 33% of LVAD recipients, but similar to other definitions of AKI, incidence has declined in more recent studies [27].

The pathophysiology of post-implant AKI is likely multifactorial, with both clinical and biochemical factors acting synergistically. For example, both cardiopulmonary bypass time and number of intraoperative blood transfusions have been associated with AKI [31, 37]. Furthermore, alteration of intrarenal local hemodynamics has been hypothesized to enhance thrombogenicity and spawn microemboli to the renal cortex, a phenomenon that has been corroborated in animal models. Finally, free iron and hemoglobin generated via erythrocyte hemolysis has been demonstrated to precipitate Tamm–Horsfall protein and cause intratubular obstruction. Availability of nitric oxide also decreases, leading to renal vasoconstriction and ischemia [27].

Post-implant AKI has been clearly defined as a negative predictor of outcome, associated with both high morbidity and mortality [10]. Irrespective of pre-implant renal function, post-implant AKI confers a three-fold increased risk of 1-year mortality [37]. In a long-term follow-up study, Borgi et al. demonstrated a highly significant association between post-implant AKI and 30-day postoperative, as well as 180- and 360-day mortality [31]. In cases of post-implant AKI necessitating RRT, 180-day mortality rates have been reported to range from 57 to 93%, although much of this data is derived from earlier studies involving first generation devices and patients who were more hemodynamically unstable at time of LVAD implantation [28]. Moreover, among BTT patients who recover from post-implant AKI and survived to transplantation, long-term survival rates are similar to those patients without post-implant AKI. However, an important caveat is that at least two distinct studies have demonstrated post-implant AKI to be associated with a significantly lower rate of cardiac transplantation [23, 38].

Similar to other forms of AKI, the greater short- and long-term mortality associated with AKI following LVAD implantation may be due to the AKI itself or due to the possibility that "sicker" patients are more susceptible to AKI. In this regard, multiple risk factors associated with post-implant AKI are evident in the literature, including advanced age, poor nutritional status, elevated central venous pressure (CVP), and lower left-ventricular end-diastolic dimension before device implantation. Surgical risk factors, including preoperative use of an IABP, longer cardiopulmonary bypass time, higher intraoperative blood loss, post-cardiotomy shock, and need for reoperation have also been associated with increased incidence of post-implant AKI. Interestingly and somewhat counterintuitively, baseline KI has *not* been shown to consistently correlate with increased incidence of post-implant AKI, therein emphasizing the difficulty in identifying reliable predictors of post-implant AKI [39, 40].

Table 18.1 Incidence of AKI in selected studies

References	Enrollment period	LVAD type	Baseline characteristics	AKI definition	AKI incidence	EPPY	Comments
Frazier et al. [29]	1996–1998	HM VE	sCr 1.72 ± 1.02 BUN 37.5 ± 20.1	AKI = sCR ≥ 2.2 mg/dL or BUN ≥ 50 mg/dL	158/280 [56]	NA	
Demirozu et al. [30]	2003–2009	HM II	sCr 1.9 (±0.6)	AKI = RRT	15/107 [14]	NA	a
Borgi et al. [31]	2006–2011	HMII and HVAD	sCr 1.4	RIFLE stage II and greater	28/100 [28]	NA	b
Lok et al. [32]	2006–2011	HMII	sCr 120 μmol/L IMP I [25], II (75)	AKI = RRT	9/85 [11]	0.08	
Hasin et al. [24]	2007–2010	HMII	sCr 1.6 (±0.7) NYHA IV (62)	AKI = RRT	8/83[10]	NA	c
John et al. [33]	2008–2010	HMII	sCr 1.4 (±0.8) IMP I [17], II [45], III–VII [38]	ND	129/1496 [9]	0.14	
Aaronson et al. [34]	2008–2010	HVAD	sCr 1.3 (±0.4) IMP I [5], II [24], III [52], IV–VII [19]	ND	12/140 [9]	0.16	
Slaughter et al. [21]	2008–2012	HVAD	eGFR 87 (±39) NYHA IV (96) IMP I [6], II [40], III [42]	ND	32/332 [10]	0.13	d
Strueber et al. [35]	2009–2012	HVAD	ND	ND	10/254 [4]	0.04	

HM II HeartMate II (Thoratec Inc., Pleasanton, CA) HVAD HeartWare ventricular assist device (HeartWare Inc., Framingham, MA), IMP INTERMACS Patient Profile I-VII, NYHA New York Heart Association Class I-IV, eGFR estimated glomerular filtration rate (ml/min/1.73 m^2), sCr serum creatinine (mg/dL), AKI acute kidney injury, EPPY events per patient-year, RRT renal replacement therapy
This single center study only included patients supported for more than 30 days 32% of patients in this study received LVAD as DT. 68% of patients in this study received LVAD as DT. 140 patients included in this study were already previously reported by Aaronson et al.

Renal Recovery Versus CKD Post-LVAD

The short-term effects of LVAD therapy on renal function have been widely studied. Renal function generally improves directly after LVAD implantation, particularly if the initial insult was secondary to renal hypoperfusion from CRS, although this distinction is often difficult to make. Indeed, up to 75% of LVAD recipients with baseline KI have been reported to undergo renal recovery [28]. A recent, comprehensive analysis of the INTERMACS database revealed a median improvement in eGFR of about 50% at 1-month post implant, with 17% of LVAD recipients experiencing a doubling of their eGFR [26]. Similarly, up to 70% of patients with a pre-implant eGFR of <60 ml/min were found to regain filtration capacity to above this level within the 1-month post-implant period [24]. Studies in both animal and human models have provided mechanistic insights into the physiologic basis for this improvement, which appears to stem predominantly from improved intrarenal hemodynamics, alleviation of RAAS activation, and mitigation of sympathetic overactivity [10, 41]. Closer inspection reveals that in the majority of cases, renal recovery occurs within the first month post-implant, with no further improvement and in fact, a potential steady decline in renal function thereafter (Fig. 18.3) [27]. Hasin et al. reported on 83 patients who received a continuous-flow LVAD. Overall eGFR increased from 53 ml/min at baseline to 87 ml/min/1.73 m^2 at 1 month after implantation and then there was progressive decline to 78 and 71 ml/min/1.73 m^2 at 3 and 6 months respectively. This pattern of decline following initial improvement was observed regardless of the baseline eGFR [24].

Furthermore, and not surprisingly, the greatest degree of improvement has been observed in patients whose kidney impairment was most severe in the pre-implantation period, with less pronounced improvements observed in patients with mild pre-implant renal function. Singh et al. performed the most illustrative study to this end, categorizing 116 patients who received LVAD therapy as BTT into three tertiles according to their pre-implant CrCl: group 1 with CrCl < 45 ml/min, group 2 with CrCl between 45 and 65 ml/min, and group 3 with CrCl > 65 ml/min. The average changes in CrCl from pre-implant levels to 6 month post implant in the respective groups were 34.1 to 73.5 ml/min (group 1), 56.7 to 66.2 ml/min (group 2) and 79.4 to 78 ml/min (group 3) [9]. Beyond the initial 1–2 month

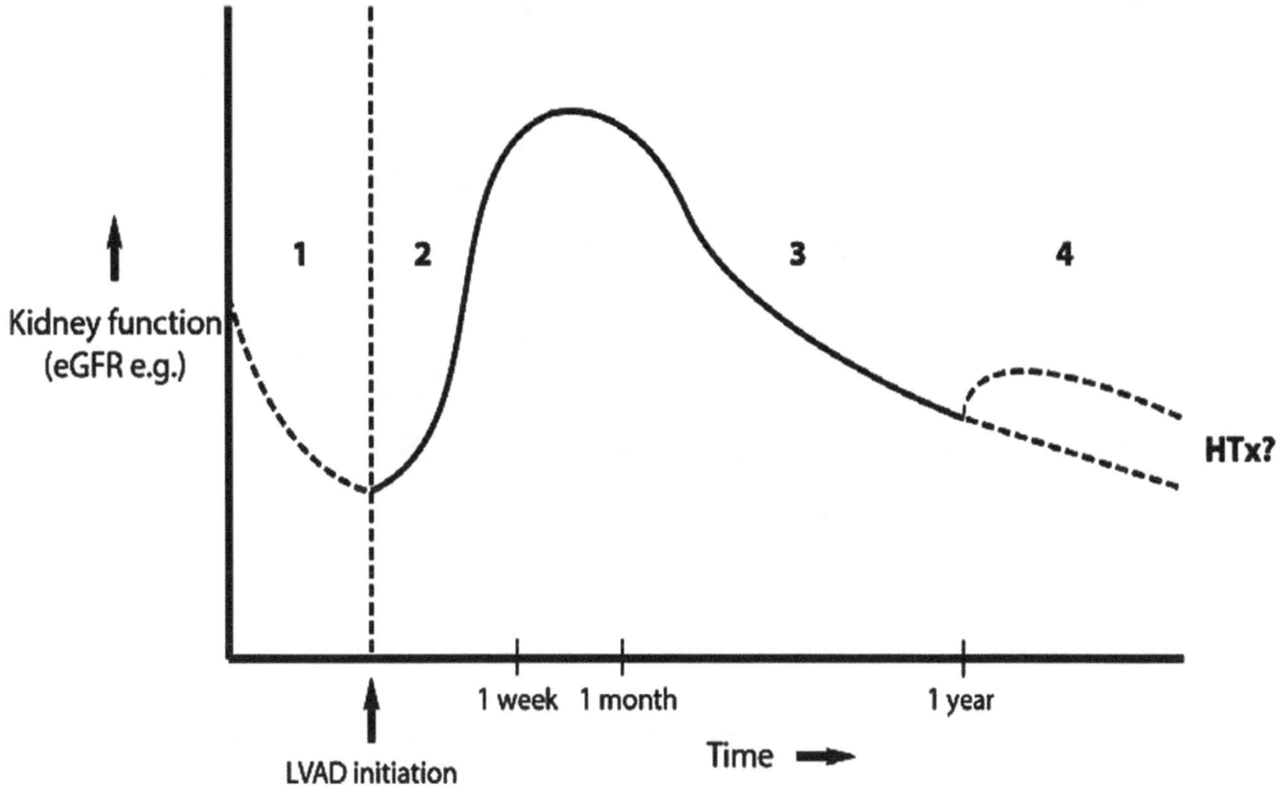

Fig. 18.3 Schematic representation of evolution in renal function over time. *Phase 1:* renal function decreases with varying degrees as a result of cardiorenal syndrome. *Phase 2:* renal function initially recovers after LVAD implantation. *Phase 3:* the functional improvement is transient, and renal function continues to decline. *Phase 4:* hypothetically, in the long term, renal function continues to decline and may necessitate RRT (*lower dotted line*). Alternatively, the patient receives a heart transplantation, which can either temporarily alleviate the downward trend (*upper dotted line*) or leave it unaltered (*lower dotted line*). Reprinted with permission from Tromp TR, de Jonge N, Joles JA. Left ventricular assist devices: a kidney's perspective. Heart Fail Rev 2015;20:524

period of improvement, data are scant regarding the overall long-term trajectory of renal function post-LVAD, with existing studies providing conflicting results. An analysis of 4000 patients reported that despite more pronounced improvements in the initial perioperative period, at 1 year post-implant, median improvement in eGFR was only 6.7% pre-implant values or by 2.6 ml/min/1.73 m^2 eGFR [26]. Another interesting observation derived from the INTERMACS registry is that patients with the largest initial increase in eGFR experienced the most substantial subsequent deterioration within 1 year of implantation, although they still maintain a higher eGFR than those recipients who did not experience significantly improved renal function following MCS (Fig. 18.4) [26]. Of importance is the observation that comparatively, the average rate of eGFR decline is more rapid than would be expected with either advancing age, CKD, or even diabetic kidney disease [27]. Of equal uncertainty is the trajectory of renal function following heart transplantation in patients receiving MCS for BTT. In one study of BTT patients consecutively undergoing MCS and then transplantation, a clear reduction of eGFR was demonstrated following transplantation, attributable primarily to post-transplant immunosuppression with calcineurin inhibitors [9]. Another noteworthy finding of that study was the dependency of post-transplant renal outcomes on renal function achieved *during* bridging therapy with MCS versus the pre-implant period, which was discussed earlier [9].

The survival benefit of improved renal function post-implant versus failed recovery from AKI has been clearly demonstrated in the previous section. Of equal importance, is the finding that compared to those patients with *no* kidney impairment pre-implant, patients who experience renal recovery post-implant have convergent 180-day post-implant survival curves. Furthermore, the similar survival rate between these two groups extends up to 1-year post cardiac transplantation [28]. As such, the precise identification of predictors of renal recovery post-LVAD is of prime importance. In one large study, although univariate analysis identified younger age, eGFR improvement on OMM pre-implant, IABP use, kidney length > 10 cm, lack of treatment with RAAS inhibitors, a higher bilirubin, and atrial fibrillation as preoperative predictors of improved renal function at 1 month; only improved eGFR on IABP remained as an independent predictor in a multivariate

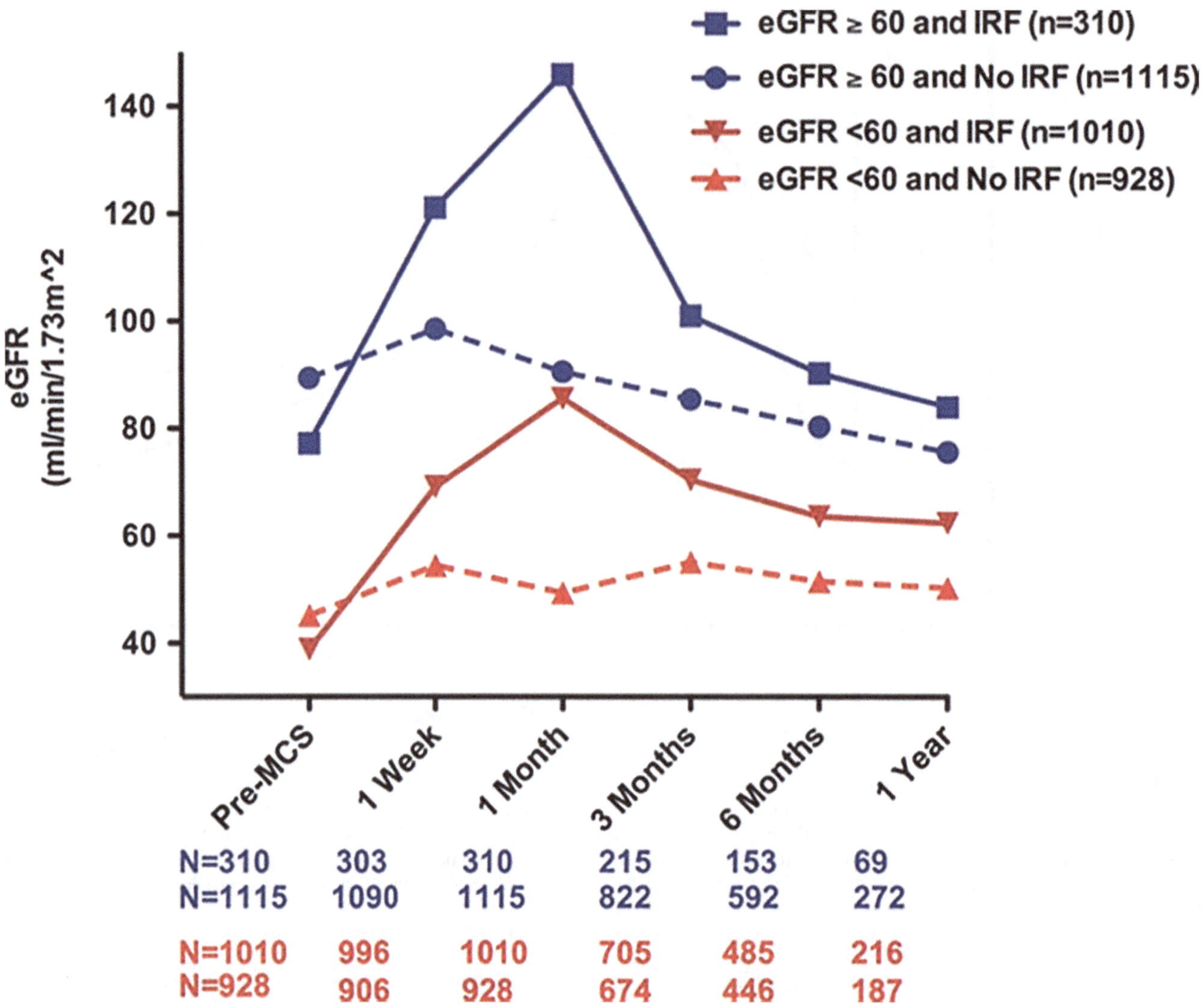

Fig. 18.4 Mean eGFR over time in patients with and without pre-MCS kidney impairment and post-MCS improvement in renal function. Mean eGFR according to presence (*red line*) or absence (*blue line*) of baseline kidney impairment further stratified by IRF (*solid line*) and no IRF (*dotted line*) at 1 month post-MCS. Kidney impairment is defined as a pre-MCS eGFR < 60 ml/min/1.73 m^2. IRF is defined as a ≥ 50% improvement in eGFR from pre-MCS to 1 month post-MCS. eGFR, estimated glomerular filtration rate; MCS, mechanical circulatory support; IRF, improvement in renal function. Reprinted with permission from Brisco MA, Kimmel SE, Coca SG, et al. Prevalence and prognostic importance of changes in renal function after mechanical circulatory support. Circ Heart Fail 2014;7:71

model [24]. A second, smaller study reported the greatest improvement in renal function in patients with the lowest pre-implant cardiac indices and those who had received inotropic support [36]. In light of these findings, it appears that the majority of positive predictors—lower cardiac indices, eGFR improvement with OMM (including inotropes), IABP utilization, higher bilirubin (indicative of congestive hepatopathy) and atrial fibrillation—insinuate that in general, pre-implant KI is likely secondary to the low output hemodynamics associated with CRS as opposed to intrinsic kidney disease, which in turn accounts for the improved renal function seen in most of these patients post-LVAD. This hypothesis is further bolstered by the observation that patients with underlying diabetes (and related kidney disease) are less likely to recover from pre-implant AKI, and supports the case for a careful assessment for other etiologies of intrinsic kidney disease among those patients whose renal function may not be responding to OMM in the pre-implant period [28].

The perpetuation of KI among some patients post-LVAD is likely multifactorial, attributable to ongoing multiorgan failure, residual damage from AKI, presence of pre-existing intrinsic renal disease from hypertension, diabetes or renovascular disease and long-standing ischemia from a protracted period of low output HF. Accounting for the progressive decline in renal function following the initial improvement in the 1–2 month post-implant time period is more nuanced. Some authors have suggested that measurement bias may be contributing, given that following LVAD therapy, patients who were primarily bed-ridden and overtly cachectic were now experiencing increased exercise capacity and muscle mass, thereby leading to physiologic increases in the serum creatinine [27]. Measuring with cystatin C, which is independent of muscle mass, may overcome this bias and provide a better assessment of renal function [27]. Another reason could be due to initiation of inhibitors of renin–angiotensin aldosterone system. The vast majority of patients with continuous-flow LVAD are started on angiotensin-converting enzyme (ACE) inhibitors or angiotensin II receptor blockers as a first-line agent for the treatment of hypertension [42]. Moreover, sub-clinical hemolysis, via similar mechanisms previously described to account for post-implant AKI, may also play a role in the long-term decline of renal function. Right ventricular (RV) failure is a serious complication of prolonged LVAD support, occurring in up to 9% of patients with an incidence of 0.10 events per patient-year [1]. Mechanistically, RV failure is thought to arise secondary to enhanced left-ventricular unloading as a normal function of LVAD support, which may in turn abruptly increase venous return and cause RV overload. Right ventricular over-distension can lead to overt RV failure which in turn can result in renal venous congestion and eventual reduction of eGFR. The reduced pulsatility of continuous-flow devices has also received considerable attention as a potential etiologic contributor to decreased long-term renal function, although comprehensive analysis of the INTERMACs registry has shown the gradual late decline of eGFR to occur with similar frequency in both pulsatile and continuous-flow devices [27]. Lastly, patients are susceptible to frequent episodes of AKI from the usual suspects such as contrast and over-diuresis. Recently there was a case report of post-infectious glomerulonephritis resulting from chronic LVAD-associated infection and bacteremia [43]. In summary, interpretation of renal function post-LVAD implantation is problematic for reasons outlined above and thus previous conclusions about the effect of LVADs on renal function need to be viewed with caution.

Renal Replacement Therapy with LVAD

Up to one-third of LVAD recipients develop AKI requiring RRT some of whom become chronically dialysis dependent [28]. More recently, the incidence of AKI necessitating RRT has been reported to decrease. Of the 4917 recipients with continuous-flow LVAD implantation between June 2006 and March 2012 in the INTERMACS registry, about 6% of patients had severe kidney impairment as defined with eGFR < 30 ml/min or requiring dialysis before implant [4]. In another study, 3% (2 of 61) of patients with LVAD required chronic RRT [25]. The primary etiology of end-stage renal disease (ESRD) following LVAD implantation was attributed to irreversible AKI occurring in the peri-implantation period [44].

Due to the high morbidity and mortality of LVAD recipients with ESRD, combined heart and kidney transplantation (HKT) is recommended in these patients. In a recent study, one year mortality rate was 100% in 22 LVAD recipients who required chronic hemodialysis without subsequent cardiac transplantation (HT) [44]. Of this group, 61% died within 30 days after LVAD implantation. The United Network for Organ Sharing Registry (UNOS) reports that from 2000 to 2010, 593 patients underwent combined HKT compared to 25,590 HT alone [45]. In recipients of combined HKT, one year survival rates are around 80%, while 5 and 10 year survival rates are 76 and 53%, respectively. Both short-and long-term survival are similar for combined HKT and HT alone [46]. Since there are fewer than 3000 donor hearts available per year, LVAD recipients with advanced CKD, or AKI which has not recovered, may require RRT chronically in the interim until the organs are available or may be deemed medically unsuitable for combined HKT [47].

In a critical care setting, RRT is often initiated as CRRT and then transitioned to intermittent hemodialysis (HD) once a patient becomes hemodynamically stable. There are several challenges of managing complex hemodynamic and volume needs of patients with LVADs requiring RRT. In particular, as a result of continuous-flow technology, in most LVAD recipients, there is an absence of pulse, precluding the standard assessment of blood pressure (BP). Blood pressure readings obtained using the automated BP devices were significantly different in systolic, diastolic, and mean arterial blood pressure readings (MAP) compared to intra-arterial catheter BP measurements, and usually these readings were consistently lower than those recorded using an arterial catheter [48]. Due to these factors BPs in LVAD recipients are often measured using nontraditional blood pressure devices, such as Doppler audible ultrasonography which provides a MAP reading. Accurate assessment of BP is crucial because patients with continuous-flow LVADs are sensitive to systemic afterload. Elevated afterload in the form of systemic hypertension can result in reduced pump flow and even retrograde flow through the LVAD due to the absence of valve [49]. Current recommendations are to target MAP between 70 and 80 mmHg and to avoid MAP above 90 mmHg to optimize cardiac output and minimize risk of stroke [50]. The issue of accurately measuring BP in continuous-flow LVAD recipients with ESRD is also important since these patients are at risk for developing hypotension during dialysis. A recent publication evaluated the relative safety of intermittent HD in 10 continuous-flow LVAD recipients [51]. Of 281 HD sessions, the mean SBP was 97 ± 18 mmHg measured using Doppler device and fluid removal ranged from 0 to 5.3 l per session with average around 2.6 ± 1.1 l per session. Only 5.3% of sessions were interrupted with 2% due to symptomatic hypotension and 1% due to asymptomatic hypotension. The remaining interruptions were due to abdominal cramps, arrhythmias, dialysis machine malfunction, and presence of hypophosphatemia. In general, intermittent HD was well tolerated in patients with Doppler MAP kept greater than 70 mmHg [51].

In addition to BP, other parameters can be used to monitor hemodynamic changes during dialysis treatment using the LVAD monitor, which displays key parameters such as pump speed, pump flow, and pulsatility index depending on the type of LVAD. Pulsatility index is a dimensionless value derived from the LVAD pump which represents the average flow pulses over 15 s intervals, indicative of the residual pulsatile activity of the native ventricle. The pulsatility index can reflect preload, and excessive fluid removal can decrease pulsatility index and thus pump flow. Because continuous-flow pumps are volume sensitive, LVAD malfunction can occur with sudden flux of intravascular volume. Excessive ultrafiltration along with increased pump speed can lead to left atrium and ventricle collapse, causing an event known as "suck-down" [28, 50, 51]. Therefore, it is critical for nephrologists and dialysis staff to have an understanding of the LVAD mechanics and the impact of dialysis on the physiology.

Peritoneal dialysis (PD) is an interesting option for RRT in LVAD recipients and has its advantages including minimizing large fluid shifts. Since older, larger pulsatile LVADs were implanted in the peritoneal cavity or abdominal wall, PD was contraindicated because of the potential for serious infection of the LVAD. However, PD can be possible with newer LVADs which are placed in the pre-peritoneal position or intrapericardially [28, 50, 52]. There have been two case reports showing the successful use of PD in these patients [52, 53]. Benefits of PD include gentle ultrafiltration, low risk of bacteremia from catheter infections, and home modality [53]. The latter is particularly important since many outpatient HD centers are not comfortable in their ability to safely dialyze a patient with an LVAD. At the present time, it is unknown which RRT modality is superior for ESRD patients with LVADs.

The choice of dialysis access is based on several factors. Initially, a temporary access with tunneled dialysis catheter is placed for patients who remain dialysis dependent. However, catheters should be avoided longterm because of

Table 18.2 Proposed nephrology pre-LVAD evaluation

History
Obtain current and previous laboratory data to determine the chronicity and progression of kidney impairment
Does the patient have a history of diabetes and/or hypertension and could either be the cause of the CKD?
Is there a history of any other systemic disease which could cause CKD?
Diagnostic Evaluation
Determination of GFR (Serum creatinine for eGFR or calculated creatinine clearance)
Urinalysis
Quantification of proteinuria (Either spot urine protein to creatinine ratio or 24 h urine collection)
Renal ultrasound for size, echogenicity, and cortical thickness
Optional testing**
Renal scan with isotope 99mTc-DTPA for GFR
Renal biopsy
Trial of ionotropes and/or intra-aortic balloon pump (If renal function remains impaired despite attaining reasonable cardiac index on medical therapy, careful assessment of intrinsic renal disease should be conducted)
Suggested criteria for dual listing for heart and kidney transplant*
1. CKD with GFR < 30–40 ml/min and/or significant proteinuria
2. AKI or cardiorenal syndrome with GFR < 30–40 ml/min for more than 8–12 weeks
3. Dialysis dependent for more than 8–12 weeks
4. Renal biopsy showing >30–75% glomerulosclerosis or >30–75% fibrosis

LVAD left ventricular assist device, *CKD* chronic kidney disease, *99mTc-DTPA* 99mTc-labeled diethylenetriaminepentacetate, *GFR* glomerular filtration rate, *eGFR* estimated glomerular filtration rate

*These criteria are opinion-based, with limited evidence on combined heart–kidney transplant [45, 54, 55]. Some of these suggestions are also based on recommendations for combined liver and kidney transplantation [56]

**Further testing should be done on case-by-case basis

their high risk for bloodstream infections. Bacteremia from central line infection can spread to the LVAD itself resulting in significant morbidity and mortality. Arteriovenous graft placement is considered the preferred long-term access for HD in these patients due to the theoretical concern for poor arteriovenous fistula maturation with reduced pulsatility [28, 29, 50]. However, there are no formal studies examining optimal HD access in LVAD recipients. Determining access patency poses a challenge since the physical findings of a palpable thrill or audible bruit are commonly absent. Doppler probes or simple needle puncture can be used to determine patency [28, 50]. Anticoagulation is generally recommended with continuous-flow LVADs due to an increased hypercoagulable state caused by these devices and theoretically may enhance vascular access patency.

Because of the challenges of monitoring hemodynamic stability and the unfamiliarity of the LVAD mechanics, placement of patients requiring HD after LVAD implantation is usually problematic. A close collaboration between nephrology and LVAD team is essential for the successful transition from inpatient to outpatient dialysis.

Conclusion

Kidney function following LVAD placement is an important determinant of clinical outcome. Patients with LVAD are at risk for developing varying forms of KI including AKI and CKD. Some develop AKI peri-implantation from acute CRS while others develop CKD from chronic CRS, irreversible AKI, and other comorbidities. Since KI is associated with high mortality, lower cardiac transplantation rate, and potential outcome for long-term dialysis, it is important to determine if pre-implantation KI is functional and potentially reversible or if it represents intrinsic renal disease which is associated with poor renal prognosis post-operatively. Table 18.2 shows our recommendations for initial nephrology assessment for patient undergoing LVAD implantation [45, 54–56]. For majority of LVAD recipients, kidney function improves following implantation. However, the initial improvement is often followed by late decline in renal function. Several reasons are proposed to explain these observations however the definitive answer remains elusive. Due to the growing number of LVAD implantations for destination therapy, it is integral to understand the cumulative impact of long-term renal function with LVAD. Those LVAD recipients who develop AKI or CKD requiring RRT provide unique challenges in their management and require an understanding of the hemodynamic and physiologic consequences of the LVAD during dialysis.

Acknowledgements This material is the result of work supported with resources and the use of facilities at the Baltimore VA Medical Center, MD.

References

1. Kirklin JK, Naftel DC, Pagani FD, Kormos RL, Stevenson LW, Blume ED, et al. Sixth INTERMACS annual report: a 10,000-patient database. J Heart Lung Transplant. 2014;33(6):555–64.
2. Park SJ, Tector A, Piccioni W, Raines E, Gelijns A, Moskowitz A, et al. Left ventricular assist devices as destination therapy: a new look at survival. J Thorac Cardiovasc Surg. 2005;129(1):9–17.
3. Patel UD, Hernandez AF, Liang L, Peterson ED, LaBresh KA, Yancy CW, et al. Quality of care and outcomes among patients with heart failure and chronic kidney disease: a get with the guidelines—Heart Failure Program study. Am Heart J. 2008;156(4):674–81.
4. Kirklin JK, Naftel DC, Kormos RL, Pagani FD, Myers SL, Stevenson LW, et al. Quantifying the effect of cardiorenal syndrome on mortality after left ventricular assist device implant. J Heart Lung Transplant. 2013;32(12):1205–13.
5. Sandner SE, Zimpfer D, Zrunek P, Rajek A, Schima H, Dunkler D, et al. Renal function and outcome after continuous flow left ventricular assist device implantation. Ann Thorac Surg. 2009;87(4):1072–8.
6. Yoshioka D, Sakaguchi T, Saito S, Miyagawa S, Nishi H, Yoshikawa Y, et al. Predictor of early mortality for severe heart failure patients with left ventricular assist device implantation: significance of INTERMACS level and renal function. Circ J. 2012;76(7):1631–8.
7. Iwashima Y, Yanase M, Horio T, Seguchi O, Murata Y, Fujita T, et al. Serial changes in renal function as a prognostic indicator in advanced heart failure patients with left ventricular assist system. Ann Thorac Surg. 2012;93(3):816–23.
8. Khot UN, Mishra M, Yamani MH, Smedira NG, Paganini E, Yeager M, et al. Severe renal dysfunction complicating cardiogenic shock is not a contraindication to mechanical support as a bridge to cardiac transplantation. J Am Coll Cardiol. 2003;41(3):381–5.
9. Singh M, Shullo M, Kormos RL, Lockard K, Zomak R, Simon MA, et al. Impact of renal function before mechanical circulatory support on posttransplant renal outcomes. Ann Thorac Surg. 2011;91(5):1348–54.
10. Mao H, Katz N, Kim JC, Day S, Ronco C. Implantable left ventricular assist devices and the kidney. Blood Purif. 2014;37(1):57–66.
11. Wilson SR, Mudge GH Jr, Stewart GC, Givertz MM. Evaluation for a ventricular assist device: selecting the appropriate candidate. Circulation. 2009;119(16):2225–32.
12. Imamura T, Kinugawa K, Shiga T, Kato N, Endo M, Inaba T, et al. How to demonstrate the reversibility of end-organ function before implantation of left ventricular assist device in INTERMACS profile 2 patients? J Artif Organs. 2012;15(4):395–8.
13. Saito S, Westaby S, Piggot D, Dudnikov S, Robson D, Catarino PA, et al. End-organ function during chronic nonpulsatile circulation. Ann Thorac Surg. 2002;74(4):1080–5.
14. Nemoto M. Experimental evaluation of the influence of complete artificial circulation on renal circulation and tissue metabolism-comparative study of pulsatile vs nonpulsatile circulation. Ann Thorac Cardiovasc Surg. 2003;9(6):355–64.

15. Kihara S, Litwak KN, Nichols L, Litwak P, Kameneva MV, Wu Z, et al. Smooth muscle cell hypertrophy of renal cortex arteries with chronic continuous flow left ventricular assist. Ann Thorac Surg. 2003;75(1):178–83 (discussion 83).
16. Ohnishi H, Itoh T, Nishinaka T, Tatsumi E, Fukuda T, Oshikawa M, et al. Morphological changes of the arterial systems in the kidney under prolonged continuous flow left heart bypass. Artif Organs. 2002;26(11):974–9.
17. Ootaki C, Yamashita M, Ootaki Y, Kamohara K, Weber S, Klatte RS, et al. Reduced pulsatility induces periarteritis in kidney: role of the local renin-angiotensin system. J Thorac Cardiovasc Surg. 2008;136(1):150–8.
18. Tromp TR, Nguyen TQ, de Jonge N, Joles JA. Absence of structural lesions in human renal arcuate arteries after LVAD implantation: response to a letter regarding "left ventricular assist devices: a kidney's perspective". Heart Fail Rev. 2015;20(6):753–4.
19. Welp H, Rukosujew A, Tjan TD, Hoffmeier A, Kosek V, Scheld HH, et al. Effect of pulsatile and non-pulsatile left ventricular assist devices on the renin-angiotensin system in patients with end-stage heart failure. Thorac Cardiovasc Surg. 2010;58(Suppl 2):S185–8.
20. Cooper TK, Griffith JW, Reibson J, Peterson R, Roush EP, Zhong Q, et al. Antibiotic-associated eosinophilic and occlusive arteritis in calves complicating preclinical studies of left ventricular assist devices. Toxicol Pathol. 2013;41(3):519–27.
21. Slaughter MS, Pagani FD, Rogers JG, Miller LW, Sun B, Russell SD, et al. Clinical management of continuous-flow left ventricular assist devices in advanced heart failure. J Heart Lung Transplant. 2010;29(4 Suppl):S1–39.
22. Miller LW, Pagani FD, Russell SD, John R, Boyle AJ, Aaronson KD, et al. Use of a continuous-flow device in patients awaiting heart transplantation. N Engl J Med. 2007;357(9):885–96.
23. Radovancevic B, Vrtovec B, de Kort E, Radovancevic R, Gregoric ID, Frazier OH. End-organ function in patients on long-term circulatory support with continuous- or pulsatile-flow assist devices. J Heart Lung Transplant. 2007;26(8):815–8.
24. Hasin T, Topilsky Y, Schirger JA, Li Z, Zhao Y, Boilson BA, et al. Changes in renal function after implantation of continuous-flow left ventricular assist devices. J Am Coll Cardiol. 2012;59(1): 26–36.
25. Deo SV, Sharma V, Altarabsheh SE, Hasin T, Dillon J, Shah IK, et al. Hepatic and renal function with successful long-term support on a continuous flow left ventricular assist device. Heart Lung Circ. 2014;23(3):229–33.
26. Brisco MA, Kimmel SE, Coca SG, Putt ME, Jessup M, Tang WW, et al. Prevalence and prognostic importance of changes in renal function after mechanical circulatory support. Circ Heart Fail. 2014;7(1):68–75.
27. Tromp TR, de Jonge N, Joles JA. Left ventricular assist devices: a kidney's perspective. Heart Fail Rev. 2015;20(4):519–32.
28. Patel AM, Adeseun GA, Ahmed I, Mitter N, Rame JE, Rudnick MR. Renal failure in patients with left ventricular assist devices. Clin J Am Soc Nephrol. 2013;8(3):484–96.
29. Amir O, Radovancevic B, Delgado RM III, Kar B, Radovancevic R, Henderson M, et al. Peripheral vascular reactivity in patients with pulsatile vs axial flow left ventricular assist device support. J Heart Lung Transplant. 2006;25(4):391–4.
30. Demirozu ZT, Etheridge WB, Radovancevic R, Frazier OH. Results of HeartMate II left ventricular assist device implantation on renal function in patients requiring post-implant renal replacement therapy. J Heart Lung Transplant. 2011;30(2):182–7.
31. Borgi J, Tsiouris A, Hodari A, Cogan CM, Paone G, Morgan JA. Significance of postoperative acute renal failure after continuous-flow left ventricular assist device implantation. Ann Thorac Surg. 2013;95(1):163–9.
32. Lok SI, Martina JR, Hesselink T, Rodermans BF, Hulstein N, Winkens B, et al. Single-centre experience of 85 patients with a continuous-flow left ventricular assist device: clinical practice and outcome after extended support. Eur J Cardiothorac Surg. 2013;44 (3):e233–8.
33. John R, Naka Y, Smedira NG, Starling R, Jorde U, Eckman P, et al. Continuous flow left ventricular assist device outcomes in commercial use compared with the prior clinical trial. Ann Thorac Surg. 2011;92(4):1406–13 (discussion 13).
34. Aaronson KD, Slaughter MS, Miller LW, McGee EC, Cotts WG, Acker MA, et al. Use of an intrapericardial, continuous-flow, centrifugal pump in patients awaiting heart transplantation. Circulation. 2012;125(25):3191–200.
35. Strueber M, Larbalestier R, Jansz P, Zimpfer D, Fiane AE, Tsui S, et al. Results of the post-market Registry to Evaluate the HeartWare Left Ventricular Assist System (ReVOLVE). J Heart Lung Transplant. 2014;33(5):486–91.
36. Sandner SE, Zimpfer D, Zrunek P, Dunkler D, Schima H, Rajek A, et al. Renal function after implantation of continuous versus pulsatile flow left ventricular assist devices. J Heart Lung Transplant. 2008;27(5):469–73.
37. Genovese EA, Dew MA, Teuteberg JJ, Simon MA, Bhama JK, Bermudez CA, et al. Early adverse events as predictors of 1-year mortality during mechanical circulatory support. J Heart Lung Transplant. 2010;29(9):981–8.
38. Hillege HL, Nitsch D, Pfeffer MA, Swedberg K, McMurray JJ, Yusuf S, et al. Renal function as a predictor of outcome in a broad spectrum of patients with heart failure. Circulation. 2006;113 (5):671–8.
39. Topkara VK, Dang NC, Barili F, Cheema FH, Martens TP, George I, et al. Predictors and outcomes of continuous veno-venous hemodialysis use after implantation of a left ventricular assist device. J Heart Lung Transplant. 2006;25(4):404–8.
40. Alba AC, Rao V, Ivanov J, Ross HJ, Delgado DH. Predictors of acute renal dysfunction after ventricular assist device placement. J Card Fail. 2009;15(10):874–81.
41. James KB, McCarthy PM, Thomas JD, Vargo R, Hobbs RE, Sapp S, et al. Effect of the implantable left ventricular assist device on neuroendocrine activation in heart failure. Circulation. 1995;92 (9 Suppl):II191–5.
42. Lampert BC, Eckert C, Weaver S, Scanlon A, Lockard K, Allen C, et al. Blood pressure control in continuous flow left ventricular assist devices: efficacy and impact on adverse events. Ann Thorac Surg. 2014;97(1):139–46.
43. Saritas T, Brandenburg V, Federico G, Grone HJ, Floege J, Moeller MJ, et al. Glomerulonephritis triggered by a chronically infected left ventricular assist device. Lancet. 2015;386 (10010):2363–4.
44. Yanagida R, Czer LS, Ruzza A, Schwarz ER, Simsir SA, Jordan SC, et al. Use of ventricular assist device as bridge to simultaneous heart and kidney transplantation in patients with cardiac and renal failure. Transplant Proc. 2013;45(6):2378–83.
45. Karamlou T, Welke KF, McMullan DM, Cohen GA, Gelow J, Tibayan FA, et al. Combined heart-kidney transplant improves post-transplant survival compared with isolated heart transplant in recipients with reduced glomerular filtration rate: analysis of 593 combined heart-kidney transplants from the United Network Organ Sharing Database. J Thorac Cardiovasc Surg. 2014;147 (1):456–61.
46. Leeser DB, Jeevanandam V, Furukawa S, Eisen H, Mather P, Silva P, et al. Simultaneous heart and kidney transplantation in patients with end-stage heart and renal failure. Am J Transplant. 2001;1(1):89–92.
47. Rose EA, Gelijns AC, Moskowitz AJ, Heitjan DF, Stevenson LW, Dembitsky W, et al. Long-term use of a left ventricular assist

device for end-stage heart failure. N Engl J Med. 2001;345 (20):1435–43.
48. Myers TJ, Bolmers M, Gregoric ID, Kar B, Frazier OH. Assessment of arterial blood pressure during support with an axial flow left ventricular assist device. J Heart Lung Transplant. 2009;28 (5):423–7.
49. Frazier OH, Myers TJ, Westaby S, Gregoric ID. Clinical experience with an implantable, intracardiac, continuous flow circulatory support device: physiologic implications and their relationship to patient selection. Ann Thorac Surg. 2004;77 (1):133–42.
50. Patel AM, Eduardo Rame J, Rudnick MR. How does the nephrologist manage an LVAD patient on chronic maintenance dialysis? Semin Dial. 2014;27(3):284–8.
51. Quader MA, Kumar D, Shah KB, Fatani YI, Katlaps G, Kasirajan V. Safety analysis of intermittent hemodialysis in patients with continuous flow left ventricular assist devices. Hemodial Int. 2014;18(1):205–9.
52. Thomas BA, Logar CM, Anderson AE. Renal replacement therapy in congestive heart failure requiring left ventricular assist device augmentation. Perit Dial Int. 2012;32(4):386–92.
53. Guglielmi AA, Guglielmi KE, Bhat G, Siemeck R, Tatooles AJ. Peritoneal dialysis after left ventricular assist device placement. ASAIO J. 2014;60(1):127–8.
54. Labban B, Arora N, Restaino S, Markowitz G, Valeri A, Radhakrishnan J. The role of kidney biopsy in heart transplant candidates with kidney disease. Transplantation. 2010;89(7):887–93.
55. Cantarovich M, Blydt-Hansen TD, Gill J, Tinckam K, Schiff J, Alwayn I, et al. Canadian forum on combined organ transplantation. Transplantation. 2015 Nov 19. 2016;100:1339–48.
56. Papafragkakis H, Martin P, Akalin E. Combined liver and kidney transplantation. Curr Opin Organ Transplant. 2010;15(3):263–8.

19 Palliation with Dual Burden of Heart and Kidney Failure: An Underutilized Strategy

Robin Turner and Hesham Shaban

Introduction

Cardiorenal syndrome (CRS) is a relatively new concept that acknowledges the complex interplay of heart failure and kidney failure. As an entity, CRS carries with it a high mortality rate and significant medical resource utilization [1, 2]. In patients with heart failure and reduced kidney function of any magnitude, there is greater hospital resources use and readmissions [2]. In patients with heart failure, creatinine clearances (CrCl) < 60 ml/min and changes in creatinine of greater than 0.3 mg/dl from baseline predict greater mortality when compared to patients with normal kidney function. A review by Bock et al. cites the ADHERE study, in which only 17% of patients with heart failure had CrCl > 90 ml/min [1]. Patients with chronic kidney disease (CKD), and/or a glomerular filtration rate (GFR) < 60 ml/min/1.73 m^2, have a higher risk of ischemic heart events, heart failure (preserved EF or reduced EF) and all cause death from cardiac causes than patients with normal GFR [1, 2].

Theories that currently exist to explain the pathophysiologic interplay between the failing heart and kidneys involve the neurohumoral systems, which affect the body's sodium and volume homeostasis [1, 3]. Clinically the vicious cycle of heart failure and kidney failure that describes CRS is manifested by volume overload and resulting symptoms related to this: dyspnea, fatigue, and discomfort. Usual management of these symptoms is far more challenging in the CRS milieu because diuretic resistance, hypotension, hyperkalemia, and decreased renal perfusion are more prevalent than in heart failure with preserved renal function [3, 4].

This scenario of high mortality, resource utilization, and high symptom burden suggests that patients with CRS would benefit from comanagement with Palliative Care. This approach to care focuses on symptom management and quality of life, and is often a part of the care of patients with heart failure or kidney failure. Symptom burden and psychosocial impact of chronic heart failure and chronic kidney disease are well defined in their individual disease territories, and less so in the overlap syndrome of CRS. Indeed, Palliative care is recommended by all of the major governing bodies of cardiology and nephrology including the American College of Cardiology, American Heart Association, European Society of Cardiology, Heart Failure Society of America, Canadian Cardiovascular Society, American Society of Nephrology, and the Renal Physicians Network. In this chapter, we will consider the role and use of palliative care services in the population of patients with joint cardiac and renal disease.

Symptom Burden and Palliative Treatment Approaches

A recent study found that the symptom burden of patients with congestive heart failure (HF) is comparable to patients with advanced lung cancer and pancreatic cancer [5]. Another study, comparing symptoms and quality of life in patients with advanced chronic kidney disease (defined as eGFR < 15 cc/min) found no difference in symptom burden when compared to a cohort with terminal malignancy [6]. Although these studies are small in size, they show that patients with heart or renal failure are highly symptomatic and warrant treatment.

The pathophysiology of CRS that results in volume overload that is resistant to usual treatments, [1, 4, 7] suggests that symptoms related to volume overload would be prevalent in these patients. This is consistent with literature in which dyspnea, pain, and fatigue are three of the most common symptoms found in the HF and CKD populations. In HF populations, some published data indicate that

R. Turner
Internal Medicine/Palliative Medicine, Duke University Health System, 2424 Erwin Road, 7206 Durham, NC 27710, USA

H. Shaban
Palliative Care, Duke University Hospital, Durham, NC 27705, USA

J. Rangaswami et al. (eds.), *Cardio-Nephrology*,
DOI 10.1007/978-3-319-56042-7_19

dyspnea is present in 69%, pain in 45–55%, fatigue in 44% and depression in 20–29% [8–10]. In a study of end stage kidney disease (ESKD) patients, 63% reported pain, 58% fatigue, 32% dyspnea, and 21% complained of edema [11]. Depression is another symptom that is highly prevalent in heart failure and ESKD.

Pain

Pain is prevalent and multifactorial in these patient populations. It is often under treated and related to poor quality of life. Pooled data from nine studies (including 2086 prevalent hemodialysis patients) consistently show that pain and overall symptom burden is strongly associated with substantially lower health related quality of life (HRQOL) [12]. Pain is predominantly musculoskeletal in origin, but neuropathic pain is also common. Chronic pain in CKD is often both nociceptive and neuropathic pain.

Increasingly, multimodal treatment strategies are recommended for these patients for chronic as well as acute pain [13]. These include the stepped approach to medication management as recommended by WHO, and attention to psychosocial contributors to perception of pain [13]. Pooled data of 42,945 patients found that the use of acetaminophen, despite its safety in CKD remains low. Non-steroidal anti-inflammatory drugs (NSAIDs) use appears inappropriately high, and despite severe pain, there appears to be a low prevalence of use of opioids. This data also shows that opioids that were prescribed are weak and often the agent selected is inappropriate for use in CKD [12].

Presence of pain should be assessed in all patients with CKD or HF, and by extrapolation, in all patients with CRS physiology. The review of systems in an initial evaluation of these patients should include a good clinical pain assessment, such as PQRST (presence of pain, quality of pain, radiation, precipitating or relieving factors, and timing). Follow up of pain can be done using a symptom assessment tool such as the modified Edmonton Symptom Assessment Scale (mESAS v2) which has been validated in both CKD and HF or the Palliative care outcome scale-renal (POS-renal) [12, 13] (Fig. 19.1).

With appropriate dose adjustment most pain medications are safe in patients despite altered metabolism and clearance of pain medications occurs in patients with CRS due to kidney failure and age related liver changes. Acetaminophen is safe in both CKD and HF, and should be considered in all pain regimens as an adjuvant (except in patients with liver impairment, and daily dose should <3.4 g in all patients). NSAIDS are contraindicated in both CKD and HF. Chronic or acute use can exacerbate CKD, cause or prolong AKI, and in HF it causes exacerbations by salt and water retention.

Morphine (and Codeine because it is metabolized to morphine) is mostly contraindicated in renal failure due to toxic cumulative side effects. Morphine is metabolized to morphine-6-glucuronide (M6G), which accumulates in CKD and can lead to neurotoxicity including confusion, delirium, sedation, myoclonus, and in large doses respiratory depression. Short term, intermittent use of morphine in early to moderate CKD (eGFR > 45 cc/min) may be safe if the patient is monitored for side effects, but should not be used for chronic pain in this population. Safer alternative opioids include hydromorphone, Oxycodone, and fentanyl. Hydromorphone is metabolized to Hydromorphone-3 glucuronide (H3G) which is better tolerated in CKD with less neurotoxic effects [12]. Oral hydromorphone is 4 times more potent than morphine which must be considered when starting this drug. Oxycodone is slightly more potent than morphine. Its metabolites are less dependent on renal clearance though no opioid is devoid of toxicity.

Both Fentanyl and Methadone are available for and useful in chronic pain. Fentanyl is a long acting opioid when used topically and is safe in kidney failure. It should only be used once a stable dose of oral opioids is achieved. The long half-life needs to be considered when switching to or from this opioid. Methadone is a long acting opioid that has both nociceptive and neuropathic pain relieving properties. Methadone should not be used in opiate naive patients, and is meant for chronic stable pain control. It should be prescribed by a provider who has experience with the drug, and understanding of its half-life and how it is titrated. Methadone can be safe in CKD and HF, however in addition to the neurotoxicity seen with other opioids; it can also cause QT prolongation [12]. An EKG before initiation and again 30 days post initiation are required to ensure safety.

Dyspnea

Causes of dyspnea, a major cause of morbidity in renal disease and HF, are multifactorial. A primary cause of dyspnea, defined as an uncomfortable abnormal awareness of breathing [14], in these diseases is volume overload. Volume overload in CRS can be more difficult to treat, and may require advanced interventions [1]. Many treatments originally tried in this patient population to manage volume, such as neseteride, have not been shown in further studies to be better than aggressive diuresis [2, 3]. Nonetheless, diuresis resistant CRS is a challenge to manage. In these patients, opioids can be a useful adjuvant [15].

Many patients feel short of breath without a fall in Sp02 or Pa02. A Cochrane review demonstrated that oxygen therapy did not help patients who were not hypoxic and is only beneficial in reducing dyspnea in those patients in

Alberta Health Services | Covenant Health

Edmonton Symptom Assessment System:
(revised version) (ESAS-R)

Please circle the number that best describes how you feel NOW:

No Pain	**0**	**1**	**2**	**3**	**4**	**5**	**6**	**7**	**8**	**9**	**10**	Worst Possible Pain
No Tiredness *(Tiredness = lack of energy)*	**0**	**1**	**2**	**3**	**4**	**5**	**6**	**7**	**8**	**9**	**10**	Worst Possible Tiredness
No Drowsiness *(Drowsiness = feeling sleepy)*	**0**	**1**	**2**	**3**	**4**	**5**	**6**	**7**	**8**	**9**	**10**	Worst Possible Drowsiness
No Nausea	**0**	**1**	**2**	**3**	**4**	**5**	**6**	**7**	**8**	**9**	**10**	Worst Possible Nausea
No Lack of Appetite	**0**	**1**	**2**	**3**	**4**	**5**	**6**	**7**	**8**	**9**	**10**	Worst Possible Lack of Appetite
No Shortness of Breath	**0**	**1**	**2**	**3**	**4**	**5**	**6**	**7**	**8**	**9**	**10**	Worst Possible Shortness of Breath
No Depression *(Depression = feeling sad)*	**0**	**1**	**2**	**3**	**4**	**5**	**6**	**7**	**8**	**9**	**10**	Worst Possible Depression
No Anxiety *(Anxiety = feeling nervous)*	**0**	**1**	**2**	**3**	**4**	**5**	**6**	**7**	**8**	**9**	**10**	Worst Possible Anxiety
Best Wellbeing *(Wellbeing = how you feel overall)*	**0**	**1**	**2**	**3**	**4**	**5**	**6**	**7**	**8**	**9**	**10**	Worst Possible Wellbeing
No __________ Other Problem *(for example constipation)*	**0**	**1**	**2**	**3**	**4**	**5**	**6**	**7**	**8**	**9**	**10**	Worst Possible __________

Patient's Name ______________________________

Date ________________ Time ________________

Completed by (check one):
- ☐ Patient
- ☐ Family caregiver
- ☐ Health care professional caregiver
- ☐ Caregiver-assisted

BODY DIAGRAM ON REVERSE SIDE

ESAS-r
Revised: November 2010

Fig. 19.1 Edmonton symptom assessment system (revised) ESAS-r: developed to assist providers in the assessment of symptoms that a patient experiences at the time of completion. Extensive instructions for use as well as references are available at www.palliative.org/NewPC/_pdfs/tools. Reprinted with permission

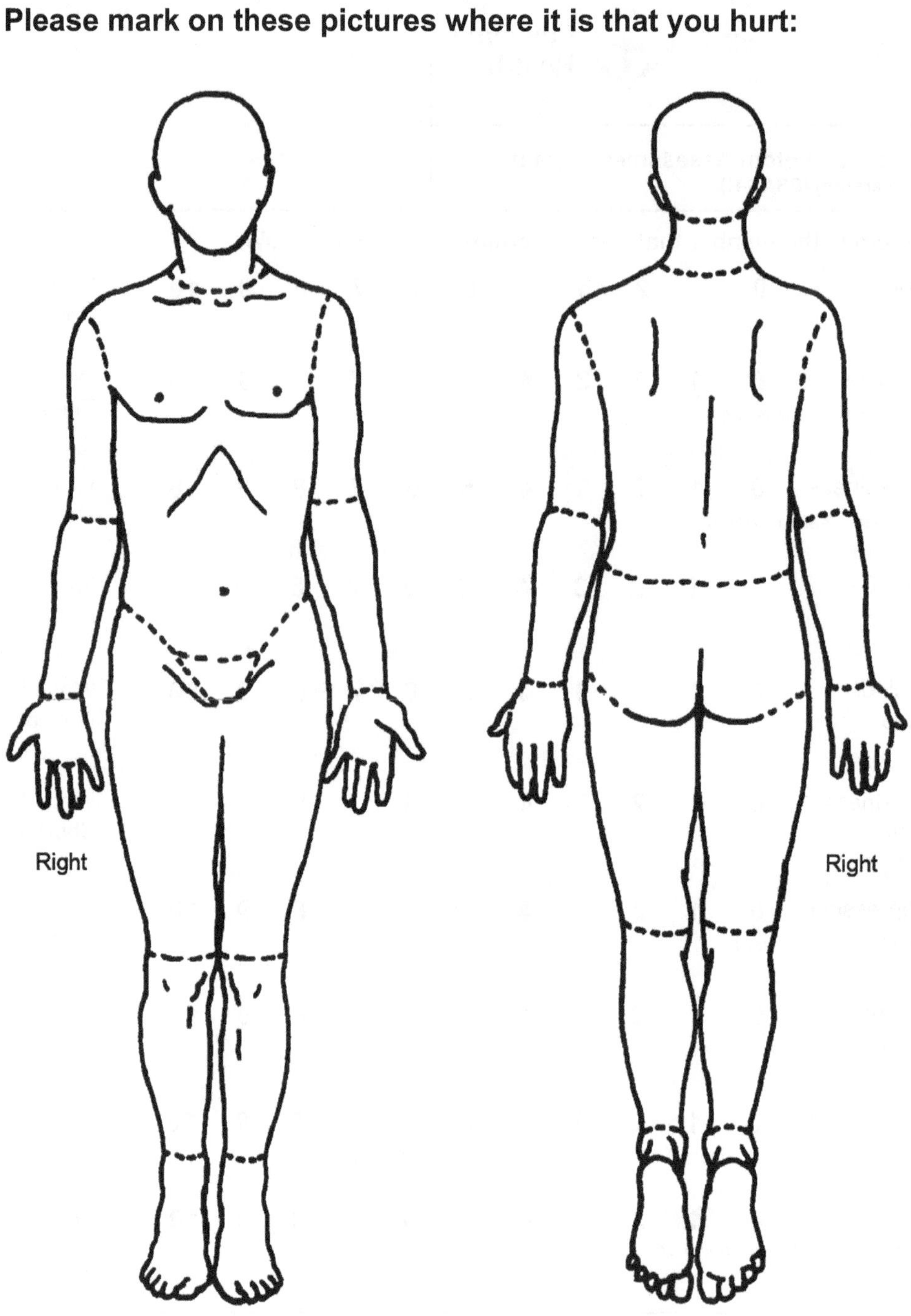

Fig. 19.1 (continued)

which hypoxia was present [16]. Early, optimization of fluid status with diuretics and optimization of heart failure medication including ACE-I, and B-Blockers are important [15]. Combination furosemide and metolazone was beneficial in improving diuresis and dyspnea even in the end of life setting [17]. A small study of 39 patients with end stage CHF and CRS type 2 showed that peritoneal ultrafiltration also provided symptom relief in volume overloaded patients [18].

Exercise is important in all stages of CKD and HF including advanced disease. A meta-analysis of 5 trials using exercise as an intervention in HF with preserved EF found that endurance exercise training improved both exercise capacity (by 6 min walk and peak V02) and quality of life (by the Minnesota living with heart failure inventory) [19]. In a single center trial, exercise improved the apnea–hypopnea index in patients with left ventricular systolic dysfunction and

A Circle Of Care
Victoria Hospice
SOCIETY

Palliative Performance Scale (PPSv2)
version 2

PPS Level	Ambulation	Activity & Evidence of Disease	Self-Care	Intake	Conscious Level
100%	Full	Normal activity & work No evidence of disease	Full	Normal	Full
90%	Full	Normal activity & work Some evidence of disease	Full	Normal	Full
80%	Full	Normal activity *with* Effort Some evidence of disease	Full	Normal or reduced	Full
70%	Reduced	Unable Normal Job/Work Significant disease	Full	Normal or reduced	Full
60%	Reduced	Unable hobby/house work Significant disease	Occasional assistance necessary	Normal or reduced	Full or Confusion
50%	Mainly Sit/Lie	Unable to do any work Extensive disease	Considerable assistance required	Normal or reduced	Full or Confusion
40%	Mainly in Bed	Unable to do most activity Extensive disease	Mainly assistance	Normal or reduced	Full or Drowsy +/- Confusion
30%	Totally Bed Bound	Unable to do any activity Extensive disease	Total Care	Normal or reduced	Full or Drowsy +/- Confusion
20%	Totally Bed Bound	Unable to do any activity Extensive disease	Total Care	Minimal to sips	Full or Drowsy +/- Confusion
10%	Totally Bed Bound	Unable to do any activity Extensive disease	Total Care	Mouth care only	Drowsy or Coma +/- Confusion
0%	Death	-	-	-	-

Instructions for Use of PPS (see also definition of terms)

1. PPS scores are determined by reading horizontally at each level to find a 'best fit' for the patient which is then assigned as the PPS% score.

2. Begin at the left column and read downwards until the appropriate ambulation level is reached, then read across to the next column and downwards again until the activity/evidence of disease is located. These steps are repeated until all five columns are covered before assigning the actual PPS for that patient. In this way, 'leftward' columns (columns to the left of any specific column) are 'stronger' determinants and generally take precedence over others.

   Example 1: A patient who spends the majority of the day sitting or lying down due to fatigue from advanced disease and requires considerable assistance to walk even for short distances but who is otherwise fully conscious level with good intake would be scored at PPS 50%.

   Example 2: A patient who has become paralyzed and quadriplegic requiring total care would be PPS 30%. Although this patient may be placed in a wheelchair (and perhaps seem initially to be at 50%), the score is 30% because he or she would be otherwise totally bed bound due to the disease or complication if it were not for caregivers providing total care including lift/transfer. The patient may have normal intake and full conscious level.

   Example 3: However, if the patient in example 2 was paraplegic and bed bound but still able to do some self-care such as feed themselves, then the PPS would be higher at 40 or 50% since he or she is not 'total care.'

3. PPS scores are in 10% increments only. Sometimes, there are several columns easily placed at one level but one or two which seem better at a higher or lower level. One then needs to make a 'best fit' decision. Choosing a 'half-fit' value of PPS 45%, for example, is not correct. The combination of clinical judgment and 'leftward precedence' is used to determine whether 40% or 50% is the more accurate score for that patient.

4. PPS may be used for several purposes. First, it is an excellent communication tool for quickly describing a patient's current functional level. Second, it may have value in criteria for workload assessment or other measurements and comparisons. Finally, it appears to have prognostic value.

Fig. 19.2 Palliative Performance Scale (PPS v2): a tool developed by Victoria Hospice and used to measure functional status and progressive decline. It is used frequently in Palliative Care as a means of communicating patient status. This tool continues to be tested for its effectiveness in prognostication in various populations. Copyright Victoria Hospice Society, BC, Canada (2001) www.victoriahospice.org. Reprinted with permission

Definition of Terms for PPS

As noted below, some of the terms have similar meanings with the differences being more readily apparent as one reads horizontally across each row to find an overall 'best fit' using all five columns.

1. Ambulation
The items '**mainly sit/lie**,' '**mainly in bed**,' and '**totally bed bound'** are clearly similar. The subtle differences are related to items in the self-care column. For example, 'totally bed 'bound' at PPS 30% is due to either profound weakness or paralysis such that the patient not only can't get out of bed but is also unable to do any self-care. The difference between 'sit/lie' and 'bed' is proportionate to the amount of time the patient is able to sit up vs need to lie down.

'**Reduced ambulation'** is located at the PPS 70% and PPS 60% level. By using the adjacent column, the reduction of ambulation is tied to inability to carry out their normal job, work occupation or some hobbies or housework activities. The person is still able to walk and transfer on their own but at PPS 60% needs occasional assistance.

2. Activity & Extent of disease
'**Some**,' '**significant**,' and '**extensive'** disease refer to physical and investigative evidence which shows degrees of progression. For example in breast cancer, a local recurrence would imply 'some' disease, one or two metastases in the lung or bone would imply 'significant' disease, whereas multiple metastases in lung, bone, liver, brain, hypercalcemia or other major complications would be 'extensive' disease. The extent may also refer to progression of disease despite active treatments. Using PPS in AIDS, 'some' may mean the shift from HIV to AIDS, 'significant' implies progression in physical decline, new or difficult symptoms and laboratory findings with low counts. 'Extensive' refers to one or more serious complications with or without continuation of active antiretrovirals, antibiotics, etc.

The above extent of disease is also judged in context with the ability to maintain one's work and hobbies or activities. Decline in activity may mean the person still plays golf but reduces from playing 18 holes to 9 holes, or just a par 3, or to backyard putting. People who enjoy walking will gradually reduce the distance covered, although they may continue trying, sometimes even close to death (eg. trying to walk the halls).

3. Self-Care
'**Occasional assistance'** means that most of the time patients are able to transfer out of bed, walk, wash, toilet and eat by their own means, but that on occasion (perhaps once daily or a few times weekly) they require minor assistance.

'**Considerable assistance'** means that regularly every day the patient needs help, usually by one person, to do some of the activities noted above. For example, the person needs help to get to the bathroom but is then able to brush his or her teeth or wash at least hands and face. Food will often need to be cut into edible sizes but the patient is then able to eat of his or her own accord.

'**Mainly assistance'** is a further extension of 'considerable.' Using the above example, the patient now needs help getting up but also needs assistance washing his face and shaving, but can usually eat with minimal or no help. This may fluctuate according to fatigue during the day.

'**Total care'** means that the patient is completely unable to eat without help, toilet or do any self-care. Depending on the clinical situation, the patient may or may not be able to chew and swallow food once prepared and fed to him or her.

4. Intake
Changes in intake are quite obvious with '**normal intake**' referring to the person's usual eating habits while healthy. '**Reduced'** means any reduction from that and is highly variable according to the unique individual circumstances. '**Minimal**' refers to very small amounts, usually pureed or liquid, which are well below nutritional sustenance.

5. Conscious Level
'**Full consciousness**' implies full alertness and orientation with good cognitive abilities in various domains of thinking, memory, etc. '**Confusion**' is used to denote presence of either delirium or dementia and is a reduced level of consciousness. It may be mild, moderate or severe with multiple possible etiologies. '**Drowsiness**' implies either fatigue, drug side effects, delirium or closeness to death and is sometimes included in the term stupor. '**Coma**' in this context is the absence of response to verbal or physical stimuli; some reflexes may or may not remain. The depth of coma may fluctuate throughout a 24 hour period.

Fig. 19.2 (continued)

sleep disordered breathing [15]. However, opioid therapy should be considered when dyspnea is refractory to maximal HF therapy, volume removal does not improve dyspnea sufficiently, and exercise therapy is both maximized and ineffective or the patient is unable to exercise.

Opioids improve the ventilator response to exercise by vasodilatation and act on opioid receptors in the brain and the lung to alter the perception of dyspnea and are also anxiolytic. In small-randomized controlled studies oral opioids improve dyspnea acutely and chronically in NYHA class II–IV patients without significant adverse effects [15]. However, when the patient has CKD as well, one must be cautious with the opioid selection, staying away from morphine and using other opioids such as oxycodone, or low dose hydromorphone.

Anemia should be worked up as it is normally done in CKD if it is found in the cardio-renal patient. Anemia is not described in heart failure; in cardio-renal patients it was present in the same rate regardless of EF and is likely a function of decreased renal function [20].

Depression is prevalent in CKD and HF and has been associated with increased morbidity and mortality. The prevalence of clinically significant depression has been reported to be greater than 20% in both the HF and CKD population, and only 2–4% in the general community, and 5–10% in the primary care setting [8, 21]. Although, there is no evidence that treating depression reduces morbidity and mortality in the context of palliative care, both pharmacotherapy as well as psychotherapy might be helpful in alleviating symptoms. In one study, patients with stage 4 CKD who were hospitalized with CHF were found to have a 12-month mortality if they were diagnosed with major depressive disorder [22]. A randomized control trial of treatment of depression in HF with sertraline (SADHART CHF), did not show a benefit with sertraline or placebo after 12 weeks [23]. SSRI's carry an increased risk of bleeding in CKD, and have higher rates of sexual dysfunction and central nervous system depression, and drug–drug interactions with MAO inhibitors, an tricyclic antidepressants [21]. A prospective cohort study of "mindfulness" support group and HF education resulted in statistically significant improvement in depression and anxiety score [15], and the role of such noninvasive and non-pharmacologic therapies should be further explored in this population.

Palliative Care

The World Health Organization (WHO) defines palliative care as "an approach that improves the quality of life of patients and their families who are facing problems associated with life-threatening illness." Palliative Care focuses on the prevention and relief of suffering "through the early identification, correct assessment and treatment of pain and other problems, whether physical, psychosocial, or spiritual." [24]. The benefits of palliative care in the cancer population are clearly demonstrated in landmark studies such as the Temel study, [25]. Studies to evaluate the benefit of palliative care to patient populations with noncancer diagnoses, including heart failure and renal failure are ongoing [11, 26]. The Palliative Care in Heart Failure study is designed as a prospective study that will assess the efficiency and cost effectiveness of Palliative Care interventions concurrently with advanced treatments for heart failure. In small studies of patients with liver and kidney disease, some benefit is shown in depression scores, resource utilization, and quality of life [11, 27]. Palliative care programs have improved symptom burden, spiritual well-being, caregiver satisfaction, and increased rates of death at home [15]. A study of palliative care patients with ESKD found that follow up with outpatient palliative care reduced ED visits and hospital readmissions, as well as decreased symptom burden [11].

Despite these results and society recommendation to involve Palliative Care, there are many barriers to its use in these patient populations. Patients and providers often misidentify palliative care as hospice, believe that employing palliative care takes away hope, and have difficulties with accepting prognostication [28]. Studies on characteristics of palliative care referrals of heart failure patients while retrospective, suggest that the patients are older, sicker, had renal failure, and have been in the ICU [29, 30]. In other words, in keeping with the prevalent notion that hospice and palliative care are the same, providers most often refer the sickest of the sick to Palliative Care. Often these referrals are often so late, that the longitudinal benefits of palliative care are unrealized. In one retrospective study, time to the palliative care consult in hospitalized patients with advanced heart failure was 21 days after hospital admission [31].

Prognostication is also a challenge. CRS, as with HF and ESKD, carries with it high morbidity and mortality. A meta-analysis of observational studies confirms that HF patients with renal dysfunction have a significant increase in relative mortality risk [31]. Statistics however, are difficult to translate to an individual patient's experience and illness trajectory. Studies that have used symptoms or clinical markers for prognosis have not necessarily predicted the individual who died soon or lived 1–2 years after diagnosis of a serious illness [15]. The course of chronic illnesses such as heart failure is undulating and punctuated by acute illness episodes, followed by periods of relative recovery. While repeated hospitalization is a poor prognostic indicator, it remains difficult to say which hospitalization will be the last. In cancer patients, the surprise question has been validated as a tool to identify patients who are at high risk for death [32]. If the answer to "Would you be surprised if your patient died in the next 6–12 months," is "No," then most likely the patient is hospice appropriate. This has been studied in ESKD, and heart failure patients and is probably a useful tool [33]. The Palliative Performance Scale (PPSv2) (Fig. 19.2) is a tool used in Palliative Care and Hospice populations. This tool allows for consistent communication about patient functional status and disease burden between providers. The PPSv2 may also have prognostic value in Palliative Care patient populations.

As an approach to care, Palliative Care provides symptom control, psychosocial support of patient and families, and help with advance care planning early in the course of a life limiting illness and importantly, parallels usual care of the underlying illness. Palliative Care unlike hospice is not prognosis dependent, and can be provided anywhere along the trajectory of illness. In its approach to care, palliative care is similar to hospice in that a team, often a physician and/or nurse practitioner, with support from social workers, chaplains and other ancillary services as might be needed provide a full spectrum of care. In large Palliative Care programs, care can be provided across the continuum, with ongoing efforts to provide care "where the patient is." Palliative Care providers comanage patients with serious illness even while treatments to prolong life or achieve cure are provided. When the patient is ready and medically appropriate, palliative care can help to refer and transition patients to hospice.

Communication

Effective communication with patients affects both their understanding and their experience throughout chronic illness, not just at the end of life [34]. The focus of communication with patients may vary throughout the course of an illness, and subjects such as medical management and self-care behaviors that affect QOL may take on a greater focus early on. However, CRS is a life limiting illness for which, at this time, there is no cure [1, 2]. In HF, patients often have little insight into the nature of their disease, or in their prognosis and rarely initiate or are offered discussion on end of life [8]. Patients and their families report that they want to have in depth discussion regarding both prognosis and end of life issues, but feel they are not given full disclosure on prognosis and the severity of illness [35]. A survey of patients enrolled in an academic HF clinic demonstrated significant discordance between patient's predicted life expectancy versus actual and model predicted life expectancy, with an average overestimation by patients of longevity by 40% [35]. Another, study found that most patients are generally comfortable discussing end of life issues, as long as information is presented honestly and balanced with hope [31].

The SUPPORT study, which was pivotal in raising awareness around end of life care in the USA, was a multicenter trial that asked among many things: if we give patients and families the information about poor prognosis, will they want aggressive care? [36] After a very specific intervention, in which a nurse provided the information about prognosis in a clear manner, patients or surrogates made no different choices than when there was no formal prognosis information. We have learned much about communication in medicine since then. There are many excellent educational programs to help providers learn techniques that improve patient satisfaction, support decision-making, and help to better elucidate goals of care (Oncotalk, Geritalk, Nephrotalk, Vitaltalk).

Nonetheless there remain physician, patient and system barriers to communication and elucidation of treatment preferences from those who are seriously ill. Patient factors include denial, and desire to protect family members [9]. Provider factors include time, comfort level and in particular, uncertainty around prognosis. A recent survey study in JAMA, identified several provider barriers including discomfort around family disagreement, and dealing with the patient/family response of denial [37]. Providers also cite that they do not receive communication skills training [37]. Discussing treatment preferences in patients with heart failure is also challenging due to the use of advanced therapies such as destination ventricular assist devices (VADs). The informed consent process for starting therapies often considers the benefits of treatment, and risks of not having treatment, but rarely includes discussion of discontinuation of therapy when it is no longer effective or meeting patient goals [38].

Communication with patients who have life limiting illnesses, in particular should be a dialog [39]. In this setting, decision-making becomes a negotiation, more so the further down the path one gets. Decision-making is always influenced by values, but this becomes more important when treatment options become more burdensome or higher risk [39]. Information giving becomes less important, and listening more important with time. Additionally, people learn differently and may want different information. For example, some people might want full disclosure, and other people might not.

However, information should always be offered, and the level of information desired by the patient should be delivered. Information that supports decision-making for patients and families includes the anticipated cause of death, discussion of treatments that are life prolonging, and the possibility of escalating symptoms and functional decline. Communication around the time of device insertion or infusions is also important. Insertion or addition of devices, use of inotropic infusions, and dialysis should only proceed after explaining the circumstances in which the patient might want these discontinued as well as other alternatives such as comfort-focused care [31]. A retrospective study based on interventions of next of kin of deceased patients who had been recipient of an ICD, deactivation of the device before insertion was discussed in only about 27% of cases. When a DNR order was in place, such discussions took place <45% of the time [8].

Advance Care Planning (ACP)

Advance Care Planning is a process that involves tools to springboard discussions around treatment preferences [40, 41]. The goal of ACP is to ensure that if a patient with a serious illness can no longer communicate treatment preferences, there is sufficient information available to provide care that is consistent with the patient's goals and values [31]. A living will is the document that outlines treatment preferences for care at the very end of life. Health Care power of attorney (HCPOA) is a document that gives a named individual(s) health care decision-making ability when a patient in incapacitated and most often requires witnesses. A patient can complete these without a lawyer, and independent of a visit with their provider. Treatment preferences change over time for many reasons, such disease severity and increased treatment burden, and treatment preferences should be reviewed on a regular basis.

Very few people have a living will even now in 2016 despite large national efforts to get people to complete them [42]. There are many potential problems with advance directives usually related to correctness and how current the information is. Since treatment preferences change over time, many question the value of a document completed previously [42]. Infrequent review by patients and providers sometimes results in incorrect information. The HCPOA may have changed for instance, over time. Many people are currently focusing on the designation of a decision maker, a HCPOA, and encourage patients to clarify wishes and preferences with that person [42].

Patients with CRS pose a particularly challenging because they can have altered mental status due to their underlying disease(s). This can wax and wane, or be an indicator of disease progression. The ACP process in these patients, especially designation of a HCPOA is critical. The recent ruling from CMS (Centers for Medicare and Medicaid) to acknowledge a provider visit to address end of life wishes is a great opportunity to put this in the forefront of care of these patients.

Hospice

Advanced Heart Failure is highly lethal, with life expectancy of less than 1 year for most patients once they enter stage D HF [19]. Studies of patient preference have noted that 90% of people would prefer to die at home as opposed to a hospital or nursing home. Yet, among patients with HF and decreased EF, 58% die in the hospital while only 29% die at home [35]. In the ESKD population, 45% die in hospital, while only 20% ever use any hospice services [43].

Hospice care is palliative care provided to patients with a life expectancy less than 6 months as defined by the rules of Medicare in the USA [44]. Hospice, as a program, was signed into Medicare law [45] in 1982.

There are many barriers to enrolling in hospice care including myths about the intent of comfort medications, including the notion of "giving up," and that the patient must have Do Not Resuscitate (DNR) Status. In fact, hospice is a comprehensive care program which provides for medications, durable medical equipment, and support services that allow medical care to be provided in the home, rather than the hospital [46, 47]. Hospice care is focused on patients with higher likelihood of dying, than the palliative care population, and specializes in care at the very end of life.

Hospice utilization has grown significantly since 1983 when the primary admission diagnosis was cancer. In 2014, only 35% of all hospice patients were cancer patients [44] while 65% were noncancer diagnoses. However, of the large group of patients who had non cancer diagnoses, only 14.7% had a diagnosis of heart failure, and 3.0% had a diagnosis of kidney failure. In the 2014 National Hospice and Palliative Care Organization (NHPCO) data [44], CRS was not a listed diagnostic code (in the list of noncancer diagnoses. Additionally, the length of stay on hospice is short. In 2014, 35.5% of patients died or were discharged within 7 days of admission to hospice. This trend is increasing [44]. In a recent study using data from the United States Renal Data System (USRDS) and the Dartmouth Atlas [43], patients with kidney failure and heart failure had more deaths in the hospital than cancer patients. Additionally, Hospice use was greater in cancer patients, less in heart failure patients and even less in patients on dialysis [43]

Families, of patients who died with hospice services were more likely to rate their dying "experience" excellent as compared with those who died in an institution or at home with only home services [48, 49]. Timing of referral to hospice is an important consideration when caring for patients who are at the end of their lives. Perception of appropriate timing of hospice care, not total length of stay correlates well with family satisfaction, where the perception of being referred "too late" was associated with greater dissatisfaction and unmet needs [48, 49].

Caregivers can be the second patient, and have a lot of stress and burden. In a study looking at caregiver burden, they found that there was no difference between caregivers of patients with the diagnosis of CHF, cancer or COPD in terms of burden, and that caregiver resources, not patient diagnosis or illness severity are the primary correlate with caregiver burden [50]. It was also found, that caregiver well-being is the most important factor in keeping a patient out of the hospital [50].

Future Directions

Further research into the etiology of symptomatology in cardio-renal syndrome are needed to see if the symptoms are indeed a combination of those seen in CKD and HF, and if their treatment follows the same general principles. Research into communication issues, and communication styles in regards to education, advanced care planning, end of life issues, and hospice referral are needed. Finally, better prognostic tools to help guide decision-making, and to better inform both the provider and the patient where the patient is at on the spectrum of disease.

Conclusion

Patients with both chronic kidney disease/Acute kidney Injury and Heart Failure are highly symptomatic, have high mortality, and high medical resource utilization. Palliative Care that includes excellent symptom management, attention to quality of life, and support of family has been shown to be beneficial in patients with heart failure as well as kidney disease but is underutilized. While more research is needed to better define these metrics in CRS, sufficient literature suggests the benefits of Palliative Care in heart failure and kidney failure. Patients want to know their prognosis, and what to expect for better or for worse, when balanced with hope. Advance Care Planning provides a tool for discussion and planning for care as treatments become more burdensome. Finally, hospice is an underutilized resource that benefits both the patient and their families at the end of life.

References

1. Bock JS, Gottlieb SS. Cardiorenal syndrome, new perspectives. Circulation. 2010;121:2592–600. doi:10.1161/CIRCULATIONAHA.109.886473.
2. Shlipak M, Massie BM. The clinical challenge of cardiorenal syndrome. Circulation. 2004;110:1514–7.
3. Liu PP. Cardiorenal syndrome in heart failure: a cardiologist's perspective. Can J Cardiol. 2008;24(Suppl B):25B–9B.
4. Liang KV, Williams AW, Greene EL, Redfield MM. Acute decompensated heart failure and the cardiorenal syndrome. Crit Care Med. 2008;36(1 Suppl):S75.
5. Bekelman DB, Rumsfeld JS, Havanek EP, Yamashita TE, Hutt E, Gottlieb SH, Dy SM, Kunther JS. Symptom burden, depression, and spiritual well-being: a comparison of heart failure and advanced cancer patients. J Gen Intern Med. 2009;24(5):592–8. doi:10.1007/s11606-009-0931-y Epub 2009 Mar 14.
6. Saini T, Murtagh FE, Dupont PJ, McKinnon PM, Hatfield P, Saunders Y. Comparative pilot study of symptoms and quality of life in cancer patients and patients with end stage renal disease. Palliat Med. 2006;20(6):631–6.
7. Testani JM, Chen J, McCauley BD, Kimmel SE, Shannon RP. Potential effects of aggressive decongestion during the treatment of decompensated heart failure on renal function and survival. Circulation 2010;122(3):265–72. doi:10.1161/CIRCULATIONAHA.109.933275 (Epub 2010 Jul 6).
8. Brown MA, Collett GK, Josland EA, Foote C, Li Q, Brennan FP. CKD in elderly patients managed without dialysis: survival, symptoms, and quality of life. CJASN. 2015;10(2):260–8. doi:10.2215/CJN.03330414.
9. Goebel JR, Doering LV, Shugarman LR, Asch SM, Sherbourne CD, Lanto AB, Evangelista LS, Nyamathi AM, Maliski SL, Lorenz KA. Heart failure: the hidden problem of pain. J Pain Symptom Manag. 2009;38(5):698–707. doi:10.1016/j.jpainsymman.2009.04.022 (Epub 2009 Sep 3).
10. Jorgenson A, Sidebottom AC, Richards H, Kirven J. A description of inpatient palliative care actions for patients with acute heart failure. Am J Hosp Palliat Care. 2016;33(9):863–70 (Epub 2015 Jun 30).
11. Chan KY, Cheng HW, Yap DY, Yip T, Li CS, Sham MK, Wong YC, Lau WK. Reduction of acute hospital admissions and improvement in outpatient attendance by intensified renal palliative care clinic follow-up: the Hong Kong experience. a description of inpatient palliative care actions for patients with acute heart failure. J Pain Symptom Manag. 2015;49(1):144–9. doi:10.1016/j.jpainsymman.2014.04.010 Epub 2014 May 23.
12. Davidson SN, Koncicki H, Brennan F. Pain in chronic kidney disease: a scoping review. Semin Dial. 2014;27(2):188–204. doi:10.1111/sdi.12196 Epub 2014 Feb 12.
13. Leung L. From ladder to platform: aew concept for pain management. J Prim Health Care. 2012;4(3):254–8.
14. Bass JB. Dyspnea. In: Walker HK, Hall WD, Hurst JW, editors. Clinical methods: the history, physical, and laboratory examinations, 3rd edition. Boston: Butterworths; 1990. Chapter 36. http://www.ncbi.nlm.nih.gov/books/NBK357/.
15. Goodlin SJ. Palliative care in congestive heart failure. J Am Coll Cardiol. 2009;54(5):386–96. doi:10.1016/j.jacc.2009.02.078.
16. Clemens KE, Quednau I, Klaschik E. Use of oxygen and opioids in the palliation of dyspnoea in hypoxic and non-hypoxic palliative care patients: a prospective study. Support Care Cancer. 2009;17:367–77.
17. Cheng HWB, Sham MW, Chan KY, Li CS, Au HY, Yip T. Combination therapy with low-dose metolazone and furosemide: a "needless" approach in managing refractory fluid overload in elderly renal failure patients under palliative care. Int Urol Nephrol. 2014;46:180. doi:10.1007/s11255-014-0724-z9-1813.
18. Frohlich H, Katus HA, Tager T, Lossnitzer N, Leonie G, Kihm L, Zeier M, Remppis A, Frankenstein L, Schwenger V. Peritoneal ultrafiltration in end-stage chronic heart failure. Clin Kindey J. 2015;8:219–25.
19. Fukuta H, Goto T, Wakami K, Ohte N. Effects exercise of drug and intervention on functional capacity and quality of life in heart failure with preserved ejection fraction: a meta-analysis of randomized controlled trials. Eur J Prev Cardiol. 2016;23(1):78–85. doi:10.1177/2047487314564729 (Epub 2014 Dec 17)
20. Cohen RS, Mubashir A, Wajahat R, Mani S, Hummel S, Maurer MS. The cardio-renal-anemia syndrom in elderly subjects with heart failure and a normal ejection fraction: a comparison with heart failure and low ejection fraction. Congest Heart Fail. 2006;12(4):186–91.
21. Hedayati SS, Finkelstein FO. Epidemiology, diagnosis, and management of depression in patients with CKD. Am J Kidney Dis. 2009;54(4):741–52. doi:10.1053/j.ajkd.2009.05.003.

22. Hedayati SS, Jiang W, O'Connor CM, et al. The association between depression and chronic kidney disease and mortality among patients hospitalized with congestive heart failure. Am J Kidney Dis. 2004;44:207–15.
23. O'Connor CM, Jiang W, Kuchibhatla M, et al. Safety and efficacy of sertraline for depression in patients with heart failure: results of the SADHART-CHF (sertraline against depression and heart disease in chronic heart failure) trial. J Am Coll Cardiol. 2010;56:692–9.
24. www.who.int/mediacenter/factsheets/fs402/en/ last updated July 2015. Accessed 12/18/15.
25. Temel JS, Geer JA, Muzikansky A, Gallagher ER, Admane A, Jackson VA, et al. Early palliatieve care for patients with metastatic non-small-cell lung cancer. NEJM. 2010;363(8):733–42.
26. Mentz R, Tulsky J, Granger B, Anstrom K, Adams P, Dodson G. The palliative care in heart failure trial: rationale and design. Am Heart J. 2014;168(5):645–51.
27. Baumann AJ, Wheeler DO, James MJ, Turner RN, Roberta MD, Siegel A, Navarro V. Benefit of early palliative care in end stage liver disease patients awaiting transplantation. JPSM. 2015;50 (6):882–6.
28. Hupcey JE. The state of palliative care and heart failure. Heart Lung J Acute Crit Care. 2012;41(6):529.
29. Bakitas M, MacMartin M, Trzepkowski K, Robert A, Jackson L, Brown J, Dionne-Odom J, Kono A. Palliative care for heart failure patients: how many, when and why? J Cardiac Fail. 2013; 19(3):193.
30. Greener DT, Quill T, Amir O, Szydlowski J, Gramling RE. Palliative care referal among patients hospitalized with advanced heart failure. J Palliat Med. 2014;17(10):1115–20. doi:10.1089/jpm.2013.0658.
31. Gallagher R, Kimel G. Letter to the editor: palliative care for heart failure: more than is written. Can J Cardiol. 2011;27:871-e7.
32. Moss AH, Lunney JR, Culp S, Auber M, Kurian S, Rogers J, Dower J, Abraham J. Prognostic significance of the "surprise" question in cancer patients. J Palliat Med. 2010;13(7):837–40.
33. Schneider N, Oster P, Hager K, Klindtworth K. Identifying elderly heart failure patients at the end of life. Int J Cardiol. 2011;153 (1):98–9. doi:10.1016/j.ijcard.2011.09.018 (Epub 2011 Oct 2)
34. Bernacki RE, Block SD. Communication about serious illness care goals a review and synthesis of best practices. JAMA Internal Med. 2014;174(12):1994–2003. doi:10.1001/jamainternmed.2014.5271.
35. Lemond L, Allen LA. Palliative care and hospice in advanced heart failure. Prog Cardiovasc Dis. 2011;54(2):168–78. doi:10.1016/j.pcad.2011.03.012.
36. Connors AF, Dawson NV, Desbiens NA, et al. A controlled trial to improve care for seriously ill hospitalized patients. The study to understand prognoses and preferences for outcomes and risks of treatments (SUPPORT). The SUPPORT principal investigators. JAMA. 1995;274(20):1591–8.
37. You J, Downar J, Fowler R, Lamontagne F, Ma I, Jayaraman D. Barriers to goals of care discussions with seriously ill hospitalized patients and their familiesa multicenter survey of clinicians. JAMA Internal Med. 2015;175(4):549–56. doi:10.1001/jamainternmed.2014.7732.
38. Cordasco KM. Obtaining informed consent from patients: brief update review. Rockville (MD): Agency for Healthcare Research and Quality (US); Making Health Care Safer II: An Updated Critical Analysis of the Evidence for Patient Safety Practices. Evidence Reports/Technology Assessments, No. 211. 2013. Chap. 39.
39. Kleinman A, Eisenberg L, Good B. Culture, illness, and care: clinical lessons from anthropologic and cross-cultural research. Ann Intern Med. 1978;88(2):251–8.
40. Pollock K. Is home always the best and preferred place of death? BMJ. 2015;351:4855. doi:10.1136/bmj.h4855.
41. Holley JL. Advance care planning in ESRD/CKD: an evolving process. Clin J Am Soc Nephrol. 2012;7:1033–8. doi:10.2215/CJN.00580112.
42. Fagerlin A, Schneider CE. Enough: the failure of the living will. Hastings Cent Rep. 2004;34(2):30–42.
43. Wong SP, Kreuter W, O'Hare AM. Treatment intensity at the end of life in older adults receiving long-term dialysis. Arch Intern Med. 2012;172(8):661–3.
44. http://www.nhpco.org/hospice-statistics-research-press-room/facts-hospice-and-palliative-care. Accessed 15 Jan 2015.
45. http://www.nhpco.org/history-hospice-care.
46. Fast Fact #82 Medicare Hospice Benefit-Part I: Eligibility and Treatment Plan www.mypcnow.org.
47. Fast Fact and concept #87 Medicare Hospice Benefit-Part II: Places of care and Funding, www.mypcnow.org.
48. Teno JM, Clarridge BR, Casey V, Welch LC, Wetle T, Shield R, Mor V. Family perspectives on end-of-life care at the last place of care. JAMA. 2004;291(1):88.
49. Wright AA, Keating NL, Balboni TA, Matulonis UA, Block SD, Prigerson HG. Place of death: correlations with quality of life of patients with cancer and predictors of bereaved caregivers' mental health. J Clin Oncol. 2010;28(29):4457.
50. Burton AM, Sautter JM, Tulsky JA, Lindquist JH, Hays JC, Olsen MK, Zimmerman SI, Steinhauser KE. Burden and well-being among a diverse sample of cancer, congestive heart failure, and chronic obstructive pulmonary disease caregivers. J Pain Symptom Manag. 2012;44(3):410–20. doi:10.1016/j.jpainsymman.2011.09.018 (Epub 2012 Jun 22).

Part IV

Cardiac Evaluation of the Renal Transplant Candidate

Screening Strategies for Coronary Artery Disease (CAD) in Candidates for Kidney Transplants

20

Guilherme Vianna Silva, John D. Allison, and Francisco Yuri Bulcao Macedo

Introduction

As the age of the American population increases, so does the incidence of many chronic medical conditions, including cardiovascular disease and chronic kidney disease. In a worrisome trend, the number of new cases of CKD among Medicare patients doubled from the year 2000–2008 [1]. And while in 2011 the number of patients enrolled in the US End Stage Kidney Disease (ESKD) program reached an all-time high of 615,899, the incidence of ESKD in the United States has levelled off at 350 cases per million since 2001 [2]. This interesting discordance is not completely understood, but improved survival from non-renal diseases, such as cardiovascular disease, has definitely played a role.

As of January, 2016, there were 100,791 people awaiting a kidney transplant in the US. While more than 17,000 transplants will be performed in 2016, unfortunately, every year, up to 9500 potential recipients die before receiving the transplant or become too sick to undergo the operation [3, 4].

Among those patients awaiting transplant, as well as all ESKD patients, coronary artery disease is a major cause of morbidity and mortality. At the time of diagnosis of ESKD, 40% of patients already have ischemic heart disease, with the incidence of acute coronary syndrome being 2.9% per year [5, 6]. Ultimately, cardiac disease accounts for 45% of all ESKD deaths.

Its no surprise that cardiovascular disease is so prevalent within the ESKD population.

Many risk factors independently predispose patients to both cardiovascular and kidney disease and include hypertension, diabetes, advanced age, sedentary lifestyle, and certain autoimmune diseases. In addition, the physiologic changes that occur when the kidneys fail, as well as when we try to replicate their function, further increase the risk for cardiovascular disease. For example, uremia and the process of hemodialysis itself, result in oxidative stress and increased levels of C-reactive protein, which indicates inflammation and has been shown to enhance risk for cardiovascular death [7]. Furthermore, dysfunction in calcium metabolism, as well as the administration of phosphate binders, causes calcium deposition in the coronary arteries and increased atherosclerosis. As such, guidelines from both the National Kidney Foundation and the American Heart Association recommend classifying ESKD as a cardiovascular disease equivalent [8, 9].

For most patients, a successful kidney transplant provides substantially longer survival and better quality of life. The adjusted risk reduction of acute myocardial infarction after a successful transplant is 17%, and the risk is further reduced among certain populations, such as recipients less than 65 years old and those that undergo transplant within 6 months of initiating dialysis [10]. This reduction in cardiac deaths has not been completely explained, but evidence exists that its in part due to improvement in left ventricular hypertrophy as well as vascular stiffness [11]. However, 30% of patients with a functioning transplant will still die of cardiovascular complications; it is the leading cause of death in the post-transplant patient [12].

Despite the heavy burden of cardiovascular disease in the pre and post-transplant patient, there are no consensus guidelines for the screening of CAD in these populations. In fact, the AHA/ACC guidelines simply conclude that "there is no strong evidence for or against routine cardiac screening of asymptomatic transplantation candidates" [13]. Screening for CAD has more uses than just determining whether it is safe to proceed with transplant. The data garnered by screening tests helps inform transplant patients of their pre and post-transplant risk for an ischemic event, as well as guide

G.V. Silva (✉) · J.D. Allison · F.Y.B. Macedo
Department of Medicine - Cardiology, Baylor College of Medicine, 6620 Main St., Houston, TX 77030, USA
e-mail: gvsilva@bcm.edu

J.D. Allison
e-mail: jallison@bcm.edu

F.Y.B. Macedo
e-mail: yuribulcao@gmail.com

J. Rangaswami et al. (eds.), *Cardio-Nephrology*,
DOI 10.1007/978-3-319-56042-7_20

medical decision-making to optimize post-transplant success. Although a universal screening algorithm does not exist, the proper risk stratification is of utmost importance for patient survival, as revascularization of patients at high risk for CAD has been shown to reduce cardiovascular events after transplant [14]. In fact, those patients found to have obstructive CAD on angiogram during the pre-transplant work-up have the same rate of cardiovascular events at 1 month AND 1 year as those with non-obstructive CAD or no angiographic evidence of CAD if revascularization is done [15]. Nearly all patients awaiting transplant have at least one cardiovascular risk factor other than CKD, usually diabetes. Combined with the universal perception that CKD patients are high risk for CAD, the randomized clinical trials necessary to create a screening protocol will likely never be performed. As such, in this chapter we explore the available CAD screening modalities as well as the evidence for their use in pre-kidney transplant evaluation.

Resting, Noninvasive Studies

History and Physical

Every initial patient–physician encounter begins with a history and physical exam. While necessary for many medical decisions, the information gathered from the H&P has shown to be limited in predicting ischemic events before and after kidney transplant. The process is made difficult by the often atypical features of ACS in ESKD patients, usually due to long-standing diabetes. For example, the most common presenting symptom of an acute myocardial infarction in ESKD patients is shortness of breath rather than chest pain [16]. Furthermore, many patients on the transplant list are too deconditioned to properly determine functional status. In one retrospective analysis of 229 patients that underwent angiography prior to kidney transplant, the only risk factor that predicted the presence of CAD was a known history of CVD [15].

Physical exam findings may also hint at CAD, but none independently predict ischemic event rates, and none can be used solely to determine whether a screening for CAD is required prior to transplant. These findings include signs of peripheral artery disease, evidence of metabolic syndrome, or new atrial fibrillation.

Risk scores can be a powerful tool for synthesizing data from the history and physical and stratifying patients to the correct risk group. When applied to potential kidney transplant recipients, the classic Framingham Heart Study score tends to underestimate the risk of ischemic events in patients on the transplant list as well as those that have undergone the operation [17]. As such, several attempts have been made to create risk scores targeted specifically at patients awaiting kidney transplant in order to determine who would benefit most from CAD screening. In a risk-stratification algorithm created by Lewis et al. [18], low-risk patients underwent no further cardiac testing prior to transplant while those with ≥ 1 risk factor (age > 50, insulin-dependent diabetes, abnormal ECG, or a history of either angina or congestive heart failure) were deemed high-risk and underwent stress testing and possible angiography. There was only one cardiac death in the low-risk group, and cardiac mortality was significantly lower in the low-risk group when compared with the high-risk group (1 vs. 17%, $p < 0.001$).

The history and physical are part of the basic patient evaluation that will be done on every initial encounter. The information gathered will help guide all clinical decisions, but more information is usually needed before deciding whether a pre-transplant patient requires CAD screening. Only in a very specific, low-risk, group as described above, can CAD screening be forgone with data from just the H&P.

Electrocardiogram

The resting 12-lead electrocardiogram is a simple, noninvasive, inexpensive test that has been used in pre-operative cardiac assessment for decades. Several studies have identified factors that have varying abilities at predicting CAD. In one study of asymptomatic, diabetic patients undergoing an ischemic cardiac work-up (that did not specifically look at ESKD or pre-transplant patients), Q waves on ECG were found to be strongly associated with a high-risk SPECT score (chi-square = 38.3, OR 3.92, 95% CI 2.54–6.04, $p < 0.001$) [19]. In type-1 insulin-dependent diabetic patients awaiting transplant, abnormal ST-T segments (defined as ST-T segment elevation or depression >1 mm, or inverted T-waves in any lead where the QRS-complex had a net positive deflection), were independently predictive of CAD when confirmed by angiography (OR 5.7, 95% CI 1.5–21.5, $p < 0.05$) [14].

Although an abnormal ECG is capable of predicting CAD in pre-transplant patients to some degree, a normal ECG can be used to help exclude CAD in certain patients. In fact, in type-1 diabetic patients awaiting transplant that are less than 45 years old, have no smoking history, and have had diabetes less than 25 years, the absence of ST-T wave changes predicts that there will be no evidence of CAD on angiogram with a sensitivity of 97% and a negative predictive value of 96% [14].

Additionally, because the ECG is so widely available and easy to perform on almost all patient populations, this simple test can be done serially during the pre-transplant work-up, and continue while the patient awaits the operation. If changes are detected, the course of the ischemic evaluation may be altered.

A resting ECG is a reasonable test to perform on all patients awaiting kidney transplant. Signs of ischemia as defined above will likely necessitate more advanced or invasive testing for confirmation, but a normal ECG, when combined with other clinical factors, can suggest that no further testing is needed, and the transplant can proceed.

Transthoracic Echocardiogram

The transthoracic echocardiogram (TTE) is a more cumbersome test than the ECG and is not typically used as a screening tool for CAD. Nonetheless, many ESKD patients already have a TTE simply because the National Kidney Foundation recommends that it be performed within several months of starting dialysis [20]. Unfortunately, due to a long history of diabetes and/or hypertension, many ESKD patients can have abnormal TTE findings, such as left ventricular hypertrophy or increased LV size, that do not necessarily indicate coronary artery disease. In diabetic patients, resting wall motion abnormalities (WMAs) are associated with more ischemic events, and in patients without a known history of CAD, resting WMAs often correlate with abnormal stress imaging [21, 22].

However, currently, no studies exist that compare TTE findings suggestive of ischemia in potential kidney transplant recipients with confirmed CAD on angiography or with pre or post-transplant coronary events. However, in one study of liver transplant recipients, increased pulmonary artery systolic pressure was associated with significantly increased risk of hospitalization for myocardial infarction or heart failure (subhazard ratio per 5 mm Hg increase in PASP, 1.79; 95% CI 1.48–2.17; $p < 0.001$), but it is unclear how, or if, this information can be used to guide CAD screening in patients awaiting kidney transplant [23].

The resting echocardiogram can be used to assess change in clinical status of those awaiting transplant, such as new onset shortness of breath, but there is no evidence for its use as a CAD screening modality prior to kidney transplant. More data is needed, but it is unlikely that the TTE will replace more sophisticated stress testing or angiography when screening for coronary artery disease in patients undergoing kidney transplant work-up.

Coronary Artery Calcium Score

In the general population, long-standing diabetes and hypertension results in the build-up of calcium containing atherosclerotic plaques within the intima of the coronary arteries. Since the 1980s, electron-beam CT, and now non-contrast multidetector CT, has been used to measure this calcium to create a coronary artery calcium (CAC) score. Multiple studies have shown that CAC is proportional to adverse cardiovascular events [24, 25].

As discussed previously, however, traditional risk factors for CAD are not the only proposed culprits for the higher prevalence of ischemic heart disease among patients with ESKD. Dysfunctional calcium and phosphate metabolism results in abnormal deposition of calcium in not only the intima, but also the media of the coronary arteries which is not seen in patients with intact renal function [26]. It follows, then, that while the CAC is higher for patients with ESKD than with age and sex matched controls [27], some of the calcium is deposited within the media and, thus, not necessarily contributing to occlusive plaques. As such, while some studies have correlated CAC with cardiovascular events in patients with ESKD, the CAC cutoff required to predict these outcomes was substantially higher than the generally accepted normal values [28, 29]. Conversely, a CAC of zero in patients with ESKD has a negative predictive value of 88% for significant luminal stenosis on coronary angiography [30].

Attempts to demonstrate a relationship between CAC and degree of ischemic disease in ESKD patients have produced inconsistent results. In one study that included dialysis patients as well post-transplant patients, CAC was proportional to extent of plaque burden on angiography, but the mean CAC in patient with an abnormal angiogram was 2870 U [31]. Ultimately, large clinical trials in the ESKD population need to be performed to determine CAC score cutoffs that optimize the sensitivity and specificity of this test by correlating the results with angiography, stress testing, or ischemic events.

It is important to note that while CAC may be able to predict cardiovascular events, there is no data to support that screening for CAD with CAC improves cardiac outcomes, particularly in patients with ESKD that are awaiting transplant. A low CAC (<20) can help exclude significant ischemic disease, but given pathophysiology of ESKD, very few patients on the transplant list are likely to have such little calcium deposition. CAC alone is not an effective method to screen for CAD in the pre-transplant patient, but combination with other modalities, such as SPECT, may increase its sensitivity and specificity.

Coronary Computed Tomographic Angiography

Historically, the utility of coronary computed tomographic angiography (CCTA) has been limited by the technology behind it. Older detectors were limited by high rates of artifact due to fast heart rates, inadequate breath holding, or extensive calcification that deemed many coronary segments "non-evaluable." The new generation of machines, however, addresses these concerns, and a recent study suggests that the specificity of detecting obstructive CAD in the intermediate risk group of the general population is the same as other noninvasive tests such as SPECT and stress echocardiogram (83%), while the sensitivity is higher (95%) [32].

When applied to patients with ESKD, though, the same characteristic that limits the use of CAC in those awaiting kidney transplant also limits the use of CCTA: increased calcium burden. Dialysis patients are more likely to have diffuse coronary calcification than control groups with intact renal function, but these calcifications are not necessarily occlusive; they may be located in the vessel media [33]. While the significance of the location of the calcium is debatable, most studies that the evaluate the use of CCTA in dialysis patients conclude that the sensitivity is on par with non-dialysis patients, but the specificity is lower, likely related to higher rates of false-positive results that is due to increased non-occlusive calcium [34, 35].

Nonetheless, in one small study, among patients with ESKD, extensive CAD by CCTA was associated with a 36% chance of experiencing a cardiovascular event, while none of the patients without significant CAD by CCTA reached that endpoint [36]. No studies have been done that review how CCTA affects rates of ACS following a kidney transplant.

Given the high sensitivity of CCTA in patients on dialysis, its role in screening for CAD during pre-transplant work-up is likely limited to the low-risk group. However, the necessity of intravenous contrast and risk of damaging any residually functioning nephrons in the already tenuous pre-transplant patient may make this testing modality less attractive than similarly accurate SPECT or stress echocardiogram.

Cardiac MRI

Cardiac magnetic resonance imaging (CMR) is quickly becoming a popular and powerful tool to assess cardiac chamber sizes and function. The addition of contrast enhancement allows healthy myocardium to be distinguished from fibrotic tissue, and increasingly well described patterns of gadolinium extravasation can be used to define the myocardial viability, which correlates to the likelihood of functional recovery after revascularization [37]. In particular, isolated subendocardial late gadolinium enhancement (LGE) is more likely to indicate reversible ischemia than transmural LGE [38].

Unfortunately, it is this same property of gadolinium extravasation that has the potential to induce nephrogenic systemic fibrosis (NSF), particularly in ESKD patients. This process is irreversible and potentially fatal. Although rare, the risk of NSF has precluded any large studies of contrast enhanced CMR being done in pre-transplant patients. Despite the risk, one study of pre-transplant ESRD patients that was focused on further classification of uremic cardiomyopathy found that subendocardial LGE was linked to cardiovascular risk factors, a history of CAD, and depressed ejection fraction [39]. Only a small portion of these patients had angiography, as it was not part of the study protocol, but subendocardial LGE appeared to be more strongly associated with a heavy burden of CAD than diffuse LGE [40].

Cardiac MRI is capable of detecting coronary artery disease in the general population, but it is not widely available, and thus, not routinely used for screening. More data would be needed to determine whether this technology is applicable to patients awaiting kidney transplant as there are no studies dedicated to correlating CMR findings suggestive of CAD to positive stress tests or angiography, but these studies cannot be recommended routinely at this time, given the risk of gadolinium induced nephrogenic systemic fibrosis and the potential to compromise the status of their transplant. Recent data looking at global, septal and mid-septal T1 relaxation times showed that these correlated with left ventricular mass indices in patients on hemodialysis when compared to controls [41]. Septal T1 times correlated with troponin levels and electrocardiogram corrected Qt intervals [41]. Similarly, peak global longitudinal strain correlated with left ventricular mass indices in the hemodialysis group, thus opening up alternate options in estimating myocardial fibrosis with cardiac MRi without the use of gadolinium.

Cardiac Biomarkers

Cardiac biomarkers are traditionally used to evaluate acute cardiac events (troponin for ACS and brain natriuretic peptide for heart failure exacerbations), but there is growing interest concerning their role in assessing cardiac status of asymptomatic patients, particularly for cardiac troponin in patients waiting for renal transplant.

In the asymptomatic potential transplant recipient, data supporting the use cardiac troponin T (cTnT) is inconsistent. In one study, cTnT was worse at detecting CAD than dobutamine stress echocardiogram, and when used in combination with DSE, lowered the sensitivity and specificity [42]. However, patients that had baseline elevation in cTnT had worse cardiac outcomes before and after transplant. In another study, increased cTnT not only correlated with mortality, but magnitude of elevation correlated with mortality rates [43]. Also notable was that only 2% of patients with normal cTnT level died during the follow-up period, and some classically high-risk patients had a normal cTnT, including patients with age > 50, diabetes, stress-induced myocardial ischemia, or depressed ejection fraction.

Cardiac biomarkers will continue to play an important role in assessing cardiac status in patients presenting with acute symptoms such as chest pain or shortness of breath. There are promising developments for the use of cardiac troponin T in the asymptomatic potential renal transplant recipient, but more studies need to be done with the goal of comparing this simple blood test to accepted screening modalities. Fortunately, the ease, availability, and cost of this test should make clinical trials feasible.

Stress, Noninvasive Studies

Exercise Stress Test

Despite its robust use in the general population, the exercise stress test (EST) has struggled to find significance in screening for CAD prior to kidney transplant. Many patients awaiting transplant are not candidates for the EST due to a very poor functional status and inability perform the required mets. Additionally, a long history of cardiovascular risk factors, or a personal history of CAD may have deemed the exercise ECG uninterpretable. Studies that have attempted to prognosticate exercise stress test results in the pre-transplant patient are limited by very high incomplete test rates due to failure to reach target heart rates, usually around 45% [44, 45]. Only 2 studies, with a total of 129 patients, have compared EST results to angiography in patients screened for CAD prior to kidney transplant, and these demonstrated a very wide range of sensitivity and specificity, 36–100% and 0–91%, respectively. The inconsistent results were likely due to failure to meet criteria for a diagnostic test [46, 47].

The exercise stress test is a simple test that can provide valuable information regarding CAD risk if done properly and to completion. There is scant evidence to support its use when screening for CAD in potential kidney transplant recipients, though, and the large studies necessary to determine its efficacy are likely not practical given the baseline characteristics of patients on the transplant list, most notably poor exercise tolerance.

Myocardial Perfusion Scintigraphy/Spect

There is a plethora of data regarding the efficacy of myocardial perfusion scintigraphy (MPS) at diagnosing coronary artery disease in potential kidney transplant recipients as well as its ability to predict adverse cardiovascular events both before and after transplant.

In one meta-analysis of 9 studies with 582 participants awaiting kidney transplant comparing MPS to angiography, there was a pooled sensitivity of 74% and specificity 70% [48]. Importantly, among diabetic kidney transplant recipients, a PPV and NPV of 34 and 96%, respectively, meant that 1 year after transplant, the group with positive stress results experienced more ischemic events (22.4 vs. 3.4%) than those with negative stress results. Rates of all cardiovascular events as well as all-cause mortality were also statistically significantly higher in the positive stress group [49].

And while the diagnostic accuracy of MPS appears to be moderately inferior to dobutamine stress echocardiography, the difference may not translate to a difference in cardiac outcomes. A recent large meta-analysis concluded that the relative risk of cardiovascular mortality did not vary between studies using MPS, DSE, or coronary angiography, though there was some weak evidence that angiography was better at predicting all-cause mortality [50].

The difficulty of interpreting the meta-analyses rises from the high disparity among the patient populations; little mention was made of how participants were chosen for the studies. In an attempt to further define who should be candidates for MPS versus other methods of screening, one study found that the only potential kidney transplant recipients to gain any benefit from the MPS results were those in the "intermediate risk" group [51]. These patients had ESRD plus one of the following risk factors: age $\geq$ 50, diabetes, or clinical CV disease. Patients with none of the above risk factors did well regardless of the results, while those with two or three risk factors had a higher rate of cardiac events independent of the MPS results. Using this risk-stratification strategy, it's estimated that roughly only 40% of patients on the transplant list qualify for MPS, and the remaining 60% can either forgo any further testing or go straight to angiography.

The chief concern for using MPS to screen for CAD prior to kidney transplant is the risk for false negative results. Should global ischemia be present, a significant possibility given the high prevalence of CAD and extensive personal history of risk factors in this population, there will be no discernible perfusion defect due to the universally decreased uptake throughout the entire myocardium. Additionally, patients with CKD have higher baseline levels of native adenosine that can potentially attenuate any difference in isotope perfusion [52].

There is strong evidence to support the use of myocardial perfusion scintigraphy when screening for coronary artery disease in patients awaiting kidney transplant. It can be effective at detecting CAD and predicting ischemic events following transplant. However, it performs best when used in the correctly risk-stratified patient, and caution must be applied as there is a risk for false negative results.

Dobutamine Stress Echocardiogram

The increasing prevalence of the use of dobutamine stress echocardiography (DSE) during the CAD work-up prior to kidney transplant is supported by a significant amount of literature that suggests DSE is not inferior to myocardial perfusion scintigraphy (MPS) in both detecting CAD and predicting cardiac outcomes in potential transplant recipients.

A meta-analysis of 13 studies (745 participants) that compared DSE to MPS and angiography found a pooled sensitivity of 79% and specificity of 89% [48]. While the sensitivity is not significantly higher for DSE than MPS, the improved specificity is likely because DSE does not depend on heterogeneity of myocardial perfusion to detect CAD, nor does it rely on human interpretation of perfusion defects.

Not only can DSE detect CAD with accuracy comparable to other methods, such as MPS, but an abnormal DSE is an independent predictor of cardiac events following transplant [53]. In fact, increased numbers of abnormal segments seen on DSE reflect increased risk of cardiovascular mortality after transplant. When compared to MPS and angiography, DSE was not inferior an inferior prognosticator of cardiac death in transplant recipients [50].

While DSE may perform similarly to MPS when screening for CAD in potential kidney transplant recipients, it can also provide additional information that is not available with MPS, such as left ventricular wall thickness, the presence of atrial fibrillation, and pulmonary pressures, which may help predict non-ischemic cardiac deaths. DSE can also be an attractive choice for stress testing over MPS due to its lack of ionizing radiation, particularly since many potential transplant recipients are on the waiting list for significant amounts of time and may end up getting several repeat studies. However, some patients are not candidates for DSE due to poor echocardiographic windows, and others are unable to reach target heart rate, which deems the test incomplete.

It is clear that DSE is an effective method of screening for CAD in patients awaiting kidney transplant, though currently available data does not suggest any obvious superiority of DSE versus MPS. Most likely, the decision to perform either test will rely on the capabilities of the transplant center as well as specific patient characteristics that may make either test not feasible.

Stress Cardiac MRI (Dobutamine and Adenosine)

The advantage of stress CMR over resting CMR is the ability to detect dynamic changes and see reversible areas of ischemia in real time. This relatively new technology can be performed with two different techniques. Adenosine stress CMR causes coronary vasodilation that allows myocardial perfusion defects to be visualized. Gadolinium is required, which limits its use in the CKD population due to the risk of nephrogenic sclerosing fibrosis as discussed earlier. Consequently, this section will focus on dobutamine stress cardiac MRI (DSCMR) which does not require gadolinium contrast.

In patients with normal renal function, DSCMR is an effective means of detecting CAD in the moderate risk group. One meta-analysis of 14 studies demonstrated a sensitivity of 83% and specificity of 86%, which is better than SPECT and similar to DSE [54]. Only one study has been done to test the feasibility and safety of DSCMR in patients awaiting kidney transplant, and the sensitivity and specificity were similar to that of the general population [55]. Furthermore, there was no significant difference in safety profile or inadequate results.

Dobutamine stress echocardiography and nuclear myocardial perfusion studies are less expensive and more available than DSCMR. Moreover, there is an abundance of data that correlates positive results in the two former tests to adverse cardiovascular events following kidney transplantation. Unlike MPS, though, DSCMR does not require ionizing radiation; and additional information gained from DSCMR but not available with MPS, such as LV wall thickness and valve function, may be predictive of non-ischemic cardiac mortality in patients with ESKD [56]. The results of DSCMR are also not effected by poor echocardiographic windows, as is the case with DSE.

Ultimately, DSCMR has the potential to be a powerful tool at screening for CAD in the moderate risk group of patients awaiting renal transplant. However, its limited availability and the lack of long term data demonstrating that screening with DSCMR can improve outcomes following transplant restricts its routine use.

Invasive Studies

Coronary Angiography

It is assumed that coronary angiography remains the gold standard for detecting coronary artery disease prior to kidney transplantation. Direct visualization of the plaque, quantification of the degree of stenosis, as well as the option for therapeutic intervention are comforting characteristics for the clinician. Data describing the benefit of angiography, though, is inconsistent. One study in pre-transplant patients found that the only predictor of cardiac death was coronary stenosis >70% [57]. Two other studies, however, both larger and more recent than the study just described, found that there was no survival difference between patients that underwent angiography and those that did not [58, 59]. An additional meta-analysis also found that angiography was not better at predicting cardiovascular death than MPS or DSE [50]. These seemingly contradictory results are likely due to patient disparity among, as well as unclear status at follow-up. Without guidelines, there was no agreement as to which risk factors qualified for angiography. Additionally, in de Lima et al. [57], there is no mention of how many patients underwent transplant during the follow-up period, which undoubtedly affects survival rates.

Prior to committing a patient to angiography, there needs to be a serious discussion of potential risks to the patient. The immediate risks of invasive angiography include stroke, dissection, arrhythmia, and possibly death. Perhaps most worrisome to the patient that is about to undergo potentially life-saving renal transplant, though, is the discovery of an occlusive lesion that requires intervention, and thus, the need for dual antiplatelet therapy (DAPT), and subsequent delay of surgery up to 1 year.

Historically, angiography has been the gold standard for detecting CAD. Improved imaging modalities and risk-stratification, however, may be equally effective in patients awaiting kidney transplant. The true benefit of invasive coronary angiography lies in its ability to perform simultaneous intervention on occlusive lesions. More studies need to be done to determine if revascularization improves survival while patients are awaiting transplant, as well as after the operation is completed.

Conclusion

Despite alarmingly high incidence of ischemic heart disease before and after kidney transplant, current guidelines for the screening of CAD in asymptomatic, potential kidney transplant recipients are limited to expert opinion and tend to be based on observational studies. The results of studies examining the usefulness of almost all screening modalities have been inconsistent, but the necessary clinical trials are not feasible due to the very high rates of cardiac death in this population. As new screening modalities come on the market, and older tests improve, we may become better at predicting cardiac deaths in this high-risk population. But no screening test can be recommended until a method of screening and intervention proves to decrease rates of ischemic events in patients awaiting transplant, which has yet to be done. Until that time, perhaps the best course of action is aggressive cardiovascular risk-reduction with measures such as blood pressure control, diabetes management, and weight loss.

References

1. National Institute of Diabetes and Digestive and Kidney Diseases. Kidney disease statistics for the United States [Internet] 2016 [cited 2016 May 22]. http://www.niddk.nih.gov/health-information/health-statistics/Pages/kidney-disease-statistics-united-states.aspx#23.
2. United States Renal Data System. USRDS 2013 annual data report: atlas of chronic kidney disease and end-stage renal disease in the United States. National Institutes of Health. National Institute of Diabetes and Digestive and Kidney Diseases. Bethesda, MD, 2013.
3. United Network for Organ Sharing. Data [Internet]. 2015 [cited 2016 May 22]. https://www.unos.org/data/.
4. Organ Procurement and Transplant Network. Data [Internet] 2016 [cited 2016 May 22]. |FCO|Hyperlink https://optn.transplant.hrsa.gov/data/.
5. Cheung AK, Sarank MJ, Yan G, Berkoben M, Heyka R, Kaufman A, Lewis J, Rocco M, Toto R, Windus D, Ornt D, Levey AS. Cardiac diseases in maintenance hemodialysis patients: results of the HEMO Study. Kidney Int. 2004;65(6):2380–9.
6. Trespalacios FC, Taylor AJ, Agodoa LY, Abbott KC. Incident of acute coronary syndromes in chronic dialysis patients in the United States. Kidney Int. 2002;62(5):1799–805.
7. Zimmermann J, Herrlinger S, Pruy A, Metzger T, Wanner C. Inflammation enhances cardiovascular risk and mortality in hemodialysis patients. Kidney Int. 1999;55(2):648–58.
8. Levey AS, Coresh J, Balk E, Kausz AT, Levin A, Steffes MW, Hogg RJ, Perrone RD, Lau J, Eknoyan G. National Kidney Foundation practice guidelines for chronic kidney disease: evaluation, classification, and stratification. Ann Intern Med. 2003;139 (2):137–47.
9. Antman EM, Anbe DT, Armstrong PW, Bates ER, Green LA, Hand M, Hochman JS, Krumholz HM, Kushner FG, Labas GA, Mullany CJ, Ornato JP, Pearle DL, Sloan MA, Smith SC Jr. ACC/AHA guidelines for the management of patients with ST-elevation myocardial infarction—executive summary: a report of the American College of Cardiology/American Heart Association Task Force on Practice Guidelines (Writing Committee to revise the 1999 Guidelines for the Management of Patients with Acute Myocardial Infarction). J Am Coll Cardiol. 2004;44(4):671–719.
10. Kasiske BL, Maclean JR, Snyder JJ. Acute myocardial infarction and kidney transplantation. J Am Soc Nephrol. 2006;17(3):900–7.
11. Ali A, Macphee I, Kaski JC, Banerjee D. Cardiac and vascular changes with kidney transplantation. Indian J Nephrol. 2016;26 (1):1–9.
12. Delos Santos RB, Gmurczyk A, Obhrai JS, Watnick SG. Cardiac evaluation prior to kidney transplantation. Semin Dial. 2010;23 (3):324–9.
13. Lentine KL, Costa SP, Weir MR, Robb JF, Fleisher LA, Kasiske BL, Carithers RL, Ragosta M, Bolton K, Auerbach AD, Eagle KA. Cardiac disease evaluation and management among kidney and liver transplantation candidates: a scientific statement from the American Heart Association and the American College of Cardiology Foundation. J Am Coll Cardiol. 2012;60(5):434–80.
14. Manske CL, Thomas W, Wang Y, Wilson RF. Screening diabetic transplant candidates for coronary artery disease: identification of a low risk subgroup. Kidney Int. 1993;44(3):617–21.
15. Lindley EM, Hall AK, Hess J, Abraham J, Smith B, Hopkins PN, Shihab F, Welt F, Owan T, Fang JC. Cardiovascular risk assessment and management in prerenal transplantation candidates. Am J Cardiol. 2016;117(1):146–50.
16. Sosnov J, Lessard D, Goldberg RJ, Yarzebski J, Gore JM. Differential symptoms of acute myocardial infarction in patients with kidney disease: a community-wide perspective. Am J Kidney Dis. 2006;47(3):378–84.
17. Kasiske BL, Chakkera HA, Roel J. Explained and unexplained ischemic heart disease risk after renal transplantation. J Am Soc Nephrol. 2000;11(9):1735–43.
18. Lewis MS, Wilson RA, Walker K, Wilson DJ, Norman DJ, Barry JM, Bennett WM. Validation of an algorithm for predicting cardiac events in renal transplant candidates. J Cardiovasc Risk. 2002;1(89):847–50.
19. Rajagopalan N, Miller TD, Hodge DO, Frye RL, Gibbons RJ. Identifying high-risk asymptomatic diabetic patients who are candidates for screening stress single-photon emission computed tomography imaging. J Am Coll Cardiol. 2005;45(1):43–9.
20. K/DOQI Workgroup. K/DOQI clinical practice guidelines for cardiovascular disease in dialysis patients. Am J Kidney Dis. 2005;45(4 suppl 3):S1–153.
21. Innocenti F, Bartalucci F, Boni V, Vicidomini S, Mannucci E, Monami M, Pini R. Coronary artery disease screening in type II

diabetic patients: prognostic value of rest and stress echocardiography. Diabetes Metab Syndr. 2014;8(1):18–23.
22. Elhendy A, van Domburg RT, Bax JJ, Roelandt JR. Significance of resting wall motion abnormalities in 2-dimensional echocardiography in patients without previous myocardial infarction referred for pharmacologic stress testing. J Am Soc Echocardiogr. 2000;13 (1):1–8.
23. Bushyhead D, Kirckpatrick JN, Goldberg D. Pretransplant echocardiographic parameters as markers of posttransplant outcomes in liver transplant recipients. Liver Transpl. 2016;22 (3):316–23.
24. Pletcher MJ, Tice JA, Pignone M. Using coronary artery calcium score to predict coronary artery disease events: a systematic review and meta-analysis. Arch Intern Med. 2004;28(164):1285–92.
25. Blaha MJ, Budoff MJ, DeFilippis AP, Blankstein R, Rivera JJ, Agatston A, O'Leary DH, Lima J, Blumenthal RS, Nasir K. Associations between C-reactive protein, coronary artery calcium, and cardiovascular events: implications for the JUPITER population from MESA, a population-based cohort study. Lancet. 2011;378(9792):684–92.
26. Bashir A, Moody WE, Edwards NC, Ferro CJ, Townend JN, Steeds RP. Coronary artery calcium assessment in CKD: utility in cardiovascular disease risk assessment and treatment? Am J Kidney Dis. 2015;65(6):937–48.
27. Braun J, Oldendorf M, Moshage W, Heidler R, Zeitler E, Luft FC. Electron beam computed tomography in the evaluation of cardiac calcification in chronic dialysis patients. Am J Kidney Dis. 1996;27(3):394–401.
28. Ohtake T, Ishioka K, Honda K, Oka M, Maesato K, Mano T, Ikee R, Moriva H, Hidaka S, Kobayashi S. Impact of coronary artery calcification in hemodialysis patients: Risk factors and associations with prognosis. Hemodial Int. 2010;14(2):218–25.
29. Drozdz M, Krasniak A, Podolec P, Chmiel G, Kowalczyk-Michalek M, Pasowicz M, Konieczynska M, Wicher-Muniak E, Tracz W, Sulowicz W. Cardiovascular calcification and five-years mortality in patients on maintenance hemodialysis. Przegl Lek. 2011;68:1162–5.
30. Sharples E, Pereira D, Summers S, Cunningham J, Rubens M, Goldsmith D, Yaqoob MM. Coronary artery calcification measured with electron-beam computerized tomography correlates poorly with coronary artery angiography in dialysis patients. Am J Kidney Dis. 2004;43(2):313–9.
31. Haydar AA, Hujairi NM, Covic AA, Pereira D, Rubens M, Goldsmith D. Coronary artery calcification is related to coronary atherosclerosis in chronic renal disease patients: a study comparing EBCT-generated coronary artery calcium scores and coronary angiography. Nephrol Dial Transplant. 2004;19 (9):2307–12.
32. Budoff MJ, Dow D, Jollis J, Gitter M, Sutherland J, Halamert E, Scherer E, Bellinger R, Martin A, Benton R, Delago A, Min JK. Diagnostic performance of 64-multidetector row coronary computed tomographic angiography of coronary artery stenosis in individuals without known coronary artery disease: results from the prospective multicenter ACCURACY (Assessment by Coronary Computed Tomographic Angiography of Individuals Undergoing Invasive Coronary Angiography) trial. J Am Cardiol. 2008;52(21):1724–32.
33. Jug B, Kadakia J, Gupta M, Papazian J, Derakhshani A, Koblik S, Karlsberg RP, Budoff MJ. Coronary calcifications and plaque characteristics in patients with end-stage renal disease: a computed tomographic study. Coron Artery Dis. 2013;24(6):501–8.
34. Park MY, Choi SJ, Kim JK, Hwang SD, Suh J, Seo HS, Kim DH. Use of multidetector computed tomography for evaluating coronary artery disease in patients undergoing dialysis. Nephrol (Carlton). 2011;16(3):285–9.
35. Winther S, Svensson M, Jorgensen HS, Bouchelouche K, Gormsen LC, Pedersen BB, Holm NR, Bøtker HE, Ivarsen P, Bøttcher M. Diagnostic performance of coronary CT angiography and myocardial perfusion imaging in Kidney Transplantation candidates. JACC Cardiovasc Imaging. 2015;8(5):553–62.
36. de Bie MK, Buiten MS, Gaasbeek A, Boogers MJ, Roos CJ, Schuijf JD, Krol MJ, Rabelink TJ, Bax JJ, Schalij MJ, Jukema JW. CT coronary angiography is feasible for the assessment of coronary artery disease in chronic dialysis patients, despite high average calcium scores. PLoS ONE. 2013;8(7):e67936. doi:10.1371/journal.pone.0067936.
37. Selvanayagam JB, Kardos A, Francis JM, Wiesmann F, Petersen SE, Taggart DP, Neubauer S. Value of delayed-enhancement cardiovascular magnetic resonance imaging in predicting myocardial viability after surgical revascularization. Circulation. 2004;110(12):1535–41.
38. Pfeiffer MP, Beiderman RW. Cardiac MRI: a general overview with emphasis on current use and indications. Med Clin North Am. 2015;99(4):849–61.
39. Mark PB, Johnston N, Groenning BA, Foster JE, Blyth KG, Martin TN, Steedman T, Dargie HJ, Jardine AG. Redefinition of uremic cardiomyopathy by contrast-enhanced magnetic resonance imaging. Kidney Int. 2006;69(10):1839–45.
40. Hakeem A, Bhatti S, Chang SM. Screening and risk stratification of coronary artery disease in end-stage renal disease. JACC Cardiovasc Imaging. 2014;7(7):715–28.
41. Rutherford E, Talle MA, Mangion K. Defining myocardial tissue abnormalities in end stage renal failure with cardiac magnetic resonance imaging using native T1 mapping. Kidney Int. 2016;90:845–52.
42. Sharma R, Pellerin D, Gaze DC, Shah JS, Streather CP, Collinson PO, Brecker SJ. Dobutamine stress echocardiography and cardiac troponin T for the detection of significant coronary artery disease and predicting outcomes in renal transplant candidates. Eur J Echocardiogr. 2005;6(5):327–35.
43. Hickson LJ, Cosio FG, El-Zoghby ZM, Gloor JM, Kremers WK, Stegall MD, Griffin MD, Jaffe AS. Survival of patients on the kidney transplant wait list: relationship to cardiac troponin T. Am J Transplant. 2008;8(11):2352–9.
44. Langford EJ, de Belder AJ, Cairns H, Hendry BM, Wainwright RJ. Non-invasive cardiac investigations in patients awaiting renal transplantation. J R Soc Med. 1997;90(3):136–7.
45. Ma MK, Zuo ML, Yap DY, Mok MM, Kwan LP, Chan GC, Siu DC, Chan TM. Chronotropic incompetence, echocardigraphic abnormalities and exercise intolerance in renal transplant recipients. J Nephrol. 2014;27(4):451–6.
46. Sharma R, Pellerin D, Gaze DC, Gregson H, Streather CP, Collinson PO, Brecker SJ. Dobutamine stress echocardiography and the resting but not exercise electrocardiograph predict severe coronary artery disease in renal transplant candidates. Nephrol Dial Transplant. 2005;20(10):2207–14.
47. Bennett WM, Kloster F, Rosch J, Barry J, Porter GA. Natural history of asymptomatic coronary arteriographic lesions in diabetic patients with end-stage renal disease. Am J Med. 1978;65(5):779–84.
48. Wang LW, Fahim MA, Hayen A, Mitchell RL, Baines L, Lord S, Craig JC, Webster AC. Cardiac testing for coronary artery disease in potential kidney transplant recipients. Cochrane Database Syst Rev. 2011;7(12):CD008691. doi:10.1002/14651858.CD008691.pub2.
49. Singh N, Parikh S, Bhatt U, Vonsiger J, Nori U, Hasan A, Samavedi S, Andreoni K, Henry M, Pelletier R, Rajab A,

Elkhammas E, Pesavento T, Vonsiger J. Cardiac stress as a risk-stratification tool for posttransplant cardiac outcomes in diabetic kidney transplant recipients. Transplantation. 2012;94 (12):1224–9.

50. Wang LW, Masson P, Turner RM, Lord SW, Baines LA, Craig JC, Webster AC. Prognostic value of cardiac tests in potential kidney transplant recipients: a systematic review. Transplantation. 2015;99(4):731–45.
51. De Lima JJG, Gowdak HHW, de Paula FJ, Ramires JAF, Bortolotto LA. The role of myocardial scintigraphy in the assessment of cardiovascular risk in patients with end-stage chronic kidney disease on the waiting list for renal transplantation. Nephrol Dial Transplant. 2012;27(7):2979–84.
52. Marwick TH, Steinmuller DR, Underwood DA, Hobbs RE, Go RT, Swift C, Braun WE. Ineffectiveness of dipyrimadole SPECT thallium imaging as a screening technique for coronary artery disease in patients with end-stage renal failure. Transplantation. 1990;49(1):100–3.
53. Bergeron S, Hillis GS, Haugen EN, Oh JK, Bailey KR, Pellikka PA. Prognostic value of dobutamine stress echocardiography in patients with chronic kidney disease. Am Heart J. 2007;153(3):385–91.
54. Nandalur KR, Dwamena BA, Choudhri AF, Nandalur MR, Carlos RC. Diagnostic performance of stress cardiac magnetic resonance imaging in the detection of coronary artery disease: a meta-analysis. J Am Coll Cardiol. 2007;50(14):1343–53.
55. Ripley DP, Kannoly S, Gosling OE, Hossain E, Chawner RR, Moore J, Shore AC, Bellenger NG. Safety and feasibility of dobutamine stress cardiac magnetic resonance for cardiovascular assessment prior to renal transplantation. J Cardiovasc Med. 2014;15(4):288–94.
56. Foley RN, Parfrey PS, Harnett JD, Kent GM, Murray DC, Barre PE. The prognostic importance of left ventricular geometry in uremic cardiomyopathy. J Am Soc Nephrol. 1995;5(12):2024–31.
57. De Lima JJ, Sabbaga E, Vieira ML, de Paula FJ, Ianhez LE, Krieger EM, Ramires JA. Coronary angiography is the best predictor of events in renal transplant candidates compared with noninvasive testing. Hypertension. 2003;42(3):263–8.
58. Hage FG, Smalheiser S, Zoghbi GJ, Perry GJ, Deierhoi M, Warnock D, Iskandrian AE, de Mattos AM, Aqel RA. Predictors of survival in patients with end-stage renal disease evaluated for kidney transplantation. Am J Cardiol. 2007;100(6):1000–5.
59. Patel RK, Mark PB, Johnston N, McGeoch R, Lindsay M, Kingsmore DB, Dargie HJ, Jardine AG. Prognostic value of cardiovascular screening in potential renal transplant recipients: a single-center prospective observational study. Am J Transplant. 2008;8(8):1673–83.

21 Cardiac Pre-operative Evaluation as an Opportunity to Optimize Risk Factors in Kidney Transplant Candidates

Amer Kasim Ardati

Introduction

Chronic kidney disease (CKD) is an independent predictor of death and major adverse cardiovascular events. Nearly half of all deaths in ESKD patients are due to cardiovascular causes. While renal transplantation clearly improves mortality and morbidity in ESKD patients, cadaveric waiting lists remain long and patients spend a considerable amount of time at high risk for CV events. Many patients considered for renal transplantation are referred for pre-operative cardiovascular risk assessment under the care of a cardiologist. While cardiology, nephrology, and transplantation societies have provided guidance on how to evaluate for s peri-operative risk and stratification, little emphasis is placed on what if any steps the risk assessor should take to address long-term cardiovascular threats. In this chapter we will review opportunities for intervention that may contribute to improved long-term cardiovascular health in patients awaiting renal transplantation.

Lifestyle Interventions

Modifiable life style factors are thought to contribute up to 90% of the population attributable risk of myocardial infarction [1]. Simple interventions to address diet, obesity, smoking status, and physical activity have conclusively shown to improve outcomes in the general population. Efforts to replicate the impact of life style changes in the CKD patient population have also shown promise.

A.K. Ardati (✉)
Department of Medicine, Jesse Brown Veterans Affairs Medical Center, University of Illinois- Chicago, 840 S Wood St M/C 715, 934 CSB, Chicago, IL, USA
e-mail: aardati@gmail.com

J. Rangaswami et al. (eds.), *Cardio-Nephrology*,
DOI 10.1007/978-3-319-56042-7_21

Obesity, Diet and Bariatric Interventions

The prevalence of obesity in patients awaiting kidney transplantation is 25% and rising [2]. While obese patients that receive a transplant enjoy a survival benefit compared to those who do not receive an organ, obesity has been associated with adverse post-transplant outcomes [3–6]. Moreover, being overweight or obese prior to transplantation is a strong predictor of increased weight following transplant [7]. Many transplant centers will defer renal transplantation in recipients with BMI > 40 kg/m2. Analytic modeling suggests that bariatric surgery may be more effective than diet and exercise alone in helping patients lose enough weight to achieve a BMI that allows for transplant [8]. A systematic review of weight loss interventions in patients with CKD shows that nonsurgical interventions can improve proteinuria, blood pressure, and renal function and that bariatric surgery can reduce glomerular hyper-filtration and improve hypertension control [9]. The pre-operative risk assessment visit is a good opportunity to address obesity and weight loss with the transplant candidate. Ideally, that management of obesity would be incorporated into the work-up and wait list protocol of the transplant program. Care should be taken to consider the unintended consequences of bariatric surgery. Malabsorptive interventions like the Rou-en Y gastric bypass may result in hyperoxaluria which can be nephrotoxic. Considerations should also be made for the impact of bariatric interventions on the pharmacokinetics of immunosuppressive agents [10].

Exercise

Chronic kidney disease and need for renal replacement therapy have been associated with reductions in exercise capacity and muscle mass. Reduced exercise capacity has been shown to be an independent predictor of death in patients on dialysis and appears to predict the need for post-transplantation ICU care [11, 12]. Predictors of poor exercise capacity include age, gender, hemoglobin, and diabetes [13]. Organized efforts to improve exercise capacity have shown benefit in both pre-dialysis CKD patients and those on renal replacement therapy [14–16]. Most striking is the finding that even low-functioning dialysis patients stand to benefit from exercise training [17]. While controversy exists as to which parameter of exercise capacity is the best predictor of events, it is universally established that interventions to improve physical stamina are safe and effective in this patient population [18]. While KDOQI guidelines recommend that patients perform 30 min of aerobic exercise almost every day of the week, hemodialysis providers are unable or are un-incentivized to provide structured counseling and interventions to promote regular activity [19, 20].

Patients being evaluated for renal transplantation should be counseled on the critical importance of regular physical activity. Transplant candidates with marginal functional capacity may be referred for formal cardiopulmonary exercise testing. Patients with severely impaired functional capacity should receive structured physical therapy and rehabilitation in order to improve their ability to survive the waitlist and succeed after transplant.

Smoking Cessation

Smoking is a known risk factor for cardiovascular disease, cancer, and death in the general population. Active smoking is an independent predictor of death in patients on renal replacement therapy awaiting transplant [21]. While active smoking also predicts graft failure or death in patients that achieve transplant, patients that have managed to quit smoking have similar graft survival to those that never smoked [22]. Tobacco abuse following transplant is also associated with markedly higher risk of malignancy compared to patients that never smoked and those that quit prior to transplant [23].

Active smokers should be explicitly counseled on the risk of continued smoking. Transplant programs should partner with smoking cessation counselors in order to optimize the chances of quitting. Former smokers should be congratulated on their hard work to quit and encouraged to maintain abstinence.

Recommendations

The pre-operative visit is an excellent opportunity to advocate for the institution of life-style interventions to improve outcomes. Transplant centers should consider the codevelopment of comprehensive wellness programs that incorporate cardiologists, bariatric specialists, dietitians, physical therapists, and smoking cessation counselors. The consulting cardiologist should take advantage of the preoperative visit to advocate for interventions to control weight, increase exercise, and quit smoking

Medical Interventions

Progressive CKD has been associated with the accumulation of concomitant traditional cardiovascular risk factors. Patients with moderate chronic renal disease (CKD Stage 3) are more likely to suffer a major adverse cardiovascular event such as stroke, myocardial infarction, or heart failure than they are to develop frank ESKD [24]. Real-world utilization of guideline recommended cardiac prevention strategies are grossly sub-optimal in the general CKD population and in dialysis patients in particular [24, 25]. The specter of cardiovascular morbidity and mortality in patients being considered for renal transplant should trigger aggressive efforts by the consulting cardiologist to take ownership of managing modifiable risk factors.

Dyslipidemia

Dyslipidemia is common in patients with CKD. Typical features include a reduction in HDL levels and HDL operating efficiency along with an increase in triglycerides [26]. Exposure to dialysis also appears reduce LDL particle size and intensify their pro-inflammatory tendencies [27, 28]. While lipids have been a clear culprit in accelerating cardiovascular disease in patients with ESKD, the ability to mitigate their effect has been elusive. Two contemporary randomized clinical trials have failed to show the efficacy of statin therapy to reduce cardiovascular events or death in patients on hemodialysis [29, 30]. The 4D trial, which involved diabetic patients on hemodialysis randomized to atorvastatin 20 mg or placebo was negative for its primary end-point of cardiovascular death, nonfatal MI, or stroke. A subsequent post hoc analysis of this trial suggested that patients differed significantly in their intestinal absorption of cholesterol and that patients with low cholesterol absorption enjoyed a significant hazard reduction while on statin therapy [31]. Overall, it appears that statins have little or no beneficial effect in unselected dialysis patients [32].

Clinical trials that included patients with advanced CKD but not yet on dialysis have shown that lipid treatment can positively impact cardiovascular events [33, 34]. Additionally, fluvastatin has been shown to be effective in reducing cardiovascular death in otherwise low cardiovascular risk kidney transplant recipients [35].

The overall message on lipid interventions in renal transplant candidates is that those that have not yet transitioned to needing renal replacement therapy should be offered statins aggressively given the demonstrated outcome benefits. Patients currently on dialysis should be treated with caution, reserving statin therapy as a secondary prevention measure in those that have demonstrated active arterial disease. Finally, those patients who do achieve transplant should be offered statin therapy with careful consideration to drug–drug interactions between different statins and immune-suppressive therapies.

Hypertension

Hypertension is a powerful independent contributor to cardiovascular morbidity and mortality in the ESKD patient population. Despite the clear evidence of hypertension's deleterious role, hypertension recognition and management is sub-optimal in patients with advanced CKD. In a random sample from the NHANES prospective cohort of all-comers in the United States 17% of patients with Stages 3–5 CKD had undiagnosed hypertension, and only 44% of those diagnosed had achieved adequate blood pressure control with treatment [24]. In the CRIC prospective cohort of CKD patients only 64% of those with an eGFR of <30 ml/min/1.73 m^2 had been treated to a blood pressure of <140/90 mmHg and only 45% had reached the more stringent target of <130/80 mmHg. Age, black race, and high urine albumin excretion were predictive of sub-optimal blood pressure control, while treatment with ACE inhibitors was associated with an increased likelihood of being on target [36].

The impact of the anti-hypertensive therapy demonstrated in the general population appears to apply to those with CKD. In a meta-analysis of 26 randomized trials on the impact of anti-hypertensives in over 150,000 patients, the presence of renal insufficiency did not impact the 13% hazard reduction obtained for each 5 mmHg of reduction of systolic blood pressure. When looking at dialysis patients specifically studies have shown that use of blood pressure reducing agents in hypertensive patients is associated with a robust halving of the hazard of major adverse cardiovascular events [37]. Another meta-analysis of 1571 dialysis patients randomized to blood pressure treatment versus controls has shown that treatment was associated with a 29% relative reduction of cardiovascular mortality risk [38].

Blood pressure control in ESKD patients can be challenging due to changes in vascular biology resulting in increased arterial stiffness, a marker of which is independently associated with mortality [39]. Additionally, poor vascular compliance and inadequate sympathetic response can result in the inability to adequately compensate for volume shifts during dialysis resulting in symptomatic intra-dialytic hypotension [40]. Nephrology professional societies have provided valuable guideline recommendations on the goals of blood pressure control in patients on dialysis [19, 41]. Blood pressure targets should be <140/90 mmHg pre-dialysis and <130/80 mmHg post-dialysis. The initial target of therapy should be to optimize volume and sodium balance by helping the patient commit to salt restriction and water intake control. The dialysis center should work with the patient to reach and consistently maintain their dry weight. Possible interventions include more frequent or longer dialysis sessions. In the absence of a comorbidity, requiring the use of a specific anti-hypertensive ACE inhibitors or ARB are the recommended first-line agents, followed by calcium channel blockers. Third line agents include beta-blockers and clonidine. Dosing of anti-hypertensives at bedtime may help eliminate intra-dialytic hypotension. Notably, a recent prospective randomized clinical trial has found that spironolactone 25 mg daily can reduce major adverse cardiac events by over 50% in Japanese hemodialysis patients [42].

Antiplatelet Therapy

The impact of ESKD and dialysis on hemostasis is complex and associated with both an increased risk of bleeding and thrombosis [43]. Aspirin is underused in dialysis patients that carry either primary or secondary prevention indications for anti-platelet therapy [25, 44, 45]. Randomized clinical trials have not focused on the utility of aspirin for prevention of cardiovascular events in patients on renal replacement therapy. At this time the best data to support the safety and efficacy of anti-platelet therapies for cardiovascular risk reduction comes from pooled analysis of clinical trials that included patients with CKD and ESKD [46]. A pooled analysis of CKD patients included in anti-platelets clinical trials showed sizeable reductions in all-cause mortality, cardiovascular death, and myocardial infarction at the cost of an increase in the risk of bleeding complications. One contemporary randomized clinical trial that focused on the impact of aspirin in hypertensive patients with CKD showed reductions in major adverse cardiovascular events in general and myocardial infarction in particular and also suggested a magnification of benefits in those with eGFR < 45 ml/min/1.73 m^2 [47].

Anti-platelet therapies have consistently been shown to be effective in prolonging dialysis graft function [48–50]. Aspirin mono-therapy in particular was found to be a highly cost-effective measure to improve dialysis graft patency [51].

The risk of bleeding on aspirin is not negligible and may be as high as 4.4% per person per year of aspirin exposure [52]. Mechanisms to reduce the risk of aspirin related bleeding might include limiting the aspirin dose to 81 mg daily and concomitant use of a proton pump inhibitor [53, 54]. The impact of anti-platelet therapies on transplant related bleeding complications is less clear; however, one small study did suggest that use of ticlopidine or clopidogrel (often in concert with aspirin) did not impact the rate of bleeding during renal transplant [55].

In general, it is reasonable to recommend aspirin 81 mg daily for the promotion of hemodialysis access patency in all recipients who do not have a contra-indication to anti-platelet therapy. Renal transplant candidates with an indication for primary or secondary risk reduction with aspirin should be treated regardless of dialysis modality and advised of the risks and benefits at the time of pre-operative risk consultation.

Conclusions

The pre-operative consultation is a valuable opportunity for the renal transplant candidate and cardiologist to invest in long-term strategies to promote cardiovascular health. The dividends of investing in prevention appear to pay off while the patient is on the wait-list and extend beyond transplantation. Current data show gross under-utilization of preventive measures in ESKD patients. Future study should focus on documenting the efficacy of prevention strategies and optimizing the use of guideline supported intervention to reduce cardiovascular risk in this highly vulnerable patient population.

References

1. Yusuf S, Hawken S, Ôunpuu S, Dans T, Avezum A, Lanas F, et al. Effect of potentially modifiable risk factors associated with myocardial infarction in 52 countries (the INTERHEART study): case-control study. Lancet. 2004;364(9438):937–52.
2. Friedman AN, Miskulin DC, Rosenberg IH, Levey AS. Demographics and trends in overweight and obesity in patients at time of kidney transplantation. Am J Kidney Dis. 2003;41(2):480–7.
3. Bardonnaud N, Pillot P, Lillaz J, Delorme G, Chabannes E, Bernardini S, et al. Outcomes of renal transplantation in obese recipients. Transplant Proc. 2012;44(9):2787–91.
4. Gill JS, Lan J, Dong J, Rose C, Hendren E, Johnston O, et al. The survival benefit of kidney transplantation in obese patients. Am J Transplant. 2013;13(8):2083–90.
5. Grosso G, Corona D, Mistretta A, Zerbo D, Sinagra N, Giaquinta A, et al. The role of obesity in kidney transplantation outcome. Transplant Proc. 2012;44(7):1864–8.
6. Naik AS, Sakhuja A, Cibrik DM, Ojo AO, Samaniego-Picota MD, Lentine KL. The impact of obesity on allograft failure after kidney transplantation: a competing risks analysis. Transplantation 2016;100:1963–9.
7. Cofan F, Vela E, Cleries M, Registry CR. Obesity in renal transplantation: analysis of 2691 patients. Transplant Proc. 2005;37(9):3695–7.
8. Choudhury RA, Murayama KM, Abt PL, Glick HA, Naji A, Williams NN, et al. Roux-en-Y gastric bypass compared with aggressive diet and exercise therapy for morbidly obese patients awaiting renal transplant: a decision analysis. Surg Obes Relat Dis. 2014;10(1):79–87.
9. Navaneethan SD, Yehnert H, Moustarah F, Schreiber MJ, Schauer PR, Beddhu S. Weight loss interventions in chronic kidney disease: a systematic review and meta-analysis. Clin J Am Soc Nephrol: CJASN. 2009;4(10):1565–74.
10. Chan G, Garneau P, Hajjar R. The impact and treatment of obesity in kidney transplant candidates and recipients. Can J Kidney Health Dis. 2015;2:26.
11. Sietsema KE, Amato A, Adler SG, Brass EP. Exercise capacity as a predictor of survival among ambulatory patients with end-stage renal disease. Kidney Int. 2004;65(2):719–24.
12. Ting SM, Iqbal H, Hamborg T, Imray CH, Hewins S, Banerjee P, et al. Reduced functional measure of cardiovascular reserve predicts admission to critical care unit following kidney transplantation. PLoS ONE. 2013;8(5):e64335.
13. Sietsema KE, Hiatt WR, Esler A, Adler S, Amato A, Brass EP. Clinical and demographic predictors of exercise capacity in end-stage renal disease. Am J Kidney Dis. 2002; 39(1):76–85.
14. Deligiannis A, Kouidi E, Tourkantonis A. Effects of physical training on heart rate variability in patients on hemodialysis. Am J Cardiol. 1999;84(2):197–202.
15. Heiwe S, Jacobson SH. Exercise training in adults with CKD: a systematic review and meta-analysis. Am J Kidney Dis. 2014; 64(3):383–93.
16. Howden EJ, Coombes JS, Isbel NM. The role of exercise training in the management of chronic kidney disease. Curr Opin Nephrol Hypertens. 2015;24(6):480–7.
17. Painter P, Carlson L, Carey S, Paul SM, Myll J. Low-functioning hemodialysis patients improve with exercise training. Am J Kidney Dis. 2000;36(3):600–8.
18. Reboredo MM, Neder JA, Pinheiro BV, Henrique DM, Faria RS, Paula RB. Constant work-rate test to assess the effects of intradialytic aerobic training in mildly impaired patients with end-stage renal disease: a randomized controlled trial. Arch Phys Med Rehabil. 2011;92(12):2018–24.
19. K/DOQI Workgroup. K/DOQI clinical practice guidelines for cardiovascular disease in dialysis patients. Am J Kidney Dis. 2005;45:16–153.
20. Painter P, Clark L, Olausson J. Physical function and physical activity assessment and promotion in the hemodialysis clinic: a qualitative study. Am J Kidney Dis. 2014;64(3):425–33.
21. van Walraven C, Austin PC, Knoll G. Predicting potential survival benefit of renal transplantation in patients with chronic kidney disease. CMAJ. 2010;182(7):666–72.
22. Agarwal PK, Hellemons ME, Zelle DM, van Ree RM, van den Born J, van der Heide JJ, et al. Smoking is a risk factor for graft failure and mortality after renal transplantation. Am J Nephrol. 2011;34(1):26–31.
23. Opelz G, Dohler B. Influence of current and previous smoking on cancer and mortality after kidney transplantation. Transplantation. 2016;100(1):227–32.
24. Foster MC, Rawlings AM, Marrett E, Neff D, Willis K, Inker LA, et al. Cardiovascular risk factor burden, treatment, and control among adults with chronic kidney disease in the United States. Am Heart J. 2013;166(1):150–6.
25. Gowdak LH, Arantes RL, de Paula FJ, Krieger EM, De Lima JJ. Underuse of American College of Cardiology/American Heart Association Guidelines in hemodialysis patients. Ren Fail. 2007;29(5):559–65.
26. Harper CR, Jacobson TA. Managing dyslipidemia in chronic kidney disease. J Am Coll Cardiol. 2008;51(25):2375–84.
27. Vaziri ND, Navab K, Gollapudi P, Moradi H, Pahl MV, Barton CH, et al. Salutary effects of hemodialysis on low-density lipoprotein proinflammatory and high-density lipoprotein anti-inflammatory properties in patient with end-stage renal disease. J Natl Med Assoc. 2011;103(6):524–33.

28. O'Neal D, Lee P, Murphy B, Best J. Low-density lipoprotein particle size distribution in end-stage renal disease treated with hemodialysis or peritoneal dialysis. Am J Kidney Dis. 1996; 27(1):84–91.
29. Fellstrom BC, Jardine AG, Schmieder RE, Holdaas H, Bannister K, Beutler J, et al. Rosuvastatin and cardiovascular events in patients undergoing hemodialysis. N Engl J Med. 2009;360(14):1395–407.
30. Wanner C, Krane V, Marz W, Olschewski M, Mann JF, Ruf G, et al. Atorvastatin in patients with type 2 diabetes mellitus undergoing hemodialysis. N Engl J Med. 2005;353(3):238–48.
31. Silbernagel G, Fauler G, Genser B, Drechsler C, Krane V, Scharnagl H, et al. Intestinal cholesterol absorption, treatment with atorvastatin, and cardiovascular risk in hemodialysis patients. J Am Coll Cardiol. 2015;65(21):2291–8.
32. Palmer SC, Navaneethan SD, Craig JC, Johnson DW, Perkovic V, Nigwekar SU, et al. HMG CoA reductase inhibitors (statins) for dialysis patients. Cochrane Database Syst Rev. 2013;9:CD004289.
33. Baigent C, Landray MJ, Reith C, Emberson J, Wheeler DC, Tomson C, et al. The effects of lowering LDL cholesterol with simvastatin plus ezetimibe in patients with chronic kidney disease (Study of Heart and Renal Protection): a randomised placebo-controlled trial. Lancet. 2011;377(9784):2181–92.
34. Palmer SC, Navaneethan SD, Craig JC, Johnson DW, Perkovic V, Hegbrant J, et al. HMG CoA reductase inhibitors (statins) for people with chronic kidney disease not requiring dialysis. Cochrane Database Syst Rev. 2014;5:CD007784.
35. Holdaas H, Fellstrom B, Jardine AG, Holme I, Nyberg G, Fauchald P, et al. Effect of fluvastatin on cardiac outcomes in renal transplant recipients: a multicentre, randomised, placebo-controlled trial. Lancet. 2003;361(9374):2024–31.
36. Muntner P, Anderson A, Charleston J, Chen Z, Ford V, Makos G, et al. Hypertension awareness, treatment, and control in adults with CKD: results from the Chronic Renal Insufficiency Cohort (CRIC) Study. Am J Kidney Dis. 2010;55(3):441–51.
37. Agarwal R, Sinha AD. Cardiovascular protection with antihypertensive drugs in dialysis patients: systematic review and meta-analysis. Hypertension. 2009;53(5):860–6.
38. Heerspink HJ, Ninomiya T, Zoungas S, de Zeeuw D, Grobbee DE, Jardine MJ, et al. Effect of lowering blood pressure on cardiovascular events and mortality in patients on dialysis: a systematic review and meta-analysis of randomised controlled trials. Lancet. 2009;373(9668):1009–15.
39. Blacher J, Guerin AP, Pannier B, Marchais SJ, Safar ME, London GM. Impact of aortic stiffness on survival in end-stage renal disease. Circulation. 1999;99(18):2434–9.
40. Palmer BF, Henrich WL. Recent advances in the prevention and management of intradialytic hypotension. J Am Soc Nephrol JASN. 2008;19(1):8–11.
41. Jindal K, Chan CT, Deziel C, Hirsch D, Soroka SD, Tonelli M, et al. Chapter 2: management of blood pressure in hemodialysis patients. J Am Soc Nephrol. 2006;17(3 suppl 1):S8–10.
42. Matsumoto Y, Mori Y, Kageyama S, Arihara K, Sugiyama T, Ohmura H, et al. Spironolactone reduces cardiovascular and cerebrovascular morbidity and mortality in hemodialysis patients. J Am Coll Cardiol. 2014;63(6):528–36.
43. Lutz J, Menke J, Sollinger D, Schinzel H, Thurmel K. Haemostasis in chronic kidney disease. Nephrol Dial Transplant. 2014; 29(1):29–40.
44. Dempster DW, Rosenstock JL, Schwimmer JA, Panagopoulos G, DeVita MV, Michelis MF. Underutilization of aspirin in hemodialysis patients for primary and secondary prevention of cardiovascular disease. Clin Nephrol. 2005;64(5):371–7.
45. Chow FY, Polkinghorne KR, Chadban SJ, Atkins RC, Kerr PG. Cardiovascular risk in dialysis patients: a comparison of risk factors and cardioprotective therapy between 1996 and 2001. Nephrology (Carlton, Vic). 2003;8(4):177–83.
46. Palmer SC, Di Micco L, Razavian M, Craig JC, Perkovic V, Pellegrini F, et al. Effects of antiplatelet therapy on mortality and cardiovascular and bleeding outcomes in persons with chronic kidney disease: a systematic review and meta-analysis. Ann Intern Med. 2012;156(6):445–59.
47. Jardine MJ, Ninomiya T, Perkovic V, Cass A, Turnbull F, Gallagher MP, et al. Aspirin is beneficial in hypertensive patients with chronic kidney disease: a post-hoc subgroup analysis of a randomized controlled trial. J Am Coll Cardiol. 2010;56(12):956–65.
48. Dixon BS, Beck GJ, Vazquez MA, Greenberg A, Delmez JA, Allon M, et al. Effect of dipyridamole plus aspirin on hemodialysis graft patency. N Engl J Med. 2009;360(21):2191–201.
49. Harter HR, Burch JW, Majerus PW, Stanford N, Delmez JA, Anderson CB, et al. Prevention of thrombosis in patients on hemodialysis by low-dose aspirin. N Engl J Med. 1979;301(11): 577–9.
50. Hasegawa T, Elder SJ, Bragg-Gresham JL, Pisoni RL, Yamazaki S, Akizawa T, et al. Consistent aspirin use associated with improved arteriovenous fistula survival among incident hemodialysis patients in the dialysis outcomes and practice patterns study. Clin J Am Soc Nephrol CJASN. 2008;3(5):1373–8.
51. Nee R, Parker AL, Little DJ, Yuan CM, Himmelfarb J, Lowe SR, et al. Cost-effectiveness of antiplatelet therapy to prolong primary patency of hemodialysis graft. Clin Nephrol. 2014;81(1):38–51.
52. Holden RM, Harman GJ, Wang M, Holland D, Day AG. Major bleeding in hemodialysis patients. Clin J Am Soc Nephrol CJASN. 2008;3(1):105–10.
53. Hiremath S, Holden RM, Fergusson D, Zimmerman DL. Antiplatelet medications in hemodialysis patients: a systematic review of bleeding rates. Clin J Am Soc Nephrol CJASN. 2009;4(8): 1347–55.
54. Lim H, Kim JH, Baik GH, Park JW, Kang HS, Moon SH, et al. Effect of low-dose proton pump inhibitor on preventing upper gastrointestinal bleeding in chronic kidney disease patients receiving aspirin. J Gastroenterol Hepatol. 2015;30(3):478–84.
55. Benahmed A, Kianda M, Ghisdal L, Broeders N, Massart A, Lemy A, et al. Ticlopidine and clopidogrel, sometimes combined with aspirin, only minimally increase the surgical risk in renal transplantation: a case-control study. Nephrol Dial Transplant. 2014;29(2):463–6.

Revascularization in Patients on the Renal Transplant List: When and What Is Appropriate?

22

Pablo Rengifo-Moreno, Alexandre C. Ferreira, and Eduardo de Marchena

Background

According to the United States Renal Data System (USRDS) [1] cardiovascular disease is the leading cause of mortality in dialysis patients, accounting for 53% of all deaths. The presence of chronic kidney disease (CKD) or end-stage kidney disease (ESKD) contributes to worsening of other CVD risk factors, such as hypertension and dyslipidemia, leading to progression of coronary atherosclerosis. Moreover, diabetes, another major CVD risk factor, is one of the most important causes of CKD and ESKD in the United States [2]. The development of endothelial dysfunction combined with increased inflammatory mediators contributes to the accelerated atherosclerosis observed in CKD [3]. Also, an impaired calcium–phosphate metabolism contributes to the heavy calcification and worsening vascular injury, characteristic of these patients [4].

It has been well established that CVD continues to be the leading cause of mortality and morbidity following renal transplantation [5]. The mortality rate is higher than in patients on dialysis for the first 3 months, with the highest risk being during the first 2 weeks [6]. The fact that CVD is the main cause of mortality in the pre-transplant, peri-transplant and late post transplant period, underscores the importance of appropriate assessment of cardiovascular risk, pre-operative diagnosis of CVD and careful selection of patients who might benefit from revascularization prior to transplant.

Evaluation Prior to Revascularization for Patients in the Kidney Transplant List

Noninvasive Testing

The clinician should assess CVD risk during the initial evaluation and before anticipated transplantation, to determine interval changes in CVD conditions. "Active" conditions such as unstable angina, severe angina, recent myocardial infarction (MI), decompensated heart failure and significant arrhythmias are associated with high rates of perioperative cardiovascular morbidity and mortality. The presence of these conditions may require more investigation, and possible revascularization prior to transplantation [7].

Exercise endurance may predict cardiovascular events prior to non-cardiac surgery. In a cohort of 600 patients undergoing cardiovascular assessment, prior non-cardiac surgery subjects were asked to describe the number of blocks they could walk. Patients who failed to walk 4 blocks or climb 2 flights of stairs were considered to have poor exercise tolerance. Patients reporting poor exercise tolerance had more perioperative complications (20.4 vs. 10.4%; $p < .001$). Specifically, they had more myocardial ischemia, and more cardiovascular and neurologic events [8]. There is limited data available about the use of exercise capacity in combination to clinical findings and different study modalities as myocardial perfusión scintigraphy (MPS) and dobutamine stress echocardiography (DSE), to better risk stratify patients considered for kidney transplantation.

Despite inconsistent reports regarding the clinical utility of DSE and MPS in patients with ESKD (sensitivities between 0.44–0.89 and 0.29–0.92 and specificities ranging from 0.71 to 0.94 and 0.67 to 0.89, respectively) for

P. Rengifo-Moreno (✉)
Department of Medicine Phoebe Memorial Hospital, Medical College of Georgia, Augusta University, Albany, GA, USA
e-mail: Pablo.rengifo@gmail.com

A.C. Ferreira
Jackson Memorial Hospital, 3801 Biscayne Blvd Ste 230, 33137 Miami, USA
e-mail:aferreir@med.miami.edu

E. de Marchena
University of Miami Hospital, 1295 NW 14th St, South Bldg, Ste a, 33125 Miami, USA
e-mail:emarchen@med.miami.edu

J. Rangaswami et al. (eds.), *Cardio-Nephrology*,
DOI 10.1007/978-3-319-56042-7_22

identifying 1 or more coronary stenoses >70% [7], a meta-analysis of 12 studies involving either thallium-201 scintigraphy or DSE, found that patients with ESKD with inducible ischemia had approximately 6 times the risk of MI and 4 times the risk of cardiac death as patients without inducible defects [9]. Furthermore, those with fixed defects had 5 times the risk of cardiac death.

Although screening asymptomatic patient with CKD remains unproven, silent ischemia may be highly prevalent in CKD patients. In a study reporting symptoms during 256 percutaneous coronary interventions (PCI), silent myocardial ischemia, defined as the absence of chest pain in response to angioplasty, was present in 59.1% of the sample with CKD (defined as estimated glomerular filtration rate [eGFR] < 60 mL/min/1.3 m^2) compared with 29.1% without CKD [10]. Further, the symptoms of acute and chronic ischemia may differ in patients with ESKD compared with non-CKD patients. In the third National Registry of Myocardial Infarction, chest pain at presentation was reported less commonly among patients on dialysis compared with non–dialysis-dependent patients (44.4 vs. 68.3%) [11].

Diabetes, a major risk factor for CKD in pre and post transplant patients significantly increases the risk for CAD. Screening of asymptomatic diabetic patients may be challenging. The DIAD (Detection of Ischemia in Asymptomatic Diabetics) trial randomized 1123 asymptomatic patients with type 2 diabetes to MPS versus medical management without stress testing [12]. After a follow-up of over 5 years, the use of MPS screening had no effect on cardiac event rates.

Invasive Testing

There are multiple angiographic studies reporting a high incidence of significant coronary artery stenosis among patients undergoing long-term dialysis. In a prospective study of a group of 106 moderate-to-high risk patients, all of whom underwent coronary angiography prior to kidney transplant, the prevalence of CAD was 42% [13]. The probability of reaching the endpoint (major adverse cardiovascular events (MACE) defined as sudden death, MI, life threatening arrhythmia, heart failure, unstable angina and myocardial revascularization) at 1, 2, and 4 years was higher with angiographic CAD (13, 39, and 46%) versus (2, 6, and 6%) in the absence of CAD ($p = 0.001$). In a different cohort of 301 patients with ESKD on hemodialysis, significant CAD was identified in 136 individuals (45.2%). The presence of diabetes, peripheral artery disease (PAD) and previous MI were predictors of both CAD and MACE, defined as death, stroke, MI, and heart failure. The prevalence of significant CAD increased with the number of clinical predictors from 26% (absent risk factors) to 100% (all risk factors present) ($p < 0.0001$). The incidence of fatal/nonfatal MACE increased two, four, and sixfold in those with diabetes, PAD, or previous MI, respectively ($p < 0.0001$) [14].

However, other clinical studies have shown conflicting results in a similar population of patients. In a retrospective single-center study of 260 patients referred for kidney transplant evaluation studied by angiography, the presence and severity of CAD were not associated with crude survival among those who underwent angiography. The 2-year survival at follow-up was 80, 88, 86, and 78% for 0-, 1-, 2-, and 3-vessel disease ($p = 0.6$) [15]. Similarly, Patel et al., also in a single-center study, reported 99 patients who had angiography from a cohort of 300 subjects referred for kidney transplant evaluation. In the angiography sample, CAD prevalence was 57.6% (57 of 99), Obstructive CAD was found in 34.3% (34 of 99), including one, two and three-vessel CAD in 13, 15, and 6%, respectively. Revasculariation was performed in 17% (17 of 99) of the patients. Non-obstructive CAD was found in 23%. There was no difference in crude 4-year survival in patients found to have CAD and revascularized, compared with those who underwent angiography without revascularization [16]. Therefore, the benefit of coronary angiography and revascularization is still a matter of debate.

The lack of benefit of revascularization, at least in the non-CKD patient, has been associated to the challenging task of identifying flow limiting lesions and vulnerable plaque through angiography alone. The FAME 2 trial studied 1220 patients with stable coronary artery disease and ischemia, as shown by the presence of at least one stenosis with a fractional flow reserve (FFR) of 0.80 or less in a large epicardial artery. There was improvement in clinical outcome at 2 years by FFR-guided PCI with second-generation drug eluting stents plus the best available medical therapy, as compared with medical therapy alone. In patients without hemodynamically significant stenosis, best available medical therapy alone was associated with excellent 2-year clinical outcomes, regardless of the angiographic appearance of the stenoses [17]. Unfortunately, once more, CKD was under represented constituting only 3.5% of the total number of patients in the trial. Moreover, there are concerns that CKD/ESKD may be associated not only with impaired microcirculation, limiting the accuracy of FFR measurement, but also with rapid progression of CAD. Whether the presence of CKD may limit FFR accuracy is still unknown. An Italian sub-study of the FREAK trial, with 1004 patients undergoing FFR evaluation for intermediate stenosis, found FFR-positive measurement in 395 (39%) patients. Overall, 131 (13%) patients had CKD. Patients with CrCl $\leq$ 45 ml/min showed significantly higher FFR values as compared to the others (0.84 ± 0.07 vs. 0.81 ± 0.08, $p < 0.001$). Positive FFR occurrence was lower in patients with CrCl $\leq$ 45 ml/min (27 vs. 41%, $p < 0.01$). After multivariable analysis, diabetes (HR 1.07, 95% CI 1.008–

1.13, $p = 0.03$), left anterior descending artery (HR 1.35, 95% CI 1.27–1.43, $p < 0.001$) and CrCl $\leq$ 45 ml/min (HR 0.92, 95% CI 0.87–0.97, $p = 0.005$) emerged as independent predictors of FFR measurement [18]. These findings suggest a different response to vasodilation in patients with CKD when compared to controls. It is still unclear if a different protocol of vasodilation should be used in this population.

Intravascular ultrasound (IVUS) has been extensively used for plaque characterization and for identification of vulnerable atherosclerotic plaques. A gray scale IVUS study reported that hemodialysis patients have larger lesion plaque mass and more lesion site calcification, when compared with non-dialysis CKD patients [19]. An IVUS-Virtual histology (VH) study of 134 stable angina patients, suggested that declining renal function strongly affects plaque composition in diabetic patients [20]. Plaque characterization was compared between diabetics ($n = 65$) and nondiabetic group. Diabetic patients were further divided into four groups according to estimated glomerular filtration rate (eGFR, ml/min): eGFR $\geq$ 70 ($n = 20$), 50 $\leq$ eGFR < 70 ($n = 19$), GFR < 50 ($n = 18$), and ESKD on hemodialysis (HD) ($n = 11$). In this study there was no significant difference in plaque composition between the diabetic and the nondiabetic patients except for the percentage of dense calcium (8.9 vs. 6.2%; $p < 0.05$). In diabetic patients, the percent volume of necrotic core was 9.6, 11.4, 14.8, and 20.8% in the eGFR 70, 50 $\leq$ eGFR < 70, eGFR < 50, and the ESKD on HD groups, respectively, showing significantly higher percentage volume of necrotic core in eGFR < 50 ($p < 0.05$ vs. eGFR $\geq$ 70) and ESRD on HD group ($p < 0.001$). They concluded that diabetic patients have significantly larger amount of dense calcium than nondiabetic patients in non-culprit coronary artery segments, and the plaque components of non-culprit lesions in diabetics are significantly different according to the decline in renal function.

Optical coherence tomography (OCT) has recently been demonstrated to have higher resolution than IVUS. A recent post-mortem studied compared virtual histology alone with a hybrid method of invasive imaging that combines VH-IVUS and OCT, and found that the combination may be better than either modality alone at correctly identifying advanced atherosclerotic coronary plaques [21]. However, this method would consume more resources with only minimal improvement in the information obtained.

New imaging modalties continue to be developed to fulfill the unmet need of identifying vulnerable atherosclerotic plaques. Near-infrared spectroscopy (NIRS) is capable of identifying lipid core-containing plaques, which can subsequently be quantified as a lipid core burden index (LCBI). The ATEROMO-NIRS study sought to determine the long-term prognostic value of intracoronary NIRS as assessed in a nonculprit vessel in patients with CAD [22]. In this prospective, observational study, NIRS imaging was performed in a nonculprit coronary artery in 203 patients referred for angiography due to stable angina or acute coronary syndrome (ACS). The primary endpoint for this study was the composite of all-cause mortality, nonfatal ACS, stroke, and unplanned coronary revascularization, with the 1-year cumulative incidence of the primary endpoint being 10.4%. Cumulative 1-year rates in patients with an LCBI $\geq$ the median versus those with LCBI values below the median were 16.7 versus 4.0% (adjusted HR 4.04; 95% CI 1.33–12.29; $p = 0.01$). The relation between LCBI and the primary endpoint was similar in stable angina and ACS patients. Unfortunately, the prevalence of kidney disease in this study was only 6%, making it difficult to extend the conclusions of this study to the CKD and ESKD population.

In summary, the ESKD population has been underrepresented in contemporary trials addressing optimal revascularization strategies. New ongoing trials such as ISCHEMIA-CKD (see Chap. 30) addressing this specific question in patients with CKD and ESKD, will help fill this unmet need. Until robust data in this target population is available, patient selection for revascularization must be done after careful review of the clinical scenario, noninvasive and invasive data, ischemic burden, coronary anatomy, complexity of CAD and cardiac function, and the relative risks and benefits of guideline-directed medical therapy, CABG, and PCI.

Revascularization Strategies for Patients on the Kidney Transplant List

Current guidelines recommend revascularization with coronary artery bypass grafting in patients with multivessel disease, diabetics with multivessel CAD and unprotected left main [7]. There are no randomized clinical trials (RCTs) investigating revascularization strategies in patients with advanced kidney disease published at this time. Moreover, ESKD patients have been significantly underrepresented in revascularization trials. Therefore, currently, most of the evidence regarding revascularization for patients with ESKD, and patients on the kidney transplant list, comes from RCTs in patients with normal kidney function and from registry data.

In an early revascularization experience, a small cohort of 14 patients who underwent surgical revascularization from a large population of individuals with a functioning kidney transplant, found that surgical revascularization on these patients occurred at intervals of 9–144 months (mean 67 months) following their transplant. All patients had functioning renal allografts with preoperative serum creatinine levels ranging from 1.0 to 1.8 mg/100 ml (mean 1.4 mg/100 ml). Twelve patients underwent aorta-coronary saphenous vein bypass grafting. Two patients (14%) died perioperatively and one died at 45 months. Postoperative serum creatinine levels at hospital discharge averaged 1.6 mg/100 ml, not significantly changed from preoperative levels [23].

In a larger population of 45 patients (33 male and 12 female) who underwent open heart operations after previous renal transplantation, from which 31 patients received coronary artery bypass grafting, the interval between renal transplantation and cardiac operation was 57 ± 39 months (range 5 days–174 months). All patients had functioning renal allografts with preoperative serum creatinine levels ranging from 100 to 338 mol/mL (mean ± standard deviation, 195 ± 86). Early operative mortality (30 days) was 8.8%. Four patients had returned to hemodialysis at intervals of 27–83 months (mean 51 months) because of renal transplant failure [24].

Ono et al. reported another series of 46 patients with previous functioning kidney transplant who required surgical revascularization. Postoperative kidney dysfunction occurred in seven patients, three of them required temporary hemodialysis. No allograft loss was seen in early postoperative period but there was a statistically insignificant prolongation of hospitalization. By univariate analysis the factors found to adversely affect postoperative renal function included pulmonary hypertension, preoperative creatinine level, and non-elective surgery [25].

A registry analysis of kidney transplant recipients hospitalized from 1995 to 1999 for the first coronary revascularization procedure was retrospectively identified from the USRDS [26]. Their primary end points were event-free survival for all-cause death, cardiac death, MI, and the combined end point of cardiac death or MI. The outcomes were reported in 2661 renal transplant recipients hospitalized for the first coronary revascularization procedure (excluding concomitant valvular surgery) occurring after initiation of renal replacement therapy from January 1995 to December 1999, with follow-up through June 30, 2000. In the 2661 renal transplant recipients studied, the coronary revascularization procedures were as follows: bare-metal stent (BMS), 909; percutaneous transluminal balloon angioplasty (PTCA), 652; and CABG, 1100. Of those having CABG surgery, 288 had CABG without internal mammary grafts (CABG [IMG–]), and 812 had CABG with internal mammary grafts (CABG [IMG+]). All groups studied were similar in prior ESKD duration and time to revascularization after renal transplantation. In-hospital deaths occurred in each group: BMS, 21 (2.3%); PTCA, 28 (4.3%); CAB (IMG−), 27 (9.4%); and CABG (IMG+), 41 (5.0%). There was no statistically significant difference in survival related to type of coronary revascularization. However, a trend toward increased mortality rates was observed in CAB (IMG−) patients. Patients in the CABG group, particularly CAB (IMG+) patients, were less likely than other patients to reach the combined end point of cardiac death or MI. This more favorable outcome after surgery appears to be predominantly attributable to a reduced risk of MI. The most powerful predictors of death were older age (>75 years) (relative risk [RR] 2.10; 95% CI 1.19–3.70), diabetic ESKD (RR 1.72; 95% CI 1.42–2.08), congestive heart failure (RR 1.59; 95% CI 1.33–1.89). Both cerebrovascular and peripheral vascular diseases were associated with a 31% increased risk of death. There was a trend toward decreased risk for cardiac death and MI in CABG (IMG+) patients relative to CABG (IMG–) patients (RR 0.72; 95% CI 0.49–1.06; $p = 0.10$). In this study there was no difference in survival after surgical or percutaneous coronary revascularization procedures. The data also suggest that the most favorable long-term outcome (after adjustment for comorbid conditions) is associated with CABG, particulary with CABG (IMG+). However, this study compared CABG with BMS, which has a higher incidence of in-stent restenosis (ISR) [27].

Another study from the USRDS reported a cohort of 21,981 patients on maintenance dialysis with multivessel CAD who received initial coronary revascularization with CABG or PCI between 1997 and 2009 [28]. The primary outcome was death from any cause, and the secondary outcome was a composite of death or myocardial infarction. Overall survival rates were consistently poor during the study period, with unadjusted 5-year survival rates of 22–25% irrespective of revascularization strategy. Using multivariable- adjusted proportional hazards regression, they found that CABG compared with PCI was associated with significantly lower risks for both death and the composite of death or MI.

Drug eluting stents may offer some advantages over BMS in the CKD population. A systematic review of the literature and a meta-analysis of five studies comparing the outcomes of PCI with DES and BMS for ESKD patients on dialysis was performed between January 2002 and January 2009 [29]. The primary endpoints were mortality, myocardial infarction (MI) and target lesion revascularization (TLR), and the secondary endpoint was late luminal loss. In-hospital mortality and MI were also assessed. A total of 641 patients (279 DES, and 362 BMS) were included in the analysis. In-hospital clinical outcomes were similar between the two groups. At follow-up there was a trend toward lower TLR and decreased late luminal loss in patients undergoing PCI with implantation of DES. There was no difference in the rates of all-cause mortality, and MI between the two groups. They concluded that in ESKD patients on dialysis undergoing PCI, DES are safe and might reduce repeat revascularizations. Moreover, a larger meta-analysis of a similar but larger population of ESKD patients found significant reduction of combined TLR and target vessel revascularization (TVR) when using DES versus BMS [30].

In a recent study [31], a propensity-score matched population of patients with CKD who underwent PCI using everolimus-eluting stents were compared to patients who underwent isolated CABG for multivessel coronary disease in New York. The primary outcome was all-cause mortality with a secondary outcomes of MI, stroke, and repeat revascularization. From the entire cohort of 11,305 patients with CKD, a total of 5920 patients were propensity-score matched. The short term outcome revealed that PCI was associated with a lower risk of death, stroke, and repeat revascularization compared with CABG. A long-term analysis demonstrated that PCI was associated with a similar risk of death, higher risk of MI, a lower risk of stroke, and a higher risk of repeat revascularization. However, in the 243 matched pairs of patients with end-stage renal disease on hemodialysis, PCI was associated with significantly higher risk of death (HR 2.02; 95% CI 1.40–2.93) and repeat revascularization (HR 2.44; 95% CI 1.50–3.96) compared with CABG.

The SYNTAX trial randomly assigned 1800 patients to receive DES or CABG [32, 33]. Major adverse cardiac events (MACE), a composite of death, stroke, MI, or repeat revascularization during the 3 years after randomization, occurred in 20.2% of CABG patients and 28.0% of those undergoing DES implantation ($p < 0.001$). The rates of death and stroke were similar; however, MI (3.6% for CABG, 7.1% for DES) and repeat revascularization (10.7% for CABG, 19.7% for DES) were more likely to occur with DES implantation. In SYNTAX, outcomes were associated with the extent of CAD as assessed using the SYNTAX score, which is based on the location, severity, and extent of coronary stenoses, with a low score indicating less complicated anatomic CAD. The SYNTAX score predicted the occurence of MACE for DES patients, but not for those undergoing CABG. At 12-month follow-up, the primary endpoint was similar for CABG and DES in those with a low SYNTAX score. In contrast, MACE occurred more often after DES implantation than after CABG in those with an intermediate or high SYNTAX score. At 3 years of follow-up, the mortality rate was greater in subjects with 3-vessel CAD treated with PCI than in those treated with CABG (6.2 vs. 2.9%). The differences in MACE between those treated with PCI or CABG increased with an increasing SYNTAX score. The importance of the SYNTAX score for selection of CKD patients for surgical revascularization strategy is underscored in a retrospective analysis in which the SYNTAX score was calculated for 87 of 110 dialysis patients after coronary angiography. The SYNTAX score was found to be a powerful predictor of mortality and MACEs in dialysis patients undergoing percutaneous coronary intervention or coronary artery bypass graft during a 3-year follow-up [34].

Diabetes is one of the most important causes of CKD and ESKD in the United States [2]. The Future Revascularization Evaluation in Patients with Diabetes Mellitus: Optimal Management of Multivessel Disease (FREEDOM) trial was a prospective, randomized, multicenter superiority trial that compared the safety and efficiency of multivessel PCI with first-generation DES compared with CABG in 1900 diabetic patients [35]. The primary end point was a composite of all-cause death, nonfatal MI, and stroke. Three-vessel CAD was present in 83% of patients and the median SYNTAX score was 26, consistent with an anatomical complex population. PCI was performed with first-generation DES and 94.4% of patients assigned to CABG received a IMA graft. At 5-year follow-up, the primary composite end point occurred in 26.6% of patients randomly assigned to PCI compared to 18.7% of patients randomly assigned to CABG ($p = 0.005$), driven by differences in mortality (16.3 vs. 10.9%; $p = 0.49$) and MI (13.6 vs. 6.0%; $p < 0.001\%$). However, CABG was associated with an increased risk of stroke (2.4 vs. 5.2%; $p = 0.03$). It is unclear if this benefit of surgical revascularization persists or is augmented in the advanced stage diabetic population with CKD or dialysis.

In summary, revascularization decision for patients on a kidney transplant list represents a vexing problem. Surgical and clinical management relies heavily on trials designed to investigate revascularization on non-CKD populations or on retrospective analysis, underscoring the importance of designing trials investigating this question in CKD or CKD inclusive populations. Currently, guidelines recommend a heart team approach for deciding revascularization strategies on an individualized basis [7].

The vast majority of cardiovascular events happen during the first three months of kidney transplantation. Therefore, revascularization in high risk patients prior to transplant seems to be the most appropriate strategy. Even though multiple reports indicate that revascularization can be done safely after transplant, the current pre-operative cardiovascular protocols allows for early identification of CAD and treatment, avoiding the transplanted kidney to be exposed to nephrotoxic contrast, and ischemia due to hemodynamic instability. Based on the best data available, diabetic patients with multivessel CAD and patients with intermediate and high SYNTAX score, should undergo surgical revascularization, unless the surgical risk is prohibitive. As newer data on optimal revascularization strategies emerge, more specific patient selection for revascularization pre-transplant will hopefully optimize transplant potential, and contribute to superior short and long-term post transplant outcomes.

References

1. United States Renal Data System. 2015 USRDS annual data report: epidemiology of kidney disease in the United States. [Internet]. National Institutes of Health, National Institute of Diabetes and Digestive and Kidney Diseases. http://www.usrds.org/2015/view/v2_06.aspx.
2. Schiffrin EL, Lipman ML, Mann JFE. Chronic kidney disease: effects on the cardiovascular system. Circulation. 2007;116(1):85–97.
3. Amann K, Wanner C, Ritz E. Cross-talk between the kidney and the cardiovascular system. J Am Soc Nephrol JASN. 2006;17(8):2112–9.
4. Qunibi WY. Reducing the burden of cardiovascular calcification in patients with chronic kidney disease. J Am Soc Nephrol. 2005;16(11 suppl 2):S95–102.
5. Israni AK, Snyder JJ, Skeans MA, Peng Y, Maclean JR, Weinhandl ED, et al. Predicting coronary heart disease after kidney transplantation: Patient Outcomes in Renal Transplantation (PORT) Study. Am J Transplant. 2010;10(2):338–53.
6. Wolfe RA, Ashby VB, Milford EL, Ojo AO, Ettenger RE, Agodoa LY, et al. Comparison of mortality in all patients on dialysis, patients on dialysis awaiting transplantation, and recipients of a first cadaveric transplant. N Engl J Med. 1999;341(23):1725–30.
7. Lentine KL, Costa SP, Weir MR, Robb JF, Fleisher LA, Kasiske BL, et al. Cardiac disease evaluation and management among kidney and liver transplantation candidates: a scientific statement from the American Heart Association and the American College of Cardiology Foundation. J Am Coll Cardiol. 2012;60(5):434–80.
8. Reilly DF, McNeely MJ, Doerner D, et al. Self-reported exercise tolerance and the risk of serious perioperative complications. Arch Intern Med. 1999;159(18):2185–92.
9. Rabbat CG, Treleaven DJ, Russell JD, Ludwin D, Cook DJ. Prognostic value of myocardial perfusion studies in patients with end-stage renal disease assessed for kidney or kidney-pancreas transplantation: a meta-analysis. J Am Soc Nephrol JASN. 2003;14(2):431–9.
10. Almehmi A, Broce M, Wetmore J. Silent myocardiac ischemia is more prevalent in CKD patients undergoing multi-vessel coronary angioplasty (abstr). J Am Soc Nephrol JASN. 2009;20(Suppl):370A.
11. Herzog CA, Littrell K, Arko C, Frederick PD, Blaney M. Clinical characteristics of dialysis patients with acute myocardial infarction in the United States: a collaborative project of the United States Renal Data System and the National Registry of Myocardial Infarction. Circulation. 2007;116(13):1465–72.
12. Young LH, Frans JT, Chyun DA, Davey JA, Barrett EJ, Taillefer R, et al. Cardiac outcomes after screening for asymptomatic coronary artery disease in patients with type 2 diabetes: the DIAD study: a randomized controlled trial. JAMA. 2009;301(15):1547–55.
13. De Lima JJ, Sabbaga E, Vieira ML, de Paula FJ, Ianhez LE, Krieger EM, et al. Coronary angiography is the best predictor of events in renal transplant candidates compared with noninvasive testing. Hypertension. 2003;42(3):263–8.
14. Gowdak LH, de Paula FJ, Cesar LA, Martinez Filho EE, Ianhez LE, Krieger EM, et al. Screening for significant coronary artery disease in high-risk renal transplant candidates. Coron Artery Dis. 2007;18(7):553–8.
15. Hage FG, Smalheiser S, Zoghbi GJ, Perry GJ, Deierhoi M, Warnock D, et al. Predictors of survival in patients with end-stage renal disease evaluated for kidney transplantation. Am J Cardiol. 2007;100(6):1020–5.
16. Patel RK, Mark PB, Johnston N, McGeoch R, Lindsay M, Kingsmore DB, et al. Prognostic value of cardiovascular screening in potential renal transplant recipients: a single-center prospective observational study. Am J Transplant. 2008;8(8):1673–83.
17. De Bruyne B, Fearon WF, Pijls NH, Barbato E, Tonino P, Piroth Z, et al. Fractional flow reserve-guided PCI for stable coronary artery disease. N Engl J Med. 2014;371(13):1208–17.
18. Tebaldi M, Biscaglia S, Fineschi M, Manari A, Menozzi M, Secco GG, Di Lorenzo E, D'Ascenzo F, Fabbian F, Tumscitz C, Ferrari R. and Campo G. Fractional flow reserve evaluation and chronic kidney disease: analysis from a multicenter Italian registry (the FREAK Study). Cathet. Cardiovasc. Intervent. 2016; 88: 555–562.
19. Gruberg L, Rai P, Mintz GS, Canos D, Pinnow E, Satler LF, et al. Impact of renal function on coronary plaque morphology and morphometry in patients with chronic renal insufficiency as determined by intravascular ultrasound volumetric analysis. Am J Cardiol. 2005;96(7):892–6.
20. Ogita M, Funayama H, Nakamura T, Sakakura K, Sugawara Y, Kubo N, et al. Plaque characterization of non-culprit lesions by virtual histology intravascular ultrasound in diabetic patients: Impact of renal function. J Cardiol. 2009;54(1):59–65.
21. Brown AJ, Obaid DR, Costopoulos C, Parker RA, Calvert PA, Teng Z, et al. Direct comparison of virtual-histology intravascular ultrasound and optical coherence tomography imaging for identification of thin-cap fibroatheroma. Circ Cardiovasc Imaging. 2015;8(10):e003487.
22. Oemrawsingh RM, Cheng JM, García-García HM, van Geuns R-J, de Boer SPM, Simsek C, et al. Near-infrared spectroscopy predicts cardiovascular outcome in patients with coronary artery disease. J Am Coll Cardiol. 2014;64(23):2510–8.
23. Bolman RM 3rd, Anderson RW, Molina JE, Schwartz JS, Levine B, Simmons RL, et al. Cardiac operations in patients with functioning renal allografts. J Thoracic Cardiovasc Surg. 1984;88(4):537–43.
24. Dresler C, Uthoff K, Wahlers T, et al. Open heart operations after renal transplantation. The Annals of Thoracic Surgery. 1997;63(1):143–6.
25. Ono M, Wolf RK, Angouras DC, Brown DA, Goldstein AH, Michler RE. Short- and long-term results of open heart surgery in patients with abdominal solid organ transplant. Eur J Cardiothorac Surg. 2002;21(6):1061–72.
26. Herzog CA, Ma JZ, Collins AJ. Long-term outcome of renal transplant recipients in the United States after coronary revascularization procedures. Circulation. 2004;109(23):2866–71.
27. Morice MC, Serruys PW, Sousa JE, Fajadet J, Ban Hayashi E, Perin M, et al. A randomized comparison of a sirolimus-eluting stent with a standard stent for coronary revascularization. N Engl J Med. 2002;346(23):1773–80.
28. Chang TI, Shilane D, Kazi DS, Montez-Rath ME, Hlatky MA, Winkelmayer WC. Multivessel coronary artery bypass grafting versus percutaneous coronary intervention in ESRD. J Am Soc Nephrol JASN. 2012;23(12):2042–9.
29. Athappan G, Ponniah T. Clinical outcomes of dialysis patients after implantation of DES: meta analysis and systematic review of literature. Minerva Cardioangiol. 2009;57(3):291–7.
30. Abdel-Latif A, Mukherjee D, Mesgarzadeh P, Ziada KM. Drug-eluting stents in patients with end-stage renal disease: meta-analysis and systematic review of the literature. Catheter Cardiovasc Interv. 2010;76(7):942–8.
31. Bangalore S, Guo Y, Samadashvili Z, Blecker S, Xu J, Hannan EL. Revascularization in patients with multivessel coronary artery disease and chronic kidney disease: everolimus-eluting stents versus coronary artery bypass graft surgery. J Am Coll Cardiol. 2015;66(11):1209–20.

32. Serruys PW, Morice MC, Kappetein AP, Colombo A, Holmes DR, Mack MJ, et al. Percutaneous coronary intervention versus coronary-artery bypass grafting for severe coronary artery disease. N Engl J Med. 2009;360(10):961–72.
33. Kappetein AP, Feldman TE, Mack MJ, Morice MC, Holmes DR, Stahle E, et al. Comparison of coronary bypass surgery with drug-eluting stenting for the treatment of left main and/or three-vessel disease: 3-year follow-up of the SYNTAX trial. Eur Heart J. 2011;32(17):2125–34.
34. Tomaszuk-Kazberuk A, Kozuch M, Malyszko J, Bachorzewska-Gajewska H, Kobus G, Dobrzycki S, et al. Angiographically-derived SYNTAX score and its prognostic value in dialysis patients: comparison with the Khan index. Can J Cardiol. 2012;28(4):450–7.
35. Farkouh ME, Domanski M, Sleeper LA, Siami FS, Dangas G, Mack M, et al. Strategies for multivessel revascularization in patients with diabetes. N Engl J Med. 2012;367(25):2375–84.

23 Pulmonary Hypertension in the Potential Kidney Transplant Recipient

Sourin Banerji and Anjali Vaidya

Introduction

Pulmonary hypertension (PH), as defined by the World Symposium on Pulmonary Hypertension, is the mean pulmonary artery pressure (mPAP), obtained by right heart catheterization (RHC), of at least 25 mmHg at rest. Further classification of PH can subsequently be achieved with the evaluation of hemodynamic measurements, including pulmonary vascular resistance (PVR) and pulmonary artery wedge pressure (PAWP), as well as the identification of comorbidities including connective tissue diseases, HIV, cirrhosis, left heart pathology, and chronic pulmonary artery thromboembolism among others [1]. Etiologies of PH can be further delineated based on these findings into five general groups (Dana Point classification): Group I—pulmonary arterial hypertension (PAH) due to proliferative vasculopathy; Group 2—PH due to left heart disease; Group 3—PH due to lung disease and/or hypoxia; Group 4—PH due to chronic thromboembolism (CTEPH); and Group 5—PH with unclear multifactorial mechanisms (Table 23.1) [2]. In patients with chronic kidney disease (CKD) and particularly end stage kidney disease (ESKD), PH may manifest due to one or multiple mechanisms, and classifying the underling etiology into one of the above groups may not always prove straightforward. In this chapter, we will review the prevalence and prognosis of PH in patients with ESRD, the various and coexisting mechanisms of PH in these patients and the considerations for evaluation of those considered for renal transplant.

S. Banerji (✉)
Division of Cardiology, Department of Medicine, Christiana Care Medical Center, 4755 Ogletown-Stanton Road, Ste 1070, Newark, DE 19718, USA
e-mail: Sourin.banerji@christianacare.org

A. Vaidya
Advanced Heart Failure and Cardiac Transplant, Division of Cardiology, Department of Medicine, Temple University Lewis Katz School of Medicine, 9th Floor Parkinson Pavilion, 3401 North Broad Street, Philadelphia, PA 19140, USA
e-mail: Anjali.vaidya@tuhs.temple.edu

J. Rangaswami et al. (eds.), *Cardio-Nephrology*,
DOI 10.1007/978-3-319-56042-7_23

Epidemiology

Prevalence

Understanding the true prevalence of PH in patients with ESKD has proven difficult to ascertain due to varied criteria for defining PH in past studies as well as the various subgroups of patients with ESKD that have been analyzed including patients with advanced CKD not on hemodialysis (HD), and patients with ESKD on hemodialysis (HD) or peritoneal dialysis (PD). Though invasive hemodynamic assessment with right heart catheterization is instrumental in current evaluation of patients with PH, many prior studies evaluating PH in patients with ESKD have predominantly used echocardiographic assessments particularly in epidemiologic evaluations [3–19]. In these patients, pulmonary artery systolic pressure (PASP) was assessed with the modified Bernoulli equation: PASP (mmHg) = 4 × (Tricuspid Regurgitation (TR) jet velocity) 2 + right atrial pressure (estimated by inferior vena cava diameter and collapsibility) [20]. In one study identified, echocardiographic parameters were utilized to identify the mean PA pressure (mPAP) using the Mahan's equation: mPAP (mmHg) = 79—[0.45 × Acceleration Time (time to peak velocity of right ventricular outflow tract flow by Doppler imaging)] [8].

Studies evaluating the prevalence of PH in patients with CKD have largely targeted patients with ESKD on HD with arteriovenous fistulas (AVF). As noted above, the majority of these studies used echocardiographic parameters to determine the presence of PH with varied criteria including PASP > 30–40 mmHg, mean PAP > 25 mmHg, and TR jet velocity > 2.5 m/s. The prevalence of PH in these studies is wide-ranging from 19 to 56% [3–17]. A preponderance of these studies excluded patients (44–87% in studies with provided data) [3, 5, 7, 14] with comorbid conditions associated with pulmonary hypertension as defined in the Dana Point classification above, including those with left ventricular ejection fraction <50%, parenchymal lung disorders, pulmonary embolism, left-to-right cardiac shunting, and

Table 23.1 Dana Point 2008 classification of pulmonary hypertension

Group I: Pulmonary arterial hypertension	Includes: idiopathic, HIV, CTD, portal hypertension and congenital heart disease including left-to-right shunts
Group II: PH due to left sided heart disease	Includes: left ventricle systolic/diastolic dysfunction, and valvular disease (e.g., mitral stenosis/regurgitation, aortic stenosis/regurgitation)
Group III: PH due to lung diseases and/or hypoxia	Includes: COPD, interstitial lung disease, and obstructive sleep apnea
Group IV: CTEPH	Chronic pulmonary thromboembolism
Group V: Mixed etiologies	Includes: hematologic disorders (i.e., chronic hemolytic anemia), systemic disorders (i.e., sarcoidosis), and chronic renal failure

connective tissue diseases. However, the criteria used to define these conditions were not uniform and may contribute to the variance in prevalence seen. In the few studies that did not exclude patients on HD with other comorbidities that may contribute to PH, the prevalence of PH in these studies was not appreciably different [13, 15]. Furthermore, the largest of these studies in terms of sample size by Bozbas et al. yielded the lowest prevalence of PH (19%) in a cohort of ESKD patients on HD being evaluated for renal transplant [9]. However, this was a retrospective study and the timing of the echocardiogram with respect to dialysis was not defined. Other factors including small sample size, inconsistent duration of HD in patients studied, reliance on echocardiogram to identify PH, and timing of study with respect to HD session all may contribute to the distribution of prevalence observed. Studies evaluating prevalence of PH in patients with ESKD on PD or advanced CKD are much less robust. While rates of PH in patients requiring PD demonstrate similar variance from 0 to 42% [3, 9, 12, 14, 17–19], the prevalence is overall lower compared patients on HD when excluding studies with secondary causes of pulmonary hypertension. Furthermore, the rates of PH in patients on PD are on average less compared to those on HD when analyzed within the same study [9, 12, 14], with the study by Alhamad et al. [17] being an exception to this trend. However, it is difficult to draw conclusions with respect to differences in prevalence of PH in those requiring PD owing to similar inconsistencies in analysis of PH as noted above in HD patients as well as generally a younger and healthier population of patients requiring PD. Studies analyzing the prevalence of PH in patients with advanced CKD not on HD range from 8 to 39% [3, 7, 10]. These studies are few and small in sample size to draw any certain conclusion. However, in the three studies that evaluated patients with advanced CKD not on HD (non-HD) versus patients with ESKD on HD, rates of PH were consistently less in the non-HD groups [3, 7, 10] (Table 23.2). While invasive hemodynamic evaluation is necessary for defining and evaluating all patients with PH, only one study has presented RHC interrogation of patients with ESKD with PH. The PEPPER study evaluated patients with advanced CKD with unexplained dyspnea after excluding for secondary causes of PH. RHC was performed before and after initiation of HD (Group I) and in patients with advanced CKD non-HD (Group 2). Prevalence of PH in this select group of patients, as defined by a mPAP > 25 mmHg was 77% in patients on HD versus 71% in patients with CKD non-HD [21].

Incidence

Owing to a paucity of prospective case-control studies, the incidence of PH in patients with advanced CKD and ESKD is less clear. Yigla et al. evaluated 12 patients with ESKD and pre-dialysis without PH (as defined by PASP > 35 mmHg by echocardiogram) and without comorbidities associated with known etiologies of PH. Repeat PASP evaluation obtained 3–7 months post development of AVF revealed PASP > 35 mmHg in 5/12 patients [22]. In another study, evaluating 127 patients with ESKD predialysis (but after AVF creation) and followed an average of 4.7 years on HD, prevalence of PH (as defined by a PASP > 45 mmHg by echocardiogram) increased from 13% in the predialysis cohort to 29% in those on HD. In patients who developed PH after initiation of HD, 75% developed PH in 1 year and 25% developed PH in years 1–5. Moderate-severe mitral valve regurgitation and left ventricular systolic dysfunction were associated with PH in predialysis patients [23].

Prognosis

Survival in patients with ESKD on HD with PH is markedly reduced. Yigla et al. observed a 30.4% mortality rate in patients with unexplained PH (in a cohort of 58 patients with ESRD on HD) compared to 8.5% without PH [3]. In a larger study of a similar cohort, Yigla et al. observed significantly lower 1-, 3-, and 5-year survival rates in patients with ESKD on HD and PH versus those without PH (79 vs. 97%, 43 vs. 79%, and 25 vs. 66%, respectively). PH persisted as an independent predictor of all-cause mortality after

Table 23.2 Summary of reported prevalence of pulmonary hypertension in patients with chronic kidney disease

Reference	Population	Modality	Definition of PH (mmHg)	Sample Size	Prevalance (%)
Yigla [3]	HD	Echo	PASP > 35	58	40
Amin [4]	HD	Echo	PASP > 35	51	29
Nakhoul [5]	HD	Echo	PASP > 35	42	48
Tarrass [6]	HD	Echo	PASP > 35	86	27
Havlucu [7]	HD	Echo	PASP > 35	25	56
Acarturk [8]	HD	Echo	PASP > 25	32	44
Bozbas [9]	HD	Echo	PASP > 30	432	19
Abdelwhab [10]	HD	Echo	PASP > 35	45	44
Dagli [11]	HD	Echo	PASP > 30	116	21
Fabbian [12]	HD	Echo	PASP > 35	29	59
Ramasubbu [13]	HD	Echo	TR jet > 2.5 m/s	90	47
Etemadi [14]	HD	Echo	PASP > 35	34	41
Agarwal [15]	HD	Echo	PASP > 35	288	38
Mukhtar [16]	HD	Echo	PASP > 30	88	56
Alhamad [17]	HD	Echo	PASP > 40	55	22
Yigla [3]	PD	Echo	PASP > 35	5	0
Bozbas [9]	PD	Echo	PASP > 30	68	6
Kumbar [18]	PD	Echo	PASP > 35	36	42
Unal [19]	PD	Echo	PASP > 35	135	13
Fabbian [12]	PD	Echo	PASP > 35	27	19
Etemadi [14]	PD	Echo	PASP > 35	32	19
Alhamad [17]	PD	Echo	PASP > 40	17	24
Yigla [3]	CKD (predialysis)	Echo	PASP > 35	12	8
Havlucu [7]	CKD (predialysis)	Echo	PASP > 35	23	39
Abdelwhab [10]	CKD (predialysis)	Echo	PASP > 35	31	32

multivariate analysis with an adjusted hazard ratio of 3.6 in predialysis patients and 2.1 for those who developed PH after initiation of HD [23]. Agarwal et al. followed 288 patients on HD for a median duration of 2.15 years. 38% of these patients had PH as defined by a PASP > 35 mmHg by echocardiogram. Of 97 deaths in this time period, 58 occurred in those with PH. After multivariate analysis, PH persisted as an independent predictor of all-cause mortality with a hazard ratio of 2.2 [15]. Similarly, Ramasubbu et al. identified a 1 year mortality rate of 26% in HD patients with PH (defined as a TR jet velocity > 2.5 m/s) versus 6% in HD patients without PH [13].

Mortality data in patients with PH on PD is sparse. Kumbar et al. retrospectively evaluated a cohort of 36 patients on PD and identified 42% with PH as defined by a PASP > 35 mmHg by echocardiogram in a 3-year period. Mortality rates trended higher for PD patients with PH compared to those without (60 vs. 38%) although this was not statistically significant ($p = 0.31$) [18].

Mortality data of patients with PH undergoing renal transplant is also limited. Issa et al. retrospectively assessed for pretransplant PH (right ventricular systolic pressure >35 mmHg by echocardiogram) in 215 renal transplant recipients. In this instance, right ventricular systolic pressure (RVSP) was assumed equal to PASP when no evidence of pulmonic stenosis existed. 47 patients were found to have mild-moderate PH as defined by RVSP > 35 but < 50 mmHg and 22 had severe PH (RVSP > 50 mmHg). Severe PH as defined by this study was associated with hazard ratio for mortality of 3.75, although only a univariate analysis could be performed. However, there was no association of mortality with less severe RVSP. Additionally, graft survival was not associated with any level of PH [24]. Zlotnick et al. retrospectively evaluated graft survival in renal transplant patients over a 3-year period who had pre-transplant PH by echocardiogram (PASP > 35 mmHg). PH was associated with decreased graft survival of deceased donor kidney transplant recipients only [25]. Conversely, a few small single-centered studies have shown improvement, and in some instances, resolution of PH with transplantation [3, 26, 27]. The limitations of these studies as outlined above and lack of hemodynamic classification of the etiology of PH in these patients have contributed to the conflicting data on mortality and graft survival post-transplant.

Etiology and Pathogenesis

In patients with ESKD, the development of PH may be a consequence of the underlying etiology of renal failure. Yet, in other instances, PH may alternately be exacerbated or initiated by the downstream effects of ESKD itself. As noted above, approximately 40–80% of patients with ESKD were excluded in evaluation of PH due to the presence of one or more comorbid conditions that may have predisposed them to PH including connective tissue diseases (CTD), pulmonary disorders, history of pulmonary embolus, and the presence of cardiac diseases including left ventricular ejection fraction (LVEF) < 50%, left-to-right intracardiac shunts, and the mitral and/or aortic valve disorders [3, 5, 7, 14].

However, the above comorbidities are not always present in patients with ESKD and PH prompting consideration and evaluation for other etiologies discussed below (Fig. 23.1).

Arteriovenous Fistulae

Given the overall higher prevalence of PH in patients with HD compared to those on PD and CKD non-HD, arteriovenous fistulae (AVF) have been suspected to contribute to PH in ESKD patients particularly given reports of reduction in PAP following compression and/or ligation of AVF [3, 28]. However, available data evaluating PH in pre- and post-HD patients has been conflicting. In 12 pre-dialysis patients with no PH, Yigla et al. identified the development of PH (by echocardiography) in 5 of these patients after initiation of HD [22]. Unal et al. however reported a reduction in PH prevalence after initiation of HD in a cohort of 20 patients [29]. Furthermore, in a more symptomatic cohort, Pabst et al. reported the reduction in prevalence of PH after initiation of HD (by RHC evaluation) [21]. Both AVF flow rate and duration of AVF have been associated with PH in various studies [5, 7, 10–12, 15, 16]. However, this association has not been consistently demonstrated. Similarly, while brachiocephalic AVF are associated with more flow compared to radial AVF access, this difference has not been convincingly shown to contribute to higher prevalence of PH [6]. Anemia related to decreased erythropoietin has also been identified as contributor to increased cardiac output (and PH) in ESKD patients both pre-dialysis and on hemodialysis, but this association is sparsely reported [14]. While, individually, these variables associated with AVF have not been reliably proven to contribute to PH in patients with ESKD, it is perhaps the combination of all of these factors, particularly in the presence

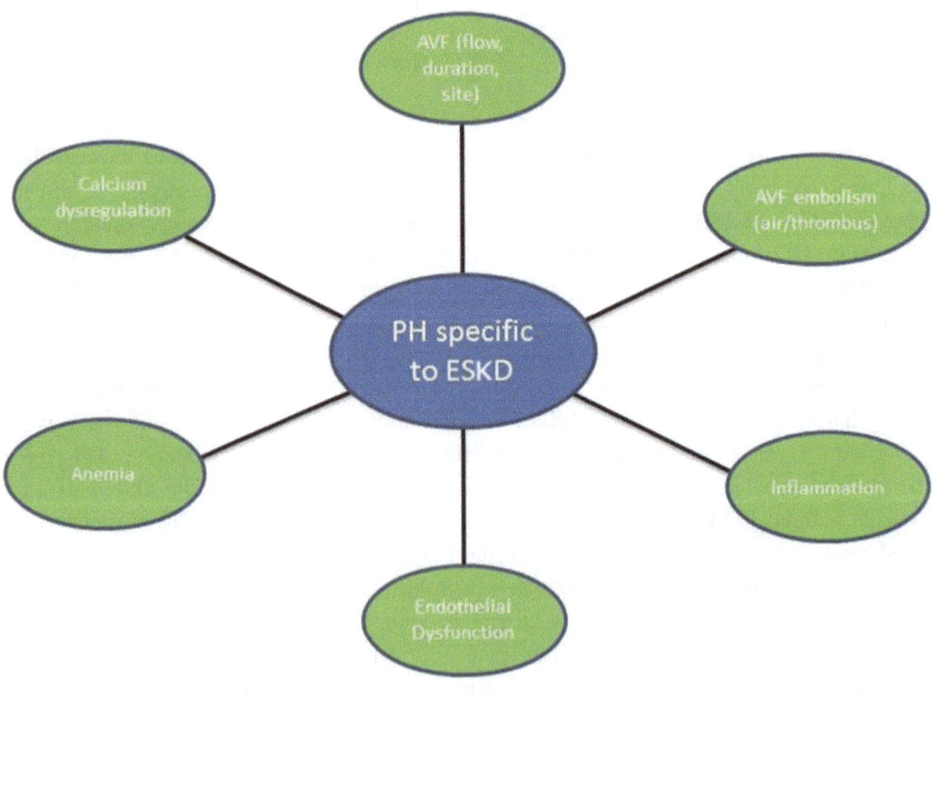

Fig. 23.1 Pathophysiology of pulmonary hypertension in patients with end stage kidney disease

of left sided heart disease that may prove a more consistent relationship with PH. Raza et al. presented a case series of 5 patients with ESKD and concomitant PH, left ventricular hypertrophy, AVF of greater than 4 years duration and with high output who all had symptoms of heart failure. Surgical ligation and/or banding resulted in significant decrease in mPAP with associated improvement in symptoms [30].

Pulmonary Vascular Remodeling—Endothelial Dysfunction

Besides enhanced cardiac output, AVF formation may contribute to PH with pulmonary vascular remodeling. As noted previously, in a cohort of ESKD with dyspnea, Pabst et al. demonstrated unexplained elevated pulmonary vascular resistance and PH ("precapillary PH") in 10% of dialysis patients as opposed to none in CKD non-HD patients, suggesting increased endothelial dysfunction in HD patients. Endothelial dysfunction has been reported in patients with CKD due to reduced production of L-Arginine which serves as a precursor to nitric oxide (NO)—a potent vasodilator and regulator of endothelial function. Additionally, dialysis is associated with accumulation of naturally occurring inhibitors of nitric oxide production [31]. Furthermore, enhanced shear stress in the pulmonary vasculature (as can be seen in HD patients with AVF flow) has been shown to increase Endothelin (ET)—a potent vasoconstrictor and regulator of endothelial function—by upregulating gene expression [32]. Nakhoul et al. assessed endothelin and nitric oxide levels in HD patients with and without PH. HD patients, regardless of PH presence, demonstrated increased ET levels compared with normal control subjects. Basal levels of NO were significantly decreased in HD patients with PH compared to those without PH and normal controls, and HD patients with PH showed a blunted rise of NO after HD therapy. Abdelwhab et al. further demonstrated the contribution of HD to endothelium dysfunction by reporting an increase in thromboxane (a potent vasoconstrictor and regulator of endothelial function) in patients with PH on HD compared to CKD patients not on HD [10]. All of this suggests impaired pulmonary vasculature endothelium—in ESKD patients on HD—that may contribute to PH.

Pulmonary Vascular Remodeling—Parathyroid Hormone and Calcium Regulation

Dysregulation in parathyroid hormone (PTH) and calcium handling is a known complication of advanced CKD and ESKD. Chronically elevated PTH levels are associated with increased calcium deposition in tissues and have been postulated to contribute to pulmonary artery calcification seen routinely in patients who have received regular hemodialysis [33]. Faubert et al. analyzed 23 patients with ESRD on HD and found 61% demonstrated pulmonary artery calcification by technetium-99 m diphosphate scanning [34]. However, in two subsequent studies assessing pulmonary hypertension (established by echocardiography) in ESKD on HD, there was no significant association with pulmonary artery calcification. Furthermore, there was no significant difference in calcium, phosphorus, or PTH levels between those with and without PH [4, 35]. However, in a larger study of patients with CKD non-HD (190 patients), elevated PTH levels were significantly associated with PH defined by echocardiography, yet pulmonary artery calcification was not assessed [36]. Limitations of these studies included evaluation of pulmonary pressures by echocardiography only, and inherent limitations of noninvasive imaging modalities to accurately assess pulmonary artery calcification burden. Additionally, there are no reported studies evaluating pulmonary artery calcification in ESKD on PD. The limited studies reporting the association of calcium, phosphorus, and PTH levels with PH in PD patients are conflicting [18, 19]. Therefore, the role of calcium and PTH dysregulation affecting PH development in patients with ESKD remains unclear.

Pulmonary Vascular Remodeling—Thromboembolism

While chronic venous thromboembolism is established as an etiologic agent for PH, the association with thromboembolism from AVF is less certain. Harp et al. identified a trend toward more PH (as defined by echocardiography) in patient with ESKD on HD undergoing one or more HD graft thrombectomy procedures (OR 1.5). However, this was not statistically significant [37]. Hsieh et al. evaluated PH more accurately with RHC assessment but also found no association with PH and number of thrombectomy procedures in ESKD patients on HD [38]. Gas microemboli occurring in hemodialysis has also been postulated to contribute to PH. These microemboli are suspected to develop during turbulent flow around the venous access site. Current HD machines are equipped with ultrasonic detectors of larger air emboli, but smaller emboli frequently evade alarm. Recurrent emboli can affect pulmonary vasculature via mechanical obstruction with subsequent complement and clotting activation and increased inflammatory response. Repeated dialysis and gas microemboli formation in the venous system leads to chronic microvascular trauma in the pulmonary arteries that may simulate thromboembolism [39]. While animal studies have shown PH and increased pulmonary vasoreactivity with repeated micro air embolism, this association has not been studied in humans [40].

Inflammation

Inflammatory cytokines including TNF-alpha, IL-1, and IL-6 have been associated with PH in animal and human studies [41, 42]. Increased inflammatory cytokines have been reported in patients with uremia and have been suspected as a contributing factor in the development of PH in ESKRD. Yu et al. analyzed inflammatory cytokine levels in patients with ESRD with and without PH on HD. TNF-alpha, Interleukin-1 Beta, Interleukin 6, and high sensitivity C-reactive protein were significantly higher in patients with PH suggesting an etiologic role. However, further longitudinal studies are lacking to provide a more definitive causal relationship.

Management of PH in Candidates for Renal Transplant

As noted previously, mortality and graft survival in patients with renal transplant and pre-existing PH has not been consistent in the few studies published. While limitations in these studies, including small sample sizes, single-center analyses, and retrospective cohorts have contributed to these conflicting findings, the multiple and varied mechanisms of PH described above have also played a role. The most recent American Heart Association/American College of Cardiology Foundation (AHA/ACCF) scientific statement on the evaluation and management of pulmonary hypertension in kidney transplant candidates recommends confirming PH and clarifying hemodynamics with RHC in patients screened with echocardiography demonstrating an RVSP > 45 mmHg [43]. The use of RHC to establish Group I PH, also referred to as pulmonary arterial hypertension (PAH) or precapillary PH (defined as mPAP > 25 mmHg, PCWP < 15 mmHg and PVR > 3 WU), is paramount given the growth of pharmaceutical therapies for this subset of PH. These therapies generally target three pathways implicated in the proliferative vasculopathy of PAH: (a) nitric oxide, (b) endothelin, and (c) prostacyclin. Phosphodiesterase type 5 inhibitors (Tadalafil, Sildenafil) and soluble guancylate cyclase stimulators (Riociguat) enhance nitric oxide pulmonary artery vasodilation. Endothelin receptor antagonists (Bosentan, Ambrisentan, Macitentan) impair endothelin vasoconstriction of pulmonary arteries. Finally, prostanoids (Epoprostenol, Trepostinil, Iloprost, and Selexipag) enhance prostacyclin mediated pulmonary artery vasodilation. These medicines are available in oral form and, in the case of prostacyclins, can be delivered via inhaled, subcutaneous or intravenous routes as well [44]. Side effects of these medications are numerous, and caution should be taken in utilizing these medications in patients with evidence of left sided heart disease or evidence of pulmonary parenchymal disorders as pulmonary edema and ventilation-perfusion mismatching can occur respectively. In PAH patients with World Health Organization I or II functional class and response to vasoreactivity testing on RHC evaluation (using inhaled NO or inhaled epoprostenol), dihydropyridine calcium channel blocker use has been demonstrated to yield some improvement [45]. Additionally, limited studies have identified the benefit of anticoagulation in Group I PH patients—particularly those with no identifiable provocateur of PAH [46]. The AHA/ACCF scientific statement also recommends screening and appropriate treatment for secondary causes including left sided heart disease (Group II PH), intrinsic pulmonary disorders/sleep-disordered breathing (Group III PH), and chronic pulmonary embolism (Group IV PH). Those with CTEPH (Group IV PH) should be initiated on anticoagulation promptly and be considered for pulmonary thromboendarterectomy at centers specialized for this [43]. Patients with CTEPH have also been shown to benefit from soluble guancylate cyclase stimulators (Riociguat) [45]. It should be noted that trials evaluating the above therapeutic options have excluded patients with ESKD, and the efficacy of these treatments in improving outcomes for renal transplant is unknown. Treatments targeting suspected etiologies of PH specific to ESKD are less clear. The use of erythropoietin stimulating agents on animal models have yielded conflicting effects on PH and have not been well studied for this purpose in humans much less those with ESKD [47, 48]. Patients with high AVF and PH have demonstrated improved pulmonary artery pressures with banding or ligating of the AVF. However, the available published literature of this intervention is limited to case reports and case series. Given inconsistent outcome data on patients with ESKD and PH undergoing renal transplant, the mortality and graft rejection risks of transplant should be balanced with the consistently established elevated mortality of patients with PH on dialysis. Because of the multiple etiologies implicated in PH in patients with ESKD and the complexity of treatment, it is recommended that experienced providers evaluate and manage PH in patients with ESKD particularly in those being considered for renal transplant.

Conclusion

The prevalence of PH is increasingly recognized in patients with ESKD on dialysis. The etiologies are diverse and multiple owing to the many comorbidities of patients with ESKD and renal dysfunction itself. While PH can be screened for by echocardiography, RHC is the gold standard for confirmation and for further classification. PH is associated with significantly increased mortality in patients with ESRD compared to those without, but its impact on transplant outcomes is not well established. Care should be taken to identify any of the numerous etiologies that are involved in any individual case and aggressive treatment of reversible conditions should be pursued with the assistance of a specialist with expertise in PH. Areas of future research include (1) further classification of etiologies using right heart catheterization in patients with PH and ESKD and outcomes related to these various etiologies in both those receiving and not receiving renal transplant; (2) evaluation of new drug therapies in patients with Group I PH (PAH) and ESKD on survival outcomes in both those receiving and not receiving transplant; (3) assessment of the effect of treatment of specific PH etiologies unique to those with ESKD on survival outcomes; and (4) utilization of echocardiographic features including interventricular septal positioning and spectral Doppler interrogation of the right ventricular outflow tract flow to further classify PH etiology noninvasively. Results of research in these areas may help lead to more refined decision making in selecting appropriate candidates with ESKD and PH who will benefit from renal transplantation.

References

1. Hoeper MM, et al. Definitions and diagnosis of pulmonary hypertension. J Am Coll Cardiol. 2013;62(25): Suppl D 42–50.
2. Simmonneau G, et al. Updated clinical classification of pulmonary hypertension. J Am Coll Cardiol. 2013;62(25): Suppl D 34–41.
3. Yigla M, et al. Pulmonary hypertension in patients with end-stage renal disease. Chest. 2003;123(5):1577–82.
4. Amin M, et al. Pulmonary hypertension in patients with chronic renal failure: role of PTH and pulmonary artery calcifications. Chest. 2003;124:2093–7.
5. Nakhoul F, et al. The pathogenesis of pulmonary hypertension in haemodialysis patients via arterio-venous access. Nephrol Dial Transplant. 2005;20:1686–92.
6. Tarrass F, et al. Doppler echocardiograph evaluation of pulmonary hypertension in patients undergoing hemodialysis. Hemodial Int. 2006;10:356–9.
7. Havlucu Y, et al. Pulmonary hypertension in patients with chronic renal failure. Respiration. 2007;74:503–10.
8. Acarturk G, et al. The relationship between arteriovenous fistula blood flow rate and pulmonary artery pressure in hemodialysis patients. Int Urol Nephrol. 2008;40:509–13.
9. Bozbas SS, et al. Pulmonary hypertension in patients with end-stage renal disease undergoing renal transplantation. Transpl Proc. 2009;41:2753–6.
10. Abdelwhab S, et al. Pulmonary hypertension in CRF patients. Am J Nephrol. 2008;28:990–7.
11. Dagli CE, et al. Prevalance and factors affecting pulmonary hypertension in hemodialysis patients. Respiration. 2009;78:411–5.
12. Fabbian F, et al. Pulmonary hypertension in dialysis patients: a cross-sectional italian study. Int J Nephrol. 2011;2011:283475.
13. Ramasubbu K, et al. A prospective echocardiographic evaluation of pulmonary hypertension in chronic hemodialysis patients in the United States: prevalance and clinical signficance. Int J Gen Med. 2010;3:279–86.
14. Etemadi J, et al. Unexplained pulmonary hypertension in peritoneal dialysis and hemodialysis patients. Rev Port Pneumol. 2011;18:10–4.
15. Agarwal R, et al. Prevalence, determinants and prognosis of pulmonary hypertension among hemodialysis patients. Nephrol Dial Transplant. 2012;27:3908–14.
16. Mukhtar KN, et al. Frequency of pulmonary hypertension in hemodialysis patients. Pak J Med Sci. 2014;30(6):1319–22.
17. Alhamad EH, et al. Pulmonary hypertension in end-stage renal disease and post renal transplant patients. J Thorac Dis. 2014; 6(6):606–14.
18. Kumbar L, et al. Pulmonary hypertension in peritoneal dialysis patients. Adv Perit Dial. 2007;23:127–31.
19. Unal A, et al. Pulmonary hypertension in peritoneal dialysis patients: prevalence and risk factors. Perit Dial Int. 2009;29:191–8.
20. Berger M, et al. Quantitative assessment of pulmonary hypertension in patients with tricuspid regurgitation using continuous wave Doppler ultrasound. J Am Coll Cardiol. 1985;6:359–65.
21. Pabst S, et al. Pulmonary hypertension in patients with chronic kidney disease on dialysis and without dialysis: results of the PEPPER-study. PLoS ONE. 2012;7:e35310.
22. Yigla M, et al. Arterio-venous access in end-stage renal disease patients and pulmonary hypertension. Ther Adv Respir Dis. 2008;2:49–53.
23. Yigla M, et al. Pulmonary hypertension is an independent predictor of mortality in hemodialysis patients. Kidney Int. 2009;75:969–75.
24. Issa N, et al. Pulmonary hypertension is associated with reduced patient survival after kidney transplantation. Transplantation. 2008;86:1384–88.
25. Zlotnick DM, et al. Non-invasive detection of pulmonary hypertension prior to renal transplantation is a predictor of incrweased risk for early graft dysfunction. Nephrol Dial Transplant. 2010;25:3090–6.
26. Casas-Aparicio G, et al. The effect of successful kidney transplantation on ventricular dysfunction and pulmonary hypertension. Transplant Proc. 2010;42:3524–8.
27. Reddy YN, et al. Progressive pulmonary hypertension: another criterion for expeditious renal transplantation. Saudi J Kidney Dis Transpl. 2013;24:925–9.
28. Clarkson MR, et al. Reversal of pulmonary hypertension after ligation of a brachiocephalic arteriovenous fistula. Am J Kidney Dis. 2002;40(e8):1–4.
29. Unal A, et al. The long-term effect of arteriovenous fistula creation in the development of pulmonary hypertension in hemodialysis patients. Hemodial Int. 2010;14:398–402.
30. Raza F, et al. Case series of 5 patients with end stage renal disease with reversible dyspnea, heart failure and pulmonary hypertension related to arteriovenous dialysis access. Pulm Circ. 2015;5(2): 398–406.
31. Vaziri ND. Effect of chronic renal failure on nitric oxide metabolism. Am J Kidney Dis. 2001;38:S74–9.
32. Dschietzig T, et al. Flow-induced pressure differentially regulates endothelin-1, urotensin II, adrenomedullin, and relaxin in pulmonary vascular endothelium. Crt Biochem Biophys Res Commun. 2001;289:245–61.
33. Conger JD, et al. Pulmonary calcification in chronic dialysis patients. Ann Intern Med. 1975;83:330–6.
34. Faubert PF, et al. Pulmonary artery calcification in hemodialyzed patients detected by technetium-99m diphosphate scanning. Kidney Int. 1980;18:95–102.
35. Yigla M, et al. Pulmonary calcification in hemodialysis patients: correlation with pulmonary artery pressure values. Kidney Int. 2004;66:806–10.

36. Genctoy G, et al. Secondary hyperparathyroidism is associated with pulmonary hypertension in older patients with chronic kidney disease and proteinuria. Int Urol Nephrol. 2015;47:353–8.
37. Harp RJ, et al. Pulmonary hypertension among end-stage renal failure patients following hemodialysis access thrombectomy. Cardiovasc Intervent Radiol. 2005;28:17–22.
38. Hsieh MY, et al. Pulmonary hypertension in hemodialysis patients following repeated endovascular thrombectomy. Acta Cardiol Sin. 2016;32:299–306.
39. Barak M, et al. Pathophysiology and clinical implications of microbubbles during hemodialysis. Semin Dial. 2008;21:232–8.
40. Perkett EA, et al. Continuous air embolization into sheep causes sustained pulmonary hypertension and increased pulmonary vasoreactivity. Am J Pathol. 1988;132:444–54.
41. Fujita M, et al. Overexpression of tumor necrosis factor-alpha produces an increase in lung volumes and pulmonary hypertension. Am J Physiol Lung Cell Mol Physiol. 2001;280:L39–49.
42. Humbert M, et al. Increased interleukin-1 and interleukin-6 serum concentrations in severe primary pulmonary hypertension. Am J Respir Crit Care Med. 1995;151:1628–31.
43. Lentine, et al. Cardiac disease evaluation and management among kidney and liver transplantation candidates. Circulation. 2012;126:617–63.
44. McLaughlin VV, et al. Management of pulmonary artery hypertension. J Am Coll Cardiol. 2015;65:1976–97.
45. Rich S, et al. The effect of high doses of calcium-channel blockers on survival in primary pulmonary hypertension. N Engl J Med. 1992;327:76–81.
46. Olsen KM, et al. Anticoagulation and survival in pulmonary arterial hypertension—results from the comparative, prospective registry of newly initiated therapies for pulmonary hypertension (COMPERA). Circulation. 2014;129:57–65.
47. Satoh K, et al. Important role of endogenous erythropoietin system in recruitment of endothelial progenitor cells in hypoxia-induced pulmonary hypertension in mice. Circulation. 2006;113:1442–50.
48. Hasegawa J, et al. Altered pulmonary vascular reactivity in mice with excessive erythrocytosis. Am J Resp Crit Care Med. 2004;169:829–35.

Cardiac Surveillance Whilst Listed for Renal Transplantation

24

Karen L. Keung, Madhav C. Menon, and Barbara Murphy

Introduction

Based on OPTN data as of January 11, 2016, 100,791 people were on the kidney transplant wait list in the United States. For patients newly listed in 2009 either for a first-time or for repeat kidney-alone transplant, the median time spent on the wait list was 3.6 years [1]. Annual mortality whilst listed is estimated at 5% [2], although this does not distinguish between active and inactive patients, with the latter experiencing higher mortality. Cardiovascular disease is the most common cause of death in these patients, accounting for approximately one third of cases with a documented cause [3].

The incidence and prevalence of coronary artery disease is high in the end-stage disease kidney (ESKD) population, with the cumulative incidence of acute myocardial infarction rising steadily after joining the wait list, estimated to afflict between 8.7 and 16.7% of candidates by 3 years [4, 5]. In addition, arrhythmias and decompensated heart failure, as a consequence of abnormalities including valvular disease, and left ventricular dysfunction, are also common causes of adverse cardiac outcomes in patients with ESKD.

After initial cardiac assessment and activation on the waiting list, it may be several years before the patient receives a kidney transplant. Some transplant centers review actively listed patients at regular intervals, whilst others follow-up within a year of the candidates being estimated to reach the "top" of the waiting list. In this chapter, we will discuss the role, if any, of periodic cardiac surveillance based on the current literature and recommendations from existing guidelines, specifically relating to coronary artery disease, left ventricular dysfunction, and valvular heart disease (summarized in Table 24.1).

Coronary Artery Disease

The accelerated rate of progression of coronary artery disease (CAD) in the ESKD population, compounded by increasing risk with longer duration of dialysis, means periodic surveillance for CAD following the initial assessment (discussed in an earlier chapter) whilst waitlisted would seem reasonable. There is great heterogeneity amongst published guidelines regarding the role of CAD monitoring for listed patients and a paucity of quality studies to support the utility of this strategy, let alone the optimal frequency of repeat screening for those with a negative initial test. In addition, the best modality for ongoing surveillance is unclear. The studies discussed below use varying imaging techniques, each with their limitations (reviewed in an earlier chapter).

The 2005 National Kidney Foundation/Kidney Disease Outcomes Quality Initiative (NKF/KDOQI) "Clinical Practice Guidelines for Cardiovascular Disease in Dialysis Patients" recommended repeat stress testing annually for diabetic patients with ESKD and every other year for "high risk" nondiabetic patients [7]. Several relevant studies have been published since the writing of the guidelines.

One of the largest observational studies examining cardiac events (cardiac death or nonfatal MI) following a normal myocardial perfusion scan (MPS), identified an event rate of 1.1% over the mean follow-up of 2 years in a cohort of 7376 participants [11]. This was greater in those with a

K.L. Keung
Centre for Transplant and Renal Research, The Westmead Institute for Medical Research, University of Sydney at Westmead Hospital, 176 Hawkesbury Rd., Westmead, Sydney, NSW 2145, Australia
e-mail: kkeu6183@uni.sydney.edu.au

M.C. Menon
Division of Nephrology and Recanati-Miller Transplantation Institute, Mount Sinai Hospital, One Gustave L. Levy, Place Box 1243 New York, NY 10029, USA
e-mail: madhav.menon@mssm.edu

B. Murphy (✉)
Icahn School of Medicine, Mount Sinai, One Gustave L. Levy, Place Box 1118 New York, NY 10029, USA
e-mail: Barbara.murphy@mssm.edu

J. Rangaswami et al. (eds.), *Cardio-Nephrology*,
DOI 10.1007/978-3-319-56042-7_24

Table 24.1 Recommendations on cardiac surveillance in asymptomatic transplant candidates

	2012 AHA/ACCF Scientific Statement [6]	2005 NKF/KDOQI Guidelines [7]	2007 Lisbon Conference [8]	2013 European Best Practice Guidelines [9]
Coronary Artery Disease (CAD)	The usefulness of periodically screening asymptomatic kidney transplant candidates for myocardial ischemia whilst on the transplant waiting list to reduce the risk of major adverse cardiac events (MACE) is uncertain (class IIb, level of evidence C)	The evaluation of CAD in dialysis patients depends on individual patient status (level of evidence C) For transplant candidates: 1. With diabetes who had an initial normal assessment for CAD, should have 12 monthly evaluations. 2. Without diabetes but "high risk"[a] for CAD, evaluation every 24 months. 3. Those who are not high risk for CAD should have evaluation every 36 months	For those with an expected wait of over 2 years for transplantation, assessment for cardiovascular disease (CVD) should be repeated annually in high- risk individuals, defined as those with 1. Diabetes 2. Prior CVD 3. Multiple CVD risk factors, such as more than 1 year on dialysis; left ventricular hypertrophy; age 60 years; smoking; hypertension; and dyslipidemias	No specific recommendations on surveillance
Valvular Heart Disease (VHD)	May be reasonable to consider ESRD patients with moderate aortic stenosis to be equivalent to demonstrated "rapid progressors" who warrant a yearly echocardiogram and monitoring for early symptoms (Class IIb, Level of C)	Patients should be evaluated for the presence of VHD and for follow-up of VHD in the same manner as the general population[b] except for frequency for follow-up of aortic stenosis. For asymptomatic patients on the wait list with at least moderate aortic stenosis, annual doppler echocardiogram is recommended	No specific recommendations on surveillance	No specific recommendations on surveillance
Left Ventricular Dysfunction (LVD)	Reasonable to perform preoperative assessment of left ventricular function by echocardiography in potential kidney transplant candidates (class IIa; level of evidence B). There is no evidence for or against surveillance by repeated left Ventricular function tests after listing for kidney transplantation	Echocardiograms should be performed in all patients at the initiation of dialysis (level of evidence A), and at 3 yearly intervals thereafter (level of evidence B)	No specific recommendations on surveillance	No specific recommendations on surveillance

AHA American Heart Association; *ACCF* American College of Cardiology Foundation; *NKF KDOQI* National Kidney Foundation Kidney Disease Outcomes Quality Initiative

[a]High risk was defined as more than 20% per 10 years cardiovascular event rate risk according to Framingham data includes those with two or more "traditional" risk factors, a known history of coronary disease, left ventricular ejection fraction 40%, or peripheral vascular disease

[b]2014 AHA/ACC guideline for the management of patients with valvular heart disease: a report of the American College of Cardiology/American Heart Association Task Force on Practice Guidelines [10]

history of CAD (1.3 vs. 0.7%). Patients with chronic kidney disease were not specifically evaluated in this study, and only 10% had diabetes. Given that patients with CKD or diabetes have a greater rate of CAD acceleration, it is probable that there is a shorter "warranty" period on a normal scan in these subgroups. This is supported by observations from a retrospective cohort study of the Veterans Affairs Information System Technology and Architecture database of 1747 patients with known or suspected CAD who underwent MPS with a similar mean period of follow-up. In those with normal imaging results, the annual cardiac death rate was 0.9% for those with no diabetes mellitus (DM) and no CKD (defined as eGFR > 60 mL/min/1.73 m^2), 0.5% in the DM alone group, 2.35% in CKD alone, and 2.9% in those with both DM and CKD [12]. The same authors also demonstrated that when subjects with a normal MPS, when stratified based on renal function, the yearly cardiac mortality increases steadily from 0.9% in those with eGFR > 90 mL/min/1.73 m^2 to 4.7% when eGFR falls to <30 mL [13].

The probability of coronary artery disease following reassuring cardiac investigations in the dialysis population is not well defined. A Japanese study of 100 hemodialysis patients at a single center was cleared of CAD on the basis of MPS/coronary angiography or SPECT and followed for a median period of 2 years. Only 5 patients had an adverse cardiac event in the second year post-investigation [14]. An Australian group assessed a cohort of 107 patients with either stage 4/5 CKD or dialysis dependence and normal baseline dobutamine stress echocardiogram (DSE). Of the 73/107 who underwent repeat DSE, 12% developed evidence of inducible ischemia and a further 9% had scar formation at median follow-up of 1.8 years [15]. The findings of these studies suggest there may be a role for surveillance imaging. However, authors of a large study in this area suggested otherwise [16]. This prospective cohort study of 604 patients aimed to describe CV event rates in ESRD patients awaiting cadaveric renal transplant, along with the frequency of cardiovascular investigations performed during this period and its impact on outcomes. The risk for CV events in diabetic and nondiabetic candidates was 12.7 and 4.5% per year, respectively, over a mean follow-up of 3.7 years. Interestingly, there was no difference in the frequency of major adverse cardiac events or survival when patients were divided into two groups—those who underwent periodic cardiac surveillance in keeping with guideline recommendations at the time versus those who were re-evaluated based on clinical assessment/opinion. In addition, the latter group had fewer investigations performed. The authors concluded that periodic surveillance cardiac investigation may be unnecessary, but warrants further study.

The 2007 report from the Lisbon Conference on the care of renal transplant recipients advised annual reassessment of "high risk" individuals (defined as those with DM, prior history of CAD, multiple cardiac risk factors) who are anticipated to be on the wait list for more than 2 years [8]. A specific screening modality was not recommended. The 2013 European Renal Best Practice (ERBP) guidelines on "The management and evaluation of the kidney donor and recipient" [9] did not provide recommendations on CAD surveillance after the initial evaluation in those on the waiting list. Most recently, the 2012 American Heart Association/American College of Cardiology Foundation (AHA/ACCF) released a scientific statement entitled "Cardiac Disease Evaluation and Management among Kidney and Liver Transplantation Candidates" which was endorsed by the American Society of Transplant Surgeons, American Society of Transplantation, and National Kidney Foundation. Authors concluded that the usefulness of periodic screening for cardiac ischemia to reduce the rate of major cardiac events in asymptomatic subjects awaiting transplant is uncertain (Class IIb, level of evidence C) [6].

Valvular Heart Disease

From national registry data in the US, valvular heart disease (VHD) is more prevalent in patients with pre-dialysis CKD compared to age-matched controls (13.6% compared to 4.9%) [17]. A similar breakdown from national registry data for ESRD patients is unavailable. Observational single center studies involving clinical and autopsy data reveal a high prevalence of mitral and/or aortic valvular calcification in patients with ESKD (35–60% of patients studied) [18–20]. These studies also suggest an etio-pathogenic role of ESKD on both the development and progression of valvular calcification that is linked to abnormalities in calcium–phosphate metabolism which are nearly universally present in ESKD [20, 21]. VHD contributes up to 5% of all deaths in the CKD stage-IV population [22]. While similarly crystalized national data is available from the ESKD population in CAD and atherosclerotic vascular diseases [17], the best surrogate for the contribution of VHD to mortality in ESKD, albeit incomplete, would appear to be through congestive heart failure (CHF). Similar to CKD-stage-IV, CHF contributed to 5% of all deaths in the ESRD population on dialysis. When annualized data from the national kidney transplant waitlist in the US between 2010 and 2012 were examined, waitlist death rate decreased from 6.5 to 5.8 per 100-person-years, while the proportion of patients deemed "too sick to transplant" and delisted, increased from 1.89 to 2.71 [23]. These data do not break down the causes of death on the waitlist and hence the exact contribution of VHD to these proportions nationally is undetermined. However, a retrospective study in 35,215 patients on the kidney transplant waitlist between 1994 and 1997 suggested that uncorrected VHD is a barrier to transplantation, and patients with VHD who did not undergo surgical correction had lower rates of transplantation [24]. Together these data would suggest that VHD is both prevalent and contributes to morbidity and mortality in CKD pre-ESKRD, ESKD on dialysis as well as patients on the kidney waitlist.

The 2012 ACC/ACCF guidelines for the evaluation and management of patients with cardiac disease on the kidney- and liver-transplant waitlists [6] presented recommendations for initial evaluation of other forms of CVD, and are similarly applicable to VHD. For instance, "active cardiac conditions" in candidates would need urgent management before listing. The presence of one or more of these conditions confers high rates of perioperative cardiovascular morbidity and mortality and may require delay or cancelation of surgery. These would include severe, symptomatic VHD. In asymptomatic candidates with VHD, the guidelines are generally similar to management guidelines in non-transplant candidates with VHD. These are detailed in the 2008 focused update from the AHA/ACC [10] and more recently in their 2014 guidelines on the management of VHD [25].

A thorough history and physical examination is recommended to identify cardiac conditions including moderate VHD at initial evaluation at the transplant center. Considerable focus must be placed on assessing exercise tolerance when VHD is suspected or confirmed. The ACC/AHA 2007 "Guidelines on Perioperative Cardiovascular Evaluation and Care for Noncardiac Surgery" [26] highlight the need to risk stratify patients based on functional capacity—a functional capacity ≥ 4 METS in a patient without an active cardiac condition including VHD suggests low risk and no further functional testing may be needed at initial evaluation. Even in asymptomatic patients, we perform baseline echocardiography in all candidates >40 years of age, candidates <40 years with any CVD-comorbidities, or candidates with suggestion of VHD from clinical assessment. Volume status of ESKD patients significantly impacts the echocardiographic assessment of hemodynamics in valvular lesions. For instance, the severity of mitral regurgitation may range from mild to severe on the basis of preload (volume status) and afterload (blood pressure). Thus, it is recommended that transplant candidates on dialysis be evaluated when they are at their dry weight (immediately after dialysis or the intra-dialytic day) and with optimal hemodynamics (heart rate and blood pressure control) [7]. The timing of evaluation may be less important in patients on continuous peritoneal dialysis. We refer all waitlisted patients with VHD of any severity to cardiology for further delineation of risk status.

Specific to the type of valvular disease, the management of VHD in Kidney-waitlist patients may differ. For instance, prospective studies have suggested accelerated progression of aortic stenosis (AS) in ESKD patients [27]. One study reported a twice-normal rate of progression of calcific AS in ESKD—from 0.05 to 0.1 cm^2/year in the general population to 0.23 cm^2/year in the ESKD patients [20]. While data does not exist to support serial echocardiography after initial echo for asymptomatic VHD, candidates with asymptomatic AS may be considered for serial screening for progression of AS lesion, given the higher likelihood of encountering "rapid progressors". The ACC–AHA guidelines for management of CVD in patients on the kidney transplant waitlist recommends annual echocardiographic screening in ESKD patient with moderate AS (Class IIb; Level of Evidence C) [6]. Along similar lines, the ACC–AHA in their VHD management guidelines have recommended that aortic valve replacement may be considered in asymptomatic severe AS if a high likelihood of progression was ascertained [25]. Conversely, studies have suggested that "functional" mitral regurgitation, representing ventricular dysfunction more than structural valvular disease, may be overestimated in ESKD and may improve after transplantation. If valve replacement is considered necessary for VHD, recent data suggests safety of bioprosthetic valves in ESKD patients. Two studies, involving 5858 ESRD patients and 1335 kidney transplant recipients, have suggested similar survival in the study groups within each study independent of whether a bioprosthetic or mechanical valve was used [28, 29]. When corrective surgery for VHD is performed in waitlisted patients, retrospective data suggests that waitlist times are not significantly prolonged, as opposed to leaving VHD that is uncorrected [24]. The safety and efficacy of trans-catheter angiographic procedures for treating mitral and aortic stenosis specific to the kidney-waitlist patients needs further study.

Left Ventricular Dysfunction

Systolic left ventricular dysfunction has been described to be present in 15% of patients starting dialysis, with more recent data suggesting diastolic dysfunction is even more prevalent in the CKD population [30, 31]. Both lead to the clinical syndrome of CHF, the prevalence of which is threefold higher in those with eGFR < 60 mL/min/1.73 m^2 versus those with normal kidney function [32]. Median survival in those with and without heart failure at dialysis initiation is estimated to be 36 and 62 months, respectively [33]. Measurable structural changes including elevated left ventricular mass index as a surrogate marker of left ventricular hypertrophy, often precede functional changes and have been demonstrated to be an independent predictor of cardiac outcomes [34]. There is emerging data on surveillance imaging of cardiac structure and function in the CKD population. However, in ESKD or more specifically in the transplant candidate, rigorous data on risk stratification based on cardiac structural changes is limited. Amongst the few observational or cross-sectional studies in this area, most have relatively short periods of follow-up and not all correlate the progression and/or regression of echocardiographic abnormalities with subsequent cardiac morbidity and mortality outcomes. This has made it difficult to draw firm conclusions on whether serial surveillance of LV dysfunction should be routinely performed in advanced CKD, let alone in the potential transplant recipient.

The 2005 KDOQI guidelines of ESRD recommended an evaluation of cardiac structure and function with echocardiogram in 1–3 months after the initiation of dialysis, and every 3 years thereafter, regardless of symptoms [7]. The recommendation is based on findings of cross sectional and observational studies (summarized in these guidelines) from the 1980s and 1990s, which identified increases in LV mass index and presence of systolic dysfunction in patients with ESRD as predictors of cardiovascular events. When interpreting these results one must consider that standard treatment since the period of recruitment has changed, the routine use of erythropoietin for correction of anemia in advanced CKD is one example, whilst for heart failure therapeutics including beta-blockers have altered the natural progression of disease. The KDOQI guidelines acknowledged in their recommendations that "long-term echocardiographic surveillance of dialysis patients in the modern treatment era is lacking. The appropriate time interval for re-evaluation in chronic dialysis patients is therefore uncertain" [7]. A number of these publications referenced by the KDOQI guidelines derived data from a single clinical cohort of 433 patients in a longitudinal multicenter Canadian study that followed patients from the initiation of dialysis, over a mean duration of 41 months. Patients had annual clinical assessment, with baseline and progress echocardiogram performed on average 3.3 and 17.6 months, respectively, after the initiation of dialysis. On baseline echocardiogram, LVH was identified in 73.9%, dilated LV in 35.5%, and systolic dysfunction in 14.8% [30]. Of the 299 patients without clinical evidence of congestive cardiac failure (CCF) at the initiation of dialysis, 76 (25%) developed de novo CCF at median time of 15 months, equating to a rate of 7% per year. Factors identified at initial screening, which predicted development of CCF included elevated left ventricular mass index, elevated left ventricular end-diastolic diameter, and worse LV systolic dysfunction. Cardiac failure, peripheral vascular disease, left ventricular fractional shortening, systolic dysfunction, and LV cavity volume were associated with cardiac mortality, whilst LV mass index was independently associated with death after 2 years. The same group evaluated changes between baseline and progress echocardiogram performed 1 year after the initiation of dialysis in 227 patients [35]. Of the 137 who had no history of CHF, 36 (26%) developed de novo cardiac failure after the first year following dialysis initiation. Comparing those who did and did not develop de novo cardiac failure after the first year, the mean changes in LV mass index were 17 and 0 g/m^2, respectively, and for fractional shortening −8 and 0%, respectively. The authors concluded that serial echocardiography adds prognostic information beyond what is provided from a baseline study. A self-selected subgroup of 29 patients from the original cohort had four sequential echocardiograms performed annually following the initiation of dialysis [36]. Statistically significant increases in posterior wall thickness, left ventricular end-diastolic diameter, left ventricular mass index, and cavity volume index were noted to develop over time. Most of the changes in mass and volume index occurred in the first year, but increases were still seen thereafter. These studies would suggest baseline and progress evaluation of cardiac function in dialysis patients is probably useful in identifying patients at risk of future de novo cardiac failure. Nevertheless, further studies to evaluate if progression confers a worse prognosis and/or regression improves outcomes in the modern treatment era to justify routine surveillance are needed.

More recently, studies assessing the role of surveillance imaging of LV structure/function in patients at different stages of CKD to ESKD have been published [31, 37, 38]. Zoccali et al. evaluated a subset of patients from the Cardiovascular Risk Extended Evaluation in Dialysis Patients (CREED) study [37] for progression of LV systolic dysfunction, measured by mid wall fractional shortening (mwFS). These were dialysis patients without a history of heart failure and with baseline LV ejection fraction of $\geq 35\%$ [37]. 191 patients had baseline and repeat echocardiograms performed on average 17 months apart, and were then followed for a further 27 months after the second scan. 85/191 patients had at least one CV event, and in 52 patients these were fatal. The Kaplan–Meier analysis with patients stratified by mwFS < 50th (change in mwFS $-1.3 \pm 1.2\%$), 51st–75th ($0.3 \pm 0.2\%$), and >75th percentile ($+1.4 \pm 0.7\%$), showed a 41% increase in the relative risk for fatal and nonfatal CV events for patients in the highest quartile compared to those in the lowest.

The Longitudinal Changes of Cardiac Structure and Function in CKD (CASCADE) study prospectively followed 300 patients with stage 3–5 CKD who underwent baseline echocardiogram [30]. 278 had progress imaging after 1 year where both systolic and diastolic parameters were evaluated. This is in contrast to earlier studies that focused on systolic dysfunction only. The entire cohort showed a significant increase in LV mass index with an increased prevalence of LVH and diastolic dysfunction over 1 year, along with severity of diastolic dysfunction. Stratification by CKD stage (3a, 3b, and stage 4/5) showed a greater decline in eGFR in the latter group, along with a greater increase in LV mass index and volume index, without significant difference in the change in LV function between the different CKD stages. Having stage 4/5 CKD was an independent predictor of progression in LV mass index, LV volume index and diastolic dysfunction grades, after controlling for other known factors associated with LV abnormalities. However, one of the limitations of the study was that echocardiographic findings were not correlated with clinical outcomes.

In a cross-sectional study of a subset of 190 patients from the Chronic Renal Insufficiency Cohort (CRIC) study [37] enrolled from 2003 to 2007 and followed to 2011, an echocardiogram was performed when they met criteria for advanced CKD (eGFR < 20 mL/min/1.73 m^2), and again after progression to ESKD (defined as requiring maintenance hemodialysis or peritoneal dialysis). This period is of interest since renal transplant candidates in the US may be pre-dialysis at their initial cardiac evaluation and when they are waitlisted as "active," but eventually transition to dialysis whilst awaiting transplantation. The mean duration between the echocardiograms was 2 (± 1.0) years, and the mean time between advanced CKD echocardiogram and initiation of dialysis was 1.1 (±0.9) years. There was no significant change in LV mass index over this period, but statistically significant changes in the mean LVEF declined from 53 to 50%, whilst the proportion of participants with EF $\leq 50\%$ increased from 29 to 48% [38]. Whether a fall in LVEF at this "near normal" range has prognostic implication with regards to cardiac morbidity and mortality again was not evaluated and it remains to be seen whether correlation with clinical outcomes will emerge in coming years.

It is worthwhile to highlight that there is also an increasing body of evidence that regimens of more frequent dialysis compared to conventional thrice-weekly dialysis results in a reduction in LV mass [39, 40]. The Frequent Hemodialysis Network (FHN) trial group has also shown that patients who received frequent (six times weekly) hemodialysis intervention versus conventional (thrice-weekly) hemodialysis over a 12-month period had significant improvements in both coprimary outcomes (death or 12-month change in left ventricular mass and death or 12-month change in self-reported physical health) [41], and demonstrated reduced long-term mortality with a median follow-up of 3.6 years [42]. It remains to be studied whether the difference in mortality is a consequence of the impact on cardiac indices and whether this ultimately translates to superior outcomes post-transplant.

As it stands, there are no studies that have described cardiac outcomes of transplant candidates who have and have not undergone periodic echocardiogram surveillance of LV dysfunction, hence the utility of screening for LV dysfunction is not substantiated. The 2007 Lisbon Conference document included LVH as a cardiovascular risk factor for identifying "highest risk" patients to be screened annually whilst listed. The 2012 AHA/ACCF cardiovascular guidelines for transplant candidates state it is reasonable to perform preoperative assessment of left ventricular function by echocardiography in potential kidney transplant candidates (Class IIa, Level of Evidence B); and there is no evidence for or against surveillance by repeated left ventricular function tests after listing for kidney transplantation [6]. The 2013 ACCF/AHA "Guideline for the Management of Heart Failure" also concluded that in those with LV dysfunction in the general population, unless there is a change in clinical status or treatment interventions, there is no role for routine repeat measurement of LV function assessment (Level of evidence B) [43]. However, the 2014 ACC/AHA "Guidelines on Perioperative Cardiovascular Evaluation and Management of Patients Undergoing Noncardiac Surgery" recommends reassessment of LV function in clinically stable patients with previously documented LV dysfunction may be considered if there has been no assessment within a year (Class IIb, Level of evidence C) [44].

Summary

There is little consistent, quality evidence even in advanced CKD cohorts let alone in the subgroup of renal transplant candidates, to strongly support the practice of periodic re-screening for CVD whilst listed, when initial assessment is unremarkable and clinical risk profile remains unchanged. Whether scheduled periodic screening, as opposed to re-evaluation based on clinician assessment alone, improves major cardiovascular morbidity and mortality and justifies the high costs associated with this remains to be seen. Suggestions were made by the 2012 AHA/ACCF cardiac disease guidelines for transplant candidates [6] for future study design that may help to answer these questions.

References

1. Matas AJ, Smith JM, Skeans MA, Thompson B, Gustafson SK, Stewart DE, et al. OPTN/SRTR 2013 annual data report: kidney. Am J Transplant. 2015;15(Suppl 2):1–34.
2. System USRD. USRDS annual data report: epidemiology of kidney disease in the United States. Bethesda, MD: National Institutes of Health, National Institute of Diabetes and Digestive and Kidney Diseases; 2015.
3. Davies DB, Harper A. The OPTN waiting list, 1988–2003. Clin Transpl. 2004; 19:27–40.
4. Lentine KL, Brennan DC, Schnitzler MA. Incidence and predictors of myocardial infarction after kidney transplantation. J Am Soc Nephrol. 2005;16(2):496–506.
5. Kasiske BL, Maclean JR, Snyder JJ. Acute myocardial infarction and kidney transplantation. J Am Soc Nephrol. 2006;17(3):900–7.
6. Lentine KL, Costa SP, Weir MR, Robb JF, Fleisher LA, Kasiske BL, et al. Cardiac disease evaluation and management among kidney and liver transplantation candidates: a scientific statement from the American Heart Association and the American College of Cardiology Foundation: endorsed by the American Society of Transplant Surgeons, American Society of Transplantation, and National Kidney Foundation. Circulation. 2012;126 (5):617–63.
7. Group KDW. K/DOQI clinical practice guidelines for cardiovascular disease in dialysis patients. Am J Kidney Dis. 2005;45(4 Suppl 3):S1–153.
8. Abbud-Filho M, Adams PL, Alberu J, Cardella C, Chapman J, Cochat P, et al. A report of the Lisbon Conference on the care of the kidney transplant recipient. Transplantation. 2007;83(8 Suppl): S1–22.
9. ERBP Guideline on the Management and Evaluation of the Kidney Donor and Recipient. Nephrology, dialysis, transplantation: official publication of the European Dialysis and Transplant Association—European Renal Association. 2013;28(Suppl 2):ii1–71.
10. Bonow RO, Carabello BA, Chatterjee K, de Leon AC, Jr Faxon DP, Freed MD, et al. 2008 Focused update incorporated into the ACC/AHA 2006 guidelines for the management of patients with valvular heart disease: a report of the American College of Cardiology/American Heart Association Task Force on Practice Guidelines (Writing Committee to Revise the 1998 Guidelines for the Management of Patients With Valvular Heart Disease): endorsed by the Society of Cardiovascular Anesthesiologists, Society for Cardiovascular Angiography and Interventions,

and Society of Thoracic Surgeons. Circulation. 2008;118(15): e523–661.
11. Hachamovitch R, Hayes S, Friedman JD, Cohen I, Shaw LJ, Germano G, et al. Determinants of risk and its temporal variation in patients with normal stress myocardial perfusion scans: what is the warranty period of a normal scan? J Am Coll Cardiol. 2003;41(8):1329–40.
12. Hakeem A, Bhatti S, Karmali KN, Dillie KS, Cook JR, Xu J, et al. Renal function and risk stratification of diabetic and nondiabetic patients undergoing evaluation for coronary artery disease. JACC Cardiovasc Imaging. 2010;3(7):734–45.
13. Hakeem A, Bhatti S, Dillie KS, Cook JR, Samad Z, Roth-Cline MD, et al. Predictive value of myocardial perfusion single-photon emission computed tomography and the impact of renal function on cardiac death. Circulation. 2008;118(24):2540–9.
14. Joki N, Tanaka Y, Ishikawa H, Takahashi Y, Iwakura Y, Masuda H, et al. Optimum second screening point for detection of coronary artery disease in hemodialysis patients without advanced coronary artery disease. Am J Nephrol. 2009;29(5):420–5.
15. Rakhit DJ, Marwick TH, Armstrong KA, Johnson DW, Leano R, Isbel NM. Effect of aggressive risk factor modification on cardiac events and myocardial ischaemia in patients with chronic kidney disease. Heart (British Cardiac Society). 2006;92(10):1402–8.
16. Gill JS, Ma I, Landsberg D, Johnson N, Levin A. Cardiovascular events and investigation in patients who are awaiting cadaveric kidney transplantation. J Am Soc Nephrol. 2005;16(3):808–16.
17. System USRD. USRDS annual data report: Chronic Kidney Disease in the United States. Bethesda: National Institutes of Health, National Institute of Diabetes and Digestive and Kidney Diseases; 2015.
18. Maher ER, Young G, Smyth-Walsh B, Pugh S, Curtis JR. Aortic and mitral valve calcification in patients with end-stage renal disease. Lancet. 1987;2(8564):875–7.
19. Takahashi H, Ishii H, Aoyama T, Kamoi D, Kasuga H, Ito Y, et al. Association of cardiac valvular calcifications and C-reactive protein with cardiovascular mortality in incident hemodialysis patients: a Japanese cohort study. Am J Kidney Dis. 2013;61(2):254–61.
20. Umana E, Ahmed W, Alpert MA. Valvular and perivalvular abnormalities in end-stage renal disease. Am J Med Sci. 2003;325(4):237–42.
21. Fox CS, Larson MG, Vasan RS, Guo CY, Parise H, Levy D, et al. Cross-sectional association of kidney function with valvular and annular calcification: the Framingham heart study. J Am Soc Nephrol. 2006;17(2):521–7.
22. Thompson S, James M, Wiebe N, Hemmelgarn B, Manns B, Klarenbach S, et al. Cause of death in patients with reduced kidney function. J Am Soc Nephrol. 2015;26(10):2504–11.
23. OPTN/SRTR. 2012 Annual Report of the U.S. Organ Procurement and Transplantation Network and the Scientific Registry of Transplant Recipients. Department of Health and Human Services, Health Resources and Services Administration, Healthcare Systems Bureau, Division of Transplantation, Rockville, MD; United Network for Organ Sharing, Richmond, VA; University Renal Research and Education Association, Ann Arbor, MI. 2014.
24. Abbott KC, Hshieh P, Cruess D, Agodoa LY, Welch PG, Taylor AJ, et al. Hospitalized valvular heart disease in patients on renal transplant waiting list: incidence, clinical correlates and outcomes. Clin Nephrol. 2003;59(2):79–87.
25. Nishimura RA, Otto CM, Bonow RO, Carabello BA, Erwin JP 3rd, Guyton RA, et al. 2014 AHA/ACC guideline for the management of patients with valvular heart disease: a report of the American College of Cardiology/American Heart Association Task Force on Practice Guidelines. J Thorac Cardiovasc Surg. 2014;148(1):e1–132.
26. Fleisher LA, Beckman JA, Brown KA, Calkins H, Chaikof EL, Fleischmann KE, et al. ACC/AHA 2007 guidelines on perioperative cardiovascular evaluation and care for noncardiac surgery: a report of the American College of Cardiology/American Heart Association Task Force on Practice Guidelines (Writing Committee to Revise the 2002 Guidelines on Perioperative Cardiovascular Evaluation for Noncardiac Surgery) developed in collaboration with the American Society of Echocardiography, American Society of Nuclear Cardiology, Heart Rhythm Society, Society of Cardiovascular Anesthesiologists, Society for Cardiovascular Angiography and Interventions, Society for Vascular Medicine and Biology, and Society for Vascular Surgery. J Am Coll Cardiol. 2007;50(17):e159–241.
27. Zentner D, Hunt D, Chan W, Barzi F, Grigg L, Perkovic V. Prospective evaluation of aortic stenosis in end-stage kidney disease: a more fulminant process? Nephrol Dialysis Transplant. 2011;26(5):1651–5.
28. Herzog CA, Ma JZ, Collins AJ. Long-term survival of dialysis patients in the United States with prosthetic heart valves: should ACC/AHA practice guidelines on valve selection be modified? Circulation. 2002;105(11):1336–41.
29. Sharma A, Gilbertson DT, Herzog CA. Survival of kidney transplantation patients in the United States after cardiac valve replacement. Circulation. 2010;121(25):2733–9.
30. Foley RN, Parfrey PS, Harnett JD, Kent GM, Martin CJ, Murray DC, et al. Clinical and echocardiographic disease in patients starting end-stage renal disease therapy. Kidney Int. 1995;47(1):186–92.
31. Cai QZ, Lu XZ, Lu Y, Wang AY. Longitudinal changes of cardiac structure and function in CKD (CASCADE study). J Am Soc Nephrol. 2014;25(7):1599–608.
32. Kottgen A, Russell SD, Loehr LR, Crainiceanu CM, Rosamond WD, Chang PP, et al. Reduced kidney function as a risk factor for incident heart failure: the atherosclerosis risk in communities (ARIC) study. J Am Soc Nephrol. 2007;18(4):1307–15.
33. Foley RN, Parfrey PS, Hefferton D, Singh I, Simms A, Barrett BJ. Advance prediction of early death in patients starting maintenance dialysis. Am J Kidney Dis. 1994;23(6):836–45.
34. Stack AG, Saran R. Clinical correlates and mortality impact of left ventricular hypertrophy among new ESRD patients in the United States. Am J Kidney Dis. 2002;40(6):1202–10.
35. Foley RN, Parfrey PS, Kent GM, Harnett JD, Murray DC, Barre PE. Serial change in echocardiographic parameters and cardiac failure in end-stage renal disease. J Am Soc Nephrol. 2000;11(5):912–6.
36. Foley RN, Parfrey PS, Kent GM, Harnett JD, Murray DC, Barre PE. Long-term evolution of cardiomyopathy in dialysis patients. Kidney Int. 1998;54(5):1720–5.
37. Zoccali C, Benedetto FA, Tripepi G, Mallamaci F, Rapisarda F, Seminara G, et al. Left ventricular systolic function monitoring in asymptomatic dialysis patients: a prospective cohort study. J Am Soc Nephrol. 2006;17(5):1460–5.
38. Bansal N, Keane M, Delafontaine P, Dries D, Foster E, Gadegbeku CA, et al. A longitudinal study of left ventricular function and structure from CKD to ESRD: the CRIC study. Clin J Am Soc Nephrol. 2013;8(3):355–62.
39. Culleton BF, Walsh M, Klarenbach SW, Mortis G, Scott-Douglas N, Quinn RR, et al. Effect of frequent nocturnal hemodialysis vs conventional hemodialysis on left ventricular mass and quality of life: a randomized controlled trial. JAMA. 2007;298(11):1291–9.
40. Chan CT, Greene T, Chertow GM, Kliger AS, Stokes JB, Beck GJ, et al. Determinants of left ventricular mass in patients on

hemodialysis: Frequent Hemodialysis Network (FHN) trials. Circ Cardiovasc Imaging. 2012;5(2):251–61.
41. Chertow GM, Levin NW, Beck GJ, Depner TA, Eggers PW, Gassman JJ, et al. In-center hemodialysis six times per week versus three times per week. New Engl J Med. 2010;363 (24):2287–300.
42. Chertow GM, Levin NW, Beck GJ, Daugirdas JT, Eggers PW, Kliger AS, et al. Long-term effects of frequent in-center hemodialysis. J Am Soc Nephrol. 2016;27(6):1830–6.
43. Yancy CW, Jessup M, Bozkurt B, Butler J, Casey DE Jr, Drazner MH, et al. 2013 ACCF/AHA guideline for the management of heart failure: a report of the American College of Cardiology Foundation/American Heart Association Task Force on Practice Guidelines. J Am Coll Cardiol. 2013;62(16):e147–239.
44. Fleisher LA, Fleischmann KE, Auerbach AD, Barnason SA, Beckman JA, Bozkurt B, et al. 2014 ACC/AHA guideline on perioperative cardiovascular evaluation and management of patients undergoing noncardiac surgery: a report of the American College of Cardiology/American Heart Association Task Force on practice guidelines. J Am Coll Cardiol. 2014;64(22):e77–137.

25 Post-Kidney Transplant Modification of Cardiovascular Risk

Mythili Ghanta, Swati Rao, Iris Lee, and Serban Constantinescu

Introduction

Kidney transplantation (KT) remains the optimal and most cost-effective modality of treatment for patients with end-stage renal disease (ESRD). KT offers a survival advantage compared to remaining dialysis dependent, in addition to improvement in quality of life [1]. Short-term graft survival rates after KT have considerably improved over the past decade due to advances in immunosuppressive strategies and reduction in acute rejection rates. However, there remains a lag in the improvement of long-term graft survival rates. Death with a functioning transplant contributes to majority (>50%) of late graft loss. Cardiovascular disease (CVD) is the leading cause of death after KT [2]. The risk of major adverse cardiovascular events (MACE) is highest within the immediate post-transplant period and decreases thereafter. Hence the current pre-transplant evaluation is centered on CVD risk assessment and modification to lower the incidence of immediate post-operative cardiac events. This chapter discusses the various factors that elevate post KT CVD risk, and how to optimize these to improve long-term outcomes.

M. Ghanta (✉)
Department of Internal Medicine, UT Southwestern Medical Center, 5323 Harry Hines Blvd., Dallas, TX 75390, USA
e-mail: mythili.ghanta@utsouthwestern.edu

S. Rao · I. Lee · S. Constantinescu
Department of Medicine, Section of Nephrology, Hypertension and Kidney Transplantation, Lewis Katz School of Medicine, Temple University, 3440 N Broad Street, Kresge West, Suite 100, Philadelphia, PA 19140, USA
e-mail: swati.rao@tuhs.temple.edu

I. Lee
e-mail: iris.lee@tuhs.temple.edu

S. Constantinescu
e-mail: serban.constantinescu@tuhs.temple.edu

J. Rangaswami et al. (eds.), *Cardio-Nephrology*,
DOI 10.1007/978-3-319-56042-7_25

Incidence/Prevalence of Cardiovascular Disease in Kidney Transplant Recipients

CVD accounts for 35–50% of all-cause mortality in kidney transplant recipients (KTR), and CVD mortality rates are at least twice as high in an age-matched KTR compared to the general population. However, when compared to age-matched dialysis patients, CVD risk is significantly lower post-KT. The two most likely explanations for the reduced risk in KTR compared to dialysis patients are: (1) a selection bias in favor of those undergoing KT, and (2) removal of the hemodynamic/uremic abnormalities associated with maintenance dialysis after KT [2]. An international study comprising of >20,000 KTR (Patient Outcomes in Renal Transplantation-PORT Study) reported the incidence of coronary heart disease in KTR as 3, 5, and 7% at 1, 3, and 5 years post-KT, respectively [3]. Similarly, United States Renal Data System (USRDS) registry data analysis showed post-KT acute myocardial infarction (AMI) rates as 4, 5, and 11% at 6, 12, and 36 months post-KT [4]. In this analysis older recipient and donor age, pre-transplant CVD, history of diabetes, and deceased donor transplantation were identified as risk factors for AMI. Diagnosis of post-transplantation diabetes or graft failure markedly increased the risk of AMI, and post-transplantation AMI-predicted allograft failure, and death.

Risk Factors for Cardiovascular Disease in Kidney Transplant Recipients

Risk factors for CVD in KTR are manifold and are summarized in Table 25.1. They include traditional CVD risk factors, such as hypertension, diabetes, hyperlipidemia, and smoking which are highly prevalent in KTR, and nontraditional risk factors (factors unique to transplantation itself), such as the direct effects of immunosuppressive agents, rejection, and allograft dysfunction. Several pre-transplant factors determine the risk of CVD post-KT. For example, duration of dialysis pre KT as well as preexisting CVD remains risk factors for CVD post-KT. The prevalence of traditional risk factors at the time of wait listing for KT was recently described, which identified that at the time of listing for KT, 94% were hypertensive, 81% had dyslipidemia, 45% were smokers, 23% were diabetics, and 21% of patients had preexisting CVD [5]. When this cohort of patients was followed longitudinally, 15% sustained adverse cardiovascular events. Lawrence et al. have shown that there is increased risk of major cardiovascular events in the immediate post-transplantation period in patients who have undergone coronary interventions as part of pre-transplant CVD work up, and heightened vigilance for acute coronary events is required in this subgroup of patients. However, once the immediate post-operative phase is overcome, long-term allograft and patient survival rates were comparable to the patients not requiring coronary interventions [6].

Transplant specific risk factors (both donor as well as recipient related) play an additional role in increasing CVD risk post KT. The Australian and New Zealand transplant registry data have shown that younger KTR (age <60 years old) receiving expanded criteria deceased donor KT had higher risk of all-cause mortality largely attributed to CVD, compared to recipients within the same age range receiving standard criteria deceased donor transplants [3]. Hence both recipient and donor factors should be incorporated into the algorithm for the pre-operative cardiac evaluation and post-transplant care.

Estimation of CVD Risk in Kidney Transplant Recipients

The Framingham risk score, which is widely utilized in the general population to estimate the risk of MACE, underestimates the risk of CVD in KTR [7]. This was attributed largely to the increased risk incurred by diabetes in KTR [8]. Estimated glomerular filtration rate (GFR) <50 ml/min/m^2 in KTR is also a significant risk factor for CVD in addition to traditional Framingham criteria [9]. Based on these observations, separate risk calculators for CVD were designed for KTR. Soveri et al. validated a seven variable risk calculator for KTR utilizing the study population from the Assessment of Lescol in Renal Transplantation study (ALERT) to predict CVD in this population that included age, previous history of coronary artery disease, diabetes, low-density lipoprotein, serum creatinine, number of transplants, and smoking [10]. Israni et al. validated a CVD risk calculator for KTR and identified several risk factors for CVD based on analysis of the PORT study including history of pretransplant diabetes, new onset diabetes after transplant, pretransplant CVD events, estimated GFR, delayed graft function, acute rejection, age, sex, race, and dialysis vintage [3]. In this study, the authors concluded that variables pertinent to allograft function by far explain the increased incidence of CVD in KTR [3].

Role of Traditional Risk Factors for CVD in Kidney Transplant Recipients

Age

It is a well-established fact that advanced age is a risk factor for CVD. Over the past decade there has been a considerable increase in the number of patients older than 65 years who are waitlisted for, as well as received a KT in the United States. In fact, elderly patients represent the largest proportion of increase in the wait list in the United States over the past decade with improved access to KT [11, 12]. There is

Table 25.1 Risk factors for cardiovascular disease in kidney transplant recipients

Traditional risk factors
Age, male gender, smoking, hypertension, diabetes, dyslipidemia, obesity, metabolic syndrome
Pre-transplant risk factors
Vintage of dialysis pre-transplant, preexisting cardiovascular disease, malnutrition, Hepatitis C infection, Systemic lupus erythematosus
Transplant specific risk factors
Immunosuppressive agents
Allograft dysfunction related to acute rejection, delayed graft function or chronic kidney disease from any cause, proteinuria
Donor factors: expanded criteria donors
Repeat renal transplantation
New onset diabetes post-transplantation

definitely a survival advantage in recipients aged 60–74 years with KT compared to remaining on dialysis. However, they have increased mortality at 5 years post-KT compared to recipients younger than 60 years [1]. Although studies suggest favorable outcomes of KT in the elderly, it needs to be recognized that this is a highly selective group of recipients who have passed extensive cardiac evaluation pre-transplantation. Hence thorough cardiac evaluation and careful selection of elderly dialysis patients for KT is essential to minimize cardiovascular morbidity and mortality in the immediate post-transplant period and achieve the benefits of KT.

Gender and Ethnicity

Males are at increased risk of CVD compared to females at 1 and 3 years post-KT with adjusted hazards ratio of 1.2 and 1.3, respectively [3]. It is a well-known fact that there is racial disparity in KT survival with improvement in long-term outcomes for African American's (AA) lagging behind non-AA. These have been linked to various immunological and nonimmunological factors [13]. In a cohort of approximately 1000 KTR with 50% AA, the prevalence of preexisting CVD was similar to Caucasian KTR; however, the prevalence of hypertension and diabetes were higher in AA recipients. More importantly, CVD risk factors were not effectively controlled amongst AA KTR post-transplant [14]. Several factors such as socioeconomic disparities could have contributed to these differences and should be explored to reduce racial disparities and optimize patient and allograft outcomes. Results of the PORT study, (72% Caucasian, 14% AA, 14% other ethnicities), identified Caucasians with higher adjusted hazards ratio of CVD within 3 years post-KT (1.45), followed by AA (1.16), and least in other ethnicities [3].

Tobacco Use

The prevalence of cigarette smoking at time of KT is high (25–50%) and is comparable to the general population [15]. In KTR, smoking has been associated with increased risk of CVD, malignancies, graft failure and death. In fact, the negative impact of cigarette smoking on patient survival post-KT is similar to diabetes mellitus [16]. The KDIGO 2009 guidelines recommend screening for tobacco use at initial evaluation, and annually thereafter. In a study of more than 1300 KTR, smoking history of 11–25 pack-years was associated with increased relative risk of CV events by 1.56. The relative risk increased further to 2.14 with more than 25 pack-years of smoking. The detrimental effects of smoking decreased in patients who had quit more than 5 years before KT [15]. Thus, potential KTR should be encouraged to quit smoking via nonpharmacological and pharmacological methods. Although there is limited data on the impact of smoking cessation post-KT, it is a reasonable assumption that the KTR will also benefit from smoking cessation like the general population.

Post-Transplantation Hypertension

Hypertension (HTN) after KT is common, with approximately 85% of adult KTR requiring anti-hypertensive agents. Uncontrolled HTN was identified as an important risk factor for increased CVD mortality and graft loss. A recent post hoc analysis of the Folic Acid for Vascular Outcome Reduction in Transplantation (FAVORIT trial) suggests that in KTR every 20 mm rise in systolic BP as well as every 10 mm drop in diastolic BP below 70 mm Hg is associated with increased CVD risk [17]. Several donor and recipient factors contribute to HTN post-KT and are summarized in Table 25.2. Transplant renal artery stenosis (TRAS) is an important cause of HTN post-KT with reported prevalence ranging between 1 and 25%. The most common site of TRAS is at the transplant renal artery anastomosis to the recipient's external iliac artery; however, stenosis proximal to the anastomosis within the recipient aorta-iliac system can also lead to HTN. Clinical presentation mimics renal artery stenosis in native kidneys, and could range from isolated uncontrolled HTN to graft dysfunction especially with initiation of angiotensin converting enzyme (ACE) inhibitors to recurrent flash pulmonary edema. Noninvasive Doppler ultrasonography (USG) is diagnostic in the majority of cases; however, CT/MR angiography or invasive angiogram might need to be considered in some situations when Doppler USG is inconclusive. Aggressive medical therapy might avoid intervention in some cases, however with failure of medical therapy percutaneous angioplasty with or without stenting should be considered. Surgical correction should be reserved for cases where the above interventions failed, but with advances in percutaneous endovascular procedures, surgery is rarely performed [18]. Obstructive sleep apnea is another underdiagnosed and common cause of resistant hypertension in KTR.

Immunosuppressive agents such as corticosteroids and calcineurin inhibitors (CNI) contribute to post-transplant HTN. Among the CNIs, cyclosporine exacerbates hypertension to a greater degree than tacrolimus. Both CNIs lead to glomerular afferent arteriolar vasoconstriction, in addition to salt retention leading to HTN. Corticosteroid and CNI sparing protocols show favorable BP control in KTRs. Changes to immunosuppression targeting better BP control should carefully balance the risk of allograft rejection associated with these changes. Adequate control of BP post-

Table 25.2 Risk factors for hypertension post-kidney transplantation

Risk factors
Donor factors: older age, donor hypertension, donor–recipient size mismatch (pediatric donor)
Allograft dysfunction: acute or chronic (possibly related to acute rejection, chronic allograft nephropathy, obstruction, recurrent disease or other etiologies)
Compression/stenosis of the transplant renal artery (Kink, external compression from fluid collections)
Immunosuppressive agents: corticosteroids, calcineurin inhibitors
Recipient factors: preexisting hypertension, obesity, sleep apnea, age, primary hyperaldosteronism

KT would translate into improvement of CVD-related outcomes in addition to improved graft survival. Prospective trials to establish blood pressure goals specifically in KTR would help improve outcomes.

The management of post-transplant HTN should take into account interactions between anti-hypertensive and immunosuppressive agents. Aggressive lifestyle modification with salt restriction, physical exercise, and weight loss should be implemented. No specific groups of anti-hypertensive agents are proven to be superior to others in management of post KT HTN. Clear understanding of the recipient comorbidity profile and pathophysiology of HTN will help to choose the anti-hypertensive regimen. Patient tolerability as well as potential drug interactions especially through the cytochrome P 450 pathway, also plays a role in the choice of the agents. Volume overload in the setting of delayed or slow graft function plays an important role in uncontrolled HTN within first month post-transplantation, wherein diuretics are the mainstay of treatment. Additionally, in this time frame, high dose corticosteroids are also used, which compounds sodium and water retention. Typically, ACE or angiotensin receptor blockers (ARB) are avoided during this time frame until complete recovery of renal allograft function from ischemia reperfusion injury is achieved. Calcium channel blockers are widely utilized in KTR and are shown to overcome the vaso-constrictive properties of CNIs with beneficial impact on graft function [19]. Verapamil and cardizem are inhibitors of cytochrome P 450 leading to high CNI levels, thus amlodipine and nifedipine are widely used due to lack of drug–drug interactions. Beta Blockers are well tolerated in KTR and are indicated in patients with underlying CVD. ACE and ARBs are effective in lowering BP in KTR, however their side effect profile includes anemia, hyperkalemia, and increased susceptibility to acute kidney injury (AKI), hence close monitoring is required. Current KDIGO guidelines support use of ACE/ARB in KTR with proteinuria >1 g/day.

Metabolic Syndrome

Prevalence of obesity and metabolic syndrome is high in dialysis patients and continues to increase post KT due to weight gain as well as detrimental effects of immunosuppressive agents, notably steroids. Weight gain leads to increased risk of HTN and new onset diabetes after transplantation (NODAT) and observational data support an association between obesity and increased CVD-related mortality in KTR [20]. Interventions targeting weight gain post KT would potentially lead to improved long-term outcomes by lowering comorbidities leading to CVD events. Potential risk of oxalate nephropathy in the renal allograft should be recognized in the post-transplant period in recipients of KT following bariatric surgery [21].

Diabetes

NODAT as well as preexisting diabetes contributes to increased CVD post KT. The incidence of NODAT has been reported to vary between 2 and 60% in KTR. The literature substantiates the adverse impact of NODAT on long-term kidney allograft function and patient survival, in addition to increased risk of post-transplant CVD. A case control study from Germany analyzing the long-term impact of KT on HbA1C levels in nondiabetic deceased donor KTR showed a progressive rise in glycated hemoglobin (HbA1C) levels compared to the general population over a 5-year follow up period [22]. Therefore, interventions reducing the impact of NODAT could lead to improved overall post-KT outcomes. Risk factors for NODAT can be divided into two categories: modifiable and nonmodifiable, and are summarized in Table 25.3. The American Diabetes Association (ADA) criteria are utilized in KTR for diagnosis of NODAT. These guidelines in addition to symptoms of diabetes include random plasma glucose level ≥ 200 mg/dl or fasting plasma glucose concentration >126 mg/dl or a 2-h plasma glucose concentration >200 mg/dl during an oral glucose tolerance test [23]. The 2009 KDIGO guidelines added HbA1C into the criteria [20].

Weight gain as well as immunosuppressive agents are major risk factors for NODAT. Glucocorticoids contribute to insulin resistance. CNIs, mainly tacrolimus in addition to direct toxicity on pancreatic beta cells, decrease insulin gene expression as well as reduce glucose uptake, inducing NODAT. Evidence suggests that sirolimus reduces pancreatic beta cell proliferation leading to NODAT [24]. Reddy et al. have studied risk factors for NODAT in south Asian KTR and their analysis suggests a genetic predisposition to NODAT with increased prevalence in certain HLA types [25]. Early hyperglycemia post-KT is a risk factor for NODAT and needs to be promptly treated.

Table 25.3 Risk factors for NODAT

Nonmodifiable risk factors
Older age (>40 years)
Ethnicity (African Americans and Hispanics)
HLA antigen mismatch, acute rejection episodes
Genetic factors
Autosomal dominant polycystic kidney disease
Modifiable risk factors
Immunosuppressive agents (Tacrolimus, corticosteroids, sirolimus)
Obesity (body mass index >30 kg/m^2)
Viral infections (cytomegalovirus infection and Hepatitis C)
Peritoneal dialysis

In KTR with preexisting diabetes as well as NODAT, aggressive glycemic control as well as optimal management of other CVD risk factors, such as dyslipidemia, is warranted. Immunosuppressive modification (corticosteroid and CNI sparing) should be considered weighing the risk of acute rejection. Elderly KTR are especially at increased risk of NODAT and might be more prone to islet cell toxicity related to tacrolimus compared to younger recipients [26].

Routine screening for NODAT with fasting glucose monitoring weekly for the first 4 weeks and then HbA1C levels every 3 months for the first year post-KT is recommended. Thereafter annual HbA1C monitoring is needed. Just like in the general population, aspirin use is recommended in KTR with NODAT or preexisting diabetes for preventing ischemic CVD.

Dyslipidemia

Dyslipidemia is a major risk factor for CVD in KTR, with prevalence as high as 50% within the first year of KT [27, 28]. Evaluation of causal factors, such as diabetes mellitus and weight gain, are crucial for adequate control of dyslipidemia. Allograft specific factors, such as proteinuria, allograft dysfunction, and acute rejection also influence dyslipidemia in KTR [29].

Retrospective studies have associated increased total cholesterol (TC), low-density lipid (LDL), and triglycerides (TG) with increase CVD, whereas higher levels of high density lipid (HDL) have been associated with protection from CVD in KTR [8, 30, 31]. In fact, the risk of ischemic heart disease associated with elevated TC is higher in KTR than in the general population [8]. The effect of treatment of dyslipidemia on CVD in KTR was addressed in the ALERT study, a multicenter randomized control trial of more than 2100 KTR, with a 2-year open label extension. In the ALERT study, patients were randomized to fluvastatin 40 mg/day versus placebo with a primary end point of cardiac death, nonfatal myocardial infarction (MI), or coronary intervention. At mean follow up of about 5 years, fluvastatin significantly lowered LDL (32%), total cholesterol, and TG, whereas the HDL level was similar to the placebo group. Although the risk reduction with fluvastatin for the primary endpoint was not significant, there were significantly fewer cardiac deaths or nonfatal MI (70 vs. 104, 0.65 [0.48–0.88] $p = 0.005$) in the fluvastatin arm compared to the placebo arm [27]. The ALERT study was extended for 2 years as an open labeled use of fluvastatin XL 80 mg/day in more than 1600 KTR. The improved CVD outcomes in the fluvastatin group in the original study was sustained in this extension, with a significant decrease in the primary endpoint, defined as the time to first MACE (HR 0.79, 95% CI 0.63–0.99, $p = 0.036$) and 29% reduction in cardiac death or nonfatal MI (HR 0.79, 95% CI 0.55–0.93, $p = 0.014$) compared to the patients in the placebo group in the original study. The authors concluded that the benefit of statin in KTR is similar to the general population with significant and sustained benefits achieved with earlier initiation of therapy [32].

The high prevalence of dyslipidemia, along with its association with CVD and the positive impact of treatment of dyslipidemia on CVD in KTR, supports universal screening and treatment of dyslipidemia in KTR. The 2009 KDIGO guidelines recommend that all adult KTR be screened for hyperlipidemia at 2–3 months post-KT followed by annual testing, with additional testing conducted in case of change in treatment or conditions which are known to cause dyslipidemia [20]. Ideally, the lipid profile should be checked after an overnight fast; however when it is unfeasible to obtain a fasting sample, a nonfasting sample should be obtained rather than forgoing testing [28].

All KTR should be considered similar to the CKD population and classified in the highest risk category for coronary heart disease (CHD) for risk factor management [28]. In KTR the goal is to maintain LDL at <100 mg/dl and non-HDL cholesterol at <130 mg/dl with statins as the first line of therapy [20]. Several studies have reported the efficacy of statins with significant reduction in TC, LDL, and TG along with some studies reporting an increase in HDL in

KT recipients [27, 32]. Statins have been shown to be safe in KTR without increased risk of rejection and are generally well tolerated [32]. Certain statins: simvastatin, atorvastatin, and lovastatin are primarily metabolized by the CYP3A4 iso-enzyme and are susceptible to drug–drug interactions with CNI (cyclosporine > tacrolimus). In general, a 50% dose reduction is suggested for these statins in KTR on CNIs to prevent acute toxicity especially myotoxicity. Pravastatin, fluvastatin, and rosuvastatin have alternative metabolic pathways and have less drug–drug interactions [33]. Registry data from Austria has shown significantly higher survival at 12 years post-KT in patients on statin therapy compared to without statin therapy. Although uncommon, severe hypertriglyceridemia increases the risk of pancreatitis and should be aggressively treated. Therapeutic lifestyle changes such as diet modification, weight reduction and increased physical activity along with treatment of hyperglycemia, should be initiated. If TG remain >500 mg/dl, then treatment with fibrate or nicotinic acid is indicated [28].

Immunosuppressive medications have a significant impact on the lipid profile, and in certain conditions dyslipidemia may warrant modification of immunosuppressive regimen. Thus, it is important to understand the impact of individual and combination immunosuppression regimens on dyslipidemia. A randomized control trial (RCT) with 3 arms, cyclosporine (CsA) + mycophenolate mofetil (MMF), tacrolimus + MMF, and tacrolimus + Azathioprine (AZA), showed that the CsA group had higher total cholesterol, LDL and the number of patients needing lipid-lowering therapy than the tacrolimus-based regimen [34]. At 1 year post KT, a significantly higher incidence of de novo hyperlipidemia with CsA-based regimen than tacrolimus-based regimen was reported in a retrospective study (28 vs. 8%) [35]. Conversion from CsA to tacrolimus has been suggested for management of hyperlipidemia in KTR with improvement in cardiovascular risk profile [36, 37]. Several RCT have shown higher cholesterol and triglyceride levels in KTR treated with mammalian target of rapamycin (mTOR) inhibitor agents such as sirolimus or everolimus. Approximately 60% of KTR on mTOR inhibitor-based regimen receive lipid-lowering therapy, which is about twice the number of patients receiving lipid-lowering therapy in groups without these agents [38]. A synergy between the dyslipidemic effect of mTOR inhibitors and CsA has also been reported [39]. Corticosteroids have been long established as cause of dyslipidemia in general population and KTR. In steroid withdrawal studies, the groups had similar total cholesterol and high LDL; although a decrease in TG level and a lower need for lipid-lowering therapy has been noted in the steroid-free groups compared to patients who remained on steroids. [40, 41]. MMF and AZA do not impact the lipid profile [42]. Belatacept, a novel co-stimulation blocker, has a more favorable effect on non-HDL and TG profiles compared to a CsA-based regimen [43, 44].

Abnormal Phosphate Metabolism

Abnormal phosphate metabolism with high fibroblast growth factor (FGF-23) levels plays an important role in increased CVD prevalence in CKD and ESRD. KT restores phosphate homeostasis partially, however immediately post KT hypophosphatemia is commonly encountered as a result of persistently high FGF-23 levels with restored kidney function. At 3–6 months post KT, hypophosphatemia resolves. However, phosphate homeostasis is not completely restored due to several reasons, including allograft dysfunction and tertiary hyperparathyroidism [45]. Interventions to restore phosphate homeostasis may lead to improvement in post-transplantation CVD outcomes. Correction of post-transplant tertiary hyperparathyroidism, including agents such as cinacalcet, may also prove to have a long-term beneficial impact and warrant more rigorous studies in the transplant population.

Transplant Specific Risk Factors for CVD

Allograft Dysfunction

Weiner et al. analyzed the role of kidney allograft function on CVD risk post-KT and identified that in stable KTR with GFR < 45 ml/min/m^2, every 5 ml/min/m^2 drop in GFR is associated with 15% higher rate of CVD independent of other risk factors. Hence graft dysfunction plays a key role in the pathophysiology of CVD post KT in addition to traditional risk factors [46]. It has been shown that every 1 mg/dl increase in baseline serum creatinine almost doubles the risk of CVD-related mortality [47]. Renal transplant allograft dysfunction has been shown to be a strong and independent risk factor for CVD in KTR [48, 49]. Analysis of renal injury biomarkers on samples of KTRs involved in the FAVORIT trial suggested an association between increased urinary neutrophil gelatinase-associated lipocalin (NGAL)/creatinine ratio and increased CVD prevalence [50]. Thus, any pathological process in the renal allograft leading to drop in GFR such as acute cellular rejection, delayed graft function, and recurrent glomerular disease can lead to increased CVD post-transplant.

Post-transplant proteinuria is present in 10–30% of KTR and is caused by multiple etiologies such as de novo or recurrent glomerulonephritis, acute rejection, and transplant glomerulopathy [51]. It is well established that proteinuria worsens graft survival (RR 6.4) [52]. Roodnat et al. reported that proteinuria influences the risk of death due to both cardiovascular and noncardiovascular causes in KTR [53].

Immunosuppressive Agents

Current immunosuppressive agents effectively prevent acute rejection of the allograft; however, extensive drug toxicity and adverse impact of these agents on cardiometabolic profile contribute to significant morbidity and mortality. CNIs remain the cornerstone of maintenance immunosuppression in KT due to their potency. However, their nephrotoxicity as well as adverse effects on metabolic profile contribute to increased risk of CVD in KTR. Corticosteroids and CsA are the agents with most adverse impact on weight gain, hypertension, diabetes, and dyslipidemia. Among the CNIs, tacrolimus considerably increases the risk of NODAT by direct toxic effect on islet cell function compared to CsA. Corticosteroids worsen glycemic control in preexisting diabetes as well as NODAT [37]. mTOR inhibitors have the most negative effect on dyslipidemia. mTOR inhibitors promote lipolysis with increased free fatty acid levels in addition to inhibiting the uptake of lipids into the adipose tissue by altering gene expression [54]. The adverse impact of mTOR inhibitors on lipid profiles is dose dependent. Hence minimizing the loading dose of mTOR inhibitors along with aiming for lower target trough concentrations (8–10 ng/ml), and liberal utilization of statin therapy are ways to overcome dyslipidemia involved with mTOR inhibitor use.

Strategies to Reduce CVD Risk Post-Transplantation

To achieve the greatest benefit from KT, a multifaceted approach addressing all the above risk factors should begin prior to KT. Cardio-protective strategies applicable to the general population such as smoking cessation, diet, exercise, and weight control also apply to KTR as discussed above. Although randomized controlled studies addressing these measures in KTR are lacking, clinical practice guidelines endorse the use of strategies such as aspirin, beta-blockers, and statins as recommended in the general population. KDIGO guidelines recommend target blood pressure control of <130/80 in KTR [20]. Standard therapeutic measures such as achieving target BP and lipid-lowering therapy lower the risk of CVD in KTR [55]. In addition to general cardio-protective strategies, transplant-specific interventions would also lead to improvement in overall outcomes. We focus further discussion in this review on transplant-specific cardio-protective strategies.

Immunosuppression Modification

Immunosuppression modification weighing the risks of acute rejection as well other side effects could be effective in lowering the CVD risk in KTRs. These strategies are mainly aimed at reducing corticosteroid as well CNI exposure as summarized in Table 25.4. The favorable effects of these measures are mediated by minimizing nephrotoxicity and lowering the burden of metabolic risk factors.

Choice of CNI

In a study conducted in Germany, patients randomly assigned to tacrolimus had comparatively improved lipid profiles and lower BP, compared to cyclosporine (CsA). However, incidence of NODAT was higher in the tacrolimus group. In this study, the estimated CVD risk by Framingham score was significantly lower in males treated with tacrolimus compared to CsA, but this benefit was not observed in women [56]. Similar reduction in the risk of CVD by Framingham risk score was observed in other studies including stable KTR converted from CsA to tacrolimus [57].

CNI Minimization

CNI have immensely improved allograft survival rates in KTR with effective prevention of acute rejection episodes. However, these drugs have a narrow therapeutic window and are associated with nephrotoxicity in kidney as well as other solid organ transplant recipients. This led the transplant community toward CNI minimization/avoidance protocols to overcome metabolic side effects as well as nephrotoxicity. Agents used as alternatives to CNI are mTOR inhibitors and belatacept which will be discussed below.

Mammalian Target of Rapamycin Inhibitors

mTOR inhibitors allow avoidance or minimization of CNI. Evidence from the heart transplant literature supports that mTOR inhibitors are shown to have favorable effects on progression of atherosclerosis with delay in progression of coronary artery intimal thickening and reduced incidence of cardiac allograft vasculopathy compared to CNI. Furthermore, mTOR inhibitors reduce ventricular remodeling as well as improve arterial stiffness via anti-fibrotic effects [58].

The "Spare the Nephron" trial assessed an MMF/sirolimus (SRL) -based regimen in comparison with an MMF/CNI regimen and showed improved renal function as well as survival rates with a trend toward improved graft survival in MMF/SRL regimen compared to MMF/CNI regimen at 2-year follow up [59]. The Concept study analyzed the impact of conversion from CNI to SRL at 3 months post KT and identified that SRL in combination with MMF resulted in improvement in renal function compared to CNI/MMF combination. There was no increase in acute rejection rates; however, a subset of patients in the SRL arm had adverse reactions such as apthous ulcers, diarrhea and elevated triglycerides [60]. None of these trials had cardiovascular events as their primary outcome. Although initial studies

Table 25.4 Immunosuppressive strategies to decrease cardiovascular disease risk in KTR

Choice of CNI based on side effect profile
CNI minimization and discontinuation
Corticosteroid minimization and discontinuation
CNI to Belatacept conversion
CNI to mTOR inhibitor conversion

CNI calcineurin inhibitors, *mTOR* mammalian target of rapamycin

appeared to be safe, more recent studies have raised concerns for development of donor-specific antibodies, antibody mediated rejection, and inferior recipient survival with conversion from CNI to mTOR inhibitors [61–63]. Furthermore, there is reported non-adherence with mTOR inhibitor use mostly related to the adverse effect profile. Considering these facts, the use of mTOR inhibitor has remarkably decreased in United States. Some of these obstacles could partly be overcome by dose reduction strategies aiming for lower therapeutic troughs and hence mTOR inhibitors might have salutary CVD benefits via preserving allograft function in carefully selected groups of KTR with close monitoring of DSA.

Corticosteroid Minimization/Discontinuation

The metabolic, bone, and cardiovascular adverse effect profile of corticosteroids make corticosteroid minimization strategies a cornerstone of immunosuppression modification for the future in KTR. The FREEDOM trial, a randomized multicenter trial of steroid avoidance or early steroid withdrawal showed noninferiority of steroid minimization/discontinuation regimens to the standard steroid regimen. In this study, there was increased incidence of early acute rejections, however long-term patient and graft survival were comparable [64]. The metabolic side effects of steroids were considerably reduced in this study. Patients at high risk for rejection such as re-transplants, high PRA titer, and prolonged DGF were excluded from this study. Similar results were achieved in the ATLAS study, which included a European cohort of low-immunologic risk KTR [65]. Another study from the United States analyzed a steroid-free protocol with thymoglobulin induction including immunologically high risk patients such as repeat KTR and showed comparable outcomes at short-term follow up with favorable metabolic profile [66]. However, the implications of long-term rejection risk in the setting of steroid withdrawal in high-immunologic risk recipients remain to be studied, and hence it remains unanswered if the short-term improvements in the metabolic profile with steroid withdrawal translates into overall improvement in survival.

Woodle et al. observed lower incidence of CVD events at 1 and 2 years in KTR assigned to early corticosteroid discontinuation compared to KTR remaining on chronic steroids. The incidence of new onset metabolic syndrome was also lower in the early corticosteroid discontinuation group [67]. Estimated CVD risk fell by 10% at 1-year post-KT with early corticosteroid discontinuation [68]. Hence steroid minimization in carefully selected low immunologic risk KTR offers promise to lower CVD. Whether this favorable impact translates into long-term reduced incidence of CVD remains to be studied. Further studies with corticosteroid minimization are needed in high immunologic risk KTR to widely implement steroid sparing protocols.

Belatacept

Belatacept is a immunosuppressive agent that blocks T-cell co-stimulation and is utilized in CNI free immunosuppressive protocols in KTR. In a recently published meta-analysis of five major trials comparing belatacept to CNIs in KTR, belatacept use in comparison to CNI is associated with similar patient, graft survival, and acute rejection rates at 3 year follow up. However, estimated GFR was significantly higher in the belatacept arm. Favorable cardiovascular risk factor profiles were observed in belatacept treated patients including better BP control and lipid profiles, as well as reduced risk of NODAT. Whether these short-term benefits of belatacept use translate into long-term improvement of cardiovascular outcomes in KTR remain to be studied [69]. Based on current evidence, belatacept appears to be a safer and effective alternative to CNIs; however, its long-term impact on allograft function warrants further follow-up.

Pre-emptive and Living Donor Transplantation

It is well-established fact that dialysis vintage pre-KT is a risk factor for adverse CVD outcomes. Hence minimizing or avoiding time on dialysis altogether with pre-emptive transplantation would lead to favorable CVD outcomes. Furthermore, allograft dysfunction and delayed graft function rates are risk factors for post KT CVD. Live donor transplants result in much lower delayed graft function rates as well as superior allograft function compared to deceased donor transplants and may lead to reduction in risk of CVD post KT.

Conclusion

CVD remains the leading cause of death post-KT. There is an increased prevalence of traditional CVD risk factors in KTR such as diabetes, hypertension, and metabolic syndrome, when compared to the general population. However, specific transplant-related risk factors also play an additional detrimental role in increasing overall CVD risk. Immunosuppressive agents have several adverse impacts on cardio metabolic profile. CVD reduction strategies should begin prior to KT to achieve maximal benefit. Appropriate management of evolving metabolic issues as well as optimal use of immunosuppression minimization strategies might improve long-term success of KT. An individualized approach to immunosuppression weighing the risks of rejection and recipient's cardiovascular risk factors may improve overall outcomes.

References

1. Wolfe RA, Ashby VB, Milford EL, Ojo AO, Ettenger RE, Agodoa LY, et al. Comparison of mortality in all patients on dialysis, patients on dialysis awaiting transplantation, and recipients of a first cadaveric transplant. N Engl J Med. 1999;341(23):1725–30.
2. Neale J, Smith AC. Cardiovascular risk factors following renal transplant. World J Transpl. 2015;5(4):183–95.
3. Israni AK, Snyder JJ, Skeans MA, Peng Y, Maclean JR, Weinhandl ED, et al. Predicting coronary heart disease after kidney transplantation: patient outcomes in renal transplantation (PORT) study. Am J Transpl. 2010;10(2):338–53.
4. Lentine KL, Brennan DC, Schnitzler MA. Incidence and predictors of myocardial infarction after kidney transplantation. J Am Soc Nephrol. 2005;16(2):496–506.
5. Delville M, Sabbah L, Girard D, Elie C, Manceau S, Piketty M, et al. Prevalence and predictors of early cardiovascular events after kidney transplantation: evaluation of pre-transplant cardiovascular work-up. PLoS ONE. 2015;10(6):e0131237.
6. Laurence JM, Barbas AS, Sapisochin G, Marquez MA, Bazerbachi F, Selzner M, et al. The significance of preoperative coronary interventions on outcome after pancreas transplantation. Clin Transpl. 2016;30(3): 233–40. doi: 10.1111/ctr.12681. Epub 2016 Jan 25.
7. Silver SA, Huang M, Nash MM, Prasad GV. Framingham risk score and novel cardiovascular risk factors underpredict major adverse cardiac events in kidney transplant recipients. Transplantation. 2011;92(2):183–9.
8. Kasiske BL, Chakkera HA, Roel J. Explained and unexplained ischemic heart disease risk after renal transplantation. J Am Soc Nephrol. 2000;11(9):1735–43.
9. Clayton PA, Lim WH, Wong G, Chadban SJ. Relationship between eGFR decline and hard outcomes after kidney transplants. J Am Soc Nephrol.
10. Soveri I, Holme I, Holdaas H, Budde K, Jardine AG, Fellstrom B. A cardiovascular risk calculator for renal transplant recipients. Transplantation. 2012;94(1):57–62.
11. Abecassis M, Bridges ND, Clancy CJ, Dew MA, Eldadah B, Englesbe MJ, et al. Solid-organ transplantation in older adults: current status and future research. Am J Transpl. 2012;12 (10):2608–22.
12. Knoll GA. Kidney transplantation in the older adult. Am J Kidney Dis. 2013;61(5):790–7.
13. Eckhoff DE, Young CJ, Gaston RS, Fineman SW, Deierhoi MH, Foushee MT, et al. Racial disparities in renal allograft survival: a public health issue? J Am Coll Surg. 2007;204(5):894–902 (discussion -3).
14. Taber DJ, Pilch NA, Meadows HB, McGillicuddy JW, Bratton CF, Chavin KD, et al. The impact of cardiovascular disease and risk factor treatment on ethnic disparities in kidney transplant. J Cardiovasc Pharmacol Ther. 2013;18(3):243–50.
15. Kasiske BL, Klinger D. Cigarette smoking in renal transplant recipients. J Am Soc Nephrol. 2000;11(4):753–9.
16. Cosio FG, Falkenhain ME, Pesavento TE, Yim S, Alamir A, Henry ML, et al. Patient survival after renal transplantation: II. The impact of smoking. Clin Transpl. 1999;13(4):336–41.
17. Carpenter MA, John A, Weir MR, Smith SR, Hunsicker L, Kasiske BL, et al. BP, cardiovascular disease, and death in the Folic acid for vascular outcome reduction in transplantation trial. J Am Soc Nephrol. 2014;25(7):1554–62.
18. Ali A, Mishler D, Taber T, Agarwal D, Yaqub M, Mujtaba M, et al. Long-term outcomes of transplant recipients referred for angiography for suspected transplant renal artery stenosis. Clin Transpl. 2015;29(9):747–55.
19. Cross NB, Webster AC, Masson P, O'Connell PJ, Craig JC. Antihypertensive treatment for kidney transplant recipients. Cochrane Database Syst Rev. 2009;3:CD003598.
20. Kasiske BL, Zeier MG, Chapman JR, Craig JC, Ekberg H, Garvey CA, et al. KDIGO clinical practice guideline for the care of kidney transplant recipients: a summary. Kidney Int. 2010;77 (4):299–311.
21. Troxell ML, Houghton DC, Hawkey M, Batiuk TD, Bennett WM. Enteric oxalate nephropathy in the renal allograft: an underrecognized complication of bariatric surgery. Am J Transpl. 2010;13 (2):501–9.
22. Tillmann FP, Hermsen D, Hemmrich K, Woznowski M, Rump LC, Quack I. Long-term effect of renal transplantation and aging on hemoglobin A1C levels: a case-control study in 191 non-diabetic deceased donor renal transplant recipients. Ann Transpl. 2014;20:729–33.
23. Handelsman Y, Bloomgarden ZT, Grunberger G, Umpierrez G, Zimmerman RS, Bailey TS, et al. American association of clinical endocrinologists and american college of endocrinology—clinical practice guidelines for developing a diabetes mellitus comprehensive care plan—2015. Endocr Pract. 2015;21(Suppl 1):1–87.
24. Palepu S, Prasad GV. New-onset diabetes mellitus after kidney transplantation: Current status and future directions. World J Diabetes. 2015;6(3):445–55.
25. Reddy YN, Abraham G, Sundaram V, Reddy PP, Mathew M, Nagarajan P, et al. Is there a genetic predisposition to new-onset diabetes after kidney transplantation? Saudi J Kidney Dis Transpl. 2015;26(6):1113–20.
26. Staatz CE, Tett SE. Pharmacokinetic considerations relating to tacrolimus dosing in the elderly. Drugs Aging. 2005;22(7):541–57.
27. Holdaas H, Fellstrom B, Jardine AG, Holme I, Nyberg G, Fauchald P, et al. Effect of fluvastatin on cardiac outcomes in renal transplant recipients: a multicentre, randomised, placebo-controlled trial. Lancet. 2003;361(9374):2024–31.
28. Kasiske B, Cosio FG, Beto J, Bolton K, Chavers BM, Grimm R Jr, et al. Clinical practice guidelines for managing dyslipidemias in kidney transplant patients: a report from the Managing Dyslipidemias in Chronic Kidney Disease Work Group of the National Kidney Foundation Kidney Disease Outcomes Quality Initiative. Am J Transpl. 2004;4(Suppl 7):13–53.

29. Andany MA, Kasiske BL. Dyslipidemia and its management after renal transplantation. J Nephrol. 2001;14(Suppl 4):S81–8.
30. Kasiske BL, Guijarro C, Massy ZA, Wiederkehr MR, Ma JZ. Cardiovascular disease after renal transplantation. J Am Soc Nephrol. 1996;7(1):158–65.
31. Aker S, Ivens K, Grabensee B, Heering P. Cardiovascular risk factors and diseases after renal transplantation. Int Urol Nephrol. 1998;30(6):777–88.
32. Jardine AG, Fellstrom B, Logan JO, Cole E, Nyberg G, Gronhagen-Riska C, et al. Cardiovascular risk and renal transplantation: post hoc analyses of the Assessment of Lescol in Renal Transplantation (ALERT) Study. Am J Kidney Dis. 2005;46 (3):529–36.
33. Wanner C, Kramer-Guth A, Galle J. Use of HMG-CoA reductase inhibitors after kidney and heart transplantation: lipid-lowering and immunosuppressive effects. BioDrugs. 1997;8(5):387–93.
34. Johnson C, Ahsan N, Gonwa T, Halloran P, Stegall M, Hardy M, et al. Randomized trial of tacrolimus (Prograf) in combination with azathioprine or mycophenolate mofetil versus cyclosporine (Neoral) with mycophenolate mofetil after cadaveric kidney transplantation. Transplantation. 2000;69(5):834–41.
35. Deleuze S, Garrigue V, Delmas S, Chong G, Swarcz I, Cristol JP, et al. New onset dyslipidemia after renal transplantation: Is there a difference between tacrolimus and cyclosporine? Transpl Proc. 2006;38(7):2311–3.
36. McCune TR, Thacker LR II, Peters TG, Mulloy L, Rohr MS, Adams PA, et al. Effects of tacrolimus on hyperlipidemia after successful renal transplantation: a Southeastern Organ Procurement Foundation multicenter clinical study. Transplantation. 1998;65(1):87–92.
37. Marcen R, Morales JM, del Castillo D, Campistol JM, Seron D, Valdes F, et al. Posttransplant diabetes mellitus in renal allograft recipients: a prospective multicenter study at 2 years. Transpl Proc. 2006;38(10):3530–2.
38. Kasiske BL, de Mattos A, Flechner SM, Gallon L, Meier-Kriesche HU, Weir MR, et al. Mammalian target of rapamycin inhibitor dyslipidemia in kidney transplant recipients. Am J Transpl. 2008;8 (7):1384–92.
39. Ciancio G, Burke GW, Gaynor JJ, Ruiz P, Roth D, Kupin W, et al. A randomized long-term trial of tacrolimus/sirolimus versus tacrolimums/mycophenolate versus cyclosporine/sirolimus in renal transplantation: three-year analysis. Transplantation. 2006;81 (6):845–52.
40. Woodle ES, First MR, Pirsch J, Shihab F, Gaber AO, Van Veldhuisen P. A prospective, randomized, double-blind, placebo-controlled multicenter trial comparing early (7 day) corticosteroid cessation versus long-term, low-dose corticosteroid therapy. Ann Surg. 2008;248(4):564–77.
41. Cantarovich D, Rostaing L, Kamar N, Ducloux D, Saint-Hillier Y, Mourad G, et al. Early corticosteroid avoidance in kidney transplant recipients receiving ATG-F induction: 5-year actual results of a prospective and randomized study. Am J Transpl. 2014;14(11):2556–64.
42. Akman B, Uyar M, Afsar B, Sezer S, Ozdemir FN, Haberal M. Lipid profile during azathioprine or mycophenolate mofetil combinations with cyclosporine and steroids. Transpl Proc. 2007;39(1):135–7.
43. Durrbach A, Pestana JM, Pearson T, Vincenti F, Garcia VD, Campistol J, et al. A phase III study of belatacept versus cyclosporine in kidney transplants from extended criteria donors (BENEFIT-EXT study). Am J Transpl. 2010;10(3):547–57.
44. Vincenti F, Charpentier B, Vanrenterghem Y, Rostaing L, Bresnahan B, Darji P, et al. A phase III study of belatacept-based immunosuppression regimens versus cyclosporine in renal transplant recipients (BENEFIT study). Am J Transpl. 2010;10 (3):535–46.
45. Baia LC, Heilberg IP, Navis G, de Borst MH. Phosphate and FGF-23 homeostasis after kidney transplantation. Nat Rev Nephrol. 2015;11(11):656–66.
46. Weiner J, Scalea J, Ishikawa Y, Okumi M, Griesemer A, Hirakata A, et al. Tolerogenicity of donor major histocompatibility complex-matched skin grafts in previously tolerant Massachusetts general hospital miniature swine. Transplantation. 2012;94 (12):1192–9.
47. Fellstrom B, Jardine AG, Soveri I, Cole E, Gronhagen-Riska C, Neumayer HH, et al. Renal dysfunction as a risk factor for mortality and cardiovascular disease in renal transplantation: experience from the Assessment of Lescol in Renal Transplantation trial. Transplantation. 2005;79(9):1160–3.
48. Soveri I, Holdaas H, Jardine A, Gimpelewicz C, Staffler B, Fellstrom B. Renal transplant dysfunction—importance quantified in comparison with traditional risk factors for cardiovascular disease and mortality. Nephrol Dial Transpl. 2006;21(8):2282–9.
49. Ma MK, Lim WH, Craig JC, Russ GR, Chapman JR, Wong G. Mortality among younger and older recipients of kidney transplants from expanded criteria donors compared with standard criteria donors. Clin J Am Soc Nephrol. 2016;11(1):128–36.
50. Bansal N, Carpenter MA, Weiner DE, Levey AS, Pfeffer M, Kusek JW, et al. Urine injury biomarkers and risk of adverse outcomes in recipients of prevalent kidney transplants: the folic acid for vascular outcome reduction in transplantation trial. J Am Soc Nephrol. 2015;27(7):2109–21.
51. Ponticelli C, Graziani G. Proteinuria after kidney transplantation. Transpl Int. 2012;25(9):909–17.
52. Ibis A, Akgul A, Ozdemir N, Colak T, Sezer S, Arat Z, et al. Posttransplant proteinuria is associated with higher risk of cardiovascular disease and graft failure in renal transplant patients. Transpl Proc. 2009;41(5):1604–8.
53. Roodnat JI, Mulder PG, Rischen-Vos J, van Riemsdijk IC, van Gelder T, Zietse R, et al. Proteinuria after renal transplantation affects not only graft survival but also patient survival. Transplantation. 2001;72(3):438–44.
54. Morrisett JD, Abdel-Fattah G, Hoogeveen R, Mitchell E, Ballantyne CM, Pownall HJ, et al. Effects of sirolimus on plasma lipids, lipoprotein levels, and fatty acid metabolism in renal transplant patients. J Lipid Res. 2002;43(8):1170–80.
55. Davidson J, Wilkinson A, Dantal J, Dotta F, Haller H, Hernandez D, et al. New-onset diabetes after transplantation: 2003 International consensus guidelines. In: Proc international expert panel meeting. Barcelona, Spain, 19 February 2003. Transplantation. 2003;75(10 Suppl):SS3–24.
56. Kramer BK, Zulke C, Kammerl MC, Schmidt C, Hengstenberg C, Fischereder M, et al. Cardiovascular risk factors and estimated risk for CAD in a randomized trial comparing calcineurin inhibitors in renal transplantation. Am J Transpl. 2003;3(8):982–7.
57. Baid-Agrawal S, Delmonico FL, Tolkoff-Rubin NE, Farrell M, Williams WW, Shih V, et al. Cardiovascular risk profile after conversion from cyclosporine A to tacrolimus in stable renal transplant recipients. Transplantation. 2004;77(8):1199–202.
58. Eisen HJ, Tuzcu EM, Dorent R, Kobashigawa J, Mancini D, Valantine-von Kaeppler HA, et al. Everolimus for the prevention of allograft rejection and vasculopathy in cardiac-transplant recipients. N Engl J Med. 2003;349(9):847–58.
59. Carpenter MA, Weir MR, Adey DB, House AA, Bostom AG, Kusek JW. Inadequacy of cardiovascular risk factor management in chronic kidney transplantation—evidence from the FAVORIT study. Clin Transpl. 2012;26(4):E438–46.

60. Lebranchu Y, Thierry A, Toupance O, Westeel PF, Etienne I, Thervet E, et al. Efficacy on renal function of early conversion from cyclosporine to sirolimus 3 months after renal transplantation: concept study. Am J Transpl. 2009;9(5):1115–23.
61. Liefeldt L, Brakemeier S, Glander P, Waiser J, Lachmann N, Schonemann C, et al. Donor-specific HLA antibodies in a cohort comparing everolimus with cyclosporine after kidney transplantation. Am J Transpl. 2012;12(5):1192–8.
62. Isakova T, Xie H, Messinger S, Cortazar F, Scialla JJ, Guerra G, et al. Inhibitors of mTOR and risks of allograft failure and mortality in kidney transplantation. Am J Transpl. 2013;13 (1):100–10.
63. Guerra G, Ciancio G, Gaynor JJ, Zarak A, Brown R, Hanson L, et al. Randomized trial of immunosuppressive regimens in renal transplantation. J Am Soc Nephrol. 2011;22(9):1758–68.
64. Vincenti F, Schena FP, Paraskevas S, Hauser IA, Walker RG, Grinyo J. A randomized, multicenter study of steroid avoidance, early steroid withdrawal or standard steroid therapy in kidney transplant recipients. Am J Transpl. 2008;8(2):307–16.
65. Kramer BK, Klinger M, Vitko S, Glyda M, Midtvedt K, Stefoni S, et al. Tacrolimus-based, steroid-free regimens in renal transplantation: 3-year follow-up of the ATLAS trial. Transplantation. 2012;94(5):492–8.
66. Nikkel LE, Mohan S, Zhang A, McMahon DJ, Boutroy S, Dube G, et al. Reduced fracture risk with early corticosteroid withdrawal after kidney transplant. Am J Transpl. 2012;12(3):649–59.
67. Rike AH, Mogilishetty G, Alloway RR, Succop P, Roy-Chaudhury P, Cardi M, et al. Cardiovascular risk, cardiovascular events, and metabolic syndrome in renal transplantation: comparison of early steroid withdrawal and chronic steroids. Clin Transpl. 2008;22(2):229–35.
68. Rogers CC, Alloway RR, Buell JF, Boardman R, Alexander JW, Cardi M, et al. Body weight alterations under early corticosteroid withdrawal and chronic corticosteroid therapy with modern immunosuppression. Transplantation. 2005;80(1):26–33.
69. Masson P, Henderson L, Chapman JR, Craig JC, Webster AC. Belatacept for kidney transplant recipients. Cochrane Database Syst Rev. 2014;11:CD010699.

Cardiomyopathy in the Potential Kidney Transplant Candidate

26

Burhan Mohamedali

Introduction

Chronic kidney disease (CKD), including end stage kidney disease (ESKD), is a highly prevalent cardiovascular disease risk factor affecting one in seven adults. The complex interplay between the heart and the kidney known as cardiorenal syndrome, where impairment of one organ affects the other, leads to an endless cycle of accelerated disease progression resulting in congestive heart failure (CHF). The incidence of patients with end stage kidney disease (ESKD) requiring hemodialysis (HD) continues to increase, and is projected to reach 2 million patients by 2030 [1]. In ESKD patients, cardiovascular mortality is 10–30 times higher than age and gender match controls without CKD [2–4]. Although cardiovascular diseases accounts for over 50% of deaths in patient with ESRD, only 20% of mortality can be attributed to coronary artery disease (CAD) [5]. CHF, both systolic and diastolic, is more common in patient with ESKD, and over 80% of ESKD patients with CHF will die within 3 years of this diagnosis [6]. With such high mortality, further understanding of the pathophysiology CHF in CKD patients is of utmost importance to allow for treatment of this morbid condition, and to optimize potentially transplantable patients.

Epidemiology of CHF and ESKD

United States Renal Data System (USRDS) data indicated that mortality rate for patients with ESKD is higher than age match controls with other disease such as cancer, DM, and stroke. This mortality, however, appears to be driven by cardiovascular diseases and accounts for in excess of 10–30 times higher mortality in the ESKD population [7]. Left ventricular hypertrophy (LVH) is highly prevalent in ESKD patients and is thought to be present in up to 74% of ESKD patients at the time of dialysis initiation [8]. LVH is also an independent predictor of poor survival in HD patients [9]. LVH results from a compensatory mechanism by which wall stress is maintained in the setting of pressure and/or volume overload. Continued compensatory LVH results in maladaptive cardiomyocytes damage and apoptosis, leading to left ventricular (LV) dilation, and CHF. In the dialysis population, the presence of CHF at the initiation of HD is a strong predictor of mortality.

Diagnosing CHF in End Stage Kidney Disease

CHF can be classified in two distinct groups: Systolic CHF resulting from impaired ability of the left ventricle (LV) to contract, and diastolic CHF which results from impaired relaxation properties of the LV. In ESKD patients, it is often difficult to distinguish CHF from volume overload. This is particularly true in patients with diastolic dysfunction (DD). Diastolic filling is frequently altered in ESKD patients from increased LV stiffness, which results in exaggerated hemodynamic changes in response to volume changes [10, 11]. In a stiff LV, even small increases in LV volume can lead to high LV end diastolic pressure, left atrial pressures and pulmonary pressures resulting in pulmonary congestion. On the other hand, patients with systolic dysfunction may be easier to identify based on left ventricular dysfunction (LVD). Subsequently, whether a patient is in CHF exacerbation or simply volume overloaded due to kidney disease, is often hard to clinically distinguish.

Magnetic resonance imaging (MRI) is traditionally the standard method of assessing ventricular dimensions, function as well as fibrosis. Imaging studies with cardiac MRIs have shown evidence of diffuse myocardial fibrosis in uremic patients, which is a distinctly different pattern from subendocardial fibrosis seen in ischemic heart disease [12] (see Chap. 5, CKD associated cardiomyopathy). The association of gadolinium with nephrogenic systemic fibrosis

B. Mohamedali (✉)
Department of Internal Medicine, Rush University Medical Center, 1725 West Harrison St., Suite 1159, Chicago, IL 60612, USA
e-mail: burhan_mohamedali@rush.edu

J. Rangaswami et al. (eds.), *Cardio-Nephrology*,
DOI 10.1007/978-3-319-56042-7_26

(NSF), has led to the decreased usage of this modality. Additionally, MRI cannot be used in patients with implantable devices such as internal cardioverter defibrillator (ICD) and pacemakers which are found in a significant number of patients with cardiomyopathy (CM) [13].

Due to these limitations, echocardiography, with it widespread availability and ease of administration, is often employed to evaluate myocardial properties and function in patients with a suspected cardiomyopathy. A depressed ejection fraction can clinch a diagnosis of LV dysfunction. Echocardiography can also asses LVH, LV mass index (LVMI), as well as chamber sizes and dimensions. Continuous wave Doppler and tissue Doppler measurements can be useful in determining degree of DD, as can assessment of left atrial volume index. Unfortunately, echocardiography is limited by skills of the technician, acoustic windows, poor endocardial enhancements, and interobserver reader variability [13]. Additionally, many diastolic parameters are strongly load dependent and can be challenging in dialysis patients where relative high preload can mask DD [14]. Nevertheless, despite its limitation, echocardiography remains the initial test for choice for diagnosing cardiomyopathy in CKD/ESKD patients.

The gold standard test for diagnosing DD is an invasive heart catheterization. A diagnosis can be made with elevated filling pressures with mean pulmonary capillary wedge pressure >12 or LV end diastolic pressure >16 [15]. However, since this modality is invasive and subjects patients to increased risk, it is often reserved for cases where a diagnosis cannot be made by other imaging tests.

Pathophysiology of Cardiomyopathy and ESKD

Cardiomyopathy (CM) in CKD patients is commonly attributed to comorbid conditions such preexisting coronary artery disease (CAD), hypertension, and diabetes. However, CKD is an independent risk factor for CM in patients, even in the absence of these factors [16]. Multiple pathophysiological processes are thought to be implicated in development of CM in patients with ESKD (Fig. 26.1). Increased afterload, volume overload, anemia, CAD, and uremia are all implicated in the development of CM in these patients. Nontraditional risk factors such as uremic toxins, calcium phosphate imbalance, inflammation, renin–angiotensin–aldosterone system (RAAS) activation, and oxidative stress are all implicated in the process as well. The mechanisms by which such processes induce cardiac derangement are complex and closely interwoven. The net result of these processes is the development of LVH, myocardial interstitial fibrosis, and thickening of intramural arteries and arterioles. LVH and vascular remodeling are thought to be an adaptive mechanism to pressure and volume overload, while interstitial fibrosis may be related to changes in myocardial metabolism [17].

Increased afterload is commonly encountered in ESKD patients. The pathogenesis is the result of the interaction between LV ejection and opposing factors such as peripheral resistance and impedance of aorta and large central arteries [18]. The high impedance in such arterial conduits from arteriosclerosis is frequently encountered in advanced stages of CKD and is often implicated in the development of LVH [18–21]. The increased afterload is manifested as HTN, and at a cellular level, results in elevated levels of multiple regulatory and inflammatory factors such as TGF-B, pro collagen type I, and C- reactive protein all of which can promote myocardial fibrosis [22, 23]. In a similar light, activation of RAAS in CKD patients not only contributes to increased afterload from vasoconstriction, but is also directly implicated in LVH and myocardial fibrosis [24, 25].

Patients with insufficient to absent urine output for effective diuresis are predisposed to volume overload. Although dialysis removes volume from these patients, most patients receive 3 times per week sessions. This leads to development

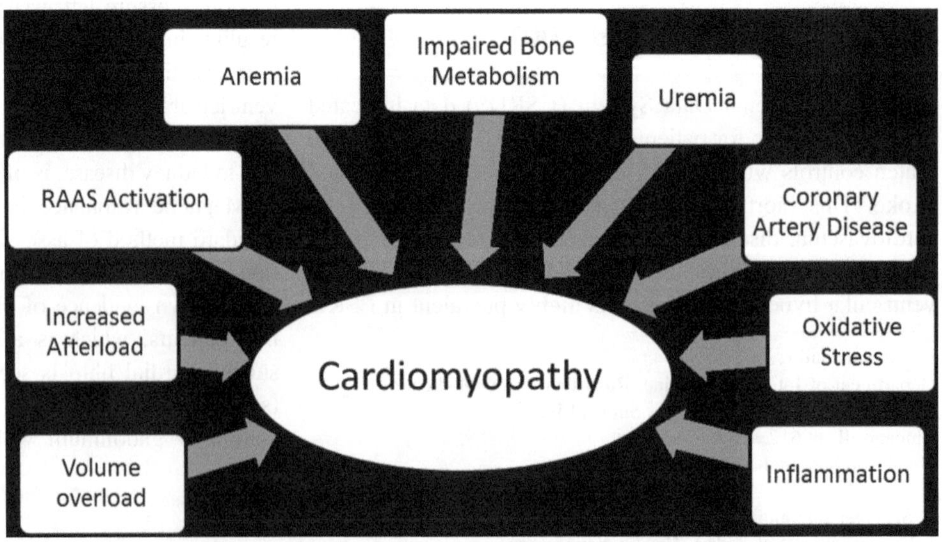

Fig. 26.1 Pathophysiology of development of cardiomyopathy in ESRD patients

of interdialysis periods of volume overload. Such body water fluctuation in HD patients can predispose patients to persistent LVH and resulting CM [26]. Although regression of LV dimensions and LVH is noted with initiation of dialysis, higher level of LVH regression was noted in patients treated with daily HD sessions presumably explained by, better blood pressure control, and reduction of both extracellular fluid volume and volume fluctuation [27, 28].

The presence of vascular access for HD can lead to increase vascular flow of up to 400–800 ml/min for forearm access and up to 800–1500 ml/min for brachial access [29]. The increase in flow initially results in increased cardiac output and ejection fraction, at the expense of decrease myocardial oxygen supply. Multiple studies have demonstrated a high BNP level in these patients after creation of vascular access [30, 31]. The resulting high-flow state may result in development or worsening of both systolic and diastolic CHF.

Anemia in CKD, particularly chronic anemia in ESKD patients due to decreased erythropoietin synthesis, is implicated in development of LVH. Anemia results in increased oxygen extraction, increased preload, and sympathetic activation leading to increased myocardial oxygen demand and progressive cardiac dysfunction and LVH [32, 33]. Hemodynamic adaptation to anemia lead to a high flow state form reduction in arterial resistance, due to arteriolar dilation and decreased blood viscosity, increased preload from increased venous return, and increased LV contractility [34]. In HD patients, erythropoietin supplementation and treatment of anemia were noted to improve both function and structure of the LV. However the optimal hemoglobin target to achieve remains controversial due to the increased cardiovascular morbidity and mortality associated with erythropoietin stimulating agents (ESAs) [35–37].

CKD-related bone and mineral abnormalities resulting in increased parathyroid hormone (PTH) production has long been thought to cause cardiovascular adverse effects leading to the induction of LVH, cardiac fibrosis, and arterial wall thickening [38–40]. LVH also appears to be accelerated by fibroblast growth factor-23, which starts rising even as early as stage 2 CKD [41]. Similarly, hyperphosphatemia is also known to promote LVH, possibly through changes in arterial stiffness, systemic vascular resistance, and direct myocardial toxicity [42]. Additionally, CKD associated vitamin D deficiency has been associated with LV dysfunction [43]. Low serum vitamin D levels stimulate RAAS, causing vasoconstriction and salt and water retention [44]. In animal models, treatment with active vitamin D analog-reduced myocardial hypertrophy and improved function, but similar outcomes in humans are controversial [45].

Uremia, independent of pressure and volume overload, can lead to development of a CM. This has been demonstrated in both human and animal studies [46, 47]. At a cellular level, the mechanism by which CM ensues is thought to be through integrin-mediated intracellular downstream responses to extracellular matrix stretch [48–50] causing increased cardiomyocyte diameter, reduced capillary length density, and increase interstitial volume [51]. Other molecules implicated in LVH from uremia include endothelin 1, tumor necrosis factor α[alpha], and endogenous digitalis like substances [52–54]. In addition to LVH, in uremia, the size of the heart is also increased from more interstitial fibrotic tissue [55, 56]. The onset of fibrosis is primarily thought to result in worsening DD in these patients [57]. As a consequence, myocardial apoptosis and intermyocardial fibrosis, DD and later systolic dysfunction develop, leading to progressive cardiac dysfunction resulting in full blown uremic CM.

Chronic Kidney Disease and Cardiac Reserve

In addition to the above-described cardiomyocyte derangements, CKD also appears to impair cardiomyocyte energetics [58]. Assessment of myocardial contractile reserve in CKD patients shows impaired contractile reserve even in the setting of normal resting parameters [59]. Similarly, peak oxygen consumption (peak V02), a surrogate for peak cardiac performance derived from cardiopulmonary stress testing (CPX), is impaired in CKD patients [60, 61]. Such peak impairment in CKD patients may be due to a multitude of comorbid factors such as CM, anemia, HTN, uremia, etc. Chinnappa et al., in a proof of concept study, demonstrated that peak cardiac power output (calculated as product of cardiac output and mean arterial pressure) in asymptomatic male patients with CKD was significantly lower than normal healthy males, implicating the effect of CKD and likely uremia on cardiac reserve [58]. This study has implication on utilizing metabolic testing in assessment of cardiac reserve in patients with ESKD and CM, especially when evaluating transplantation potential.

Treatment of Cardiomyopathy in ESKD

The current treatment of CM in ESKD patients is centered on treating underlying factors such as g pressure and volume overload, anemia, secondary parathyroidism, and uremia.

Strict blood pressure control with antihypertensive regimens as well as optimal fluid balance with HD to maintain a near euvolemic state are all the mainstay at stabilizing and preventing the progression of CM. Nonpharmacological approaches include salt and water restriction, weight loss, and smoking cessation [62]. Pharmacological treatment for HTN is similar to treatment in patients without ESKD. These medications are tailored based on the presence or absence of systolic dysfunction. Generally, evidence-based select betablocker (metoprolol XL, carvedilol, and bisoprolol) and angiotensin converting enzyme-inhibitor (ACEI) or angiotensin receptor blockers (ARBs), are usually first line in systolic dysfunction. These medications can be further complemented with vasodilators such a hydralazine and nitrates for patients with refractory HTN, especially if African American. In DD, peripheral calcium channel blockers in addition to ACEI/ARB, and/or a combination of the above medications are thought to improve symptoms and promote regression of LVH [63, 64]. The target pressure in ESKD patients is not known but the Kidney Disease Outcomes Quality Initiative (KDOQI) guidelines recommend a pre-dialysis blood pressure of less than 140/90 mmHg. Although this target may be applicable to patients with DD, in systolic dysfunction the goal blood pressure is generally as low are tolerated without symptoms.

Optimization of the dialysis prescription including more frequent HD sessions such as short daily dialysis, nocturnal dialysis, and peritoneal dialysis (PD) are known provide a more physiologic approach to volume, electrolyte, and acid-base management compared to the conventional three time a week hemodialysis schedule [65, 66]. A higher degree of LVH regression is noted in patient with daily HD compared to 3 times a week routine [27]. Prolonged HD sessions lasting 8 h (such as with nocturnal dialysis) have been shown to optimally control blood pressure and LVH [67].

Anemia therapy is centered on insufficient erythropoiesis due to ESKD. Although several randomized trials have failed to show a benefit of treatment with erythropoiesis-stimulating agents on LVH, it appears that correction of severe anemia (hemoglobin < 10 gm/dl), with erythropoiesis-stimulating agents seems beneficial, although correction above 12 mg/dl does not appears to derive additional benefits and has also shown to be associated with increased risk of myocardial infarction and thrombotic events [68–71].

Hyperparathyroidism is associated with increased cardiovascular morbidity and mortality. Parathyroid hormone appears to directly influence vascular remodeling, CM, and LVH [72, 73]. Vitamin D analogs and cinacalcet, a calcimimetic, are utilized to suppress overproduction of parathyroid hormone. Although initial animal and human studies showed a beneficial effect of this therapy through decreased progression of valvular and coronary disease, randomized controlled trials have not shown any benefits in regression of CM, or LV mass. However, the PRIMO trial demonstrated a statistically significant reduction in CHF hospitalizations in patients receiving replacement therapy [74–76].

Urema is thought to be a major contributor of CM in ESKD patients. The accumulation or "uremic toxins" is implicated in accelerated atherosclerosis and vascular calcification and mortality. In a recent study, Meduell et al. [77] demonstrated that better solute clearance and use of ultrapure diasylate as replacement fluid decreases cardiovascular mortality by 33% compared to conventional dialysis algorithms. The results of the above study suggest that further refining of the process of HD can improve solute clearance, especially with middle and large molecular weight uremic toxins, which are increasingly recognized as important mediators of vascular stiffness.

Transplant in Patients with Cardiomyopathy: Diastolic Dysfunction

DD is very frequent in patients on dialysis and is thought to result from a combination of LVH, myocardial fibrosis, and impaired myocyte relaxation. The presence of LVH or abnormal Doppler signals on echocardiogram can certainly aid in the diagnosis of DD, but, whether symptoms in these patients are from CM, volume overload, or uremia are difficult to tease out. LVMI, LVH, and left ventricular and atrial volumes are thought to regress after kidney transplantation (KT) and may allow for normalization of hemodynamics. Although such explanation may be plausible, data to support these findings have been very controversial [78–82]. The various imaging modalities used and nonstandardized definitions of what truly constitutes DD further adds an element of complexity in the interpretation of the data on DD in ESKD. Multiple studies have demonstrated a post-KT regression of LVH or LVMI [83–88], which is thought to persist through 2 years after transplant (Table 26.1) [85].

Other studies and MRI findings have refuted these assessments (Table 26.1) [89–93]. However, the field of diastology is rapidly evolving and as further knowledge about diastolic CHF is attained, more light can be shed on whether DD is completely, partially, or not at all reversed by KT.

The united network for organ sharing (UNOS) restricts heart transplantation as a last resort in patients with severe DD to individuals with hypertrophic CM, amyloidosis, and other nonreversible restrictive cardiomyopathies [94]. In most cases of patients with ESKD, the symptoms from DD are CKD mediated and can be treated. In many cases, DD can be reversed with appropriate treatment. In the absence of genetic conditions or systemic infiltrative disease, most patients with isolated DD may be listed for KT.

Kidney Transplant in Patients with Cardiomyopathy: Systolic Dysfunction

KT is the treatment of choice for patients with ESKD and is associated with improved outcomes and reduced mortality [95]. Cardiovascular deaths in these patients are lower in patients with KT compared to patients on HD, suggesting that KT does provide a protective cardiovascular effect in

Table 26.1 Selected trials evaluating LVH and LVMI

Trial	*N*	Trial design	Follow up (*M*)	Imaging modality	Variable measured	Pre-KT	Post-KT	*p* value
Himelman [83]	41	Retrospective	28	Echocardiography	WT	1.5	1.3	<0.05
Huting [91]	24	Prospective	41	Echocardiography	LVH	71	67	NS
Peteiro [84]	30	Prospective	10	Echocardiography	LVMI	201	171	<0.01
De Lima [92]	53	Prospective	30	Echocardiography	LVH	82	71	NS
Mcgregor [79]	67	Retrospective	4	Echocardiography	LVMI	143	145	NS
Rigatto [85]	143	Prospective	24	Echocardiography	LVMI	161	146	0.009
Sahugn [86]	11	Prospective	3	Echocardiography	LVH	81	18	<0.005
Ferriera [89]	12	Prospective	24	Echocardiography	LVH	75	52	0.125
Dudziak [81]	43	Prospective	30	Echocardiography	LVH	70	40	$p < 0.05$
Iqbal [87]	52	Prospective	12	Echocardiography	LVMI	275	191	<0.001
Patel [90][a]	50	Prospective	29	MRI	LVMI	64.2	66.3	0.96
					LVH	68	68	1
Dounousi [88][a]	108	Retrospective	6	Echocardiography	LVH	52	33	NS
					LVMI	103	124	0.01
Slubowska [93]	83	Prospective	12	Echocardiography	LVH	51.2	50	NS
					LVMI	106	102	NS

MRI magnetic resonance imaging, *LVH* left ventricular hypertrophy (%), *LVMI* left ventricular mass index (g/m^2), *NS* not significant, *WT* wall thickness (cm)

[a]Compared renal failure patients to kidney-transplanted patients

ESKD patients. However despite this protective effect, cardiovascular disease accounts for up to 30% of death and is an independent factor for allograft failure [96, 97].

The current management of patients with ESKD with LVD is controversial. Patients with LVD are often thought to be at high risk for KT surgery. As a result, there is reluctance by nephrologists and cardiologists to refer these patients for KT. Furthermore, due to the perceived high risk status, many centers will not consider such patients for listing. Finally, consensus is lacking whether these patients should be listed for single organ KT or double organ heart/kidney transplantation.

Left Ventricular Dysfunction and Kidney Transplantation Controversy

The issue surrounding the controversy can simply be stated as cause and effect. In patient with advanced CHF, type I and II cardio-renal syndrome is prevalent. This syndrome can often present with worsening renal failure, and can overtime lead to intrinsic renal disease and ESKD. However, in some patients, advanced renal dysfunction can lead to CM from mechanisms described above.

Often times it is difficult to determine which organ, the heart or the kidney, is the cause of the other's dysfunction. Further fueling this controversy is that the data (mostly retrospective) on survival in patients with LVD who underwent KT shows yielded mixed results. A study of 653 renal transplant patients at University of Alabama with 119 patients with LVD were followed for a mean duration of 3.0 ± 1.9 years. Multivariate analysis concluded that LVD was an independent risk factor for cardiac death with an almost fivefold increase in death (HR 4.8, 95% CI 2.09–11.21, $p \leq 0.001$). They also further demonstrated that LV systolic dysfunction was a risk factor for overall mortality and was associated with increased cardiac hospitalizations [98].

On the other hand, in a rare case report of a patient with CM and ESKD who underwent KT on two separate occasions, the effects of uremia on CM was described in detail [99]. A 27-year-old patient with IgA nephropathy with a CM with EF of 18% underwent KT. One-year post-transplantation, patient's EF was noted to be improved to 45%. However, 4 years after transplantation, patient was diagnosed with a lymphoproliferative disorder necessitating cessation of immunosuppression and subsequent graft loss. Post-nephrectomy, patients had recurrence of CHF symptoms to New York Heart Association (NYHA) class III and EF was found to be depressed again at 20%. A decision was made to re-transplant patient. Six month after re-transplantation, patient had complete resolution of CHF symptoms and was NHYA class I and normal EF. The authors serially tracked LV dimensions in this case. They showed that post index KT, in addition to improvement in EF, there was a regression of LV end diastolic dimension and grade of mitral regurgitation. All three parameters worsened after graft loss, and improved post-retransplantation [99].

Many authors have demonstrated an improvement in LV EF after KT (Fig. 26.2) [99–105]. Wali et al., in a retrospective cohort study of 103 patients with LV EF of less than 45% who underwent KT, showed that a majority of patient had improvement in symptoms and normalization of EF post-KT [101]. What was particularly interesting was that in this study, patients were stratified into three groups based on post-KT EF: Group 1; had a post-transplant EF $\geq 50\%$, Group 2; 40–50%, and Group 3; had an EF of <40%. Although the mean EF in all three groups prior to KT was around 32%, at a mean follow up of 3 years, 72/103 (70%) of patients had normalized their EF, while 16 patients had improved their EF to between 40 and 50%, and 15 patients persistent remained below 40%. There was no relationship between the degree of pre-transplant LV EF depression on post-transplant EF. Mortality in group 1 was statistically significantly lower than in group 2 and 3 (Group 1: 6/103 (8%), versus Group 2: 10/103 (62%), versus Group 3: 9/103 (62%), $p \leq 0.001$) (Fig. 26.3). Their analysis suggested that it was the post-transplant EF, not pre-transplant EF that dictated outcomes. A similar conclusion was reached by a Cleveland Clinic study that showed patients with LVD prior to renal transplant had a higher mortality rate; however after controlling for patients who improved their EF by >10%, no difference in mortality was seen [100].

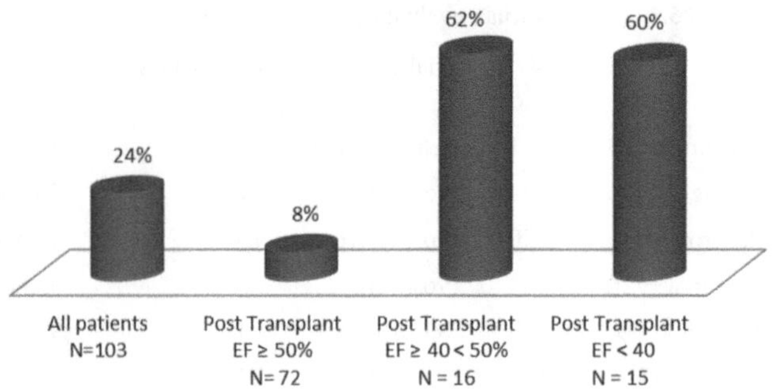

Fig. 26.3 Mortality based on post kidney transplant ejection fraction. *EF* ejection fraction [101]

It is apparent that there is a distinct phenotype of patients that will improve their ejection fraction after KT, and based on the above studies, patients who do not normalize their EF are likely the ones that have worse morbidity and mortality

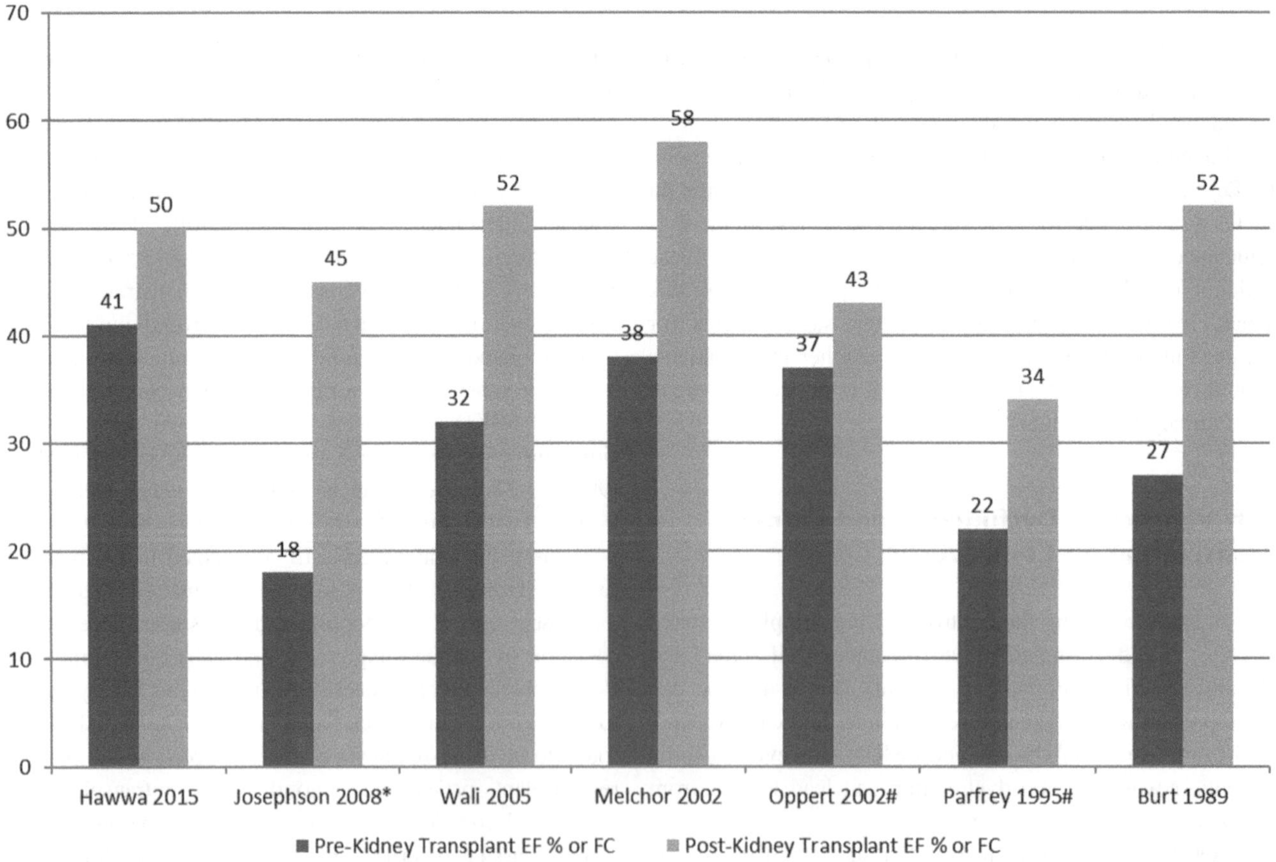

Fig. 26.2 Improvement in left ventricular ejection fraction after renal transplantation *Case report # fractional shortening. *EF* ejection fraction (%), *FC* fractional shortening (%)

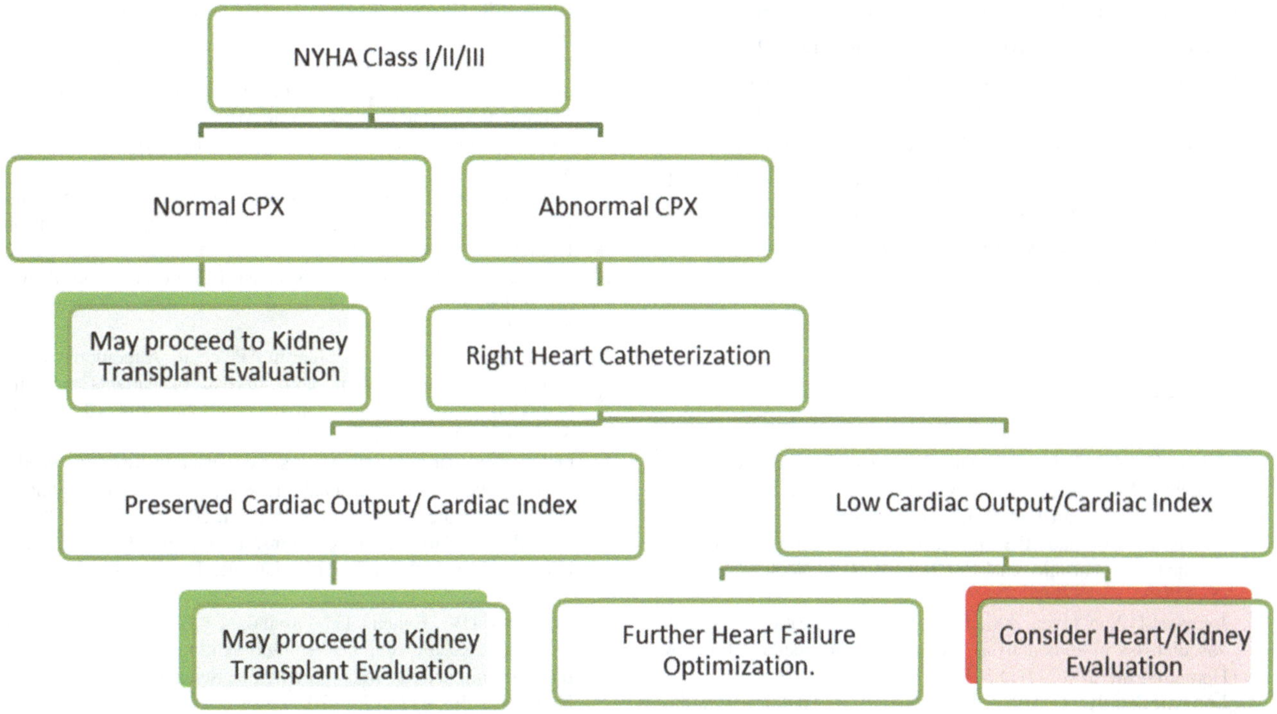

Fig. 26.4 A possible work-up for patients with cardiomyopathy being evaluated for kidney transplantation. *CPX* cardiopulmonary stress test, *NYHA* New York Heart Failure Association

after KT. Patients who have resolution of their CM after KT are likely the ones that are responsive to reversal of renal hemodynamics, metabolic and physiological derangement after KT. Unfortunately, prospective studies to identify which patients will normalize their cardiac function after transplantation are lacking.

The evidence about resolution of CM although strong, lacks the clinical tools to allow clinicians to identify patients a priori as to who will normalize their EF after KT. Such screening tools would also allow to prevent listing high risk patients who are unlikely to normalize their EF, and are at higher risk for adverse outcomes after KT. In the absence of such screening tools, both referring physicians and transplant programs are faced with a dilemma of whether they should refer patients for KT or not. Currently there is no consensus on best practice guidelines and practice patterns vary from institution to institution. Due to lack of clear consensus, some institutions refer these patients for dual heart/KT. However, given the paucity of available donors for heart transplantation, utilization of this valuable resource in a patient with reversible CM is of great concern.

The decision to list a patient with CM for either KT of dual organ heart/KT is often complex, and is based on multiple specialty and interdisciplinary committee consensus opinions. In most centers, all potential recipients with low EF and negative coronary angiography or persistent low EF after revascularization, are referred to heart failure specialists for optimization and evaluation for single or combined dual organ transplantation. Some centers employ cardiopulmonary stress testing to determine cardiac reserve, as well as right heart catheterization hemodynamic data to determine listing eligibility. Generally, patients with preserved cardiac reserve and/or preserved cardiac output may be listed for single organ kidney transplantation. A nonvalidated algorithm used at our center is outlined as an example, in Fig. 26.4.

Conclusion

The understanding of CM in ESKD patients is in its infancy, but is rapidly evolving. Confounding our understanding of this complex condition is the intricate interplay between the heart and the kidney, commonly referred as cardio-renal syndrome. The exact mechanism for development of CM in CKD/ESKD patients is not well known, but thought to be multifactorial, centered around development and progression of LVH, LVD and myocardial fibrosis. CKD, and ultimately ESKD, leads to profound biochemical, hemodynamic, and physiological derangements that may be implicated in the developments of CM in these patients. Treatment is centered toward controlling pressure and volume overload, while correctly underlying pathophysiological processes to restore homeostasis. The therapeutic gold standard reverse the above derangements is kidney transplantation, which is very controversial in patients with LVD. A majority of patients with CM improve their systolic and DD after KT. However, patients with LVD overall, as a group, have poor survival in KT compared to patients without LV dysfunction. The survival disadvantage is mainly driven by patients who fail to improve their EF after KT. A validated approach to prospectively identify patients who will not recover their EF after KT is needed to further understand this complex process.

References

1. Alhaj E, Alhaj N, Rahman I, Niazi TO, Berkowitz R, Klapholz M. Uremic cardiomyopathy: an underdiagnosed disease. Congest Heart Fail. 2013;19(4):E40–5.
2. Sarnak MJ, Coronado BE, Greene T, et al. Cardiovascular disease risk factors in chronic renal insufficiency. Clin Nephrol. 2002;57(5):327–35.
3. Johnson DW, Craven AM, Isbel NM. Modification of cardiovascular risk in hemodialysis patients: an evidence-based review. Hemodial Int. 2007;11(1):1–14.
4. Longenecker JC, Coresh J, Powe NR, et al. Traditional cardiovascular disease risk factors in dialysis patients compared with the general population: the CHOICE study. J Am Soc Nephrol. 2002;13(7):1918–27.
5. Collins AJ, Foley RN, Herzog C, et al. Excerpts from the US Renal Data System 2009 Annual Data Report. Am J Kidney Dis. 2010;55(1 Suppl 1):S1–420, A426–7.
6. Trespalacios FC, Taylor AJ, Agodoa LY, Bakris GL, Abbott KC. Heart failure as a cause for hospitalization in chronic dialysis patients. Am J Kidney Dis. 2003;41(6):1267–77.
7. Nolan CR. Strategies for improving long-term survival in patients with ESRD. J Am Soc Nephrol. 2005;16(Suppl 2):S120–7.
8. Foley RN, Parfrey PS, Harnett JD, et al. Clinical and echocardiographic disease in patients starting end-stage renal disease therapy. Kidney Int. 1995;47(1):186–92.
9. Silberberg JS, Barre PE, Prichard SS, Sniderman AD. Impact of left ventricular hypertrophy on survival in end-stage renal disease. Kidney Int. 1989;36(2):286–90.
10. Periyasamy SM, Chen J, Cooney D, et al. Effects of uremic serum on isolated cardiac myocyte calcium cycling and contractile function. Kidney Int. 2001;60(6):2367–76.
11. Ritz E, Rambausek M, Mall G, Ruffmann K, Mandelbaum A. Cardiac changes in uraemia and their possible relationship to cardiovascular instability on dialysis. Nephrol Dial Transplant. 1990;5(Suppl 1):93–7.
12. Mark PB, Johnston N, Groenning BA, et al. Redefinition of uremic cardiomyopathy by contrast-enhanced cardiac magnetic resonance imaging. Kidney Int. 2006;69(10):1839–45.
13. Zoccali C, Benedetto FA, Mallamaci F, et al. Prognostic impact of the indexation of left ventricular mass in patients undergoing dialysis. J Am Soc Nephrol. 2001;12(12):2768–74.
14. Barberato SH, Mantilla DE, Misocami MA, et al. Effect of preload reduction by hemodialysis on left atrial volume and echocardiographic Doppler parameters in patients with end-stage renal disease. Am J Cardiol. 2004;94(9):1208–10.
15. Nagueh SF, Appleton CP, Gillebert TC, et al. Recommendations for the evaluation of left ventricular diastolic function by echocardiography. Eur J Echocardiogr. 2009;10(2):165–93.
16. Dhingra R, Gaziano JM, Djousse L. Chronic kidney disease and the risk of heart failure in men. Circ Heart Fail. 2011;4(2):138–44.
17. London GM. Left ventricular alterations and end-stage renal disease. Nephrol Dial Transplant. 2002;17(Suppl 1):29–36.
18. London GM, Marchais SJ, Safar ME, et al. Aortic and large artery compliance in end-stage renal failure. Kidney Int. 1990; 37(1):137–42.
19. Mourad JJ, Pannier B, Blacher J, et al. Creatinine clearance, pulse wave velocity, carotid compliance and essential hypertension. Kidney Int. 2001;59(5):1834–41.
20. Konings CJ, Dammers R, Rensma PL, et al. Arterial wall properties in patients with renal failure. Am J Kidney Dis. 2002;39(6):1206–12.
21. London GM, Pannier B, Guerin AP, et al. Alterations of left ventricular hypertrophy in and survival of patients receiving hemodialysis: follow-up of an interventional study. J Am Soc Nephrol. 2001;12(12):2759–67.
22. Ortega O, Gallar P, Munoz M, et al. Association between C-reactive protein levels and N-terminal pro-B-type natriuretic peptide in pre-dialysis patients. Nephron Clin Pract. 2004;97(4):c125–30.
23. Laviades C, Varo N, Diez J. Transforming growth factor beta in hypertensives with cardiorenal damage. Hypertension. 2000;36(4):517–22.
24. Vlahakos DV, Hahalis G, Vassilakos P, Marathias KP, Geroulanos S. Relationship between left ventricular hypertrophy and plasma renin activity in chronic hemodialysis patients. J Am Soc Nephrol. 1997;8(11):1764–70.
25. Sato A, Funder JW, Saruta T. Involvement of aldosterone in left ventricular hypertrophy of patients with end-stage renal failure treated with hemodialysis. Am J Hypertens. 1999;12(9 Pt 1): 867–73.
26. London GM. Cardiovascular disease in chronic renal failure: pathophysiologic aspects. Seminars Dial. 2003;16(2):85–94.
27. Fagugli RM, Reboldi G, Quintaliani G, et al. Short daily hemodialysis: blood pressure control and left ventricular mass reduction in hypertensive hemodialysis patients. Am J Kidney Dis. 2001;38(2):371–6.
28. Ozkahya M, Ok E, Cirit M, et al. Regression of left ventricular hypertrophy in haemodialysis patients by ultrafiltration and reduced salt intake without antihypertensive drugs. Nephrol Dial Transplant. 1998;13(6):1489–93.
29. Malik J, Tuka V, Mokrejsova M, Holaj R, Tesar V. Mechanisms of chronic heart failure development in end-stage renal disease patients on chronic hemodialysis. Physiol Res. 2009;58(5): 613–21.
30. Iwashima Y, Horio T, Takami Y, et al. Effects of the creation of arteriovenous fistula for hemodialysis on cardiac function and natriuretic peptide levels in CRF. Am J Kidney Dis. 2002;40(5):974–82.
31. Ori Y, Korzets A, Katz M, Perek Y, Zahavi I, Gafter U. Haemodialysis arteriovenous access—a prospective haemodynamic evaluation. Nephrol Dial Transplant. 1996;11(1):94–7.
32. Parfrey PS, Harnett JD, Barre PE. The natural history of myocardial disease in dialysis patients. J Am Soc Nephrol. 1991;2(1):2–12.
33. Ma JZ, Ebben J, Xia H, Collins AJ. Hematocrit level and associated mortality in hemodialysis patients. J Am Soc Nephrol. 1999;10(3):610–9.
34. London GM, Parfrey PS. Cardiac disease in chronic uremia: pathogenesis. Adv Ren Replace Ther. 1997;4(3):194–211.
35. Phrommintikul A, Haas SJ, Elsik M, Krum H. Mortality and target haemoglobin concentrations in anaemic patients with chronic kidney disease treated with erythropoietin: a meta-analysis. Lancet. 2007;369(9559):381–8.

36. Drueke TB, Locatelli F, Clyne N, et al. Normalization of hemoglobin level in patients with chronic kidney disease and anemia. N Engl J Med. 2006;355(20):2071–84.
37. Singh AK, Szczech L, Tang KL, et al. Correction of anemia with epoetin alfa in chronic kidney disease. N Engl J Med. 2006; 355(20):2085–98.
38. Amann K, Tornig J, Kugel B, et al. Hyperphosphatemia aggravates cardiac fibrosis and microvascular disease in experimental uremia. Kidney Int. 2003;63(4):1296–301.
39. Achinger SG, Ayus JC. Left ventricular hypertrophy: is hyperphosphatemia among dialysis patients a risk factor? J Am Soc Nephrol. 2006;17(12 Suppl 3):S255–61.
40. Fujii H, Kim JI, Abe T, Umezu M, Fukagawa M. Relationship between parathyroid hormone and cardiac abnormalities in chronic dialysis patients. Intern Med. 2007;46(18):1507–12.
41. Silver J, Rodriguez M, Slatopolsky E. FGF23 and PTH—double agents at the heart of CKD. Nephrol Dial Transplant. 2012; 27(5):1715–20.
42. Chue CD, Edwards NC, Moody WE, Steeds RP, Townend JN, Ferro CJ. Serum phosphate is associated with left ventricular mass in patients with chronic kidney disease: a cardiac magnetic resonance study. Heart. 2012;98(3):219–24.
43. Weishaar RE, Simpson RU. Vitamin D3 and cardiovascular function in rats. J Clin Investig. 1987;79(6):1706–12.
44. Cozzolino M, Ronco C. The impact of paricalcitol on left ventricular hypertrophy. Contrib Nephrol. 2011;171:161–5.
45. Bodyak N, Ayus JC, Achinger S, et al. Activated vitamin D attenuates left ventricular abnormalities induced by dietary sodium in Dahl salt-sensitive animals. Proc Natl Acad Sci USA. 2007;104(43):16810–5.
46. Wolf WC, Yoshida H, Agata J, Chao L, Chao J. Human tissue kallikrein gene delivery attenuates hypertension, renal injury, and cardiac remodeling in chronic renal failure. Kidney Int. 2000;58 (2):730–9.
47. Raev DC. Left ventricular function and specific diabetic complications in other target organs in young insulin-dependent diabetics: an echocardiographic study. Heart Vessels. 1994; 9(3):121–8.
48. Yamazaki T, Komuro I, Kudoh S, et al. Endothelin-1 is involved in mechanical stress-induced cardiomyocyte hypertrophy. J Biol Chem. 1996;271(6):3221–8.
49. Yamazaki T, Komuro I, Yazaki Y. Molecular mechanism of cardiac cellular hypertrophy by mechanical stress. J Mol Cell Cardiol. 1995;27(1):133–40.
50. Nielsen FS, Sato A, Ali S, et al. Beneficial impact of ramipril on left ventricular hypertrophy in normotensive nonalbuminuric NIDDM patients. Diabetes Care. 1998;21(5):804–9.
51. Amann K, Breitbach M, Ritz E, Mall G. Myocyte/capillary mismatch in the heart of uremic patients. J Am Soc Nephrol. 1998;9(6):1018–22.
52. Kennedy DJ, Vetteth S, Periyasamy SM, et al. Central role for the cardiotonic steroid marinobufagenin in the pathogenesis of experimental uremic cardiomyopathy. Hypertension. 2006; 47(3):488–95.
53. Fedorova OV, Talan MI, Agalakova NI, Lakatta EG, Bagrov AY. Coordinated shifts in Na/K-ATPase isoforms and their endogenous ligands during cardiac hypertrophy and failure in NaCl-sensitive hypertension. J Hypertens. 2004;22(2):389–97.
54. Gansevoort RT, Correa-Rotter R, Hemmelgarn BR, et al. Chronic kidney disease and cardiovascular risk: epidemiology, mechanisms, and prevention. Lancet. 2013;382(9889):339–52.
55. Mall G, Huther W, Schneider J, Lundin P, Ritz E. Diffuse intermyocardiocytic fibrosis in uraemic patients. Nephrol Dial Transplant. 1990;5(1):39–44.
56. Aoki J, Ikari Y, Nakajima H, et al. Clinical and pathologic characteristics of dilated cardiomyopathy in hemodialysis patients. Kidney Int. 2005;67(1):333–40.
57. Diez J. Mechanisms of cardiac fibrosis in hypertension. J Clin Hypertens. 2007;9(7):546–50.
58. Chinnappa S, Mooney A, Lewis NT, Goldspink D, El Nahas M, Tan LB. New evidence of cardiac dysfunction associated with renal impairment. Int J Cardiol. 2011;152(3):411–3.
59. Mitsnefes MM, Kimball TR, Witt SA, Glascock BJ, Khoury PR, Daniels SR. Left ventricular mass and systolic performance in pediatric patients with chronic renal failure. Circulation. 2003;107(6):864–8.
60. Sietsema KE, Amato A, Adler SG, Brass EP. Exercise capacity as a predictor of survival among ambulatory patients with end-stage renal disease. Kidney Int. 2004;65(2):719–24.
61. Weaver DJ Jr, Kimball TR, Knilans T, et al. Decreased maximal aerobic capacity in pediatric chronic kidney disease. J Am Soc Nephrol. 2008;19(3):624–30.
62. Reisin E. Nonpharmacologic approaches to hypertension. Weight, sodium, alcohol, exercise, and tobacco considerations. Med Clin N Am. 1997;81(6):1289–303.
63. Zazgornik J, Biesenbach G, Forstenlehner M, Stummvoll K. Profile of antihypertensive drugs in hypertensive patients on renal replacement therapy (RRT). Clin Nephrol. 1997;48(6):337–40.
64. Dyadyk AI, Bagriy AE, Lebed IA, Yarovaya NF, Schukina EV, Taradin GG. ACE inhibitors captopril and enalapril induce regression of left ventricular hypertrophy in hypertensive patients with chronic renal failure. Nephrol Dial Transplant. 1997;12 (5):945–51.
65. Ly J, Chan CT. Impact of augmenting dialysis frequency and duration on cardiovascular function. ASAIO J. 2006;52(6):e11–4.
66. Weinreich T, De los Rios T, Gauly A, Passlick-Deetjen J. Effects of an increase in time vs. frequency on cardiovascular parameters in chronic hemodialysis patients. Clin Nephrol. 2006;66(6): 433–9.
67. Chazot C, Charra B, Laurent G, et al. Interdialysis blood pressure control by long haemodialysis sessions. Nephrol Dial Transplant. 1995;10(6):831–7.
68. Ayus JC, Go AS, Valderrabano F, et al. Effects of erythropoietin on left ventricular hypertrophy in adults with severe chronic renal failure and hemoglobin <10 g/dL. Kidney Int. 2005;68(2): 788–95.
69. Parfrey PS, Lauve M, Latremouille-Viau D, Lefebvre P. Erythropoietin therapy and left ventricular mass index in CKD and ESRD patients: a meta-analysis. Clin J Am Soc Nephrol. 2009;4 (4):755–62.
70. Galetta F, Cupisti A, Franzoni F, et al. Left ventricular function and calcium phosphate plasma levels in uraemic patients. J Intern Med. 2005;258(4):378–84.
71. Li S, Collins AJ. Association of hematocrit value with cardiovascular morbidity and mortality in incident hemodialysis patients. Kidney Int. 2004;65(2):626–33.
72. Saleh FN, Schirmer H, Sundsfjord J, Jorde R. Parathyroid hormone and left ventricular hypertrophy. Eur Heart J. 2003; 24(22):2054–60.
73. Walker MD, Silverberg SJ. Cardiovascular aspects of primary hyperparathyroidism. J Endocrinol Invest. 2008;31(10):925–31.
74. Aladren Regidor MJ. Cinacalcet reduces vascular and soft tissue calcification in secondary hyperparathyroidism (SHPT) in hemodialysis patients. Clin Nephrol. 2009;71(2):207–13.
75. Thadhani R, Appelbaum E, Pritchett Y, et al. Vitamin D therapy and cardiac structure and function in patients with chronic kidney disease: the PRIMO randomized controlled trial. JAMA. 2012;307(7):674–84.

76. Investigators ET, Chertow GM, Block GA, et al. Effect of cinacalcet on cardiovascular disease in patients undergoing dialysis. N Engl J Med. 2012;367(26):2482–94.
77. Maduell F, Moreso F, Pons M, et al. High-efficiency postdilution online hemodiafiltration reduces all-cause mortality in hemodialysis patients. J Am Soc Nephrol. 2013;24(3):487–97.
78. Dzemidzic J, Rasic S, Saracevic A, et al. Predictors of left ventricular remodelling in kidney transplant recipients in the first posttransplant year. Bosnian J Basic Med Sci. 2010;10(Suppl 1): S51–5.
79. McGregor E, Stewart G, Rodger RS, Jardine AG. Early echocardiographic changes and survival following renal transplantation. Nephrol Dial Transplant. 2000;15(1):93–8.
80. Torres S, Maximino J, Pereira S, et al. Morphologic course of the left ventricle after renal transplantation. Echocardiographic study. Port J Cardiol. 1991;10(6):497–501.
81. Dudziak M, Debska-Slizien A, Rutkowski B. Cardiovascular effects of successful renal transplantation: a 30-month study on left ventricular morphology, systolic and diastolic functions. Transpl Proc. 2005;37(2):1039–43.
82. Pirat B, Bozbas H, Demirtas S, et al. Comparison of tissue Doppler echocardiography parameters in patients with end-stage renal disease and renal transplant recipients. Transpl Proc. 2008;40(1):107–10.
83. Himelman RB, Landzberg JS, Simonson JS, et al. Cardiac consequences of renal transplantation: changes in left ventricular morphology and function. J Am Coll Cardiol. 1988;12(4): 915–23.
84. Peteiro J, Alvarez N, Calvino R, Penas M, Ribera F, Castro Beiras A. Changes in left ventricular mass and filling after renal transplantation are related to changes in blood pressure: an echocardiographic and pulsed Doppler study. Cardiology. 1994;85(5):273–83.
85. Rigatto C, Foley RN, Kent GM, Guttmann R, Parfrey PS. Long-term changes in left ventricular hypertrophy after renal transplantation. Transplantation. 2000;70(4):570–5.
86. Sahagun-Sanchez G, Espinola-Zavaleta N, Lafragua-Contreras M, et al. The effect of kidney transplant on cardiac function: an echocardiographic perspective. Echocardiography. 2001;18 (6):457–62.
87. Iqbal MM, Rashid HU, Banerjee SK, Rahman MH, Mohsin M. Changes in cardiac parameters of renal allograft recipients: a compilation of clinical, laboratory, and echocardiographic observations. Transpl Proc. 2008;40(7):2327–9.
88. Dounousi E, Mitsis M, Naka KK, et al. Differences in cardiac structure assessed by echocardiography between renal transplant recipients and chronic kidney disease patients. Transpl Proc. 2014;46(9):3194–8.
89. Ferreira SR, Moises VA, Tavares A, Pacheco-Silva A. Cardiovascular effects of successful renal transplantation: a 1-year sequential study of left ventricular morphology and function, and 24-hour blood pressure profile. Transplantation. 2002; 74(11):1580–7.
90. Patel RK, Mark PB, Johnston N, McGregor E, Dargie HJ, Jardine AG. Renal transplantation is not associated with regression of left ventricular hypertrophy: a magnetic resonance study. Clin J Am Soc Nephrol. 2008;3(6):1807–11.
91. Huting J. Course of left ventricular hypertrophy and function in end-stage renal disease after renal transplantation. Am J Cardiol. 1992;70(18):1481–4.
92. De Lima JJ, Abensur H, da Fonseca JA, Krieger EM, Pileggi F. Comparison of echocardiographic changes associated with hemodialysis and renal transplantation. Artif Organs. 1995;19(3): 245–50.
93. Slubowska K, Lichodziejewska B, Pruszczyk P, Szmidt J, Durlik M. Left ventricular hypertrophy in renal transplant recipients in the first year after transplantation. Transpl Proc. 2014;46(8):2719–23.
94. Meyer DM, Rogers JG, Edwards LB, et al. The future direction of the adult heart allocation system in the United States. Am J Transplant. 2015;15(1):44–54.
95. Wolfe RA, Ashby VB, Milford EL, et al. Comparison of mortality in all patients on dialysis, patients on dialysis awaiting transplantation, and recipients of a first cadaveric transplant. N Engl J Med. 1999;341(23):1725–30.
96. West M, Sutherland DE, Matas AJ. Kidney transplant recipients who die with functioning grafts: serum creatinine level and cause of death. Transplantation. 1996;62(7):1029–30.
97. Israni AK, Snyder JJ, Skeans MA, Kasiske BL, Investigators P. Clinical diagnosis of metabolic syndrome: predicting new-onset diabetes, coronary heart disease, and allograft failure late after kidney transplant. Transpl Int. 2012;25(7):748–57.
98. Siedlecki A, Foushee M, Curtis JJ, et al. The impact of left ventricular systolic dysfunction on survival after renal transplantation. Transplantation. 2007;84(12):1610–7.
99. Josephson CB, Delgado D, Schiff J, Ross H. The effectiveness of renal transplantation as a treatment for recurrent uremic cardiomyopathy. Can J Cardiol. 2008;24(4):315–7.
100. Hawwa N, Shrestha K, Hammadah M, Yeo PS, Fatica R, Tang WH. Reverse remodeling and prognosis following kidney transplantation in contemporary patients with cardiac dysfunction. J Am Coll Cardiol. 2015;66(16):1779–87.
101. Wali RK, Wang GS, Gottlieb SS, et al. Effect of kidney transplantation on left ventricular systolic dysfunction and congestive heart failure in patients with end-stage renal disease. J Am Coll Cardiol. 2005;45(7):1051–60.
102. Melchor JL, Espinoza R, Gracida C. Kidney transplantation in patients with ventricular ejection fraction less than 50 percent: features and posttransplant outcome. Transpl Proc. 2002;34(7): 2539–40.
103. Oppert M, Schneider U, Bocksch W, et al. Improvement of left ventricular function and arterial blood pressure 1 year after simultaneous pancreas kidney transplantation. Transpl Proc. 2002;34(6):2251–2.
104. Parfrey PS, Foley RN, Harnett JD, Kent GM, Murray DC, Barre PE. Outcome and risk factors for left ventricular disorders in chronic uraemia. Nephrol Dial Transplant. 1996;11(7):1277–85.
105. Burt RK, Gupta-Burt S, Suki WN, Barcenas CG, Ferguson JJ, Van Buren CT. Reversal of left ventricular dysfunction after renal transplantation. Ann Intern Med. 1989;111(8):635–40.

Part V

Anticoagulation and Antiplatelet Therapy in CKD

Anticoagulation in Patients with Atrial Fibrillation and Chronic Kidney Disease

27

Michelle D. Carlson and Gautam R. Shroff

Epidemiological Considerations

Prevalence and Incidence of Atrial Fibrillation in CKD

Atrial fibrillation (AF) is the most frequently encountered sustained cardiac arrhythmia and represents an important modifiable risk factor for ischemic stroke. Its prevalence progressively increases with age; among United States Medicare beneficiaries the prevalence of nonvalvular AF (NVAF) among those aged 65–74, 75–84, and over 85 years was estimated at 4.5, 10, and 15%, respectively, in the year 2010 [1]. Chronic kidney disease (CKD) has increased in prevalence, affecting about 20 million Americans based on the most recent estimates by the Centers of Disease Control; the greatest increase in CKD prevalence has occurred in adults older than 60 years. Thus, there is a growing aging population with co-prevalent NVAF and CKD. Advancing CKD is independently associated with a higher risk of both prevalent and incident AF. In a large population based sample, adjusted odds for prevalent AF were 2–3 times higher among those with advancing stages of CKD compared with participants without CKD [2]. Using the Medicare 5% sample, the hazard of incident AF at a follow-up interval of 2 years was about 14% among beneficiaries with CKD stages 3–5; significantly higher compared to beneficiaries without CKD [3].

A similar theme pertaining to rising prevalence of AF is noted among patients with CKD stage 5D (end-stage kidney disease on dialysis) who constituted a prevalent population of about 661,648 in the US in the year 2013. Data from the United States Renal Data System (USRDS) indicate that the baseline prevalence of AF is markedly higher among hemodialysis patients compared to the general population. The average prevalence of AF among hemodialysis patients was estimated at about 7.7% and increased threefold from 3.5 to 10.7% between 1992 and 2006 [4]. As with the general population, the prevalence in this cohort increased with advancing age, estimated at 9.3, 13.9, and 17%, respectively, among hemodialysis patients aged 65–74, 75–84, and over 85 years. In a systematic review of 25 studies, the prevalence of AF was reported at about 11.6% among end-stage kidney disease (ESKD) patients with an overall incidence of 2.7/100 patient-years, both much higher than the general population [5]. There is wide variation in AF prevalence among hemodialysis patients in different countries, likely reflective of variations in demographics and medical comorbidities as well as socioeconomic status and healthcare delivery [6]. The prevalence of asymptomatic AF detected using implantable monitoring devices may be much higher than previously reported in this population based on emerging data.

Risks of Stroke, Bleeding, and Mortality with Atrial Fibrillation and CKD

An accurate assessment of the risks of stroke and bleeding is imperative for a decision regarding risks versus benefits of anticoagulation in this high-risk population. Compared to non-CKD patients, the risk of stroke is generally considered higher among patients with CKD and AF, but this issue is more controversial among dialysis patients. Reduced creatinine clearance (CrCl) was a strong and independent predictor of stroke and systemic embolism in large, contemporary studies [7]. Moreover, the inclusion of reduced CrCl (R2CHADS2) improved the net reclassification index for predicting future thromboembolic risk compared to the use of conventional risk calculators (CHADS2/CHA2DS2VASc). In a large Danish registry

M.D. Carlson (✉) · G.R. Shroff
Cardiology Division, Hennepin County Medical Center, 701 Park Ave, Minneapolis, MN 55415, USA
e-mail: michelle.carlson2@hcmed.org

G.R. Shroff
e-mail: shrof010@umn.edu

J. Rangaswami et al. (eds.), *Cardio-Nephrology*,
DOI 10.1007/978-3-319-56042-7_27

population, a statistically significant increase was reported in the hazard of stroke or systemic embolism among patients with CKD relative to patients without CKD [hazard ratio (HR) 1.49, $p < 0.001$] and those receiving renal replacement therapy (HR 1.8, $p < 0.001$) [8].

The risk of ischemic stroke among dialysis patients with AF is more difficult to measure accurately because of the high competing risk of mortality and other causes of stroke, and routine use of anticoagulation is controversial. In a recent propensity matched analysis of a large population identified from Taiwan's National Research Database, hemodialysis patients with AF had higher risks of ischemic stroke (adjusted HR 1.27, $p < 0.001$) compared to patients without AF [9]. However, after statistical consideration for in-hospital mortality as a competing risk, the authors reported that the risk of ischemic stroke was no longer a significant variable (AHR 1.01, $p = 0.83$).

There is general agreement in the literature that the risks of bleeding complications are higher among CKD patients treated with anticoagulation compared to the general population, and particularly so among hemodialysis patients. In a large cohort of patients with AF from the SPORTIF III and V trials, the presence of renal impairment (defined as CrCl <50 mL/min) was identified as an independent predictor of major bleeding (HR 1.98, $p < 0.001$) in multivariable analysis [10]. Bleeding complications were also significantly higher in the Danish registry among those with CKD (HR 2.24, $p < 0.001$) and those on renal replacement therapy (HR 2.7, $p < 0.001$) [8]. Among dialysis patients, the risks of bleeding with use of warfarin are significantly higher than the general population [11], but it is problematic to extrapolate these data to AF patients since most studies assessed warfarin use for graft patency and included varied INR targets.

Finally, the combination of CKD and AF is associated with a higher hazard of mortality compared to patients with either condition alone. Data from a large Medicare sample of AF patients show that worsening stages of CKD are associated with an increasing relative hazard of all-cause mortality compared to patients without CKD [3]. Among patients with incident AF, unadjusted survival at 1-year follow-up was 79, 68, and 64% for patients without CKD, with stage 1–2 CKD, and with stages 3–5 CKD, respectively. Similarly, in a large population from a health maintenance organization in the United States, incident AF was associated with a 66% increase in relative risk of mortality among patients with CKD [12]. In a systematic analysis, the mortality hazard of hemodialysis patients with AF was double that of patients without AF (26.9 vs. 13.4/100 patient-years) [5]. It is not feasible to accurately determine the precise attributable risk of AF toward mortality in the CKD population due to confounding by several contributory coexisting factors; perhaps the milieu that contributes to the development of AF (e.g., structural cardiovascular disease, neurohormonal factors)—rather than AF alone—contributes to the increased hazard of mortality. Nonetheless, the association of an increased mortality hazard in the setting of co-prevalent AF and CKD has been convincingly demonstrated in the literature. These studies underline the high-risk nature of the population with concomitant CKD and AF, with heightened risks of bleeding, stroke, and mortality, and highlight the clinical conundrum of anticoagulation, which has been likened to navigating the waters between Scylla and Charybdis [13].

Anticoagulation in Atrial Fibrillation

In the general population, the use of therapeutic anticoagulation with warfarin has been convincingly demonstrated to associate with substantial reductions in the risk of ischemic stroke and all-cause mortality. In a metaanalysis incorporating data from 29 clinical studies and 28,044 patients, anticoagulant therapy using adjusted-dose warfarin reduced the ischemic stroke risk by nearly 60% and mortality by nearly 25% [14]. For several years, vitamin K antagonists (VKAs), primarily warfarin, were the only agents available for systemic anticoagulation. Given interactions with many medications and foods, the need for frequent monitoring, and the difficulty in maintaining a therapeutic INR in many patients taking warfarin, the direct oral anticoagulants (DOACs) were greeted with enthusiasm. With the approval of DOACs, a paradigm shift has occurred in the approach toward anticoagulation. This is of particular relevance among patients with CKD, because, unlike warfarin, dosing of medications is heavily contingent upon renal clearance, and there is no approved blood test to guide dosing and ascertain therapeutic levels. Fortunately, the pivotal randomized controlled trials included patients with stage 3 CKD; therefore, representative information pertaining to this population is available to guide medical decision-making. Subgroup analyses of these trials generally compare those with an estimated CrCl (eCrCl) <50–60 mL/min (Cockcroft–Gault equation) to those with a higher eCrCl and support prior evidence that CKD is associated with an increased risk of embolic events and major bleeding. Patients with eCrCl <30 mL/min were excluded from the DOAC trials, likely both because of an increased risk of bleeding and because of the considerable renal clearance of these drugs [15].

Direct Oral Anticoagulants in Atrial Fibrillation

Summary of the Pivotal Clinical Trials

Dabigatran, a direct thrombin inhibitor, was approved in 2010 for stroke prevention in NVAF, based on the results of the RE-LY trial [16]. Rivaroxaban was the first factor Xa inhibitor to be approved for NVAF in 2011 (ROCKET AF), followed by apixaban in 2012 (ARISTOTLE and AVERROES), and most recently edoxaban in 2015 (ENGAGE AF-TIMI 48) [17–20]. These trials are summarized in Table 27.1. RE-LY, ROCKET AF, ARISTOTLE, and ENGAGE AF-TIMI 48 were randomized, controlled, noninferiority trials comparing the study drug to warfarin (goal INR of 2–3) in patients with NVAF [16–18, 20]. Dabigatran and edoxaban were both tested at high and low doses. All study drug doses were shown to be noninferior to warfarin for the primary endpoint of stroke or systemic embolism

Table 27.1 Initial randomized controlled trials of direct oral anticoagulants for nonvalvular atrial fibrillation

Trial	RE-LY	ROCKET AF	ARISTOTLE	AVERROES	ENGAGE AF-TIMI 48
n	18,113	14,264	18,201	5,599	21,105
CHADS2, mean	2.1	3.5	2.1	2.1	2.8
Age, median	71[a]	73	70	70[a]	72
Renal exclusion	eCrCl < 30	eCrCl < 30	Cr > 2.5 or CrCl < 25	Cr > 2.5 or CrCl < 25	eCrCl < 30
Subjects with renal dysfunction, *n* (%)	eCrCl < 50 = 3554 [20] eCrCl 50–80 = 8553 [47]	eCrCl < 50 = 2905 [20] eCrCl 50–80 = 6698 [47]	eCrCl < 50 = 3017 [17] eCrCl 50–80 = 7587 [42]	eCrCl < 60 = 1697 [12]	eCrCl < 50 = 4074 [19] eCrCl 50–80 = 9075 [43]
Study drug	Dabigatran 110 mg bid or 150 mg bid	Rivaroxaban 20 mg daily	Apixaban 5 mg bid	Apixaban 5 mg bid	Edoxaban 30 mg daily or 60 mg daily
Control	Warfarin, goal INR 2–3, median TTR 64%	Warfarin, goal INR 2–3, median TTR 58%	Warfarin, goal INR 2–3, median TTR 66%	ASA 81–324 mg daily	Warfarin, goal INR 2–3, median TTR 68%
Follow-up, median	2 years	1.9 years	1.8 years	1.1 years	2.8 years
Statistical design	Noninferiority	Noninferiority	Noninferiority	Superiority	Noninferiority
Primary outcome: stroke or systemic embolism					
Study drug	110 mg: 1.5%/year 150 mg: 1.1%/year[‡]	1.7%/year[b]	1.3%/year	1.6%/year	30 mg: 1.6%/year 60 mg: 1.2%/year
Control	1.7%/year	2.2%/year[b]	1.6%/year	3.7%/year (ASA)	1.5%/year
Ratio, *p* value[†]	110 mg: RR 0.91, <0.001 150 mg: RR 0.66, <0.001	HR 0.79, <0.001	HR 0.79, 0.01	HR 0.45, <0.001	30 mg: HR 1.07, 0.005 60 mg: HR 0.79, <0.001
Safety outcome: Major bleeding					
Study drug	110 mg: 2.7%/year 150 mg: 3.1%/year	3.6%/year	2.1%/year	1.4%/year	30 mg: 1.6%/year 60 mg: 2.75%/year
Control	3.3%/year	3.4%/year	3.1%/year	1.2%/year (ASA)	3.4%/year
Ratio, *p* value	110 mg: RR 0.80, 0.003 150 mg: RR 0.93, NS	HR 1.04, NS	HR 0.69, <0.001	HR 1.13, NS	30 mg: HR 0.47, <0.001 60 mg: HR 0.80, <0.001
Secondary outcome: all-cause mortality					
Study drug	110 mg: 3.8%/year 150 mg: 3.6%/year	1.9%/year	3.5%/year	3.5%/year	30 mg: 3.8%/year 60 mg: 3.99%/year
Control	4.1%/year	2.2%/year	3.9%/year	4.4%/year (ASA)	4.35%/year
Ratio, *p* value	110 mg: RR 0.91, NS 150 mg: RR 0.88, NS	HR 0.85, NS	HR 0.89, 0.047	HR 0.79, NS	30 mg: HR 0.87, 0.006 60 mg: HR 0.92, 0.08

ASA aspirin, *Cr* creatinine in mg/dL, *eCrCl* estimated creatinine clearance calculated by Cockcroft–Gault formula in mL/min, *HR* hazard ratio, *ITT* intention-to-treat, *NR* not reported, *NS* not statistically significant, *RR* relative risk, *TTR* time in therapeutic range

[a]Mean age

[†]*p* value for noninferiority for primary outcomes except for AVERROES (superiority)

[‡]RR for dabigatran 150 mg versus 110 mg 0.73, *p* value for superiority 0.005

[b]Per-protocol analysis

(SSE). High-dose dabigatran and apixaban met superiority endpoints compared to warfarin for prevention of SSE by intention-to-treat analysis; high-dose edoxaban was superior to warfarin only in the modified intention-to-treat analysis. High-dose dabigatran was shown to be superior to low-dose dabigatran in prevention of SSE with a higher risk of bleeding; low-dose versus high-dose edoxaban was not compared. Low-dose dabigatran, apixaban, and both doses of edoxaban had a statistically significantly lower risk of major bleeding compared to warfarin. In each trial, warfarin carried a significantly higher relative risk of intracranial hemorrhage relative to DOACs, while all DOACs except apixaban carried a higher risk of gastrointestinal bleeding. Apixaban and low-dose edoxaban were associated with a decreased risk of all-cause mortality compared to warfarin.

AVERROES was a randomized, controlled, superiority trial comparing apixaban to aspirin (81–324 mg) in patients with NVAF who were not candidates for anticoagulation with a VKA, either due to an increased risk of bleeding, difficulty maintaining a therapeutic INR, or a CHADS2 score of 0 [19]. This trial showed that apixaban was superior to aspirin for prevention of SSE (Table 27.1) and did not carry an increased risk of major bleeding or death.

Pharmacokinetic and Pharmacodynamic Characteristics: Practical Considerations

Each DOAC has specific characteristics that allow the choice of agent to be tailored to an individual (see Table 27.2). The DOACs are direct-acting agents with a rapid onset of action and a half-life less than 24 h, and have no associated increase in thrombotic risk with initiation (as with warfarin); thus, the DOACs can be initiated without any bridging therapy in the setting of NVAF, and routine monitoring of anticoagulation is not recommended [21]. The DOACs have more selective action on the coagulation cascade and do not exhibit the irreversible downstream effects that warfarin enacts on the clotting cascade. Warfarin must be held for several days prior to procedures to allow adequate hemostasis, while the DOACs can be held for a shorter duration, contingent upon baseline renal function.

Dabigatran, a reversible direct inhibitor of thrombin, is administered orally as a pro-drug (dabigatran etexilate) that is rapidly hydrolyzed to the active metabolite. It has a high degree of renal clearance (80%), with prolongation of the half-life with worsening renal function (from 14 h in normal subjects to 28 h in those with eCrCl ≤ 30 mL/min). Dabigatran is largely cleared by dialysis—at least 60% in one pharmacokinetic study. Given prolonged half-life with renal dysfunction, dabigatran should be held for a longer period of time pre-procedurally in those with renal dysfunction (1–2 days for eCrCl ≥ 50 mL/min, 3–5 days for eCrCl <50 mL/min).

Rivaroxaban is a reversible factor Xa inhibitor that has increased bioavailability when taken with food. Renal clearance is 35%, and, though the half-life is only slightly prolonged with impaired renal function, drug level increases significantly with progressive renal dysfunction. Based on pharmacologic data, a reduced dose of rivaroxaban of 15 mg daily was used in ROCKET AF for patients with eCrCl <50 mL/min. Rivaroxaban should be held for at least 24 h before procedures that carry an increased risk of bleeding.

Apixaban, also a reversible factor Xa inhibitor, is absorbed throughout the gastrointestinal tract, including the small bowel and ascending colon, with a half-life of about 12 h with repeat dosing. Only 25% of the drug is renally cleared. Dose adjustment on the basis of moderate renal dysfunction alone is not necessary, but for those with a creatinine ≥ 1.5 mg/dL and an additional risk factor for higher drug exposure (age ≥ 80 years or weight ≤ 60 kg), a decreased dose of 2.5 mg twice daily (BID) is recommended. Apixaban should be held for 24 h before procedures with a low risk of bleeding and 48 h before procedures with a high risk of bleeding.

Edoxaban, the most recent reversible factor Xa inhibitor, has a half-life of 10–14 h, with 40% of the drug renally cleared. Systemic exposure to the drug increases with worsening renal function. In ENGAGE AF-TIMI 48, a 50% dose reduction was used for those with eCrCl 30–50 mL/min based on pharmacokinetic modeling. Edoxaban should be held for at least 24 h before procedures that carry an increased risk of bleeding. Of note, in ENGAGE AF-TIMI 48, subjects with eCrCl >95 mL/min who were treated with edoxaban had a higher rate of stroke and systemic embolism than those treated with warfarin (1.0 vs. 0.6%/year, HR 1.87, 95% CI 1.10–3.17), driven by an increase in ischemic stroke. Edoxaban blood levels decrease with increasing renal function—about 30% less with eCrCl >80 mL/min and 40% less with eCrCl >95 mL/min—so it is not recommended for use in subjects with eCrCl >95 mL/min.

Laboratory Monitoring and Management of Bleeding for DOACs

One of the advantages of the DOACs is the lack of need for routine monitoring to ensure that therapeutic drug levels are achieved. However, there are certain clinical situations in which it can be advantageous to know the degree of anticoagulation present—for example, in the setting of an emergent surgery, when there is concern for noncompliance, prior to thrombolytic therapy for ischemic stroke, or, most

Table 27.2 Direct oral anticoagulant prescribing information and characteristics

DOAC	Dabigatran	Rivaroxaban	Apixaban	Edoxaban
Mechanism of action	Direct thrombin inhibitor	Factor Xa inhibitor	Factor Xa inhibitor	Factor Xa inhibitor
Dosing for NVAF	eCrCl > 30: 150 mg bid eCrCl 15–30: 75 mg bid eCrCl < 15 or dialysis: not recommended	eCrCl > 50:20 mg daily eCrCl 15–50: 15 mg daily eCrCl < 15 or dialysis: not recommended	5 mg bid 2.5 mg bid if 2 of the following: Cr $\geq$ 1.5 age $\geq$ 80 weight $\leq$ 60 kg Cr > 2.5, eCrCl < 15 or dialysis: use based on pharmacokinetics	eCrCl > 95: not recommended eCrCl 51–95: 60 mg daily eCrCl 15–50: 30 mg daily eCrCl < 15 or dialysis: not recommended
Geriatric use	Increased risk of bleeding with age; risk-benefit profile still favorable	Increased risk of bleeding with age; risk-benefit profile still favorable	Age $\geq$ 80: see above	Similar efficacy and safety in elderly patients (>65 years old)
Extremes in body weight		<50 kg or >120 kg: <25% change in exposure	Weight $\leq$ 60 kg: see above	Dose reduction for weight $\leq$ 60 kg only recommended for VTE
Administration	Do not crush or chew Take with or without food	Can be crushed Take with largest meal (food increases bioavailability)	Can be crushed Take with or without food	No data regarding crushing Take with or without food
Converting from warfarin	Start when INR < 2	Start when INR < 3	Start when INR < 2	Start when INR < 2.5
Discontinuing before procedures	CrCl $\geq$ 50 mL/min: 1–2 days CrCl < 50 mL/min: 3–5 days	24 h	48 h if moderate/high risk of bleeding 24 h if low risk of bleeding	24 h
Metabolism	Liver; pro-drug converted to dabigatran	Liver; CYP450—3A4/5, 2J2	Liver; CYP450—primarily 3A4	Minimal; CYP450–3A4
T_{max} (h)	1–3	2–4	3–4	1–2
Half-life (h)	12–17	5–9	~12	10–14
Renal clearance	80%	35%	25%	40%
Side effects	Bleeding Gastrointestinal: dyspepsia, abdominal pain	Bleeding	Bleeding	Bleeding
Drug interactions[a]	P-gp inducers decrease exposure P-gp inhibitors increase exposure	Combined P-gp and CYP3A4 inducers decrease exposure Combined P-gp and CYP3A4 inhibitors increase exposure	Combined P-gp and CYP3A4 inducers decrease exposure Combined P-gp and CYP3A4 inhibitors increase exposure	P-gp inducers decrease exposure P-gp inhibitors increase exposure
Management of bleeding	Idaracizumab Charcoal within 2 h of last ingestion Dialyzable (60% in 2–3 h) Life-threatening bleed: PCC, aPCC	Andexanet and ciraparantag under investigation Charcoal within 2 h of last ingestion Not dialyzable Life-threatening bleed: PCC, aPCC	Andexanet and ciraparantag under investigation Charcoal within 6 h of last ingestion Not dialyzable Life-threatening bleed: PCC, aPCC	Andexanet and ciraparantag under investigation No information on charcoal Not dialyzable Life-threatening bleed: PCC, aPCC
Laboratory monitoring†	Dabigatran level Thrombin time	Anti-Xa level	Anti-Xa level	Anti-Xa level

aPCC active prothrombin complex concentrate (Feiba), *Cr* creatinine in mg/dL, *eCrCl* estimated creatinine clearance in mL/min calculated by Cockcroft–Gault equation, *NVAF* nonvalvular atrial fibrillation, *PCC* four-factor prothrombin complex concentrate (Kcentra), *P-gp* P-glycoprotein, *VTE* venous thromboembolism

[a]P-gp inducers include rifampin. P-gp inhibitors include azithromycin, clarithromycin, erythromycin, itraconazole, ketoconazole, quinidine, and verapamil. Combined P-gp and CYP3A4 inducers include carbamazepine, phenytoin, rifampin, and St. John's wort. Combined P-gp and CYP3A4 inhibitors include clarithromycin, erythromycin, fluconazole, itraconazole, ketoconazole, and ritonavir

†Generally only indicated in the setting of major or life-threatening bleed

importantly, in the setting of bleeding [22]. Thrombin time (TT) is exquisitely sensitive to dabigatran, and a normal TT essentially rules out the presence of the drug [23]. The activated partial thromboplastin time (aPTT) may be elevated in the setting of dabigatran but can be normal at trough drug levels, and the prothrombin time/international normalized ratio (PT/INR) is even less sensitive [22]. If a more exact quantification of dabigatran level is required, the dilute TT or ecarin clotting time may be used, although these are not widely available. For patients on rivaroxaban or edoxaban, a prolonged PT can indicate the drug's presence, but a normal PT does not exclude the possibility of a clinically significant drug level. PT is less sensitive to apixaban, and aPTT is even less sensitive to all three anti-Xa agents. The chromogenic anti-factor Xa assay is most sensitive for ruling out the presence of rivaroxaban, apixaban, or edoxaban, as well as for providing a quantitative evaluation of drug level.

Kcentra® is a 4-factor prothrombin complex concentrate (PCC) that contains coagulation factors II, VII, IX, and X as well as antithrombotic proteins C and S. It is approved for reversal of warfarin in the setting of life-threatening bleeding, with a dose based on the INR [24]. The 2012 Antithrombotic Guidelines suggest using PCC rather than FFP for patients with a life-threatening bleed while on VKA therapy, given the higher risk of allergic reaction, prolonged preparation time, and greater volume with FFP [25]. It is reasonable to use 4-factor PCC in the setting of life-threatening DOAC-associated bleeding, although there are no randomized data for its use in this setting. Pro-hemostatic agents including activated PCC and recombinant factor VIIa (rFVIIa) have weak supporting evidence and may be an option if PCC is not available, with the knowledge that pro-hemostatic agents are associated with an increased risk of thrombosis.

Dabigatran, which is 35% protein bound, can be cleared by hemodialysis if needed. In one study, 60% of dabigatran was cleared with a 4-h run of hemodialysis at 400 mL/min targeted blood flow [26]. The factor Xa inhibitors are insufficiently protein bound to be effectively cleared by dialysis. Activated charcoal may be effective in the setting of an overdose within 2 h of ingestion for dabigatran or rivaroxaban or within 6 h of ingestion for apixaban.

Idarucizimab, a monoclonal antibody fragment that binds and neutralizes both free and thrombin-bound dabigatran, normalizes coagulation parameters in healthy volunteers [27]. The agent was approved by the United States Food and Drug Administration (FDA) under the accelerated approval program, which allows approval of drugs based on surrogate endpoints for situations in which no other therapy is available. Further clinical data will need to be collected in post-marketing analysis [28]. Idarucizumab is approved for reversal of dabigatran anticoagulation in the setting of emergent surgery, an urgent procedure, or life-threatening or uncontrolled bleeding [29]. Andexanet alfa is an inactive recombinant factor Xa protein that acts as a "decoy" to bind factor Xa inhibitors with a high affinity and allow endogenous factor Xa to function [30]. Andexanet has been shown to be effective in reversing the anticoagulant effects of rivaroxaban and apixaban in healthy volunteers. An open-label prospective trial employing andexanet in patients with factor Xa inhibitor-associated major bleeding is underway [31]. Ciraparantag, a cationic molecule originally designed to bind unfractionated and low-molecular weight heparin, has been shown to also bind factor Xa inhibitors in a similar fashion [32]. Additional clinical evidence is awaited.

Anticoagulation for Atrial Fibrillation in Advanced CKD

Anticoagulation in CKD Stage 3 Patients with AF

Warfarin

Patients with stage 3 CKD were represented in the Stroke Prevention in Atrial Fibrillation (SPAF) III trial, which randomized high-risk participants to adjusted-dose warfarin versus fixed-dose warfarin plus 325 mg aspirin [33]. In a post hoc analysis, among patients with stage 3 CKD ($n = 516$) included in the trial, adjusted-dose warfarin-reduced clinical events (ischemic stroke and systemic embolism) by 76% compared to fixed low-dose warfarin plus aspirin, with no increase in major bleeding events.

DOACs

Prespecified subgroup analyses of patients with renal dysfunction in RE-LY, ROCKET AF, and ARISTOTLE consistently demonstrate that the rates of stroke, systemic embolism, and major bleeding increase as renal function decreases, independent of treatment arms. The specific event rates for stroke/systemic embolism, major bleeding, and all-cause mortality for each DOAC are summarized in Table 27.3.

A prespecified subgroup analysis of RE-LY compared 3554 subjects (20% of study cohort) with eCrCl <50 mL/min to those with mild renal dysfunction and normal renal function [34]. In those with eCrCl <50 mL/min, the rate of stroke or systemic embolism was higher compared to patients with eCrCl >50 mL/min; reported as 2.3%/year with dabigatran 110 mg BID, 1.5%/year with dabigatran 150 mg BID, and 2.7%/year with warfarin (Table 27.3). The rate of major bleeding in those with eCrCl <50 mL/min was 5.5%/year, higher compared to patients with normal renal function. Dabigatran 150 mg BID met the superiority endpoint for decreased risk of stroke or systemic embolism (HR 0.56 [95% CI 0.37–0.85]) compared to warfarin in

Table 27.3 Subjects with renal dysfunction in initial randomized controlled trials of direct oral anticoagulants for nonvalvular atrial fibrillation

Trial	RE-LY	ROCKET AF	ARISTOTLE	AVERROES	ENGAGE AF-TIMI 48
Definition of renal dysfunction	eCrCl 30–50 mL/min	eCrCl 30–50 mL/min	eCrCl 25–50 mL/min	eCrCl 25–60 mL/min	eCrCl 30–50 mL/min
n (% of study cohort)	3554 (20%)	2950 (21%)	3017 (15%)	1697 (30%)	4074 (19%)
CHADS2, mean	2.5	3.7	2.6	2.4	NR
Age, mean	75	79	78	75	NR
Study drug	Dabigatran 110 mg bid or 150 mg bid	Rivaroxaban 15 mg daily (reduced dose for renal dysfunction)	Apixaban 5 mg bid (25% received 2.5 mg bid)	Apixaban 5 mg bid (12% received 2.5 mg bid)	Edoxaban 30 mg daily for eCrCl 15–50 mL/min
Control	Warfarin, goal INR 2–3	Warfarin, goal INR 2–3	Warfarin, goal INR 2–3	ASA 81–324 mg daily	Warfarin, goal INR 2–3
Statistical design	Noninferiority	Noninferiority	Noninferiority	Superiority	Noninferiority
Primary outcome: stroke or systemic embolism					
Study drug	110 mg: 2.3%/year 150 mg: 1.5%/year	2.3%/year	2.1%/year	1.8%/year	2.3%/year
Control	2.7%/year	2.8%/year	2.7%/year	5.6%/year (ASA)	2.7%/year
HR (95% CI)	110 mg: 0.85 (0.59–1.24) 150 mg: 0.56 (0.37–0.85)[‡]	0.84 (0.57–1.23)	0.79 (0.55–1.14)	0.57 (0.37–0.87)	0.87 (0.64–1.19)
Safety outcome: major bleeding					
Study drug	110 mg: 5.5%/year 150 mg: 5.5%/year	4.5%/year	3.2%/year	2.5%/year	3.8%/year
Control	5.5%/year	4.7%/year	6.4%/year	2.2%/year (ASA)	5.1%/year
HR (95% CI)	110 mg: 0.99 (0.77–1.28) 150 mg: 1.01 (0.79–1.30)	0.95 (0.72–1.26)	0.50 (0.38–0.66)	1.2 (0.65–2.1)	0.76 (0.58–0.99)
Secondary outcome: all-cause mortality					
Study drug	110 mg: 7.9%/year 150 mg: 6.8%/year	NR	7.1%/year	6.2%/year	NR
Control	6.8%/year	NR	8.3%/year	7.1%/year (ASA)	NR
HR (95% CI)	110 mg: 1.16 (0.93–1.44) 150 mg: 1.00 (0.80–1.25)	NR	0.86 (0.70–1.05)	0.86 (0.61–1.2)	NR

ASA aspirin, *eCrCl* estimated creatinine clearance calculated by Cockcroft–Gault formula in mL/min, *HR* hazard ratio, *NR* not reported, *NS* not statistically significant

[†]*p* value for superiority

[‡]HR for dabigatran 150 mg versus 110 mg 0.66 (95% CI 0.43–1.01)

those with eCrCl <50 mL/min, without an associated increase in the risk of major or life-threatening bleeding. Dabigatran 110 mg BID and warfarin were similarly effective in preventing stroke and systemic embolism across all levels of renal function.

In ROCKET AF, subjects with eCrCl 30–49 mL/min (n = 2950; 21% of study cohort) received a reduced dose of rivaroxaban (15 mg daily) based on pharmacokinetic modeling [35]. Patients with eCrCl 30–49 mL/min had a rate of stroke or systemic embolism of 2.3%/year in those treated with rivaroxaban and 2.8%/year in those treated with warfarin (compared to 1.6 and 2.0%/year, respectively, in those with eCrCl $\geq$50 mL/min). The treatment effect with rivaroxaban was similar for those with and without renal dysfunction. The risk of major bleeding was similar between rivaroxaban and warfarin, although fatal bleeding occurred less frequently with rivaroxaban.

In a prespecified subgroup analysis of ARISTOTLE, 3017 subjects with eCrCl <50 mL/min (15% study cohort) were compared to those with mild renal dysfunction and normal renal function [36]. A reduced dose of apixaban (2.5 mg BID) was used for those with two or more of the following characteristics: age $\geq$80 years, weight $\leq$60 kg, and Cr $\geq$1.5 mg/dL. Of those with eCrCl <50 mL/min, 25% received the reduced dose of apixaban. The rate of stroke or systemic embolism was 2.1%/year with apixaban and 2.7%/year with warfarin (compared to 0.99 and 1.1%/year, respectively, in those with normal renal function) (see Table 27.3). Apixaban and warfarin were similarly efficacious in preventing stroke and systemic embolism, irrespective of the degree of renal dysfunction. Apixaban carried a lower risk of major bleeding compared to warfarin, and this decreased risk of bleeding was statistically significant in those with eCrCl <50 mL/min (HR 0.50, 95% CI 0.38–0.66, $p < 0.005$).

In AVERROES, 1697 subjects with eCrCl <60 mL/min (30% of study cohort) were more likely to receive a decreased dose of apixaban than those with eCrCl >60 mL/min [37]. Apixaban was superior to aspirin for reduction of stroke and systemic embolism in patients with stage 3 CKD (HR 0.32; 95% CI 0.18–0.55; $p < 0.001$). The risk of major bleeding increased with kidney dysfunction in both treatment arms, with no significant interaction between apixaban versus aspirin on major bleeding based on CKD status.

In the ENGAGE AF-TIMI 48 trial, 4074 of those enrolled (19% of study cohort) had eCrCl 30–50 mL/min and received half dose edoxaban (either 15 mg or 30 mg daily) versus warfarin [20]. The edoxaban package insert recommends a reduction in dose to 30 mg once daily in patients with creatinine clearance 15–50 mL/min and reports event rates by renal subgroup (rate of stroke or systemic embolism in those with eCrCl 30–50 mL/min of 2.3 and 2.7%/year for edoxaban and warfarin, respectively [HR 0.87, 95% CI 0.64–1.19] compared to a rate of 1.3%/year with edoxaban and 0.97%/year with warfarin for those with eCrCl 80–95 mL/min) [38]. In patients with eCrCl 30–50 mL/min, the risk of major bleeding was lower with edoxaban compared to warfarin (3.8 vs. 5.1%/year [HR 0.76, 95% CI 0.58–0.99]).

Nielsen et al. performed a systematic review and meta-analysis of DOACs versus warfarin in patients with varying degrees of renal dysfunction (none, mild, or moderate) [39]. They found that the DOACs had similar efficacy and safety compared to warfarin across different strata of renal dysfunction. Indirect comparisons between drugs seemed to favor edoxaban 30 mg daily and apixaban when considering safety pertaining to bleeding risk in those with moderate renal dysfunction (eCrCl 30–49 mL/min). Harel et al. performed a similar comparison of DOACs versus VKAs among patients with CKD (eCrCl 30–50 mL/min) including patients with both AF and venous thromboembolism, prior to the approval of edoxaban [40]. In this analysis, the risk of stroke/systemic thromboembolism as well as the risk of major or clinically relevant nonmajor bleeding was similar between the DOACs and VKAs. Any indirect comparisons of drugs evaluated in different trials is problematic due to differences in inclusion criteria, trial conduction, etc., and while these data may be considered by clinicians, they should not solely guide clinical practice.

Anticoagulation in Stage 4 CKD Patients with AF

No randomized data pertaining to patients with stage 4 CKD and AF exists with warfarin. Patients with eCrCl <30 mL/min were excluded from the RE-LY trial [16], but a decreased dose of dabigatran (75 mg BID) is FDA-approved for those with eCrCl 15–30 mL/min based on a pharmacokinetic modeling [41]. Given the moderate increase in rivaroxaban drug levels with reduced renal function, only a small dose adjustment is recommended for patients with stage 4 CKD [42]. In ROCKET AF, patients with eCrCl <30 mL/min were excluded, but the reduced dose of rivaroxaban (15 mg daily) used for those with eCrCl <50 mL/min is approved for eCrCl as low as 15 mL/min based on pharmacokinetic data [17, 43]. The ARISTOTLE and AVERROES trials excluded patients with a Cr >2.5 mg/dl or eCrCl <25 mL/min [18, 19]. However, apixaban is approved for use in patients with eCrCl <15 mL/min based on pharmacokinetic studies, without any dose adjustment (unless additional criteria for dosage adjustment are met) [44]. Only 25% of apixaban is cleared renally, and there appears to be only a small increase in levels when used in patients with severely reduced renal function. Those with eCrCl <30 mL/min were excluded from the ENGAGE AF-TIMI 48 trial, but a reduced dose of edoxaban 30 mg daily is recommended for those with eCrCl between

15–50 mL/min [20, 38]. This is based on pharmacokinetic modeling that predicted a similar drug exposure for patients with severely reduced renal function who received half the dose of those with normal renal function [45, 46].

Anticoagulation in Stage 5D CKD Patients with AF

Warfarin

There are no randomized trials to provide guidance in the use of warfarin for patients with ESKD and AF; clinicians are relegated to evaluating the strengths and weaknesses of observational data to guide management in this high-risk population. As outlined previously, the risks of stroke and bleeding are both higher, and the use of warfarin in this population is controversial. In a retrospective analysis of a cohort of 1671 incident hemodialysis patients with AF from a large dialysis facility in the US, warfarin use was associated with a significantly higher risk for all-cause stroke (HR 1.93, 95% CI 1.29–2.90) but not all-cause mortality [47]. On further analysis, compared to nonwarfarin users, the AHR for ischemic stroke with warfarin use was 1.81 (95% CI 1.12–2.92) and the AHR for hemorrhagic stroke was 2.22 (95% CI 1.01–4.91). Similarly, in an analysis of the Dialysis Outcomes and Practice Patterns Study (DOPPS), use of warfarin was associated with a significant increase in stroke among patients >75 years of age (HR 2.17, 95% CI 1.04–4.53) and a nonsignificant increase in stroke among patients <75 years of age [6]. In a retrospective analysis of 1626 dialysis patients from Canada with AF, warfarin use was not associated with reduction in risk for stroke (AHR 1.14, 95% CI 0.78–1.67) but was associated with a markedly higher risk for bleeding (AHR 1.44, 95% CI 1.13–1.85) [48]. Finally, in a large cohort of 12,284 hemodialysis patients with incident AF identified from the USRDS between 2007 and 2011, warfarin use associated with a borderline but significant reduction in risk of ischemic stroke (HR 0.68, 95% CI 0.47–0.99) [49]. Thus, the available evidence from observational studies is extremely conflicted, with studies variably demonstrating harm, no benefit, or marginal benefit from the use of warfarin in dialysis patients with AF. Expert recommendations in this matter are also discrepant. The Kidney Disease: Improving Global Outcomes (KDIGO) consensus states that the existing evidence is insufficient for firm recommendations regarding routine anticoagulation for primary prevention of stroke in this group, whereas the societal guidelines recommend that warfarin is reasonable for CKD 5D patients with NVAF and conventional risk factors [50, 51]. Randomized trials are urgently needed to evaluate the risks versus benefits of therapeutic anticoagulation in this high-risk population [52].

DOACs

Patients with ESKD were excluded from all the DOAC trials. Observational trials of DOACs in patients with dialysis have been performed involving small numbers of patients in order to study pharmacokinetics and pharmacodynamics, from which meaningful clinical conclusions cannot be derived. Apixaban is approved by the FDA for use in patients with CKD stage 5D based on the results of pharmacokinetic studies. No dose adjustment for apixaban is recommended for patients on dialysis, unless additional criteria for dosage adjustment are met, as outlined above. Owing to the complexities involved pertaining to ischemic stroke and bleeding rates in dialysis patients, randomized controlled trials are necessary, as outlined previously.

Pragmatic Clinical Considerations for Anticoagulation in CKD Patients

Although warfarin has been in wide use for anticoagulation, there are two specific clinical concerns pertaining to its use that merit mention among patients with CKD. Warfarin use has been associated with the development of accelerated vascular calcification in multiple studies [53], hypothesized due to inhibition of the vitamin K-dependent matrix Gla protein. Among patients with ESKD who have evidence for secondary hyperparathyroidism, accelerated vascular calcification can be particularly problematic. The other entity is warfarin-related nephropathy, which is most notable among CKD patients and associated with worsening renal function and higher risk of mortality [54]. Several putative mechanisms are proposed including glomerular hemorrhage and oxidative stress. In a post hoc analysis of the RE-LY trial, temporal reduction in eGFR was shown among all three arms receiving oral anticoagulation but was greatest with warfarin versus dabigatran, raising concern about the potential for warfarin-related nephropathy [55]. The clinical significance of these findings will hopefully become evident in longer term follow-up among patients receiving DOACs. For further reading on anticoagulation-related nephropathy (ARN), the reader is referred to Chap. 28 of this textbook.

It is clear that patients receiving DOACs need significant dose adjustments in the context of fluctuating renal function, with attendant risk of significant bleeding complications. It deserves emphasis that in the pivotal randomized controlled trials comparing DOACs to warfarin, cut-offs based on eCrCl (Cockcroft–Gault equation) were utilized to define inclusion and exclusion criteria. Thus, FDA labels for these agents are also based on eCrCl values. However, estimated glomerular filtration rate (eGFR), calculated using the Modification of Diet in Renal Disease (MDRD) equation or the Chronic Kidney Disease Epidemiology Collaboration

(CKD-EPI) equations, is generally used routinely by most clinicians. A recent study emphasizes the significant discordance in DOAC doses based on the different equations used for estimating GFR, particularly among elderly patients with impaired renal function [56]. The discordance in doses was higher for dabigatran and rivaroxaban (13–30%) and lowest for apixaban (<5%).

It also deserves mention that about 6% of hemodialysis patients were initiated on either dabigatran or rivaroxaban in the US according to a study from a large dialysis population published in 2015 [57]. The use of these agents occurred despite their use being contraindicated due to lack of inclusion of hemodialysis patients in the RCTs. Importantly, use of dabigatran or rivaroxaban among dialysis patients in this study was associated with a significantly higher risk of death from bleeding or hospitalization relative to warfarin. This fact illustrates concerns pertaining to the dissemination of DOACs in the clinical realm and association of adverse events related to renal clearance. Clinicians need to note that it is recommended that the development of acute kidney injury among patients on direct oral anticoagulants is an indication for (temporary) discontinuation of these agents. The rapid onset and offset of action of these agents requires very close considerations pertaining to monitoring of therapeutic effects and corresponding decisions about whether bridging with parenteral agents is necessary.

The authors believe that the already established paradigm of anticoagulation clinics for warfarin may be considered to follow patients receiving DOACs with any underlying degree of renal impairment [58]. Particularly among patients with CKD, the regular monitoring of eCrCl would be highly recommended because of direct implications pertaining to dose adjustment and bleeding complications; the frequency of monitoring should be contingent upon the baseline level of renal insufficiency.

Acknowledgments The authors would like to acknowledge and greatly appreciate the editorial assistance provided by Michelle Flemming.

References

1. Shroff GR, Solid CA, Herzog CA. Atrial fibrillation, stroke, and anticoagulation in medicare beneficiaries: trends by age, sex, and race, 1992–2010. J Am Heart Assoc. 2014;3(3):e000756.
2. Baber U, Howard VJ, Halperin JL, Soliman EZ, Zhang X, McClellan W, et al. Association of chronic kidney disease with atrial fibrillation among adults in the United States: REasons for Geographic and Racial Differences in Stroke (REGARDS) Study. Circ Arrhythm Electrophysiol. 2011;4(1):26–32.
3. Nelson SE, Shroff GR, Li S, Herzog CA. Impact of chronic kidney disease on risk of incident atrial fibrillation and subsequent survival in medicare patients. J Am Heart Assoc. 2012;1(4): e002097.
4. Winkelmayer WC, Patrick AR, Liu J, Brookhart MA, Setoguchi S. The increasing prevalence of atrial fibrillation among hemodialysis patients. J Am Soc Nephrol. 2011;22(2):349–57.
5. Zimmerman D, Sood MM, Rigatto C, Holden RM, Hiremath S, Clase CM. Systematic review and meta-analysis of incidence, prevalence and outcomes of atrial fibrillation in patients on dialysis. Nephrol Dial Transplant. 2012;27(10):3816–22.
6. Wizemann V, Tong L, Satayathum S, Disney A, Akiba T, Fissell RB, et al. Atrial fibrillation in hemodialysis patients: clinical features and associations with anticoagulant therapy. Kidney Int. 2010;77(12):1098–106.
7. Piccini JP, Stevens SR, Chang Y, Singer DE, Lokhnygina Y, Go AS, et al. Renal dysfunction as a predictor of stroke and systemic embolism in patients with nonvalvular atrial fibrillation: validation of the R(2)CHADS(2) index in the ROCKET AF (Rivaroxaban Once-daily, oral, direct factor Xa inhibition Compared with vitamin K antagonism for prevention of stroke and Embolism Trial in Atrial Fibrillation) and ATRIA (AnTicoagulation and Risk factors In Atrial fibrillation) study cohorts. Circulation. 2013;127(2):224–32.
8. Olesen JB, Lip GY, Kamper AL, Hommel K, Kober L, Lane DA, et al. Stroke and bleeding in atrial fibrillation with chronic kidney disease. N Engl J Med. 2012;367(7):625–35.
9. Shih CJ, Ou SM, Chao PW, Kuo SC, Lee YJ, Yang CY, et al. Risks of death and stroke in patients undergoing hemodialysis with new-onset atrial fibrillation: a competing-risk analysis of a nationwide cohort. Circulation. 2016;133(3):265–72.
10. Lip GY, Frison L, Halperin JL, Lane DA. Comparative validation of a novel risk score for predicting bleeding risk in anticoagulated patients with atrial fibrillation: the HAS-BLED (Hypertension, Abnormal Renal/Liver Function, Stroke, Bleeding History or Predisposition, Labile INR, Elderly, Drugs/Alcohol Concomitantly) score. J Am Coll Cardiol. 2011;57(2):173–80.
11. Elliott MJ, Zimmerman D, Holden RM. Warfarin anticoagulation in hemodialysis patients: a systematic review of bleeding rates. Am J Kidney Dis. 2007;50(3):433–40.
12. Bansal N, Fan D, Hsu CY, Ordonez JD, Go AS. Incident atrial fibrillation and risk of death in adults with chronic kidney disease. J Am Heart Assoc. 2014;3(5):e001303.
13. Krüger T, Brandenburg V, Schlieper G, Marx N, Floege J. Sailing between Scylla and Charybdis: oral long-term anticoagulation in dialysis patients. Nephrol Dial Transplant. 2013;28(3):534–41.
14. Hart RG, Pearce LA, Aguilar MI. Meta-analysis: antithrombotic therapy to prevent stroke in patients who have nonvalvular atrial fibrillation. Ann Intern Med. 2007;146(12):857–67.
15. Hart RG, Eikelboom JW, Ingram AJ, Herzog CA. Anticoagulants in atrial fibrillation patients with chronic kidney disease. Nat Rev Nephrol. 2012;8(10):569–78.
16. Connolly SJ, Ezekowitz MD, Yusuf S, Eikelboom J, Oldgren J, Parekh A, et al. Dabigatran versus warfarin in patients with atrial fibrillation. N Engl J Med. 2009;361(12):1139–51.
17. Patel MR, Mahaffey KW, Garg J, Pan G, Singer DE, Hacke W, et al. Rivaroxaban versus warfarin in nonvalvular atrial fibrillation. N Engl J Med. 2011;365(10):883–91.
18. Granger CB, Alexander JH, McMurray JJ, Lopes RD, Hylek EM, Hanna M, et al. Apixaban versus warfarin in patients with atrial fibrillation. N Engl J Med. 2011;365(11):981–92.
19. Connolly SJ, Eikelboom J, Joyner C, Diener HC, Hart R, Golitsyn S, et al. Apixaban in patients with atrial fibrillation. N Engl J Med. 2011;364(9):806–17.
20. Giugliano RP, Ruff CT, Braunwald E, Murphy SA, Wiviott SD, Halperin JL, et al. Edoxaban versus warfarin in patients with atrial fibrillation. N Engl J Med. 2013;369(22):2093–104.
21. Eikelboom JW, Weitz JI. New anticoagulants. Circulation. 2010;121(13):1523–32.

22. Cuker A, Siegal DM, Crowther MA, Garcia DA. Laboratory measurement of the anticoagulant activity of the non-vitamin K oral anticoagulants. J Am Coll Cardiol. 2014;64(11):1128–39.
23. Cuker A. Laboratory measurement of the non-vitamin K antagonist oral anticoagulants: selecting the optimal assay based on drug, assay availability, and clinical indication. J Thromb Thrombolysis. 2016;41(2):241–7.
24. Kcentra® Prescribing Information [package insert]. Kankakee, IL; CSL Behring LLC.; 2014.
25. Holbrook A, Schulman S, Witt DM, Vandvik PO, Fish J, Kovacs MJ, et al. Evidence-based management of anticoagulant therapy: Antithrombotic Therapy and Prevention of Thrombosis, 9th ed: American College of Chest Physicians Evidence-Based Clinical Practice Guidelines. Chest. 2012;141(2 Suppl): e152S–84S.
26. Khadzhynov D, Wagner F, Formella S, Wiegert E, Moschetti V, Slowinski T, et al. Effective elimination of dabigatran by haemodialysis. A phase I single-centre study in patients with end-stage renal disease. Thromb Haemost. 2013;109(4):596–605.
27. Pollack CV, Reilly PA, Eikelboom J, Glund S, Verhamme P, Bernstein RA, et al. Idarucizumab for dabigatran reversal. N Engl J Med. 2015;373(6):511–20.
28. FDA approves Praxbind, the first reversal agent for the anticoagulant Pradaxa. FDA News Release. 2015 Oct 19; cited 2016 Jan 28. Silver Spring (MD), U.S.Food and Drug Administration. http://www.fda.gov/newsevents/newsroom/pressannouncements/ucm467300.htm.
29. Praxbind® (idarucizumab) Prescribing Information [package insert]. Ridgefield, CT; Boehringer Ingelheim Pharmaceuticals, Inc.; 2015.
30. Siegal DM, Curnutte JT, Connolly SJ, Lu G, Conley PB, Wiens BL, et al. Andexanet alfa for the reversal of factor Xa inhibitor activity. N Engl J Med. 2015;373(25):2413–24.
31. A Study in Patients With Acute Major Bleeding to Evaluate the Ability of Andexanet Alfa to Reverse the Anticoagulation Effect of Direct and Indirect Oral Anticoagulants. 2016; cited 2016 Jan 28. Portola Pharmaceuticals, editor. https://clinicaltrials.gov/ct2/show/NCT02329327?term=NCT02329327&rank=1.
32. Ansell JE, Bakhru SH, Laulicht BE, Steiner SS, Grosso M, Brown K, et al. Use of PER977 to reverse the anticoagulant effect of edoxaban. N Engl J Med. 2014;371(22):2141–2.
33. Hart RG, Pearce LA, Asinger RW, Herzog CA. Warfarin in atrial fibrillation patients with moderate chronic kidney disease. Clin J Am Soc Nephrol. 2011;6(11):2599–604.
34. Hijazi Z, Hohnloser SH, Oldgren J, Andersson U, Connolly SJ, Eikelboom JW, et al. Efficacy and safety of dabigatran compared with warfarin in relation to baseline renal function in patients with atrial fibrillation: a RE-LY (Randomized Evaluation of Long-term Anticoagulation Therapy) trial analysis. Circulation. 2014;129 (9):961–70.
35. Fox KA, Piccini JP, Wojdyla D, Becker RC, Halperin JL, Nessel CC, et al. Prevention of stroke and systemic embolism with rivaroxaban compared with warfarin in patients with non-valvular atrial fibrillation and moderate renal impairment. Eur Heart J. 2011;32(19):2387–94.
36. Hohnloser SH, Hijazi Z, Thomas L, Alexander JH, Amerena J, Hanna M, et al. Efficacy of apixaban when compared with warfarin in relation to renal function in patients with atrial fibrillation: insights from the ARISTOTLE trial. Eur Heart J. 2012;33 (22):2821–30.
37. Eikelboom JW, Connolly SJ, Gao P, Paolasso E, De CR, Husted S, et al. Stroke risk and efficacy of apixaban in atrial fibrillation patients with moderate chronic kidney disease. J Stroke Cerebrovasc Dis. 2012;21(6):429–35.
38. SAVAYSA (edoxaban) Prescribing Information [package insert]. Parsippany, NJ; Daiichi Sankyo, Inc.; 2015.
39. Nielsen PB, Lane DA, Rasmussen LH, Lip GY, Larsen TB. Renal function and non-vitamin K oral anticoagulants in comparison with warfarin on safety and efficacy outcomes in atrial fibrillation patients: a systemic review and meta-regression analysis. Clin Res Cardiol. 2015;104(5):418–29.
40. Harel Z, Sholzberg M, Shah PS, Pavenski K, Harel S, Wald R, et al. Comparisons between novel oral anticoagulants and vitamin K antagonists in patients with CKD. J Am Soc Nephrol. 2014;25 (3):431–42.
41. Hariharan S, Madabushi R. Clinical pharmacology basis of deriving dosing recommendations for dabigatran in patients with severe renal impairment. J Clin Pharmacol. 2012;52(1 Suppl):119S–25S.
42. Girgis IG, Patel MR, Peters GR, Moore KT, Mahaffey KW, Nessel CC, et al. Population pharmacokinetics and pharmacodynamics of rivaroxaban in patients with non-valvular atrial fibrillation: results from ROCKET AF. J Clin Pharmacol. 2014;54 (8):917–27.
43. Xarelto® (rivaroxaban) Prescribing Information [package insert]. Titusville, NJ; Janssen Pharmaceuticals, Inc.; 2015.
44. Eliquis® (apixaban) Prescribing Information [package insert]. Princeton, NJ; Bristol-Myers Squibb Company; 2015.
45. Yin OQ, Tetsuya K, Miller R. Edoxaban population pharmacokinetics and exposure-response analysis in patients with non-valvular atrial fibrillation. Eur J Clin Pharmacol. 2014;70 (11):1339–51.
46. Jonsson S, Simonsson US, Miller R, Karlsson MO. Population pharmacokinetics of edoxaban and its main metabolite in a dedicated renal impairment study. J Clin Pharmacol. 2015;55 (11):1268–79.
47. Chan KE, Lazarus JM, Thadhani R, Hakim RM. Anticoagulant and antiplatelet usage associates with mortality among hemodialysis patients. J Am Soc Nephrol. 2009;20(4):872–81.
48. Shah M, Avgil TM, Jackevicius CA, Essebag V, Eisenberg MJ, Rahme E, et al. Warfarin use and the risk for stroke and bleeding in patients with atrial fibrillation undergoing dialysis. Circulation. 2014;129(11):1196–203.
49. Shen JI, Montez-Rath ME, Lenihan CR, Turakhia MP, Chang TI, Winkelmayer WC. Outcomes after warfarin initiation in a cohort of hemodialysis patients with newly diagnosed atrial fibrillation. Am J Kidney Dis. 2015;66(4):677–88.
50. Herzog CA, Asinger RW, Berger AK, Charytan DM, Diez J, Hart RG, et al. Cardiovascular disease in chronic kidney disease. A clinical update from Kidney Disease: Improving Global Outcomes (KDIGO). Kidney Int. 2011;80(6):572–86.
51. January CT, Wann LS, Alpert JS, Calkins H, Cigarroa JE, Cleveland JC Jr, et al. 2014 AHA/ACC/HRS guideline for the management of patients with atrial fibrillation: executive summary: a report of the American College of Cardiology/American Heart Association Task Force on practice guidelines and the Heart Rhythm Society. Circulation. 2014;130 (23):2071–104.
52. Granger CB, Chertow GM. A pint of sweat will save a gallon of blood: a call for randomized trials of anticoagulation in end-stage renal disease. Circulation. 2014;129(11):1190–2.
53. Brimble KS, Ingram AJ, Eikelboom JW, Hart RG. Anticoagulants in patients with atrial fibrillation and end-stage renal disease. Postgrad Med. 2012;124(6):17–25.

54. Yang Y, Liu T, Zhao J, Li G. Warfarin-related nephropathy: prevalence, risk factors and prognosis. Int J Cardiol. 2014; 176(3):1297–8.
55. Bohm M, Ezekowitz MD, Connolly SJ, Eikelboom JW, Hohnloser SH, Reilly PA, et al. changes in renal function in patients with atrial fibrillation: an analysis from the RE-LY trial. J Am Coll Cardiol. 2015;65(23):2481–93.
56. Manzano-Fernandez S, Andreu-Cayuelas JM, Marin F, Orenes-Pinero E, Gallego P, Valdes M, et al. Comparison of estimated glomerular filtration rate equations for dosing new oral anticoagulants in patients with atrial fibrillation. Revista Espanola de Cardiologia (English Version). 2015;68(06):497–504.
57. Chan KE, Edelman ER, Wenger JB, Thadhani RI, Maddux FW. Dabigatran and rivaroxaban use in atrial fibrillation patients on hemodialysis. Circulation. 2015;131(11):972–9.
58. Barnes GD, Nallamothu BK, Sales AE, Froehlich JB. Reimagining anticoagulation clinics in the era of direct oral anticoagulants. Circ Cardiovasc Qual Outcomes. 2016;9(2):182–5.

28 Anticoagulation-Related Nephropathy: Tip of the Iceberg

David S. Wheeler

Introduction and Importance

Anticoagulation-related nephropathy (ARN) is an under-recognized complication of anticoagulation that is associated with both irreversible kidney injury and increased mortality [1, 2]. The simplicity of ARN's diagnostic criteria—acute kidney injury (AKI) in the setting of over anticoagulation without other identifiable etiology—camouflages a complex disease state with an unclear molecular mechanism, nuanced epidemiologic profile and multiple clinical manifestations. The only aspect of ARN that is clear is that as the total number of patients started on anticoagulation, both warfarin and direct oral anticoagulants (DOACs) continues to increase, the healthcare burden and costs associated with ARN will rise as well. In this chapter, we seek to review the epidemiology, pathogenesis, clinical feature, treatment and prevention of ARN.

Historical Perspective

While warfarin has been in use since 1954, its harmful effects on the kidneys have only recently been fully recognized [3, 4]. In the 1960s, Reilly and colleagues reported unexplained hematuria in 35 out of 200 patients on warfarin, however no association between hematuria, prothrombin time, and kidney function was observed [5]. Over the next 50 years, isolated case studies of patients with unexplained AKI associated with hematuria, usually in the presence of a supratherapeutic international normalized ratio (INR) were reported. However, the cases were attributed to underlying kidney disease (i.e., IgA nephropathy, lupus nephritis, etc.) and the role of anticoagulation was unknown [6–9]. In 2009, Brodsky and colleagues described nine patients without underlying kidney disease who developed unexplained AKI associated with elevated INRs [3]. Kidney biopsies from those nine patients showed glomerular hemorrhage and tubular injury associated with obstructive red blood cell casts. This clinic-pathologic constellation of AKI sans alternate etiology with these biopsy findings was termed "warfarin-related nephropathy" (WRN). This disease was thought to be exclusive to warfarin until 2013 when it was shown to occur in both rats and humans taking dabigatran [10, 11]. It has subsequently been renamed anticoagulant-related nephropathy (ARN) to reflect its wider association.

Epidemiology

The incidence of ARN is difficult to determine due to its changing definition and diagnostic criteria. Originally, ARN was a pathologic diagnosis defined by (a) dysmorphic red blood cells (RBCs) implying injury to the glomerular filtration barrier, (b) uniform hemorrhage through all fields as to exclude biopsy artefact, (c) the presence of obstructive tubular RBC casts, and (d) absence of glomerulonephritis or other inflammatory changes that could account for glomerular hemorrhage (Fig. 28.1) [3]. However, given the risk of renal biopsies in the setting of anticoagulation, most cases of ARN are not biopsy-proven but presumptively diagnosed in patients who develop an unexplained AKI (increase in serum creatinine of more than 0.3 mg/dl or 1.5-fold greater than baseline) in the setting of warfarin use with an INR greater than 3.0, or use of a direct oral anticoagulant (DOAC) [2]. It is important to note that while the

D.S. Wheeler (✉)
Department of Internal Medicine, Einstein Medical Center Philadelphia, 5001 Old York Rd, Philadelphia, PA 19141, USA
e-mail: wheelerd@einstein.edu

J. Rangaswami et al. (eds.), *Cardio-Nephrology*,
DOI 10.1007/978-3-319-56042-7_28

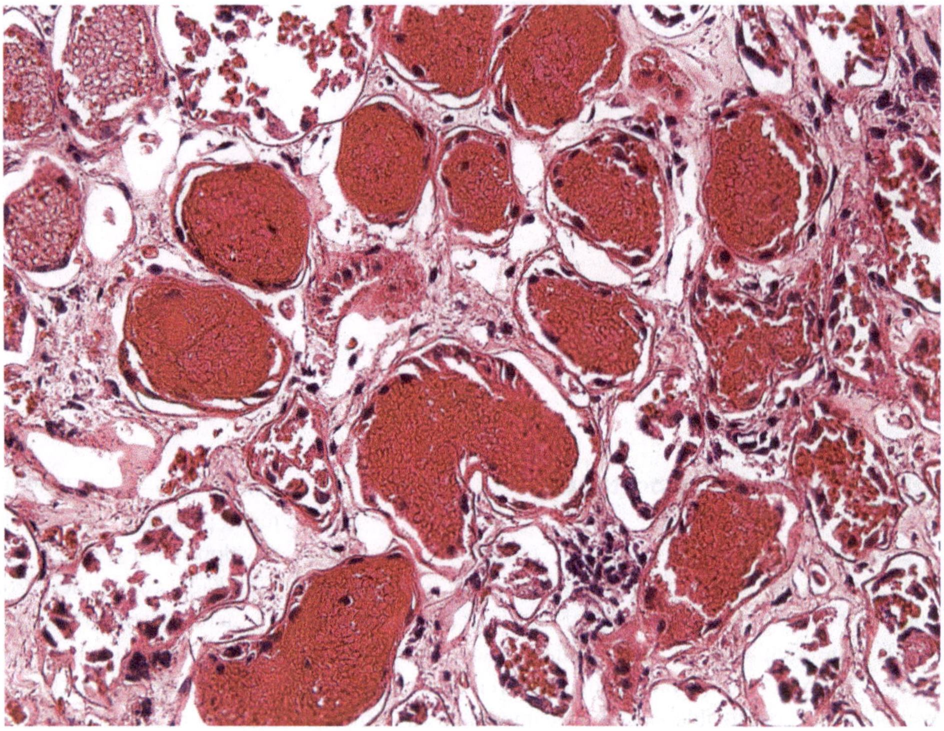

Fig. 28.1 Microscopy pathology associated with ARN. RBCs and RBC occlusive casts in a patient with anticoagulation-related nephropathy. Image provided by Surya Seshan, Chief of the Division of Renal Pathology, Weill Cornell Medical Center, NY

majority of the seminal work in ARN identified patients based on hematuria, the current definition does not require patients to have hematuria to be classified as ARN.

Using this definition, between 17 and 20.5% of all patients on warfarin develop at least one episode of ARN during treatment [1, 12]. This incidence rate should be interpreted with caution for several reasons. First, ARN may be incorrectly diagnosed if the true underlying cause of the AKI is not identified (such as concomitant chronic kidney disease, heart disease, medications, etc.). Furthermore, the reported incidence is likely affected by sampling bias since the detection of AKI is dependent on measuring serum creatinine which is much more likely to occur in more ill patients who are at higher risk to develop ARN. Finally, since ARN can spontaneously resolve the incidence is likely much higher than the prevalence.

To date, only two cases of ARN have been reported in a patient using DOACs. In both cases, patients on dabigatran developed an unexplained AKI and were found to have diffuse interstitial hemorrhage and obstructing intratubular RBC casts consistent with ARN [13, 14]. While there are currently no epidemiologic studies investigating the rate of ARN in patients on DOACs, most studies record and publish rates of acute kidney injury, a prerequisite for ARN. A formal post hoc analysis of the RE-LY trial comparing two therapeutic doses of dabigatran (110 and 150 mg) and warfarin found that both doses of dabigatran were associated with smaller estimated glomerular filtration rate (eGFR) reductions at 12 and 24 months when compared with warfarin [15]. A recent meta-analysis of RE-LY (dabigatran vs. warfarin), ROCKET (rivaroxaban vs. warfarin) and ENGAGE AF (edoxaban vs. warfarin) trials and supplementary FDA data showed no significant difference in the rates of acute renal failure between the DOAC and warfarin arms [2]. Taken together this evidence suggest that the incidence of ARN associated with DOACs less than or equal to that of warfarin but further studies are needed to measure the true incidence.

The main risk factor for ARN associated with either warfarin or DOACs appears to be chronic kidney disease (CKD). Patients with documented CKD had twice the incidence of ARN compared to normal controls [1]. 5/6-nephrectomized rats, a well-established model for chronic kidney disease, treated with either warfarin or dabigatran, developed ARN like pathology at much greater frequency than control animals [10, 16]. Limited clinical evidence suggests that age, diabetes mellitus, and hypertension are also independent predictors of increased ARN risk [1, 17].

Pathophysiology and Mechanism

Based upon histologic analysis of kidney tissue obtained from patients and experimental animal models, the macroscopic pathophysiology of ARN is well understood. Disruption of the glomerular filtration barrier leads to hemorrhage into Bowman's space and renal tubules.

Underlying structural abnormalities in the glomerular basement membrane likely predispose kidneys to this anticoagulation-mediated hemorrhage consistent with the observation that patients with underlying chronic kidney disease are more likely to develop ARN [8, 9, 13]. As red blood cells from the glomerular hemorrhage reach the tubules, they coalesce into RBC casts, the hallmark feature of ARN [3] (Fig. 28.1). These RBC casts induce tubular injury and obliteration through multiple mechanisms including ischemia and oxidative stress due to free hemoglobin [18, 19].

In contrast, the molecular mechanism of ARN is very poorly understood. Thrombin, the only vitamin K-dependent coagulation factor known to stimulate signaling cascades, binds and activates a family of proteinase-activated receptors (PARs) expressed on all endothelial cells including those within the glomeruli of the kidney [20]. It is hypothesized that reduction in thrombin levels by anticoagulation decreases PAR signaling which triggers the breakdown of endothelial cell-cell adhesions thus allowing glomerular hemorrhage. This hypothesis is supported by the observation that glomerular hemorrhage can be triggered in animal models of CKD by administration of PAR antagonists [10]. While appealing, this hypothesis fails to explain why in most epithelial model systems activation, not inhibition, of PAR results in endothelium retractions and increased paracellular flow [21, 22]. Furthermore, PAR knock-out mice do not have glomerular hemorrhage or other obvious renal phenotype [23]. Finally, the use of PAR antagonist voraxapar is not associated with higher rates of AKI or other renal effects when compared to placebo in initial clinical trials [24]. Taken together this data strongly suggest that anticoagulants are functioning through a non-PAR related mechanism. One potential mechanism could be the depletion of activated protein C, a potent but often less considered target of warfarin therapy, which is known to have trophic and anti-apoptotic effects in cultured podocytes [25, 26].

Diagnosis and Work-Up

ARN should be considered in the differential diagnosis of any patient on anticoagulation presenting with AKI especially in the setting of excessive anticoagulation (i.e., supratherapeutic INR or excessive DOAC dose). The initial work-up should consist of a clinical exam, careful medication history and urinalysis to assess for hematuria (Fig. 28.2). Subsequent diagnostic tests such as urine electrolytes, kidney ultrasound and renal biopsy may be need to exclude other causes of AKI or confirm the diagnosis in high risk individuals.

The presence of hematuria (gross or microscopic), dysmorphic RBC cells or RBC casts in the urinalysis support a diagnosis of ARN but are not definitive. Glomerulonephritides, vacuities, urinary tract infections, and nephrolithiasis can all manifest with hematuria and must be excluded prior to the diagnosis of ARN being made. Since a sizable percentage of patients with ARN do not develop hematuria patients with an inactive urine sediment should still undergo further work-up to exclude ARN. Volume depletion or treatment with medications (e.g., angiotensin-converting enzyme/angiotensinogen receptor blocker) are often

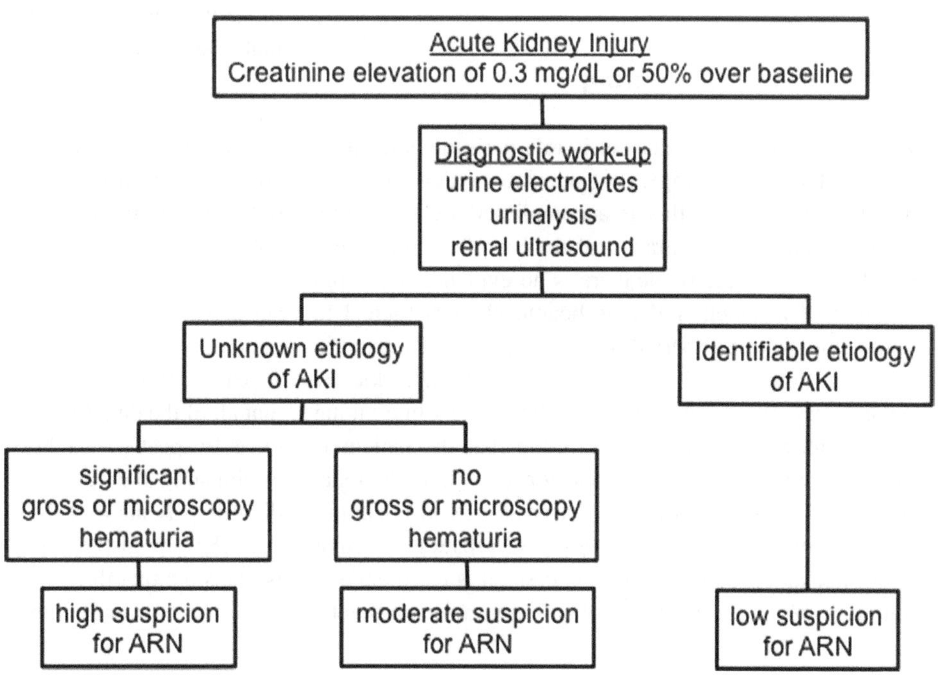

Fig. 28.2 Clinical diagnostic algorithm for suspected ARN

Table 28.1 Recommended frequency of renal monitoring for patients on anticoagulation

	Initiation	Maintenance		
	(3 months)	eGFR > 60	eGFR 30–60	eGFR < 30
Warfarin	3–4 weeks	6 months	2–3 months	2–3 months
DOAC	3–4 weeks	12 months	6 months	3 months

identified by a through clinical history, corroborated by pre-renal azotemia on urine electrolytes and proven to be the cause with a trial of volume repletion or medication abstinence. Urinary tract obstruction can be excluded via renal ultrasound. Other causes of AKI such as acute phosphate nephropathy, high-dose nonsteroidal anti-inflammatory drug (NSAID) use, crystal-induced nephropathy, myeloma cast nephropathy, acute tubular necrosis, and acute interstitial nephritis also should be considered and evaluated.

After excluding all other potential causes of renal dysfunction, a presumptive diagnosis of ARN can be made. A definitive diagnosis could be made using a renal biopsy, however this is often not performed due to the high risk of bleeding associated with renal biopsy in a patient on anticoagulation. However, there are two clinical scenarios where a biopsy would be indicated. First, if the patient's creatinine remained elevated or continued to increase despite appropriate treatment a biopsy is indicated. The serum creatinine in patients with ARN improves within the first 1–2 weeks of reversing the coagulopathy, and persistent elevated or continually rising creatinine is highly suspicious for an alternative cause of kidney injury, which likely requires a biopsy for diagnosis. Second, persistent hematuria is uncommon in ARN and therefore patients with persistent hematuria after correction of their coagulopathy should undergo renal biopsy, after urologic causes have been excluded.

Treatment and Monitoring

The mainstay of ARN treatment is returning the anticoagulation to a therapeutic range. For patients who develop ARN while taking warfarin, this is accomplished by frequently monitoring and careful titration of their warfarin dose until the INR is below 3.0. While there is no evidence that rapid correction of a patient's INR is beneficial, it is logical to assume that prolonged periods of elevated INR will result in continued glomerular hemorrhage and additional kidney tubular injury. For patients who develop ARN while taking DOACs, treatment involves confirming that the patient is taking the correct dose, adjusted for the patient's renal function. Given that elevated blood pressure and concomitant antiplatelet use are both likely to exacerbate glomerular hemorrhage and production of RBC casts, it is reasonable to obtain tight blood pressure control and minimize antiplatelet therapy when feasible. Finally, anticoagulation levels and renal function should be closely monitored for the duration of the patient's treatment.

Early detection and prompt treatment are critical to minimize kidney damage. For patients on both warfarin and DOACs, kidney function should be monitored regularly throughout treatment and with increased frequency during the first 3 months when patients are at the highest risk (Table 28.1). Any patient with a supratheurapeutic INR should have their renal function assessed as soon as possible and renal function should be closely monitored until the INR returns to the therapeutic range. There is some evidence that having an episode of ARN increases the likelihood of subsequent episodes of ARN so more frequent kidney function monitoring (i.e., every 2–3 months) after an initial episode of ARN is prudent.

Clinical Consequences

ARN is independently associated with renal morbidity and overall mortality [1]. Even if the renal function returns to baseline following the ARN episode, some of the renal tubules will have been destroyed by the obstructive RBC casts thus permanently decreasing the nephron mass of the kidney. The tubules that do survive the ischemic and oxidative insult will likely manifest hyperfiltration injury that leads to accelerated CKD progression [27]. Brodsky and colleagues clearly demonstrated that patients who developed ARN had a serum creatinine level approximately 30% greater than matched patient 1 year following the ARN episode [17]. In the same study, 1-year mortality rates were 65% greater in patients with ARN compared to a match cohort (31.1% vs. 18.9% respectively). This association between increased mortality and ARN was confirmed in a subsequent study in Korean patients, which found that patients who developed ARN were at a twofold increased 1-year mortality (32.4% vs. 15.9%) [12]. It must be noted that all of the data linking ARN and mortality has been based on retrospective studies and there is currently no data establishing the causality. In fact, clinical factors that predispose patients to ARN such as age, diabetes, heart failure, and CKD are also associated with increased mortality, and it is plausible that the impact of ARN on all-cause mortality is reflective of a more chronically ill patient population.

Prevention

Despite the importance of prevention of ARN, there is currently no evidence to guide our interventions. Likely the most important measure to prevent ARN is correct dosing and titration of anticoagulants. Warfarin doses should be titrated judiciously to avoid rapid increases in INR and the dose of each DOACs should adjusted for renal function. Furthermore, it is logical to assume that optimization of a patient's kidney function and co-morbid conditions, such as diabetes mellitus and hypertension, would decrease the risk of ARN.

Conclusions and Recommendations

The use of anticoagulation with warfarin and the new DOAC agents is increasing exponentially and thus the incidence and morbidity of ARN is only going to increase in the coming years. Given the significant impact of even a subtle decline in GFR on overall mortality, cardiovascular events and quality of life, it is imperative that all clinicians prescribing anticoagulants rigorously monitor and aggressively treat ARN to preserve kidney function. Joint collaborative efforts between cardiologists, nephrologists and hematologists will help elucidate the clinical and pathophysiological aspects of anticoagulation related nephropathy and help personalize anticoagulation to the individual patient for the future.

References

1. Brodsky SV, Nadasdy T, Rovin BH, Satoskar AA, Nadasdy GM, Wu HM, et al. Warfarin-related nephropathy occurs in patients with and without chronic kidney disease and is associated with an increased mortality rate. Kidney Int. 2011;80(2):181–9.
2. Wheeler DS, Giugliano RP, Rangaswami J. Anticoagulation-related nephropathy. J Thromb Haemost. 2016;14(3):461–7.
3. Brodsky SV, Satoskar A, Chen J, Nadasdy G, Eagen JW, Hamirani M, et al. Acute kidney injury during warfarin therapy associated with obstructive tubular red blood cell casts: a report of 9 cases. Am J Kidney Dis. 2009;54(6):1121–6.
4. Holbrook AM, Pereira JA, Labiris R, McDonald H, Douketis JD, Crowther M, et al. Systematic overview of warfarin and its drug and food interactions. Arch Intern Med. 2005;165(10):1095–106.
5. Reilly EB, Perry A, Fujita K, Nakamura RM. Haematuria and anticoagulants. Lancet. 1964;1(7332):554.
6. Praga M, Gutierrez-Millet V, Navas JJ, Ruilope LM, Morales JM, Alcazar JM, et al. Acute worsening of renal function during episodes of macroscopic hematuria in IgA nephropathy. Kidney Int. 1985;28(1):69–74.
7. Kincaid-Smith P, Bennett WM, Dowling JP, Ryan GB. Acute renal failure and tubular necrosis associated with hematuria due to glomerulonephritis. Clin Nephrol. 1983;19(4):206–10.
8. Kabir A, Nadasdy T, Nadasdy G, Hebert LA. An unusual cause of gross hematuria and transient ARF in an SLE patient with warfarin coagulopathy. Am J Kidney Dis. 2004;43(4):757–60.
9. Abt AB, Carroll LE, Mohler JH. Thin basement membrane disease and acute renal failure secondary to gross hematuria and tubular necrosis. Am J Kidney Dis. 2000;35(3):533–6.
10. Ryan M, Ware K, Qamri Z, Satoskar A, Wu H, Nadasdy G, et al. Warfarin-related nephropathy is the tip of the iceberg: direct thrombin inhibitor dabigatran induces glomerular hemorrhage with acute kidney injury in rats. Nephrol Dial Transplant. 2014 Dec;29 (12):2228–34.
11. Moeckel GW, Luciano RL, Brewster UC. Warfarin-related nephropathy in a patient with mild IgA nephropathy on dabigatran and aspirin. Clin Kidney J. 2013;6(5):507–9.
12. An JN, Ahn SY, Yoon CH, Youn TJ, Han MK, Kim S, et al. The occurrence of warfarin-related nephropathy and effects on renal and patient outcomes in korean patients. PLoS ONE. 2013;8(4):e57661.
13. Moeckel GW, Luciano RL, Brewster UC. Warfarin-related nephropathy in a patient with mild IgA nephropathy on dabigatran and aspirin. Clin Kidney J. 2013 Oct;6(5):507–9.
14. Escoli R, Santos P, Andrade S, Carvalho F. Dabigatran-related nephropathy in a patient with undiagnosed IgA nephropathy. Case Rep Nephrol. 2015;2015:298261.
15. Bohm M, Ezekowitz MD, Connolly SJ, Eikelboom JW, Hohnloser SH, Reilly PA, et al. Changes in renal function in patients with atrial fibrillation: an analysis from the RE-LY trial. J Am Coll Cardiol. 2015;65(23):2481–93.
16. Ware KM, Vance JC, Muni N, Hebert LA, Satoskar AA, Nadasdy G, et al. Oral warfarin and the thrombin inhibitor dabigatran increase blood pressure in rats: hidden danger of anticoagulants? Am J Hypertens. 2015 Feb;28(2):182–9.
17. Brodsky SV, Collins M, Park E, Rovin BH, Satoskar AA, Nadasdy G, et al. Warfarin therapy that results in an International Normalization Ratio above the therapeutic range is associated with accelerated progression of chronic kidney disease. Nephron Clin Pract. 2010;115(2):c142–6.
18. Tracz MJ, Alam J, Nath KA. Physiology and pathophysiology of heme: implications for kidney disease. J Am Soc Nephrol. 2007;18 (2):414–20.
19. Ware K, Qamri Z, Ozcan A, Satoskar AA, Nadasdy G, Rovin BH, et al. N-acetylcysteine ameliorates acute kidney injury but not glomerular hemorrhage in an animal model of warfarin-related nephropathy. Am J Physiol Renal Physiol. 2013;304(12):F1421–7.
20. Coughlin SR. Thrombin signalling and protease-activated receptors. Nature. 2000;407(6801):258–64.
21. Malik AB, Fenton JW 2nd. Thrombin-mediated increase in vascular endothelial permeability. Semin Thromb Hemost. 1992;18(2):193–9.
22. Minami T, Sugiyama A, Wu SQ, Abid R, Kodama T, Aird WC. Thrombin and phenotypic modulation of the endothelium. Arterioscler Thromb Vasc Biol. 2004;24(1):41–53.
23. Darrow AL, Fung-Leung WP, Ye RD, Santulli RJ, Cheung WM, Derian CK, et al. Biological consequences of thrombin receptor deficiency in mice. Thromb Haemost. 1996;76(6):860–6.
24. Morrow DA, Braunwald E, Bonaca MP, Ameriso SF, Dalby AJ, Fish MP, et al. Vorapaxar in the secondary prevention of atherothrombotic events. N Engl J Med. 2012;366(15):1404–13.
25. Christiaans SC, Wagener BM, Esmon CT, Pittet JF. Protein C and acute inflammation: a clinical and biological perspective. Am J Physiol Lung Cell Mol Physiol. 2013;305(7):L455–66.
26. Madhusudhan T, Wang H, Straub BK, Grone E, Zhou Q, Shahzad K, et al. Cytoprotective signaling by activated protein C requires protease-activated receptor-3 in podocytes. Blood. 2012;119(3):874–83.
27. Venkatachalam MA, Griffin KA, Lan R, Geng H, Saikumar P, Bidani AK. Acute kidney injury: a springboard for progression in chronic kidney disease. Am J Physiol Renal Physiol. 2010;298(5): F1078–94.

Impact of Antiplatelet Therapy and Platelet Reactivity Testing on Cardiovascular Outcomes in Patients with Chronic Kidney Disease

29

Sandeep Nathan and Brian Conway

Background

While the past half-century of medical research has greatly advanced our understanding of platelet biology and its impact on cardiovascular events, the role of chronic kidney disease (CKD) on altering platelet function and platelet-mediated ischemic and bleeding events remains less well-characterized, rendering the clinical management of this growing segment of the patient population often quite challenging. In this chapter, we explore clinically relevant aspects of platelet biology in patients with and without renal dysfunction, discuss the pharmacology of the currently available oral antiplatelet agents, detail methods for assessment of platelet reactivity and explore the mechanisms responsible for poor antiplatelet response. We will also cover cardiovascular outcomes in CKD patients treated with antiplatelet therapy and review the available data on platelet function testing (PFT) to guide choice and dosing of oral antiplatelet therapy.

Fundamentals of Platelet Biology and Vascular Thrombosis

Platelets comprise an anucleate cell line, originating from megakaryoblast precursors that transform into megakaryocytes which eventually produce thrombocytes, or mature platelets [1]. Platelets circulate in an inactive state until activated by vascular endothelial damage, endogenous activators, or activation of the coagulation cascade. Once activated, platelets interact with subendothelial substrates, undergo various conformational changes, release their cytoplasmic contents and aggregate [2, 3]. These complex and interrelated processes may be broadly divided into adhesion, activation, and aggregation phases. The primary physiologic purpose of this activity is prevention of hemorrhage in the setting of vascular injury, however excessive platelet activation or activation in the setting of non-traumatic endothelial injury can precipitate pathologic thrombosis and ischemia of downstream tissue beds [4]. Platelets also contribute to localized inflammatory responses by inducing release of pro-inflammatory cytoplasmic contents from other cell lines.

Vascular injury disrupts the endothelial cell layer exposing the subendothelial matrix and triggering a cascade of events aimed ultimately at sealing the defect. An important mediator of platelet adhesion is the interaction between platelet glycoprotein (GP) Ib/IX/V and von Willebrand factor (vWF) in the exposed subendothelium. Exposed collagen binds with platelet receptors GP VI and α[alpha]2β[beta]1 following platelet capture by GP Ib/IX/V-vWF. Vascular inflammation may further promote platelet adhesion in conjunction with, or even independent of, endothelial denudation.

The process of platelet activation results in the conversion of a smooth, non-adherent platelet into a rough, spiculated particle that releases biologically active molecules and exhibits the ability to bind soluble fibrinogen. Platelet shape change is induced by numerous endogenous agonists and is driven by rapid remodeling in the platelet cytoskeleton. This follows increasing cytosolic calcium concentration in response to ligand binding to cell-surface receptors [5]. Increased cytosolic calcium also results in exocytosis of platelet storage α[alpha]- and dense granules. The released granule contents attract other platelets thus enhancing the formation of a platelet plug. Several notable activators include: adenosine diphosphate (ADP), thrombin, thromboxane A2 (TXA2), epinephrine, collagen, and shear stress.

Platelet–platelet aggregation is the necessary final step in platelet-mediated hemostasis or thrombosis. The primary

S. Nathan (✉) · B. Conway
Department of Medicine/Section of Cardiology, University of Chicago Medicine, 5841 South Maryland Avenue, MC 5076, Chicago, IL 60637, USA
e-mail: snathan@medicine.bsd.uchicago.edu

B. Conway
e-mail: bdconway34@gmail.com

J. Rangaswami et al. (eds.), *Cardio-Nephrology*,
DOI 10.1007/978-3-319-56042-7_29

membrane surface protein involved in platelet aggregation is the integrin α[alpha]IIb/β[beta]3 (also known as GP IIb/IIIa), one of the most abundant receptors found in the body. Once platelet activation occurs GP IIb/IIIa receptors undergo upregulation and conformational changes that render the integrin capable of binding divalent soluble plasma fibrinogen molecules, which in turn act as bridges between activated platelets. Activated platelets also recruit additional platelets to the growing platelet plug through a variety of amplification feedback loops.

Through adhesion, activation, and aggregation, platelets form dense plugs that trap cellular debris and ultimately form mature thrombus that limits blood loss at sites of traumatic vascular injury. This process can also engender pathological thrombosis as seen in the setting of atherosclerotic plaque rupture or iatrogenic endothelial disruption vis-à-vis vascular intervention or surgery. A variety of endogenous platelet inhibitors such as nitric oxide, endothelial derived prostacyclin (PGI2), and endothelial ecto-ADPase (CD39) as well as targeted pharmacologic agents (detailed below) are capable of modifying, or even completely abolishing, the sequence of events within the platelet cascade.

Oral Antiplatelet Agents

Over the past several decades, nearly one dozen oral and parenteral antiplatelet agents have been developed, evaluated in clinical trials and gained US and European regulatory approval for the prevention and/or treatment of atherothrombotic events following acute coronary syndromes (ACS), acute myocardial infarction (MI) and PCI. In the interest of brevity, and given the typically short duration of exposure to parenteral agents such as intravenous GP IIb/IIIa inhibitors and the cyclopentyl triazolo pyrimidine compound cangrelor, the remainder of the discussion will center on oral antiplatelet agents. These agents represent the cornerstone of therapy in the management of cardiovascular disease.

Aspirin

Acetylsalicylic acid, or aspirin, is a compound originally derived from willow bark during the time of Hippocrates, but only introduced into the pharmaceutical market in the 1890s. Its primary use was as an analgesic with the knowledge of its antiplatelet properties remaining undiscovered until almost 70 years later. Aspirin exerts its effect on platelets primarily by irreversibly blocking cyclo-oxygenase 1 (COX-1)-mediated synthesis of TXA2 from arachidonic acid (AA) precursors, thus limiting the local availability of TXA2 to bind the platelet thromboxane prostanoid receptor. Aspirin also promotes platelet inhibition through an independent neutrophil-mediated, NO/cGMP-dependent mechanism and may exert beneficial cardiovascular effects by protecting LDL from oxidative modification [6–8]. Absorption of aspirin is rapid, and quantifiable platelet inhibition occurs within 60 min of administration [9–11]. Dosing aspirin at or above 100 mg abolishes the production of TXA2 in both normal individuals as well as patients with atherosclerotic disease while doses below 100 mg have a dose-dependent effect on TXA2 production [8, 12]. Aspirin-mediated platelet inhibition is irreversible and lasts the life of the platelet (approximately 10 days). Cardiovascular benefit has been demonstrated with doses from 30 to 1500 mg/day, however higher doses do not appear to be more effective and may increase gastrointestinal (GI) side effects [9, 13–15].

Use of aspirin across a variety of acute and chronic cardiovascular disease states, and in both primary and secondary prevention capacities, has demonstrated directional consistency with respect to reduction in cardiovascular morbidity and mortality, albeit with considerable variability in effect size between the various populations studied [15–24]. The Antithrombotic Trialists' (ATT) Collaboration meta-analysis of primary (95,000 low-risk individuals, 660,000 patient-years), and secondary (7000 high-risk individuals, 43,000 patient-years) prevention of vascular events with use of low-dose aspirin confirmed significant benefit in both populations [25]. A 12% relative reduction in serious vascular events was reported in the primary prevention population (0.51% aspirin vs. 0.57% control, per year, $p = 0.0001$) and a 20% relative reduction (6.7 vs. 8.2%/year, $p < 0.0001$) in the secondary prevention population studied. In both populations, the proportional reductions in serious vascular sequelae were generally similar for men and women. The main adverse event associated with aspirin therapy was extracranial hemorrhage with a 0.03% absolute annual increase in the primary prevention cohort (0.10 vs 0.07%/year; RR 1.54 [1.30–1.82], $p < 0.0001$) [25]. Hemorrhagic stroke was also increased to a modest degree in both the primary and secondary prevention cohorts while ischemic strokes were reduced in both groups. In addition to the aforementioned hazards, GI toxicity inclusive of nausea, vomiting, heartburn, indigestion, development of peptic ulcers and GI bleeding have all been reported with generally low frequency by a variety of investigators [14, 16, 17, 23, 24, 26–28]. Aspirin may also adversely impact renal function through dose-dependent inhibition of prostaglandin synthesis and increase blood pressure. It should be noted that neither the impact of aspirin therapy on renal function nor the interaction between pre-existing CKD and cardiovascular efficacy of aspirin were reported in the ATT Collaboration meta-analysis [25, 29–31].

P2Y12 Receptor Blockers

The P2Y12 receptor is a Gi-coupled, seven-transmembrane domain, purinergic receptor found on the platelet surface [32]. Along with the P2Y1 receptor, the P2Y12 receptor modulates platelet shape change and activation and also regulates the activation state of the GpIIb/IIIa receptor. Binding of ADP to the P2Y12 receptor triggers an intracellular cascade which results in the inhibition of an adenylate cyclase-mediated signaling pathway. This results in decreased intracellular cyclic adenosine monophosphate (cAMP) levels which in turn, reduces the phosphorylation rate of vasodilator-stimulated phosphoprotein (VASP), thus activating the GpIIb/IIIa receptor and inducing platelet aggregation. The P2Y12 receptor has emerged as an important target for pharmacologic modulation. There are three commercially available oral thienopyridine P2Y12 inhibitors (ticlopidine, clopidogrel, and prasugrel) and one oral cyclopentyl triazolo pyrimidine (ticagrelor). The thienopyridine agents, though variable in potency, all irreversibly bind the P2Y12 receptor disabling this activation pathway for the life of the platelet [33]. Clopidogrel bisulfate, the most commonly prescribed thienopyridine, is an inactive pro-drug in its ingested form. Following intestinal absorption, the drug undergoes a two-step sequential biotransformation, primarily through the effects of cytochrome P450 (CYP 450) enzyme sets 2C19, 1A2, 2B6, 2C9, 3A4, and 3A5 [32]. Importantly, the CYP 2C19 enzyme set is involved in both conversion steps [34, 35]. The ultimate generation of the active thiol metabolite (R-130964) from the ingested pro-drug is a relatively inefficient process with approximately 85% of absorbed clopidogrel immediately being degraded by esterases into an inactive carboxylic acid metabolite (SR26334) [32]. Clopidogrel is indicated in the United States for reduction of MI and stroke in patients with non-ST-elevation acute coronary syndromes (NSTE-ACS) and ST-elevation myocardial infarction (STEMI) and for reduction of atherothrombotic events in patients with a recent MI, recent stroke or peripheral arterial disease. It is also commonly used for prevention of stent thrombosis after coronary and peripheral vascular stent implantation, and is most often administered in conjunction with aspirin, comprising the most widely utilized iteration of oral dual antiplatelet therapy (DAPT). Clopidogrel is typically administered as a 300 mg or 600 mg oral load (contingent on physician preference and the latter often administered in the context of percutaneous coronary intervention (PCI)) with a 75 mg daily maintenance dose thereafter.

Prasugrel is a more potent, rapid acting thienopyridine antiplatelet than clopidogrel but one that still requires hepatic biotransformation from orally ingested pro-drug to active metabolite. Prasugrel's active metabolite is detectable within 15 min after a 60 mg loading dose, achieves maximal plasma concentration at 30 min and is associated with higher levels of platelet inhibition than clopidogrel, within 2 h of loading [31]. Prasugrel (60 mg oral load, 10 mg daily) was shown to be superior to clopidogrel (300 mg oral load, 75 mg daily) with respect to reduction in ischemic events and stent thrombosis in ACS patients undergoing PCI, albeit with an increased risk of major bleeding [36]. Prasugrel should not be used in patients with a prior history of stroke or transient ischemic attacks (TIA) and should be used with caution in patients >75 years of age or <60 kg body weight. The available evidence does not support the use of prasugrel in the medical management of ACS or for primary cardiovascular prevention.

Ticlopidine is rarely used today given its lower potency, twice daily dosing and most importantly, its association with granulocytopenias and resultant need for hematologic surveillance [37].

Ticagrelor is an oral nonthienopyridine, reversible, direct-acting, selective antagonist of the P2Y12 receptor [31]. Ticagrelor has demonstrated superiority over clopidogrel with respect to reduction in the incidence of ischemic morbidity and mortality for at least 12 months following ACS without any significant increase in bleeding noted. This is presumably due in part to more rapid onset and consistently greater antiplatelet potency as compared to clopidogrel. Plasma half-life is 6–8 h following dosing, and elimination is almost entirely in the feces following liver metabolism through CYP3A4/5 isoenzymes. Thus, renal dosing is not required [31]. For treatment of ACS (inclusive of STEMI), an initial oral loading dose of 180 mg is recommended followed by 90 mg twice daily for the first year in conjunction with low-dose (<100 mg daily) aspirin. Extended DAPT with ticagrelor plus aspirin may be considered following MI at a reduced dose of 60 mg twice daily. Strict contraindications are a history of intracranial hemorrhage, active bleed or hypersensitivity to any component of ticagrelor. The most common adverse reactions are bleeding and dyspnea which occur in approximately 12 and 14% of patients, respectively.

Thrombin Receptor Antagonists (TRA)

Thrombin is a ubiquitous serine protease which serves vital roles in both hemostasis and thrombosis. Additionally, it is recognized to be the most potent endogenous activator of platelets. Stimulation of platelets by thrombin occurs through its interaction with G-protein coupled, protease-activated receptors (PARs) s[33, 38]. PAR-1, and to a lesser degree PAR-4, become activated when thrombin cleaves a portion of the amino terminal exodomain, exposing a tethered ligand which in turn binds the receptor and triggers intracellular signaling [38]. Thrombin receptor antagonists (TRA) represent a new pharmacologic class of selective antagonists of the PAR-1 receptor capable of blocking the interaction of thrombin with platelets without impacting thrombin-mediated cleavage of fibrinogen [38–40].

Vorapaxar, the only approved PAR-1 inhibitor at the time of writing, is a highly selective and potent himbacine derivative antiplatelet agent which is functionally irreversible given its long half-life of greater than 1 week. Vorapaxar sulfate is administered orally as 2.5 mg daily (yielding 2.08 mg of vorapaxar), is rapidly absorbed in the GI tract with high bioavailability and peak antiplatelet effects are typically seen within 1–2 h after loading. Metabolism is mainly via the cytochrome P450 3A4 enzyme and the compound is eliminated mainly in feces (95%) [41]. No dose adjustment is required with mild to moderate hepatic impairment or with any degree of renal impairment. Vorapaxar was evaluated in two large Phase III clinical trials. The Thrombin Receptor Antagonist for Clinical Event Reduction in Acute Coronary Syndrome (TRA-CER) trial which evaluated the role of vorapaxar in addition to standard therapies in the acute management of high-risk NSTE-ACS patients, was terminated early due to significantly increased bleeding without improvement in cardiovascular outcomes [41]. Vorapaxar was ultimately approved by the FDA on the basis of the Thrombin Receptor Antagonist in the Secondary Prevention of Atherothrombotic Ischemic Events (TRA 2° P)–TIMI 50 trial results, for the reduction of thrombotic cardiovascular events in patients with a history of MI or peripheral arterial disease (PAD) but without a history of stroke or TIA [42]. Vorapaxar increases bleeding when administered in conjunction with other antiplatelet agents, commensurate with the underlying bleeding risk of the patient. While available data suggests that vorapaxar alone has minimal impact on bleeding time, vorapaxar monotherapy has not been studied in clinical trials. Vorapaxar is contraindicated in patients with a history of stroke or TIA and short-term discontinuation in the setting of bleeding is unlikely to help given its long half-life. While the aforementioned Phase III clinical trials were not powered to detect difference between specific patient subgroups, it bears mention that in the TRA 2°P trial, major bleeding events occurred with similar frequency in patients divided by estimated GFR < 60 mL/min/1.73 m2 versus ≥ 60 mL/min/1.73 m2 [32, 41–43].

Methods for Assessment of Platelet Function

The various interrelationships between platelet function, primary hemostasis and thrombotic cardiovascular sequelae have been acknowledged for some time. This is in addition to the individual biochemical phases of platelet activation, often categorized as adhesion, activation/degranulation, and aggregation. Despite the development of increasingly sophisticated laboratory methods to probe the various aspects of platelet function, it should be noted that no single test truly quantifies the myriad complexities of physiologic hemostasis or pathologic thrombosis. Rather, these tests help approximate certain components which may contribute to aggregate risk in a given patient. Available platelet function tests are numerous and vary greatly in methodology, but they may be broadly divided into laboratory-based testing and point-of-care (POC) testing. While it is beyond the scope of this chapter to provide exhaustive detail regarding all available tests, the following discussion will introduce a select few methods which may potentially aid in clinical decision-making.

The original and most basic platelet function test, the in vivo bleeding time, roughly characterizes the mechanisms contributing to primary hemostasis [44, 45]. While an abnormal test may reflect impaired platelet function or issues of vessel wall integrity, bleeding time can also be prolonged by fibrinogen or clotting factor deficiencies [46]. Additionally, many clinical disorders can affect the test results, including uremia, hepatic failure and multiple myeloma. Bleeding time has not maintained relevance in the contemporary assessment of the cardiac patient being treated with antiplatelet therapy.

The first platelet-specific methodology for assessment of aggregation was described by G.V.R. Born in 1962 [47]. Light transmission aggregometry (LTA) equates the relative passage of light through platelet rich plasma (PRP) before and after addition of an agonist to the degree of GpIIb/IIIa receptor-mediated platelet–platelet aggregation inducible within a sample. While this has remained the de facto gold standard for platelet aggregation studies and has demonstrated its value in monitoring the therapeutic effect of a wide variety of antiplatelet agents, its practical utility is limited by cost, time and technical considerations related to sample collection and preparation.

In 1980, Cardinal and Flower described a novel device for detecting changes in electrical impedance caused by platelet deposition on electrodes and demonstrated its suitability for measurement of aggregation in either PRP or whole blood [48]. Several other iterations of the whole blood aggregometry technique were subsequently described. More recently, Multiplate Electrode Aggregometry (Dynabyte—Roche Diagnostics, Mannheim, Germany) has emerged as a POC whole blood aggregometry technology with a wide variety of applications across the spectrum of treated cardiovascular disease. This includes detection of nonresponse to oral antiplatelet therapy and prediction of bleeding risk related to excessive platelet inhibition, to name a few [49].

Perhaps the most widely utilized POC platelet function test in the antiplatelet-treated cardiac patient is the VerifyNow assay (ITC, Edison, NJ, USA). This whole blood assay rapidly and reproducibly estimates residual platelet reactivity to various reagents which corresponds to the degree of therapeutic effect associated with commonly used classes of antiplatelet agents [50–54]. The VerifyNow P2Y12 assay contains a preparation of human fibrinogen-coated microbeads, a fixed concentration of platelet agonist and PGE1 to buffer and isolate P2Y12 activity from that of P2Y1. Fixed aliquots of whole blood sample are automatically drawn into sample wells from the collection tube where platelets come in contact with agonist. Aggregation is measured as a function of platelet-microbead co-agglutination and infrared dye absorption through the sample, transformed using a proprietary algorithm, and reported as P2Y12 reaction units (PRU). Higher PRU values reflect greater P2Y12-mediated reactivity, and thus, platelet aggregation [55].

Global hemostatic function may be estimated using thromboelastography (TEG) and thromboelastometry. Several clinical instruments currently exist, all studying dynamic clot formation by measurement of the viscoelastic properties and contractile force of coagulating whole blood. Historically, the usage of these devices has been restricted to the operating room or performed in the context of solid organ transplantation, in trauma surgery where large amounts of blood products may be required or guidance needed regarding impairment of specific phases of coagulation. Platelet function-specific applications on the TEG platform now also allow for monitoring of antiplatelet therapy [56–60].

Platelet Dysfunction in CKD

While hematologic abnormalities were first described in patients with CKD over 250 years ago, the specific pathobiologic mechanisms underlying these observations remain incompletely understood [61]. Even though several potential mechanisms have been identified, aggregate derangements in primary and secondary hemostasis are often difficult to predict in the CKD population rendering cardiovascular prognostication and treatment challenging. Variability in the severity and progression of renal disease as well as the impact of renal replacement therapy further contributes to the complexity of this issue. Clinicians have long observed that CKD patients often paradoxically suffer from both bleeding and thrombotic tendencies.

Endogenous Derangements of Vascular and Hemostatic Function

Numerous mechanisms are thought to contribute to altered platelet function as well as abnormal platelet–vessel wall interactions in the uremic patient [62]. A number of studies have identified platelet-α[alpha] granule abnormalities, with reduction of the platelet granular content of adenosine diphosphate (ADP) and diminished secretion of adenosine triphosphate (ATP) in response to various agonists, as compared to normal control patients [63]. The endogenous platelet inhibitor, cyclic adenosine monophosphate (cAMP) is also often elevated in this patient population and it is postulated that relative imbalances between these agonists and inhibitors may play an important role in qualitative platelet dysfunction in CKD [62, 63]. Parathyroid hormone (PTH) has also been identified as a potential modifier of platelet function in uremic patients given that PTH is often elevated in renal dysfunction and elevated PTH results in inhibition of platelet aggregation in vitro [64]. The clinical impact of this laboratory observation remains controversial, however, coarser metrics of hemostatic function, such as bleeding time, do not correlate with PTH levels [65]. Impaired thromboxane A2 (TXA2) synthesis by platelets in response to stimulation via various agonists (collagen, arachidonic acid, ADP, thrombin, etc.) has also been described, although this issue remains controversial as the available data are not entirely consistent and, moreover, this specific abnormality may be corrected by dialysis [63, 66].

The interface of platelets and vascular endothelium serves a key component of hemostasis at the site of vascular injury and derangements of this interaction have been noted in CKD patients [62]. Platelet adhesion to vascular subendothelium is mediated primarily through the interaction of von Willebrand factor (vWF) with glycoprotein (GP) Ib and fibrinogen with the α[alpha]IIbβ[beta]3 integrin complex. Whereas normal GpIb/vWF interaction and receptor density are seen in uremic patients, CKD is associated with a decrease in platelet GpIb content and increased levels of glycocalin, representing a soluble GpIb proteolytic fragment [62]. Qualitative, but not quantitative changes in the α[alpha] IIbβ[beta]3 receptor have also been observed in renal failure with decreased binding activity thought to be ascribable to dialyzable uremic toxins which interfere with binding affinity, and/or competitive occupancy of the receptor by fibrinogen split products found in uremic serum [67–69]. Impaired hemostasis may also be related, in part, to the interplay between reduced vWF activity and qualitative changes in α[alpha]IIbβ[beta]3 activity, as it relates to thrombus formation at the site of disrupted vascular endothelium.

Potential Mechanisms for Impaired Antiplatelet Response in CKD

High Platelet Reactivity

A lower than expected inhibition of agonist-stimulated platelet aggregation in patients receiving therapeutic platelet inhibitors is generally termed "high residual platelet reactivity" (HRPR) and may result from a variety of pathophysiologic conditions. Many observational studies have shown that CKD patients being treated with antiplatelet agents exhibit HRPR and that in a broad swath of cardiovascular disease patients (not limited to those with CKD), HRPR is associated with an increased risk of adverse cardiovascular outcomes [70–76]. A collaborative meta-analysis of 6 studies including 3059 clopidogrel-treated, post-PCI patients performed by Brar, et al. found a significant association between higher quartiles of on-treatment platelet reactivity and the incidence of long-term cardiovascular events (stent thrombosis, MI, and death). Receiver-operating characteristic curve analysis found a threshold of ≥ 230 P2Y12 reaction units (PRU, measured using the point-of-care VerifyNow P2Y12 assay) to be most predictive of adverse cardiovascular outcomes [76]. A smaller body of literature also links high de novo platelet reactivity (independent of aspirin or clopidogrel use) with an increased risk for ischemic cardiovascular morbidity and mortality. Given these and other similar findings, HRPR has emerged as a conceptually attractive target for therapeutic modulation.

While advanced CKD patients have historically been underrepresented in large prospective cardiovascular trials of antiplatelet therapy, smaller studies addressing this important patient population have slowly begun to emerge. Angiolillo et al. undertook a cross-sectional analysis of 306 diabetic patients with CAD treated with aspirin and clopidogrel. The cohort was divided on the basis of presence or absence of moderate/severe CKD and multichannel platelet aggregation studies were performed [77]. Flow cytometric analysis of platelet activation and expression state of various adhesive cell surface proteins was also performed. In patients stratified by CKD severity, residual on-treatment platelet reactivity was significantly higher in diabetic CKD patients than those with normal renal function [77]. Morel et al. extended these observations in another study which prospectively enrolled 440 clopidogrel-treated patients undergoing urgent or planned PCI for symptomatic CAD who were first divided by CKD (stages 3–5 vs. no CKD) status and secondarily, by level of on-treatment platelet reactivity. These patients were followed for the occurrence of cardiovascular morbidity and mortality [78]. At a mean follow-up of 9 months, the composite rate of all-cause mortality, cardiac death, and possible stent thrombosis were significantly higher in CKD than in no-CKD patients. Furthermore, while the proportion of low antiplatelet responder patients did not differ between the CKD and no-CKD groups, low antiplatelet response was associated with differentially higher rates of each individual component of the composite endpoint in the CKD patients as compared to the no-CKD patients in whom low-responder status did not seem to impact cardiovascular outcomes [78]. While most studies, the aforementioned included, have considered on-treatment platelet reactivity as a single, static metric, others have begun to ask the important question if this variable can be materially reversed by renal replacement therapies [79].

Cytochrome P450 (CYP) Polymorphisms

As previously detailed, clopidogrel bisulfate is an oral pro-drug which must undergo multistep hepatic transformation in order to yield its active thiol metabolite. A number of CYP P450 isoenzymes including CYP1A2, 2B6, 3A4, 3A5, 2C9, and 2C19 are required for this process [78, 80]. Upwards of 25–30% of clopidogrel-treated patients in the general population and perhaps even higher proportions of racial minorities, may exhibit allelic polymorphisms which may potentially confer reduced-function status to requisite CYP isozymes. It has been shown that carriers of a single reduced-function allele of CYP2C19 had a 32.4% reduction in plasma exposure of the active clopidogrel metabolite associated with a 53% relative increase in the combined endpoint of death, MI or stroke and a threefold increase in the risk of in-stent thrombosis [80]. While large-scale comparisons of CYP reduced-function allelic prevalence in CKD versus non-CKD patients have not been performed, at least one investigation found the prevalence of CYP (CYP2C9, CYP2C19, and CYP2D6) polymorphisms to be exceedingly high (77% inclusive of homozygous and heterozygous carriers) in elderly hemodialysis patients and thus, this issue must be considered as potentially contributory to the phenomenon of reduced antiplatelet response pending additional confirmatory studies [81].

Altered Non-Renal Drug Metabolism

While dosage adjustment of renally cleared medications is common practice, less consideration is given to the impact of renal failure, specifically, uremia on non-renal metabolic pathways. Uremia may impair the biologic activity of many CYP450 isoenzymes, including some involved in the clopidogrel metabolic pathway. Renal failure also impacts the expression of various organic anion transporters requisite for entrance of drugs into hepatocytes and enterocytes [82]. Additionally, the effect size of these phenomena may be proportional to the severity of renal failure. As it relates to clopidogrel effect, progressive CKD has been shown to be associated with a progressive increase in the percentage of poor responders to clopidogrel from 20% of patients with stage 2 CKD to 38% of patients with CKD stages 4 and 5 [82].

Dysfunctional VWF

Von Willebrand factor has long been recognized as an important mediator of hemostasis and, in conditions such as CKD that are associated with decreased vWF activity, an etiology for increased bleeding risk [82]. Interestingly however, the increase in vWF expression noted in uremic patients may also promote a prothrombotic vascular milieu via interaction of vWF with platelet surface Gp Ib/IX/V, subendothelial collagen, stimulation of platelet-derived procoagulant particle generation and its role in fibrin clot formation. Thus, the simultaneous quantitative and qualitative abnormalities in vWF, which occur in patients with renal failure, has been proposed as a potential explanation for the seemingly paradoxical increase in both bleeding and atherothrombotic risk [62, 82, 83].

Cardiovascular Outcomes in CKD Patients Treated with Antiplatelet Therapy

Antiplatelet Monotherapy

The vast majority of patients being treated with antiplatelet monotherapy in primary or secondary prevention capacities receive aspirin while a small minority receives clopidogrel monotherapy and a vanishingly smaller population of patients receives one of the other oral compounds (prasugrel, ticagrelor, cilostazol) alone. While it is generally regarded that aspirin offers significant clinical benefit across the spectrum of renal function, when administered in the context of acute coronary syndromes and acute myocardial infarction, data regarding the efficacy and safety of aspirin in stable patients with CKD (inclusive of dialysis patients) is conflicting. Aspirin resistance has been shown to be more prevalent in stable CAD patients with CKD versus those with normal renal function. Blann, et al. found in 169 patients with proven CAD that aspirin resistance was over twice as prevalent in those with the most severe renal dysfunction (50% of patients) compared to those with the most preserved renal function (21.4%) [84]. Similarly, Kilickesmez et al. found in a cohort of ESRD patients, 44% were aspirin-resistant and further, that these patients experienced a greater than 2-fold increase in the risk of death, MI or CVA as compared to the aspirin-responsive ESRD patients, a hazard which persisted in a multivariate risk model [69].

Data regarding the safety and efficacy of aspirin in the CKD population are less consistent than the data on aspirin resistance [82]. The First United Kingdom Heart and Renal Protection (UK-HARP) trial studied the effect of 100 mg of aspirin versus placebo on bleeding or other adverse outcomes in 448 CKD patients (pre-dialysis CKD, hemodialysis, peritoneal dialysis or prior kidney transplant) [85]. Cardiovascular efficacy was not reported and while there was no increase in major or fatal bleeding, there was a threefold increase in minor bleeding [85]. In the Dialysis Outcomes and Practice Patterns Study (DOPPS) study, data from 28,320 randomly selected hemodialysis patients (sourced from the Dialysis Outcomes and Practice Patterns Study I and II) were analyzed to ascertain aspirin prescribing patterns and the potential impact of aspirin on cardiovascular morbidity and mortality [86]. Surprisingly, aspirin was associated with an increased risk of myocardial infarction in all patients, irrespective of CAD history. A reduction in stroke risk in all patients was also noted with no increase in gastrointestinal bleeding [86]. In contrast, Sciahbasi et al. investigated the cardioprotective role of aspirin in a community-based cohort ($N = 595$) of patients presenting with acute myocardial infarction and demonstrated that there was a lower probability of presenting with ST-segment elevation myocardial infarction (STEMI, versus non-ST-segment elevation myocardial infarction) if being treated with aspirin and further, that this benefit extended to the 32% of the cohort with CKD [87]. On balance, aspirin monotherapy is more likely to offer clinical benefit when used for the secondary prevention of cardiovascular events rather than for primary prevention in CKD patients. There is little evidence to suggest that aspirin increases the risk of major or fatal bleeding however minor bleeding is likely to be increased. It remains unknown if the lack of uniform benefit of aspirin therapy in CKD patients is primarily ascribable to the high rate of aspirin resistance in this population or rather, by differences in the biology and time course of cardiovascular events.

Dual Antiplatelet Therapy

Dual antiplatelet therapy (DAPT) usually comprises aspirin plus an oral ADP P2Y12 inhibitor, most often clopidgrel, and is utilized in the acute and long-term management of patients suffering acute coronary syndromes and acute myocardial infarction as well as those patients receiving vascular stents. As noted previously, the yield of clopidogrel's active metabolite and clopidogrel's acute antiplatelet effect may both be attenuated in CKD patients especially those with severe renal impairment and those on dialysis [77–79, 81, 88]. It is also known that CKD patients exhibit more robust expression of platelet GpIIb/III receptors in response to agonist challenge and more frequently manifest HRPR on maintenance therapy compared to non-CKD patients. A large recent investigation (Assessment of Dual Antiplatelet Therapy with Drug-Eluting Stents, ADAPT-DES) focusing on patients receiving drug-eluting stents on the backdrop of DAPT with aspirin plus clopidogrel found that HRPR on clopidogrel was strongly predictive of myocardial infarction and stent thrombosis and was inversely related to bleeding risk but did not impact mortality. In contrast, high platelet reactivity to aspirin did not impact the risks of stent thrombosis, myocardial infarction or mortality but was inversely related to bleeding risk [89].

As stated previously, patients with severe CKD have largely been excluded from major prospective randomized trials of oral DAPT, however a number of post hoc analyses have been published offering disparate messages regarding the value of clopidogrel-based DAPT in patients with mild-moderate CKD. In the Clopidogrel in Unstable Angina to Prevent Recurrent Events (CURE) trial, patients presenting with non-ST elevation ACS were randomized to receive either aspirin/clopidogrel or aspirin/placebo in addition to other standard of care therapies. When patients were stratified by GFR, both the primary outcome of cardiovascular death/MI/CVA as well as bleeding occurred more frequently in the lowest tertile of GFR [90]. The clinical benefit of oral DAPT with clopidogrel, seen in the overall trial population, also extended to all 3 tertiles of renal function although, as in the overall trial results, no standalone mortality benefit was seen. In a retrospective analysis of the Clopidogrel for the Reduction of Events During Observation (CREDO) trial, mild-moderate CKD patients undergoing elective PCI with 1 year of oral DAPT (aspirin/clopidogrel) did not evidence the same beneficial reduction in the composite ischemic endpoint (death, myocardial infarction, or stroke) seen in the patients with normal renal function [91]. In a post hoc analysis of the Clopidogrel for High Atherothrombotic Risk and Ischemic Stabilization, Management, and Avoidance (CHARISMA) trial, diabetic nephropathy patients randomized to long-term oral DAPT (versus aspirin and placebo) experienced significantly increased rates of cardiovascular and overall mortality with no differences in bleeding [92]. These and other antiplatelet studies were analyzed in the context of a systematic review and meta-analysis by Palmer et al. which included 9 trials involving 9,969 ACS or PCI patients and 31 trials involving 11,701 patients with stable CAD or no CAD [70]. The authors concluded that in patients with ACS, DAPT (including use of parenteral glycoprotein inhibitors) did not decrease mortality or myocardial infarction but did increase major bleeding. In stable CAD/no CAD patients however, antiplatelet therapy decreased the risk of MI, had an uncertain effect on mortality and increased the risk of minor bleeding. These results should be interpreted with caution, however, as the quality of the source data was reportedly low and/or heterogeneous and also because a significant proportion of included studies were post hoc subgroup analyses of CKD patients [93, 94].

With growing worldwide adoption of the newer, more potent oral P2Y12 inhibitors, data with use of these compounds in the CKD population have begun to emerge and have offered some encouraging signals. In the PROMETHEUS study, a retrospective multicenter observational analysis comparing clopidogrel to prasugrel in patients undergoing ACS PCI, a sub-analysis stratifying for presence of renal disease found prasugrel to be more efficacious than clopiodgrel in CKD and non-CKD subgroups without any increase in bleeding [95]. A mechanistic comparison of prasugrel versus clopidogrel was published by Nishi el al. who performed a prospective switching study on 53 Japanese patients with CAD and found that the antiplatelet effect of clopidogrel, but not prasugrel, was decreased in patients with mild-moderate CKD versus those with normal renal function. Furthermore, prasugrel consistently produced lower platelet reactivity compared with clopidogrel, irrespective of CKD status [96].

The Platelet Inhibition and Patient Outcomes (PLATO) Trial, randomized 18,624 patients presenting with ACS (inclusive of STEMI) to treatment with aspirin/clopidogrel versus aspirin/ticagrelor and followed these subjects for the occurrence of major adverse cardiovascular events. In a prespecified subgroup analysis of patients stratified by presence of CKD (creatinine clearance <60 mL/min; $n = 3{,}237$ of 15,802 patients with baseline creatinine levels), ticagrelor versus clopidogrel significantly reduced the occurrence of the primary ischemic end point with greater risk reduction seen in CKD patients than those with normal renal function [97]. Mortality was also significantly reduced in ticagrelor-treated CKD patients and the incidence of major bleeding did not differ significantly between the ticagrelor and clopidogrel groups irrespective of presence or absence of CKD.

In summary, while no adequately powered prospective study has yet evaluated the risks and benefits of oral DAPT in CAD patients with CKD, available retrospective data suggest more consistent benefit in high-risk (versus low-risk) patients treated with clopidogrel/aspirin and perhaps greater benefit still with use of the more potent P2Y12 inhibitors, prasugrel and ticagrelor.

Platelet Function Testing in Cardiovascular Disease: Summary of the Available Data

As detailed in the preceding sections, there is a strong and consistent relationship in the published observational literature between high residual (on-treatment) platelet reactivity and adverse cardiovascular outcomes in patients with CAD or following PCI. There is a more modest inverse relationship between platelet reactivity and the risk of bleeding. Given these observations and the enormous toll that cardiovascular disease and bleeding exact on patients, independently and in concert with one another, it is tempting to infer that platelet reactivity may be therapeutically modulated or "tailored" for purposes of cardiovascular risk reduction and mitigation of bleeding risk. Solid evidence to support tailoring of antiplatelet therapy in the majority of patients using platelet function testing has been elusive however. Furthermore, virtually no data exists in this regard for specific high-risk groups such as the CKD population.

The Gauging Responsiveness with A VerifyNow assay—Impact on Thrombosis And Safety (GRAVITAS) study was a randomized, double-blind, active-control trial designed to evaluate the effect of high-dose compared with standard-dose clopidogrel, in patients with high on-treatment platelet reactivity after PCI, as determined by point-of-care (Accumetrics VerifyNow) platelet function testing. Although platelet function testing-guided use of high-dose clopidogrel resulted in significantly lower levels of on-treatment platelet reactivity at 30 days and 6 months versus standard-dose clopidogrel, the authors concluded that the positive pharmacodynamic effect of this strategy did not translate to a lower incidence of cardiovascular death, nonfatal MI or stent thrombosis [98]. The Testing platelet Reactivity In patients underGoing elective stent placement on clopidogrel to Guide alternative thErapy with pRasugrel (TRIGGER-PCI) study attempted to demonstrate that prasugrel could improve HRPR on clopidogrel and therefore improve cardiovascular outcomes post-PCI with implantation of at least 1 drug-eluting stent. This study also employed the point-of-care Accumetrics VerifyNow system and used a cutoff value of >208 P2Y12 reaction units to define HRPR with reassessment of platelet reactivity at 3 and 6 months. While switching from clopidogrel to prasugrel increased platelet inhibition as expected, the clinical utility of this approach was not demonstrable due to very low adverse event rates in both groups and therefore the study was terminated prematurely for futility [99]. The Assessment by a Double Randomization of a Conventional Antiplatelet Strategy versus a Monitoring-guided Strategy for Drug-Eluting Stent Implantation and of Treatment Interruption versus Continuation One Year after Stenting (ARCTIC) study evaluated a strategy of systematic platelet function testing to guide treatment adjustments in PCI patients with poor response to aspirin, P2Y12 inhibitors (clopidogrel or prasugrel), or both, as compared with a conventional approach without use of platelet function testing. Despite a large number of patients recruited ($N = 2440$) there was no demonstrable advantage of a platelet function guided approach to antiplatelet therapy with respect to ischemic events or bleeding [100].

Whereas prediction and mitigation of de novo/spontaneous bleeding is fraught with unpredictable event rates and logistical challenges, there may yet be value for platelet function testing to guide the timing of major surgery in patients receiving DAPT. The Timing Based on Platelet Function Strategy to Reduce Clopidogrel-Associated Bleeding Related to CABG (TARGET-CABG) Study used thromboelastography (TEG)-derived metrics of clopidogrel response to guide the timing of on-pump coronary artery bypass graft surgery. Using this strategy, bleeding (as determined by chest tube output and transfusion requirements) was comparable between clopidogrel naïve patients and DAPT-treated/TEG-guided patients with a nearly 50% reduction in the waiting time to surgery than current guideline recommendations would have mandated for DAPT-treated patients [101].

Conclusions

Chronic kidney disease represents a spectrum of illness affecting approximately 14% of the United States population but exacting a disproportionately high toll in cardiovascular morbidity and mortality [102]. Unfortunately, cardiovascular research trials have systematically excluded patients with moderate to severe CKD and thus, there is a paucity of data-driven recommendations regarding treatment in this important patient segment. Oral antiplatelet therapy represents one of the cornerstones of treatment for patients with manifest atherothrombotic conditions and is also used for primary prevention in patients at high risk for developing atherosclerotic disease. Conflicting data exist with respect to the utility and safety of oral antiplatelet monotherapy (most often aspirin) as well as dual antiplatelet therapy (most often aspirin plus clopidogrel). It should be noted however that most information in this regard has been sourced from retrospective analyses of registries or non-prespecified subgroup analyses of prospective trials and the resulting observations are largely limited to patients with mild to moderate CKD. Patients with CKD often paradoxically display simultaneous propensities for both bleeding and thrombotic complications, rendering decisions regarding use, intensity and duration of antiplatelet therapy still more challenging. Based on the available data, aspirin monotherapy is more appropriate for secondary prevention of cardiovascular events rather than for primary prevention in CKD patients and is associated with an increase in the risk of minor bleeding. The effectiveness of DAPT with aspirin and clopidogrel for secondary cardiovascular prevention in CKD patients remains uncertain and DAPT is not recommended for primary prevention in this patient population. Dual antiplatelet therapy in CKD with aspirin plus either prasugrel or ticagrelor has shown promise in some small prospective series and retrospective analyses but remains to be prospectively validated. While tailoring of antiplatelet regimens based on platelet function testing has not shown broad clinical applicability largely due to lower than anticipated event rates, the high prevalence of on-treatment high residual platelet reactivity combined with a high risk of recurrent atherothrombotic events in CKD patients (at least those on aspirin/clopidogrel regimens) creates a potential, if untested, therapeutic niche in this high risk population.

References

1. Gresele P, Fuster V, Lopez JA, Page CP, Vermylen J. Platelets in hematologic and cardiovascular disorders: a clinical handbook. Cambridge: Cambridge University Press; 2007.
2. Carlsson L, Markey F, Blikstad I, Persson T, Lindberg U. Reorganization of actin in platelets stimulated by thrombin as measured by the DNAse I inhibition assay. Proc Natl Acad Sci USA. 1979;76:6373–80.
3. Karlsson F, Lassing I, Hoglund AS, Lindberg U. The organization of microfilaments in spreading platelets: a comparison with fibroblasts and glial cells. J Cell Physiol. 1984;121:96–113.
4. Quinn M, Fitzgerald D, Cox D. Platelet function: assessment, diagnosis, and treatment. Totowa: Springer Science & Business Media; 2007.
5. Nachmias VT, Kavaler J, Jacubowitz S. Reversible association of myosin with the platelet cytoskeleton. Nature. 1985;313:70–2.
6. Lopez-Farre A, Caramelo C, Esteban A, Alberola ML, Millas I, Monton M, Casado S. Effects of aspirin on platelet-neutrophil interactions: role of nitric oxide and endothelin-1. Circulation. 1995;91:2080–8.
7. Steer KA, Wallace TM, Bolton CH, Hartog M. Aspirin protects low density lipoprotein from oxidative modification. Heart. 1997;77(4):333–7.
8. Husain S, Andrews NP, Mulcahy D, Panza JA, Quyyumi AA. Aspirin improves endothelial dysfunction in atherosclerosis. Circulation. 1998;97(8):716–20.
9. Patrono C, Coller B, FitzGerald GA, Hirsh J, Roth G. Platelet-active drugs: the relationships among dose, effectiveness, and side effects: the Seventh ACCP Conference on Antithrombotic and Thrombolytic Therapy. Chest. 2004;126(3 Suppl): 234S–64S.
10. Jimenez AH, Stubbs ME, Tofler GH, Winther K, Williams GH, Muller JE. Rapidity and duration of platelet suppression by enteric-coated aspirin in healthy young men. Am J Cardiol. 1992;69(3):258–62.
11. FitzGerald GA, Oates JA, Hawiger J, Maas RL, Roberts LJ 2nd, Lawson JA, Brash AR. Endogenous biosynthesis of prostacyclin and thromboxane and platelet function during chronicadministration of aspirin in man. J Clin Invest. 1983;71(3):676–88.
12. Patrignani P, Filabozzi P, Patrono C. Selective cumulative inhibition of platelet thromboxane production by low-dose aspirin in healthy subjects. J Clin Invest. 1982;69:1366–72.
13. Antiplatelet Trialists' Collaboration. Collaborative overview of randomised trials of antiplatelet therapy—I: prevention of death, myocardial infarction, and stroke by prolonged antiplatelet therapy in various categories of patients. BMJ. 1994;308 (6921):81–106.
14. UK-TIA Study Group. United Kingdom transient ischaemic attack (UK-TIA) aspirin trial: interim results. Br Med J (Clin Res Ed). 1988;296(6618):316–20.
15. Lembo NJ, Black AJ, Roubin GS, Wilentz JR, Mufson LH, Douglas JS Jr, King SB 3rd. Effect of pretreatment with aspirin versus aspirin plus dipyridamole on frequency and type of acute complications of percutaneous transluminal coronary angioplasty. Am J Cardiol. 1990;65(7):422–6.
16. Cairns JA, Gent M, Singer J, Finnie KJ, Froggatt GM, Holder DA, Jablonsky G, Kostuk WJ, Melendez LJ, Myers MG, Sackett DL, Sealey BJ, Tanser PH. Aspirin, sulfinpyrazone, or both in unstable angina: results of a Canadian multicenter trial. N Engl J Med. 1985;313:1369–75.
17. The RISC Group. Risk of myocardial infarction and death during treatment with low dose aspirin and intravenous heparinin men with unstable coronary artery disease. Lancet. 1990;336 (8719):827–30.
18. Lewis HD Jr, Davis JW, Archibald DG, Steinke WE, Smitherman TC, Doherty JE 3rd, Schnaper HW, LeWinter MM, Linares E, Pouget JM, Sabharwal SC, Chesler E, DeMots H. Protective effects of aspirin against acute myocardial infarction and death in men with unstable angina. Results of a Veterans Administration Cooperative Study. N Engl J Med. 1983;309 (7):396–403.
19. Théroux P, Ouimet H, McCans J, Latour JG, Joly P, Lévy G, Pelletier E, Juneau M, Stasiak J, deGuise P, Pelletier G, Rinzler D, Waters D. Aspirin, heparin, or both to treat acute unstable angina. N Engl J Med. 1988;319(17):1105–11.
20. Wallentin LC. Aspirin (75 mg/day) after an episode of unstable coronary artery disease: long-term effects on the riskfor myocardial infarction, occurrence of severe angina and the need for revascularization. Research Group on Instability in Coronary Artery Disease in Southeast Sweden. J Am Coll Cardiol. 1991;18 (7):1587–93.
21. de Feyter PJ, van den Brand M, Laarman GJ, van Domburg R, Serruys PW, Suryapranata H. Acute coronary artery occlusion during and after percutaneous transluminal coronary angioplasty. Frequency, prediction, clinical course, management, and follow-up. Circulation. 1991;83(3):927–36.
22. Schwartz L, Bourassa MG, Lespérance J, Aldridge HE, Kazim F, Salvatori VA, Henderson M, Bonan R, David PR. Aspirin and dipyridamole in the prevention of restenosis after percutaneous transluminal coronary angioplasty. N Engl J Med. 1988;318 (26):1714–9.
23. Steering Committee of the Physicians' Health Study Research Group. Final report on the aspirin component of the ongoing Physicians' Health Study. N Engl J Med. 1989;321(3):129–35.
24. Peto R, Gray R, Collins R, Wheatley K, Hennekens C, Jamrozik K, Warlow C, Hafner B, Thompson E, Norton S, Gilliland J, Doll R. Randomised trial of prophylactic daily aspirin in British male doctors. Br Med J (Clin Res Ed). 1988;296 (6618):313–6.
25. Spaulding C, Charbonnier B, Cohen-Solal A, Juillière Y, Kromer EP, Benhamda K, Cador R, Weber S. Acute hemodynamic interaction of aspirin and ticlopidine with enalapril: results of a double-blind, randomized comparative trial. Circulation. 1998;98(8):757–65.

26. The Aspirin Myocardial Infarction Study Research Group. The Aspirin Myocardial Infarction Study: final results. Circulation. 1980;62(suppl V):V79–84.
27. The Swedish Cooperative Study Group. High-dose acetylsalicylic acid after cerebral infarction: a Swedish cooperative study. Stroke. 1986;18:325–34.
28. Awtry EH, Loscalzo J. Aspirin. Circulation. 2000;101(10):1206–18.
29. Hall D, Zeitler H, Rudolph W. Counteraction of the vasodilator effects of enalapril by aspirin in severe heart failure. J Am Coll Cardiol. 1992;20(7):1549–55.
30. Al-Khadra AS, Salem DN, Rand WM, Udelson JE, Smith JJ, Konstam MA. Antiplatelet agents and survival: a cohort analysis from the Studies of Left Ventricular Dysfunction(SOLVD) trial. J Am Coll Cardiol. 1998;31(2):419–25.
31. Baigent C, Blackwell L, Collins R, Emberson J, Godwin J, Peto R, Buring J, Hennekens C, Kearney P, Meade T, Patrono C, Roncaglioni MC, Zanchetti A, Antithrombotic Trialists' (ATT) Collaboration. Aspirin in the primary and secondary prevention of vascular disease: collaborative meta-analysis of individual participant data from randomised trials. Lancet. 2009;373(9678):1849–60.
32. Kalantzi KI, Tsoumani ME, Goudevenos IA, Tselepis AD. Pharmacodynamic properties of antiplatelet agents current knowledge and future perspectives. Expert Rev Clin Pharmacol. 2012;5(3):319–36.
33. Angiolillo DJ. Variability in responsiveness to oral antiplatelet therapy. Am J Cardiol. 2009;103(3 Suppl):27A–34A.
34. Mega JL, Close SL, Wiviott SD, Shen L, Hockett RD, Brandt JT, Walker JR, Antman EM, Macias W, Braunwald E, Sabatine MS. Cytochrome p-450 polymorphisms and response to clopidogrel. N Engl J Med. 2009;360(4):354–62.
35. Simon T, Verstuyft C, Mary-Krause M, Quteineh L, Drouet E, Méneveau N, Steg PG, Ferrières J, Danchin N, Becquemont L. French Registry of Acute ST-Elevation and Non-ST-Elevation Myocardial Infarction (FAST-MI) Investigators. Genetic determinants of response to clopidogrel and cardiovascular events. N Engl J Med. 2009;360(4):363–75.
36. Wiviott S, Trenk D, Frelinger AL, O'Donoghue M, Neumann FJ, Michelson AD, Angiolillo DJ, Hod H, Montalescot G, Miller DL, Jakubowski JA, Cairns R, Murphy SA, McCabe CH, Antman EM, Braunwald E, PRINCIPLE-TIMI 44 Investigators. Prasugrel compared with high loading- and maintenance-dose clopidogrel in patients with planned percutaneous coronary intervention: the prasugrel in comparison to clopidogrel for inhibition of platelet activation and aggregation-thrombolysis in myocardial infarction 44 trial. Circulation. 2007;116(25):2923–32.
37. Quinn MJ, Fitzgerald DJ. Ticlopidine and clopidogrel. Circulation. 1999;100(15):1667–72.
38. Duvernay M, Young S, Gailani D, Schoenecker J, Hamm HE. Protease-activated receptor (PAR) 1 and PAR4 differentially regulate factor v expression from human platelets. Mol Pharmacol. 2013;83(4):781–92.
39. Liu LW, Vu TK, Esmon CT, Coughlin SR. The region of the thrombin receptor resembling hirudin binds to thrombin and alters enzyme specificity. J Biol Chem. 1991;266:16977–80.
40. Vu TK, Wheaton VI, Hung DT, Charo I, Coughlin SR. Domains specifying thrombin-receptor interaction. Nature. 1991;353: 674–7.
41. TRA*CER Executive and Steering Committees. The thrombin receptor antagonist for clinical event reduction in acute coronary syndrome (TRA*CER) trial: study design and rationale. Am Heart J. 2009;158:327–34.
42. Bonaca MP, Scirica BM, Creager MA, Olin J, Bounameaux H, Dellborg M, Lamp JM, Murphy SA, Braunwald E, Morrow DA. Vorapaxar in patients with peripheral artery disease: results from TRA2°P-TIMI 50. Circulation. 2013;127(14):1522–9, 1529e1–6.
43. Abdulsattar Y, Ternas T, Garcia D. Vorapaxar: targeting a novel antiplatelet pathway. Pharm Ther. 2011;36(9):564–8.
44. Hoffman M, Monroe DM. Coagulation 2006: a modern view of hemostasis. Hematol Oncol Clin North Am. 2007;21(1):1–11.
45. Cawthern KM, van't Veer C, Lock JB, DiLorenzo ME, Branda RF, Mann KG. Blood coagulation in hemophilia A and hemophilia C. Blood. 1998;91(12):4581–92.
46. Von dem Borne PA, Bajzar L, Meijers JC, Nesheim ME, Bouma BN. Thrombin-mediated activation of factor XI results in a thrombin-activatable fibrinolysis inhibitor-dependent inhibition of fibrinolysis. J Clin Invest. 1997;99(10):2323–7.
47. Born GV, Cross MJ. The aggregation of blood platelets. J Physiol. 1963;168:178–95.
48. Cardinal DC, Flower RJ. The electronic aggregometer: a novel device for assessing platelet behavior in blood. J Pharmacol Methods. 1980;3(2):135–58.
49. Tóth O, Calatzis A, Penz S, Losonczy H, Siess W. Multiple electrode aggregometry: a new device to measure platelet aggregation in whole blood. Thromb Haemost. 2006;96(6):781–8.
50. Cox D. Methods for monitoring platelet function. Am Heart J. 1998;135(5 Pt 2 Su):S160–9.
51. The EPIC Investigation. Use of a monoclonal antibody directed against the platelet glycoprotein IIb/IIIa receptor in high-risk coronary angioplasty. N Engl J Med. 1994;330(14):956–61.
52. Frelinger AL, Hillman RS. Novel methods for assessing platelet function. Am Heart J. 1998;135(5 Pt 2 Su):S184–6.
53. Smith JW, Steinhubl SR, Lincoff AM, Coleman JC, Lee TT, Hillman RS, Coller BS. Rapid platelet-function assay: an automated and quantitative cartridge-based method. Circulation. 1999;99(5):620–5.
54. Kereiakes DJ, Mueller M, Howard W, Lacock P, Anderson LC, Broderick TM, Roth EM, Whang DD, Abbottsmith CW. Efficacy of abciximab induced platelet blockade using a rapid point of care assay. J Thromb Thrombolysis. 1999;7:265.
55. Lordkipanidzé M, Pharand C, Nguyen TA, Schampaert E, Diodati JG. Assessment of VerifyNow P2Y12 assay accuracy in evaluating clopidogrel-induced platelet inhibition. Ther Drug Monit. 2008;30(3):372–8.
56. Carr ME Jr. In vitro assessment of platelet function. Transfus Med Rev. 1997;11(2):106–15.
57. Trentalange MJ, Walts LF. A comparison of thromboelastogram and template bleeding time in the evaluation of platelet function after aspirin ingestion. J Clin Anesth. 1991;3(5):377–81.
58. Orlikowski CE, Payne AJ, Moodley J, Rocke DA. Thromboelastography after aspirin ingestion in pregnant and non-pregnant subjects. Br J Anaesth. 1992;69:159.
59. Blais N, Pharand C, Lordkipanidzé M, Sia YK, Merhi Y, Diodati JG. Response to aspirin in healthy individuals. Cross-comparison of light transmission aggregometry, VerifyNow system, platelet count drop, thromboelastography (TEG) and urinary 11-dehydrothromboxane B(2). Thromb Haemost. 2009;102(2):404–11.
60. Kehrel BE, Brodde MF. State of the art in platelet function testing. Transfus Med Hemother. 2013;40(2):73–86.
61. Morgagni GB. Opera Omnia. Ex Typographia Remondiniana. Venezia, Italy, 1764.
62. Boccardo P, Remuzzi G, Galbusera M. Platelet dysfunction in renal failure. Semin Thromb Hemost. 2004;30(5):579–89.
63. Di Minno G, Martinez J, McKean ML, La De, Rosa J, Burke JF, Murphy S. Platelet dysfunction in uremia. Multifaceted defect partially corrected by dialysis. Am J Med. 1985;79(5):552–9.
64. Benigni A, Livio M, Dodesini P, Schieppati A, Panigada M, Mecca G, de Gaetano G, Remuzzi G. Inhibition of human platelet

aggregation by parathyroid hormone. Is cyclic AMP implicated? Am J Nephrol. 1985;5(4):243–7.

65. Viganò G, Gotti E, Comberti E, Giangrande A, Trevisan R, Remuzzi G. Hyperparathyroidism does not influence the abnormal primary haemostasis in patients with chronic renal failure. Nephrol Dial Transplant. 1989;4(11):971–4.
66. Winter M, Frampton G, Bennett A, Machin SJ, Cameron JS. Synthesis of thromboxane B2 in uraemia and the effects of dialysis. Thromb Res. 1983;30(3):265–72.
67. Kilickesmez KO, Kocas C, Abaci O, Okcun B, Gorcin B, Gurmen T. Follow-up of aspirin-resistant patients with end-stage kidney disease. Int Urol Nephrol. 2013;45(4):1097–102.
68. Palmer SC, Di Micco L, Razavian M, Craig JC, Perkovic V, Pellegrini F, Copetti M, Graziano G, Tognoni G, Jardine M, Webster A, Nicolucci A, Zoungas S, Strippoli GF. Effects of antiplatelet therapy on mortality and cardiovascular and bleeding outcomes in persons with chronic kidney disease: a systematic review and meta-analysis. Ann Intern Med. 2012;156(6):445–59.
69. Muller C, Caillard S, Jesel L, El Ghannudi S, Ohlmann P, Sauleau E, Hannedouche T, Gachet C, Moulin B, Morel O. Association of estimated GFR with platelet inhibition in patients treated with clopidogrel. Am J Kidney Dis. 2012;59(6):777–85.
70. Kilickesmez KO, Kocas C, Okcun B, Abaci O, Kaya A, Arat A, Gorcin B, Gurmen T. Laboratory signs of aspirin response in haemodialysis patients. Scand J Clin Lab Invest. 2011;71(5):426–31.
71. Baber U, Mehran R, Kirtane AJ, Gurbel PA, Christodoulidis G, Maehara A, Witzenbichler B, Weisz G, Rinaldi MJ, Metzger DC, Henry TD, Cox DA, Duffy PL, Mazzaferri EL Jr, Xu K, Parise H, Brodie BR, Stuckey TD, Stone GW. Prevalence and impact of high platelet reactivity in chronic kidney disease: results from the Assessment of Dual Antiplatelet Therapy with Drug-Eluting Stents registry. Circ Cardiovasc Interv. 2015;8(6):e001683.
72. Htun P, Kan T, Mueller E, Pohle C, Schindler R, Geisler T, Gawaz M, Bocksch W, Fateh-Moghadam S. Haemodialysis impairs clopidogrel but not aspirin responsiveness in patients with end-stage renal disease. Results of a pilot study. Thromb Haemost. 2014;111(4):662–9.
73. Gremmel T, Müller M, Steiner S, Seidinger D, Koppensteiner R, Kopp CW, Panzer S. Chronic kidney disease is associated with increased platelet activation and poor response to antiplatelet therapy. Nephrol Dial Transplant. 2013;28(8):2116–22.
74. Aradi D, Komócsi A, Vorobcsuk A, Rideg O, Tokés-Füzesi M, Magyarlaki T, Horváth IG, Serebruany VL. Prognostic significance of high on-clopidogrel platelet reactivity after percutaneous coronary intervention: systematic review and meta-analysis. Am Heart J. 2010;160(3):543–51.
75. Buonamici P, Marcucci R, Migliorini A, Gensini GF, Santini A, Paniccia R, Moschi G, Gori AM, Abbate R, Antoniucci D. Impact of platelet reactivity after clopidogrel administration on drug-eluting stent thrombosis. J Am Coll Cardiol. 2007;49 (24):2312–7.
76. Brar SS, ten Berg J, Marcucci R, Price MJ, Valgimigli M, Kim HS, Patti G, Breet NJ, DiSciascio G, Cuisset T, Dangas G. Impact of platelet reactivity on clinical outcomes after percutaneous coronary intervention. A collaborative meta-analysis of individual participant data. J Am Coll Cardiol. 2011;58(19): 1945–54.
77. Angiolillo DJ, Bernardo E, Capodanno D, Vivas D, Sabaté M, Ferreiro JL, Ueno M, Jimenez-Quevedo P, Alfonso F, Bass TA, Macaya C, Fernandez-Ortiz A. Impact of chronic kidney disease on platelet function profiles in diabetes mellitus patients with coronary artery disease taking dual antiplatelet therapy. J Am Coll Cardiol. 2010;55(11):1139–46.
78. Morel O, El Ghannudi S, Jesel L, Radulescu B, Meyer N, Wiesel ML, Caillard S, Campia U, Moulin B, Gachet C, Ohlmann P. Cardiovascular mortality in chronic kidney disease patients undergoing percutaneous coronary intervention is mainly related to impaired P2Y12 inhibition by clopidogrel. J Am Coll Cardiol. 2011;57(4):399–408.
79. Aksu HU, Oner E, Celik O, Isiksacan N, Aksu H, Uzun S, Yavuz D, Ozturk S, Gul M, Uslu N. Aspirin resistance in patients undergoing hemodialysis and effect of hemodialysis on aspirin resistance. Clin Appl Thromb Hemost. 2015;21(1):82–6.
80. Mega JL, Close SL, Wiviott SD, Shen L, Hockett RD, Brandt JT, Walker JR, Antman EM, Macias W, Braunwald E, Sabatine MS. Cytochrome p-450 polymorphisms and response to clopidogrel. N Engl J Med. 2009;360(4):354–62.
81. Parker K, Aasebø W, Haslemo T, Stavem K. Relationship between cytochrome P450 polymorphisms and prescribed medication in elderly haemodialysis patients. SpringerPlus. 2016;5:350.
82. Jain N, Hedayati SS, Sarode R, Banerjee S, Reilly RF. Antiplatelet therapy in the management of cardiovascular disease in patients with CKD: what is the evidence? Clin J Am Soc Nephrol. 2013;8(4):665–74.
83. Spiel AO, Gilbert JC, Jilma B. Von Willebrand factor in cardiovascular disease: focus on acute coronary syndromes. Circulation. 2008;117(11):1449–59.
84. Blann AD, Kuzniatsova N, Velu S, Lip GY. Renal function and aspirin resistance in patients with coronary artery disease. Thromb Res. 2012;130(3):e103–6.
85. Baigent C, Landray M, Leaper C, Altmann P, Armitage J, Baxter A, Cairns HS, Collins R, Foley RN, Frighi V, Kourellias K, Ratcliffe PJ, Rogerson M, Scoble JE, Tomson CR, Warwick G, Wheeler DC. First United Kingdom Heart and Renal Protection (UK-HARP-I) study: biochemical efficacy and safety of simvastatin and safety of low-dose aspirin in chronic kidney disease. Am J Kidney Dis. 2005;45(3):473–84.
86. Ethier J, Bragg-Gresham JL, Piera L, Akizawa T, Asano Y, Mason N, Gillespie BW, Young EW. Aspirin prescription and outcomes in hemodialysis patients: the Dialysis Outcomes and Practice Patterns Study (DOPPS). Am J Kidney Dis. 2007;50 (4):602–11.
87. Sciahbasi A, Arcieri R, Quarto M, Pendenza G, Lanzillo C, Summaria F, Romagnoli E, Commisso C, Penco M, Lioy E. Impact of chronic aspirin and statin therapy on presentation of patients with acute myocardial infarction and impaired renal function. Prev Cardiol. 2010;13(1):18–22.
88. Leng WX, Ren JW, Cao J, Cong YL, Cui H, Hu GL, Hu QQ, Niu H, Fan L. Chronic kidney disease—is it a true risk factor of reduced clopidogrel efficacy in elderly patients with stable coronary artery disease? Thromb Res. 2013;131(3):218–24.
89. Stone GW, Witzenbichler B, Weisz G, Rinaldi MJ, Neumann FJ, Metzger DC, Henry TD, Cox DA, Duffy PL, Mazzaferri E, Gurbel PA, Xu K, Parise H, Kirtane AJ, Brodie BR, Mehran R. Stuckey TD; ADAPT-DES Investigators. Platelet reactivity and clinical outcomes after coronary artery implantation of drug-eluting stents(ADAPT-DES): a prospective multicentre registry study. Lancet. 2013;382(9892):614–23.
90. Keltai M, Tonelli M, Mann JF, Sitkei E, Lewis BS, Hawken S, Mehta SR. Yusuf S; CURE Trial Investigators. Renal function and outcomes in acute coronary syndrome: impact of clopidogrel. Eur J Cardiovasc Prev Rehabil. 2007;14(2):312–8.
91. Best PJ, Steinhubl SR, Berger PB, Dasgupta A, Brennan DM, Szczech LA, Califf RM, Topol EJ, CREDO Investigators. The efficacy and safety of short- and long-term dual antiplatelet therapy in patients with mild or moderate chronic kidney disease: results from the Clopidogrel for the Reduction of Events During Observation(CREDO) trial. Am Heart J. 2008;155(4):687–93.
92. Dasgupta A, Steinhubl SR, Bhatt DL, Berger PB, Shao M, Mak KH, Fox KA, Montalescot G, Weber MA, Haffner SM,

Dimas AP, Steg PG, Topol EJ, CHARISMA Investigators. Clinical outcomes of patients with diabetic nephropathy randomized to clopidogrel plus aspirin versusaspirin alone (a post hoc analysis of the clopidogrel for high atherothrombotic risk and ischemicstabilization, management, and avoidance [CHARISMA] trial). Am J Cardiol. 2009;103(10):1359–63.

93. Robey RB, O'Rourke DJ. Effects of antiplatelet therapy on mortality and cardiovascular and bleeding outcomes in persons with chronic kidney disease. Ann Intern Med. 2012;157(4):302–3 author reply 303–4.
94. Kussmaul W. Effects of antiplatelet therapy on mortality and cardiovascular and bleeding outcomes in persons with chronic kidney disease. Ann Intern Med. 2012;157(4):302 author reply 303–4.
95. Chandrasekhar J, Dangas G, Baber U, Sartori S, Aquino M, Kini A, Muhlestein B, Strauss C, Henry T, Defranco A, Toma C, Kapadia S, Rao S, Weiss S, Weintraub W, Effron M, Keller S, Baker B, Pocock S, Mehran R. Impact of prasugrel vs. clopidogrel in the presence of chronic kidney disease in ACS PCI: results from the PROMETHEUS study [Abstract]. In: EuroPCR 2016; 2016, May 6. Paris, France.
96. Nishi T, Ariyoshi N, Nakayama T, Fujimoto Y, Sugimoto K, Wakabayashi S, Hanaoka H, Kobayashi Y. Impact of chronic kidney disease on platelet inhibition of clopidogrel and prasugrel in Japanese patients. J Cardiol. 2016. pii: S0914–5087(16) 30171-X.
97. James S, Budaj A, Aylward P, Buck KK, Cannon CP, Cornel JH, Harrington RA, Horrow J, Katus H, Keltai M, Lewis BS, Parikh K, Storey RF, Szummer K, Wojdyla D, Wallentin L. Ticagrelor versus clopidogrel in acute coronary syndromes in relation to renal function: results from the Platelet Inhibition and Patient Outcomes (PLATO) trial. Circulation. 2010;122 (11):1056–67.
98. Price MJ, Berger PB, Teirstein PS, Tanguay JF, Angiolillo DJ, Spriggs D, Puri S, Robbins M, Garratt KN, Bertrand OF, Stillabower ME, Aragon JR, Kandzari DE, Stinis CT, Lee MS, Manoukian SV, Cannon CP, Schork NJ, Topol EJ, GRAVITAS Investigators. Standard- vs high-dose clopidogrel based on platelet function testing after percutaneous coronary intervention: the GRAVITAS randomized trial. JAMA. 2011;305(11):1097–105.
99. Trenk D, Stone GW, Gawaz M, Kastrati A, Angiolillo DJ, Müller U, Richardt G, Jakubowski JA, Neumann FJ. A randomized trial of prasugrel versus clopidogrel in patients with high platelet reactivity on clopidogrelafter elective percutaneous coronary intervention with implantation of drug-eluting stents: results of the TRIGGER-PCI (Testing Platelet Reactivity In Patients Undergoing Elective Stent Placement on Clopidogrel to Guide Alternative Therapy With Prasugrel) study. J Am Coll Cardiol. 2012;59(24):2159–64.
100. Collet JP, Cuisset T, Rangé G, Cayla G, Elhadad S, Pouillot C, Henry P, Motreff P, Carrié D, Boueri Z, Belle L, Van Belle E, Rousseau H, Aubry P, Monségu J, Sabouret P, O'Connor SA, Abtan J, Kerneis M, Saint-Etienne C, Barthélémy O, Beygui F, Silvain J, Vicaut E, Montalescot G, ARCTIC Investigators. Bedside monitoring to adjust antiplatelet therapy for coronary stenting. N Engl J Med. 2012;367(22):2100–9.
101. Mahla E, Suarez TA, Bliden KP, Rehak P, Metzler H, Sequeira AJ, Cho P, Sell J, Fan J, Antonino MJ, Tantry US, Gurbel PA. Platelet function measurement-based strategy to reduce bleeding and waiting time in clopidogrel-treated patients undergoing coronary artery bypass graft surgery: the timing based on platelet function strategy to reduce clopidogrel-associated bleeding related to CABG (TARGET-CABG) study. Circ Cardiovasc Interv. 2012;5(2):261–9.
102. National Institute of Diabetes and Digestive and Kidney Diseases Kidney Disease Statistics for the United States https://www.niddk.nih.gov/health-information/health-statistics/Pages/kidney-disease-statistics-united-states.aspx. Accessed 20 January 2017.

Part VI

Interventional Strategies in Cardiovascular Disease in CKD

Revascularization Strategies in Chronic Kidney Disease: Percutaneous Coronary Intervention Versus Coronary Artery Bypass Graft Surgery

30

Amit V. Patel and Sripal Bangalore

CAD in CKD: Why Is CAD a Problem in Patients with CKD?

Statistics and Background

There has been an explosion in the prevalence of patients with chronic kidney disease (CKD) in the past decades and this is projected to increase further as obesity and its metabolic sequelae including diabetes mellitus increases [1]. According to the Centers for Disease Control's National Health and Nutrition Examination Survey (NHANES), there are over 20 million adults with CKD in the United States, and this is predicted to increase, from 13.2% currently to 16.7% by 2030 [1]. In addition, the number of patients with end-stage kidney disease (ESKD) on renal replacement therapy in the U.S. is expected to increase from 330,000 in 2007 to 534,000 by 2020 [2, 3]. Cardiovascular disease (CVD) is the leading cause of morbidity and mortality in patients with CKD and accounts for 44% of all-cause mortality [4]. Most patients with CKD succumb to cardiovascular death rather than develop ESKD [5]. However, even among those who develop ESKD and eventually have renal transplant, CVD has surpassed infection as the leading cause of death [6].

Patients with CKD have a high prevalence of coronary artery disease (CAD), and the American College of Cardiology (ACC)/American Heart Association (AHA) task force and National Kidney Foundation have proposed CKD as a coronary heart disease equivalent [7]. In addition to a high prevalence of traditional atherosclerotic risk factors, such as hypertension and diabetes mellitus, patients with CKD also have increased inflammation, oxidative stress, and anemia which may further accelerate atherosclerosis and contribute to the high prevalence of CAD [8]. Patients with CKD have an increased risk of CV events and all-cause mortality, which increases exponentially with lower eGFR (Table 30.1) [9]. Patients with CKD not on dialysis have a much higher contribution of atherosclerosis to cardiovascular mortality than patients who are ESKD, who have an increase in cardiovascular mortality from nonatherosclerotic mechanisms such as arrhythmia and sudden cardiac death (Fig. 30.1) [10].

CAD in CKD: Treatment Options

In patients with CAD and CKD, optimal medical therapy, percutaneous coronary intervention (PCI), and coronary artery bypass graft surgery (CABG) are treatment options.

Despite the high prevalence of CAD and its associated high morbidity and mortality, the majority of cardiovascular clinical trials comparing treatment options have routinely excluded patients with CKD (Fig. 30.2) [11]. As such, data on outcomes with treatment of CAD in CKD comes from observational studies or from extrapolation of results from randomized trials done predominantly in the non-CKD cohort. Observational studies have selection and ascertainment bias and there is heterogeneity in the study design with only a few studies reporting outcomes by level of kidney function, others having small sample size, using different definitions of CKD, including limited spectra of CKD, or not reporting on the severity of pre-revascularization CAD

A.V. Patel
Department of Medicine, Division of Cardiology, NYU Langone Medical Center, 550 1st Avenue, New York, NY 10016, USA
e-mail: Amit.Patel@nyumc.org

S. Bangalore (✉)
Department of Medicine, Division of Cardiology, New York University School of Medicine, 530 First Avenue, SKI 9R/109, New York, NY 10016, USA
e-mail: Sripalbangalore@gmail.com

J. Rangaswami et al. (eds.), *Cardio-Nephrology*,
DOI 10.1007/978-3-319-56042-7_30

Table 30.1 Association of eGFR with all-cause mortality and cardiovascular events

eGFR category (mL/min/1.73 m^2)	All-cause mortality HR (95% CI)	Cardiovascular events (Hospitalization for CAD, heart failure, stroke, peripheral arterial disease) HR (95% CI)
eGFR $\geq$ 60	Reference	Reference
eGFR 45–59	1.2 (1.1–1.2)	1.4 (1.4–1.5)
eGFR 30–44	1.8 (1.7–1.9)	2.0 (1.9–2.1)
eGFR 15–29	3.2 (3.1–3.4)	2.8 (2.6–2.9)
eGFR <15	5.9 (5.4–6.5)	3.4 (3.1–3.8)

CI confidence interval, *eGFR* estimated glomerular filtration rate, *HR* hazard ratio

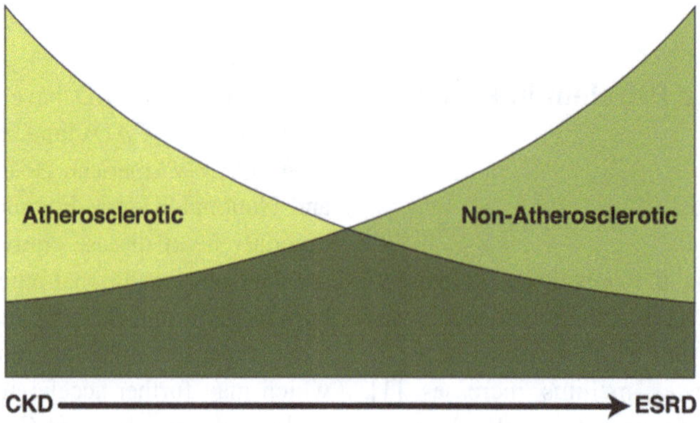

Fig. 30.1 Cardiovascular mortality in patients with chronic kidney disease versus end-stage kidney disease (Reproduced with permission from: Herzog et al. Atherosclerotic versus nonatherosclerotic evaluation: the Yin and Yang of cardiovascular imaging in advanced chronic kidney disease. JACC Cardiovascular imaging. 2014; 7(7): 729–32)

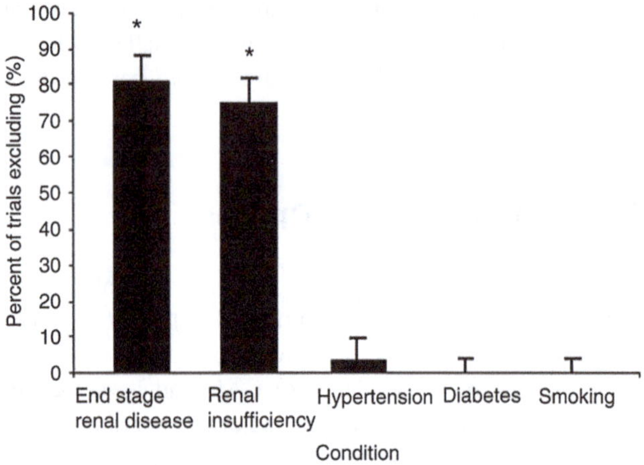

Fig. 30.2 Percentage of cardiovascular clinical trials that exclude patients with end-stage kidney disease, renal insufficiency, hypertension, diabetes, smoking (Reproduced with permission from: Charytan et al. The exclusion of patients with chronic kidney disease from clinical trials in coronary artery disease. Kidney international. 2006; 70 (11): 2021–30)

making comparisons between treatment modalities difficult. In addition, it is not known if extrapolation of data from non-CKD cohorts is justifiable.

Revascularization versus Medical Management

Contemporary randomized trials of medical therapy versus revascularization (such as COURAGE, BARI-2D, and FAME-2) have routinely excluded patients with CKD or included only a small proportion of such patients. Observational studies suggest that revascularization (PCI or CABG) is associated with lower mortality when compared with medical therapy alone [8], however patients with CKD undergo less revascularization than patients without CKD, despite being a significantly higher risk population for atherosclerotic events (Fig. 30.3) [12]. The quality of medical therapy was not reported in these observational studies and there is concern about selection and ascertainment bias. The International Study of Comparative Health Effectiveness with Medical and Invasive Approaches–Chronic Kidney Disease trial (ISCHEMIA–CKD) is an National Heart, Lung, and Blood Institute funded multicenter, international randomized clinical trial that aims to determine the best management strategy for patients with stable ischemic heart disease and advanced CKD (eGFR < 30 or on dialysis), comparing optimal medical therapy and revascularization versus optimal medical therapy alone, and will offer important insights into the treatment of such patients.

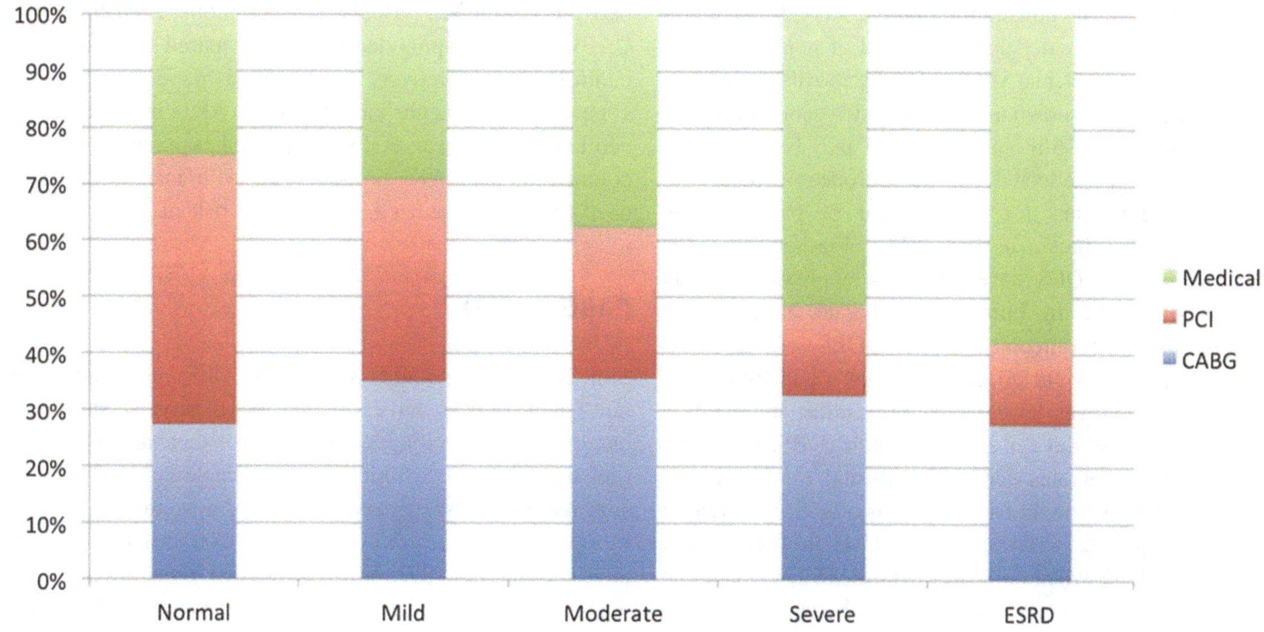

Fig. 30.3 Use of revascularization versus medical therapy as a function of baseline renal function (Adapted from Ref. [12])

Revascularization in CKD: Challenges

Patients with CKD have complex CAD with high prevalence of multivessel disease, small, heavily calcified, and diffusely diseased vessels [13], which increases the likelihood of incomplete revascularization [14]. Moreover, the presence of calcification and medial thickening of arteries increases the risk of under-expanded stents with higher risk of restenosis and stent thrombosis. In addition, the accelerated atherosclerotic process, as well as lack of response to vasoprotective medications such as statins also contributes to worse outcomes when compared with non-CKD cohorts [8, 15, 16]. Studies have therefore shown that patients with CKD have worse outcomes than non-CKD cohorts even after revascularization.

PCI in CKD

PCI has evolved from percutaneous transluminal coronary angioplasty (PTCA) to bare metal stents (BMS) to the use of drug eluting stents (DES). In a large registry study involving > 280,000 patients with a spectrum of renal function, including dialysis patients, first- generation DES use was associated with lower 30-month death rate compared to BMS in patients with normal renal function (12.2 vs. 14.7%, $p < 0.001$), mild CKD (15.1 vs. 18.6%, $p < 0.001$), moderate CKD (24.1 vs. 26.6%, $p < 0.001$), severe CKD (33.7 vs. 33.7%, $p = 0.04$) and in patients on dialysis (48.9 vs. 56.4%, $p < 0.001$). In addition, use of DES was also associated with lower adjusted 30-month myocardial infarction rates across the board, except in those on dialysis [17]. Even among DES there has been considerable progress in technology with the second-generation DES having thinner struts, thinner and more biocompatible polymers all of which reduce the risk of restenosis and stent thrombosis. As such, data from randomized trials (all-comers) have shown that the second-generation DES are associated with significantly reduced target vessel revascularization, definite stent thrombosis, MI and death compared to BMS and is the current standard for patients undergoing PCI [18, 19]. Current guidelines on the management of cardiac disease in kidney transplant candidates address stent selection in the context of transplant consideration given the general recommendations for continuation of dual antiplatelet therapy (DAPT) for at least 1 month after BMS and at least 12 months after DES [20]. For patients revascularized with PCI who need transplant surgery in the subsequent 12 months, a strategy of PTCA or BMS placement followed by 4–12 weeks of DAPT is recommended by the guidelines. However, these recommendations stem from older studies from the first-generation DES era. One recent clinical trial randomized patients deemed to be uncertain candidates for DES on the basis of high bleeding risk or high thrombotic risk (including upcoming surgery) to either second-generation DES (Zotarolimus- eluting stent) or BMS with a shorter DAPT duration (median 32 days) [21]. The study found that second-generation DES use had significantly less MI (2.9 vs. 8.1%, $p < 0.001$), target vessel revascularization (5.9 vs. 10.7%, $p = 0.001$), and definite or probable stent thrombosis (2.0 vs. 4.1%, $p = 0.019$)

compared to BMS demonstrating that the second-generation DES are potentially safer than BMS and of note ~40% of patients in this study had CrCl < 60. Moreover, other randomized trials have shown that with second- generation DES a shorter duration (3–6 months) of DAPT may be reasonable [22] and this is reflected in the European Society of Cardiology guidelines for management of patients with stable ischemic heart disease [23]. Furthermore, the second-generation DES have CE mark approval for only 1 month of DAPT in Europe. A separate, retrospective analysis evaluated outcomes between DES and BMS in patients who underwent noncardiac surgery and found that the risk of events was lowest when noncardiac surgery was performed after 90 days of implantation of DES. However, with BMS the event rates were uniformly high through 1-year post stent implantation. In fact, there was a 26% lower rate of death or MI (OR 0.74, 95% CI 0.58–0.94) at 30 days after surgery with DES when compared with BMS [24]. Thus, in patients who need renal transplant in the near future, a strategy of implantation of second- generation DES with DAPT use for a minimum of 3 months is reasonable, however further studies are needed.

Regardless of the PCI era, patients with CKD and especially those with ESKD have significant increase in the risk of restenosis, stent thrombosis, myocardial infarction, and death when compared with patients without CKD after PCI [17, 25]. In an observational study of PCI with first-generation DES, patients with a spectrum of CKD had significant higher rates of death, MI, and revascularization when compared with patients without CKD [17]. Although the outcomes have significantly improved in the second-generation DES era [18, 19], the worse outcomes in patients with CKD persist. In a small observational study with 400 patients, ~25% of whom had CKD (GFR < 60), PCI with second-generation DES in patients with CKD compared to controls demonstrated similar risk of nonfatal MI (2.08 vs. 0.98%, $p = 0.59$) and target lesion revascularization (1.04 vs. 1.97%, $p = 0.99$), but was associated with higher mortality (4.16 vs. 0.65%, $p = 0.03$) [26].

The increased risk of restenosis is likely due to under-expansion of stents secondary to calcified arteries and also rapid progression of CAD. Similarly, the increased risk of stent thrombosis has been attributed to stent mal-apposition. The increased risk of death or MI has been attributed to increased risk of restenosis and stent thrombosis but also to non-culprit lesion-related events due to rapid progression of CAD.

In the short term, PCI in patients with CKD is associated with increased peri-procedural complications including higher rates of access site and non-access site bleeding, peri-procedural MI, vascular complications, need for urgent CABG and in-hospital death when compared with non-CKD controls [14]. Moreover, in pre-dialysis patients, the risk of contrast-induced acute kidney injury (AKI) increases exponentially with lower eGFR [27]. Studies have shown that contrast-induced AKI is associated with increased risk of need for dialysis as well as increased risk of death.

CABG in CKD

Similar to PCI, patients with CKD when compared with non-CKD controls, have a higher risk of adverse short-term outcomes such as longer postoperative mechanical ventilation time, higher postoperative bleeding rates and transfusion requirements, increased length of hospital stay, sepsis, mediastinitis, myocardial infarction, AKI, stroke, and death after CABG [28, 29]. With regards to precipitating AKI, which is often a concern when performing PCI, a large retrospective analysis using Medicare claims data found that the risk of AKI was significantly higher with CABG than PCI for all-comers (OR 2.56, 95% CI 2.42–2.71) and for patients with CKD (OR 2.10, 95% CI 1.89–2.33) [27]. Operative mortality for CABG is also significantly higher for patients with ESKD than for those without, even after adjusting for confounders. In one study, early mortality was threefold higher in patients on dialysis versus not on dialysis after CABG and these findings remained significant after adjusting for age, disease severity, and comorbid conditions [30].

Long-term outcomes after CABG are also worse in patients with CKD when compared to those without CKD. In one study comparing long-term outcomes in patients with CKD to those without CKD, patients with CKD had a significantly higher rate of cardiac hospitalization at 5 years after CABG (2.48 vs. 1.77, $p < 0.001$), and the presence of CKD (defined as pre-procedure serum creatinine > 1.5 mg/dL) was an independent risk factor for all-cause mortality at 7 years following revascularization (RR 2.31, 95% CI 1.63–2.38) [31]. Despite the higher short-term and long-term morbidity and mortality in patients with CKD, saphenous vein graft (SVG) patency and internal mammary artery (IMA) patency are similar between these groups. At 1 year, SVG failure rate (OR 1.02, 95% CI 0.79–1.33) and IMA failure rate (OR 0.76, 95% CI 0.40–1.44) were similar between patients with CKD (defined as CrCl < 50) and no CKD, suggesting that other factors (such as non-culprit lesion related events or other comorbidities) are responsible for the increased adverse outcomes in patients with CKD [32].

Revascularization Options in CKD: PCI versus CABG

In patients with single vessel CAD, given the upfront risk of CABG in patients with CKD, PCI is a reasonable option. The below discussion on PCI versus CABG mainly pertains to patients with multivessel CAD.

There are several factors to consider in deciding between PCI and CABG. In addition to patient preferences and comorbidities, the extent and complexity of CAD are important (Sect. 4.1). Current ACC/AHA guidelines state that performing CABG in ESKD patients may be reasonable to improve mortality and/or relieve angina in certain anatomic subgroups (left main disease, three-vessel disease, two-vessel disease with proximal left anterior descending artery involvement) assuming life expectancy is not limited [33]. However, no specific scenarios in which PCI may be beneficial are discussed. These recommendations are echoed by the ACC/AHA guidelines for evaluation of cardiac disease in kidney transplantation candidates [20]. European Society of Cardiology and European Association of Cardiothoracic Surgery guidelines recommend CABG over PCI in patients with moderate to severe CKD whose surgical risk is acceptable, and with life expectancy >1 year [34]. If surgical risk is high and/or life expectancy is less than 1 year, PCI with DES should be considered over CABG (Table 30.2).

PTCA Versus CABG

The first PTCA was performed in 1977 and was the only form of PCI available until the late 1980s but seldom performed these days due to increased risk of complications including abrupt vessel closure and peri-procedural MI [35]. In an analysis from the United States Renal Data System (USRDS) database, there was significantly lower perioperative mortality with PTCA when compared with CABG in patients with ESKD (5.4 vs. 12.5%; $p = 0.014$). However, the survival curves crossed each other with significantly higher 2 and 5-year survival with CABG than with PTCA (56.9 vs. 52.9% at 2 years, 26.5 vs. 23.2% at 5 years) [36]. Thus, when compared with PTCA, CABG has higher upfront mortality but lower long-term mortality.

BMS Versus CABG

The next technological advance in PCI was the introduction of bare metal stents (BMS) in the late 1980s and early 1990s. BMS offered a solution to some of the problems of abrupt vessel closure and restenosis with PTCA [15].

In a subgroup analysis of the Arterial Revascularization Therapies Study there was no difference in nonfatal MI, stroke, or death with BMS versus CABG over 3 year follow-up in 290 patients with CKD (CrCl $\leq$ 50 mL/min).

Table 30.2 Major society guideline recommendations for coronary revascularization in patients with chronic kidney disease

Society	Year	Recommendations
ACCF/AHA (33)	2011	CABG to improve survival rate may be reasonable in patients with end-stage kidney disease undergoing CABG for left main coronary artery stenosis of $\geq$50% (Class IIB, LOE C) CABG to improve survival rate or to relieve angina despite guideline directed medical therapy may be reasonable for patients with end-stage kidney disease with significant stenoses ($\geq$70%) in 3 major vessels or in the proximal LAD plus 1 other major vessel, regardless of left ventricular systolic function (Class IIB, LOE B) CABG should NOT be performed in patients with end-stage kidney disease whose life expectancy is limited by noncardiac issues (Class III, LOE C)
ESC/EACTS (34)	2014	CABG should be considered over PCI in patients with moderate or severe CKD, multivessel CAD and symptoms/ischemia whose surgical risk profile is acceptable and life expectancy is beyond 1 year (Class IIA, LOE B) PCI should be considered over CABG in patients with moderate or severe CKD, multivessel CAD and symptoms/ischemia whose surgical risk profile is high or life expectancy is less than 1 year (Class IIA, LOE B) New-generation DES are recommended over BMS (Class I, LOE B)

ACCF/AHA American College of Cardiology Foundation/American Heart Association, *BMS* bare metal stents, *CABG* coronary artery bypass graft surgery, *CAD* coronary artery disease, *CKD* chronic kidney disease, *DES* drug eluting stents, *ESC/EACTS* European Society of Cardiology/European Association for Cardio-Thoracic Surgery, *LAD* Left anterior descending, *LOE* Level of evidence, *PCI* percutaneous coronary intervention

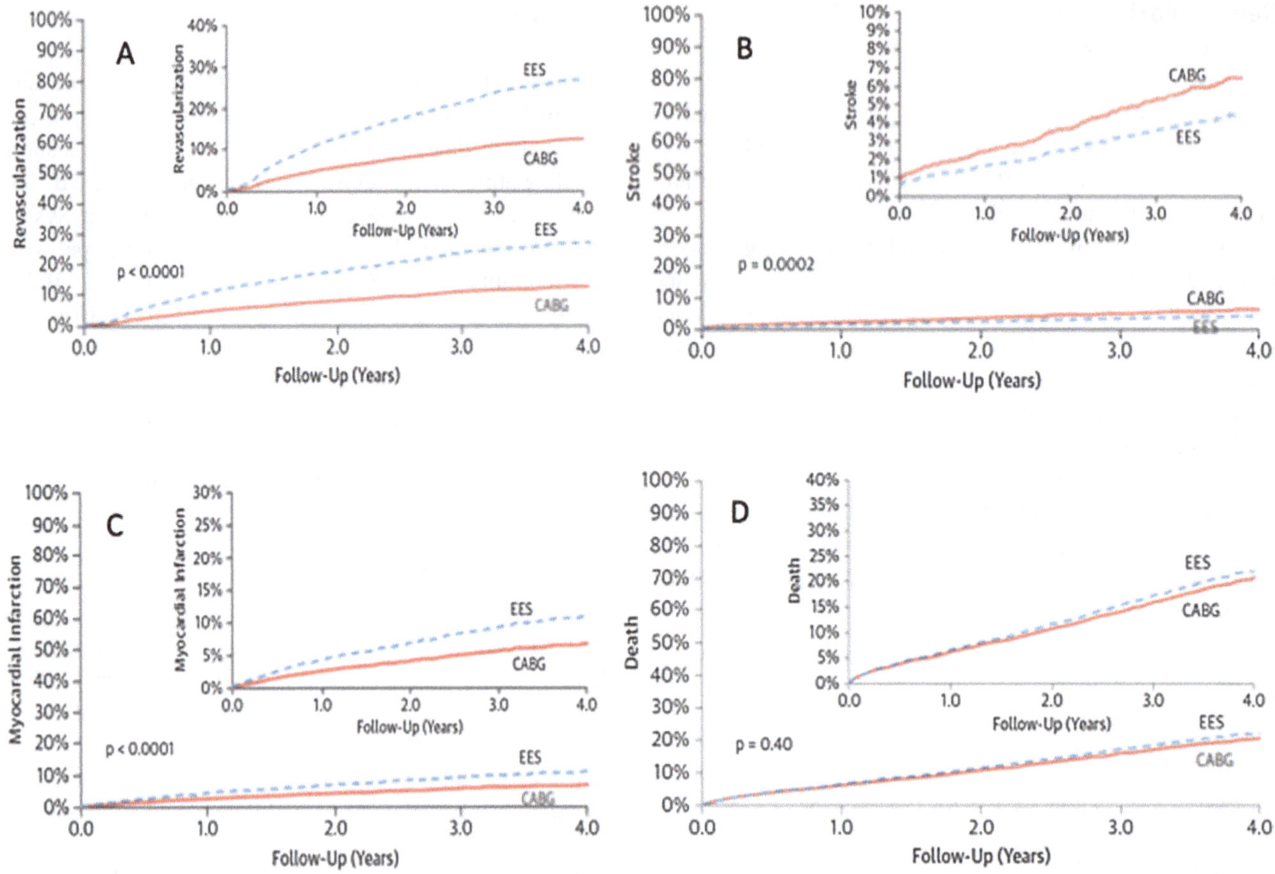

Fig. 30.4 Long-term outcomes with everolimus eluting stents (second-generation drug-eluting stent) versus coronary artery bypass graft surgery in patients with chronic kidney disease. **a** Repeat revascularization, **b** Stroke, **c** Myocardial infarction, **d** Death. (Reproduced with permission from: Bangalore et al. Revascularization in Patients with Multivessel Coronary Artery Disease and Chronic Kidney Disease: Everolimus-Eluting Stents Versus Coronary Artery Bypass Graft Surgery. J Am Coll Cardiol. 2015; 66(11): 1209–20)

However, CABG was associated with a significant reduction in repeat revascularization [37]. On the contrary, in a large observational study, CABG was associated with a significantly lower risk of death when compared to BMS (HR 0.75, 95% CI 0.56–0.99) in patients with CKD not on dialysis [8]. These findings were supported by a meta-analysis which showed significantly higher long-term mortality (OR 2.91, 95% CI 2.69–3.15) and repeat revascularization (OR 5.07, 95% CI 3.35–7.65) with BMS versus CABG in patients with CKD [38].

In patients with ESKD, among 4,280 patients who underwent PCI with BMS and 6,688 patients who underwent CABG, in-hospital death was lower for the BMS group (4.1 vs. 8.6) when compared with the CABG group. However, by 24 months ESKD patients who had undergone CABG had a significantly higher survival when compared with those who underwent BMS placement (56.4 ± 1.4 vs. 48.4 ± 2%, $p < 0.001$). Thus even when compared with BMS, CABG has higher upfront mortality but lower long-term mortality.

Drug Eluting Stents (DES) Versus CABG

The next advance in PCI was the introduction of DES in 2002. DES further improved upon BMS in that they further reduced restenosis. In the largest randomized trial comparing outcomes between CABG and first-generation DES in patients with diabetes mellitus, the FREEDOM trial, CABG reduced death and MI but increased stroke over a median of 3.8 years follow-up [39]. In addition, there was a significantly higher risk of AKI requiring hemodialysis within 30 days after the revascularization with CABG compared to those undergoing PCI (0.844 vs. 0.1%, $p = 0.02$). However, less than 10% of the patients enrolled in this trial had CKD. Thus, there is limited randomized trial data comparing CABG and DES in patients with CKD.

However, the relevance of the above studies comparing CABG with first-generation DES, to modern day practice of PCI using second-generation DES, is questionable. As outlined above, newer generation DES have been shown to be

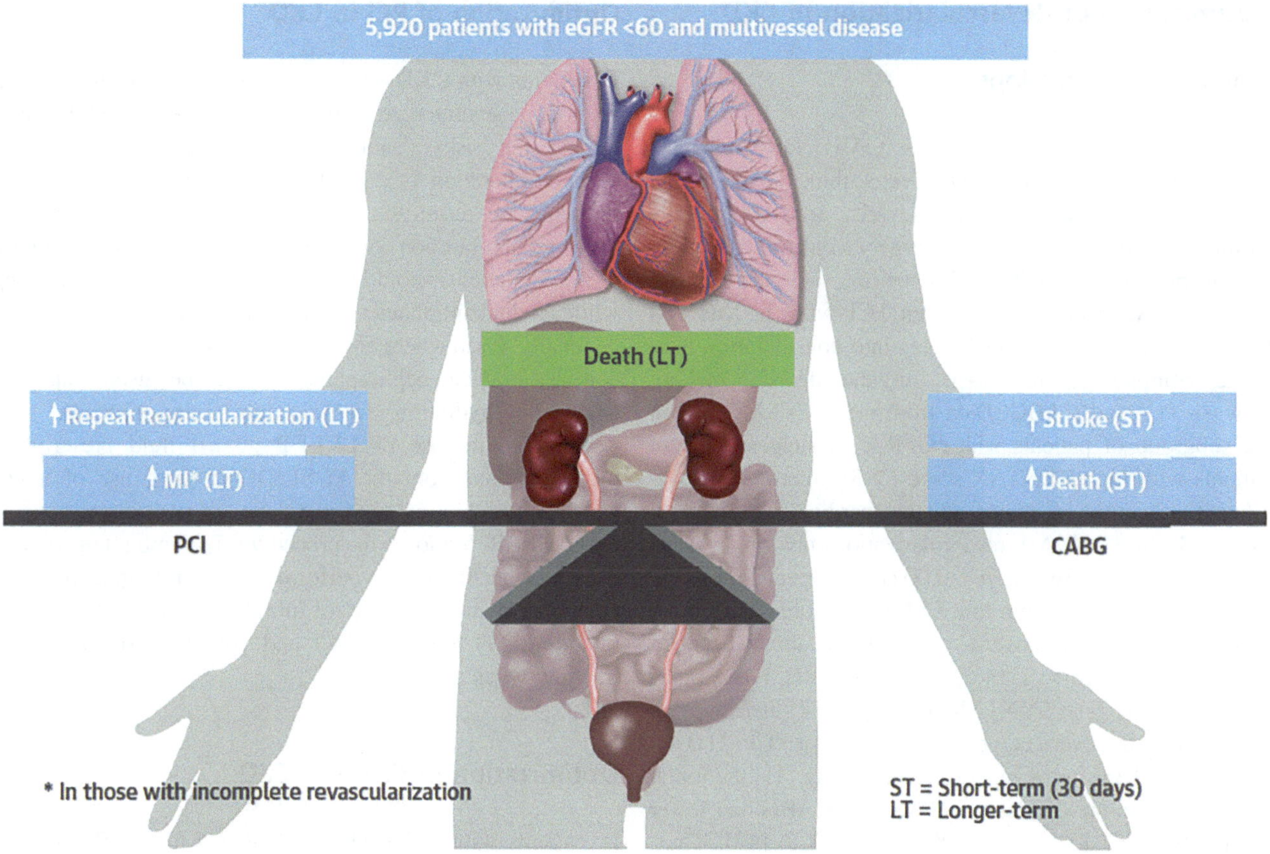

Fig. 30.5 Outcomes with second-generation drug-eluting stents versus coronary artery bypass graft surgery in patients with chronic kidney disease (Reproduced with permission from: Bangalore et al. Revascularization in Patients With Multivessel Coronary Artery Disease and Chronic Kidney Disease: Everolimus-Eluting Stents Versus Coronary Artery Bypass Graft Surgery. J Am Coll Cardiol. 2015; 66(11): 1209–20)

associated with reduction in restenosis, stent thrombosis but also death and MI, and is currently the standard of care for all patients undergoing PCI [18, 19]. Data from the New York State registries involving 2690 patients who underwent PCI with newer generation DES [everolimus-eluting stents (EES)] and propensity score matched with 2690 patients who underwent CABG showed that PCI was associated with a significantly lower short-term (within 30 days) risk of death, stroke, and repeat revascularization [40]. In the long term, PCI with second-generation DES was associated with a similar risk of death compared to CABG over an average of 2.9 years follow-up. Thus, the mortality difference between older generations of PCI versus CABG was no longer seen when PCI was performed using newer generation DES. This was consistent across anatomic subgroups based on number of diseased vessels (2-vessel vs. 3-vessel disease) and completeness of revascularization. However, in the long term, PCI was also associated with higher risk of MI and higher rate of repeat revascularization, primarily driven by those with three-vessel disease and in those who were incompletely revascularized (Fig. 30.4) [40]. The increased risk of MI with PCI was no longer significant in the subgroup of patients who underwent complete revascularization with PCI. This demonstrates that the use of second-generation DES for PCI in patients with CKD is associated with similar long-term survival as with patients undergoing CABG, thus suggesting that second-generation DES might help bridge the outcome gap between PCI versus CABG (Fig. 30.5) [40]. However, randomized trials of PCI versus CABG in patients with CKD are needed to test these associations.

In patients on dialysis, PCI was associated with a significantly higher long-term risk of death, a numerically higher risk of MI, a significantly higher risk of repeat revascularization, and no difference in stroke compared with CABG [40]. However, the dialysis subgroup was a smaller group of patients and was likely underpowered but suggests superior outcomes with CABG over PCI despite the higher upfront risk with CABG. However, randomized trials are needed to confirm these associations.

Optimization of Revascularization in CKD

General Considerations

When deciding between PCI versus CABG for revascularization in patients with CKD several things need to be considered including extent and severity of CAD, comorbidities, frailty, prior cardiac surgery, ejection fraction, patient preferences, and local expertise, amongst others. The SYNTAX (SYNergy between PCI with TAXus and Cardiac Surgery) score which takes into consideration anatomic complexity, may assist in the decision-making between PCI and CABG. Data from the SYNTAX trial in the subgroup of patients with eGFR < 60 suggests that in patients with high SYNTAX score (≥ 33) there was a significant reduction in major adverse cardiac and cerebral events (death, CVA, MI, revascularization) favoring CABG over PCI (7.4 vs. 36.6%, $p = 0.002$) at 2 years follow-up. However, for those with a low SYNTAX score (<23), there was no difference in adverse events listed above between CABG and PCI (18.4 vs. 14.6%, $p = 0.68$) [41]. For patients with an intermediate SYNTAX scores [23–34] there was no difference in the event rate between CABG or PCI (21.3 vs. 28.3%, $p = 0.35$) in the renal subgroup study [41], although at 3–4 years in the overall SYNTAX trial CABG had fewer events than PCI (21.5 vs. 32.0%, $p = 0.0006$) [42]. Thus, PCI is preferred for patients with a low SYNTAX score, CABG is preferred for those with a high SYNTAX score and either PCI or CABG for those with an intermediate SYNTAX score. In addition, if renal transplant is anticipated in the near future, the upfront risk of CABG should be weighed against the need for dual antiplatelet therapy and consequent higher bleeding risk in those who undergo PCI.

Optimization of PCI in CKD

In patients with CKD who are planned for PCI several measures can be undertaken to maximize efficacy while minimizing the risks (Table 30.3). Use of DES, especially second-generation DES, is highly recommended to reduce the risk of restenosis and potentially reduce death or myocardial infarction compared with BMS or first-generation DES. All patients should be monitored carefully for bleeding while on dual antiplatelet therapy, and all medications should be renally dosed where applicable. Measures to reduce risk of contrast-induced nephropathy should be used, such as aggressive hydration pre-procedure, intra-procedure, and post-procedure, use of LVEDP guided fluid prescription based on data from the POSEIDON study, use of iso-or low-osmolar contrast, and avoidance of nephrotoxic agents for at least 48 h prior to the procedure. The amount of contrast used can be limited by performing ischemia-guided revascularization and the use of ultralow contrast techniques including IVUS guided PCI and with the use of biplane imaging when appropriate.

Optimization of CABG in CKD

In patients with CKD who are planned for CABG several measures can be undertaken to maximize efficacy while minimizing the risks (Table 30.4). One should consider delay of surgery ≥ 7 days from time of cardiac catheterization to minimize risk of acute kidney injury. Furthermore, use of off-pump surgery and use of multiple arterial grafts for bypass should be considered. Off-pump CABG is an attractive option for surgical revascularization of CAD due

Table 30.3 Optimization of PCI in patients with chronic kidney disease

Use drug-eluting stents, new generation preferred
Monitor carefully for bleeding on dual antiplatelet therapy
Renally dose all medications
Minimize contrast-induced acute kidney injury -Pre-, intra-and post-procedure hydration -Pre-procedure high dose statins -Avoid nephrotoxic agents for at least 48 h prior -Use iso-or low-osmolar contrast agents -Limit contrast used --Ultra-low volume contrast techniques (IVUS guided PCI) --Avoid ventriculography --Use of biplane if available --Consider ischemia-guided revascularization --Consider staged PCI for complex multivessel disease

IVUS intravascular ultrasound, *PCI* percutaneous coronary intervention

Table 30.4 Optimization of CABG in patients with chronic kidney disease

Consider delay of surgery ≥ 7 days from time of cardiac catheterization to reduce risk of contrast nephropathy (33)
Use of off-pump coronary artery bypass graft surgery may be reasonable to reduce risk of serious acute kidney injury (33)
Renally dose all medications
In patients undergoing on pump CABG, maintain perioperative hematocrit >19% and mean arterial pressure >60 mmHg (33)
Use internal mammary artery bypass grafts when able

to less perioperative fluid shifts, less bleeding, and reduced need for prolonged mechanical ventilation [43]. However, patients referred for off-pump CABG need to have anatomy suitable for placement of distal anastomoses such that one is able to achieve complete revascularization [44]. The use of multiple arterial grafts when feasible during CABG is associated with reduced cardiovascular events and mortality [45]. Although there are no prospective studies comparing the use of venous and arterial grafts in patients with CKD, observational studies have demonstrated excellent 5-year survival rates when mammary grafts are used, as well as reduced in-hospital and long-term mortality in ESKD patients [44]. In a study with 7,152 ESKD patients from the STS database, the OR for 30-day mortality was lower for ESKD patients who received mammary artery grafts than for venous grafts (OR 3.6, 95% CI 3.2–4.4, vs. OR 4.3, 95% CI 3.1–6.1, $p < 0.009$) compared to patients who had normal renal function and undergoing similar procedures [29]. It is important to be aware, though, that the use of the mammary artery from the same side as an AV fistula can result in coronary steal during dialysis.

Conclusions

There are no prospective, randomized trials comparing outcomes between PCI and CABG in patients with CKD. PCI offers the advantage of being less invasive and with reduced peri-procedural morbidity and mortality compared to CABG. However, PCI is associated with increased rates of restenosis, death, and MI when compared with CABG over the long run. However, data comparing CABG to PCI using newer generation DES is promising with bridging of the mortality gap between CABG and PCI. Data suggests that the decision between PCI and CABG in patients with CKD should be based on weighing the upfront risk of death and stroke with CABG to long-term risk of repeat revascularization and myocardial infarction (in those with incomplete revascularization) with PCI using second-generation DES. In the absence of prospective, randomized trial data to help guide optimal management strategies for revascularization in patients with CKD, the choice of revascularization methodology needs to be individualized with a focus on patient comorbidities, ability to tolerate antiplatelet therapy, coronary anatomy, and balancing higher upfront mortality with potentially better long-term mortality, and likelihood for achieving complete revascularization.

References

1. Hoerger TJ, Simpson SA, Yarnoff BO, Pavkov ME, Rios Burrows N, Saydah SH, et al. The future burden of CKD in the United States: a simulation model for the CDC CKD initiative. Am J Kidney Dis. 2015;65(3):403–11.
2. Collins AJ, Foley R, Herzog C, Chavers B, Gilbertson D, Ishani A, et al. Excerpts from the United States Renal Data System 2007 annual data report. Am J Kidney Dis. 2008;51(1 Suppl 1):S1–320.
3. Coresh J, Selvin E, Stevens LA, Manzi J, Kusek JW, Eggers P, et al. Prevalence of chronic kidney disease in the United States. JAMA. 2007;298(17):2038–47.
4. NIH. USRDS 2000 Annual data report. 2000; Publication No. (NIH) 00–3176:589–684 and 69–75.
5. Charytan DM, Li S, Liu J, Herzog CA. Risks of death and end-stage renal disease after surgical compared with percutaneous coronary revascularization in elderly patients with chronic kidney disease. Circulation. 2012;126(11 suppl 1):S164–9.
6. Ojo AO, Hanson JA, Wolfe RA, Leichtman AB, Agodoa LY, Port FK. Long-term survival in renal transplant recipients with graft function. Kidney Int. 2000;57(1):307–13.
7. Sarnak MJ, Levey AS, Schoolwerth AC, Coresh J, Culleton B, Hamm LL, et al. Kidney disease as a risk factor for development of cardiovascular disease: a statement from the American Heart Association Councils on Kidney in Cardiovascular Disease, High Blood Pressure Research, Clinical Cardiology, and Epidemiology and Prevention. Circulation. 2003;108(17):2154–69.
8. Hemmelgarn BR, Southern D, Culleton BF, Mitchell LB, Knudtson ML, Ghali WA, et al. Survival after coronary revascularization among patients with kidney disease. Circulation. 2004;110(14):1890–5.
9. Go AS, Chertow GM, Fan D, McCulloch CE, Hsu CY. Chronic kidney disease and the risks of death, cardiovascular events, and hospitalization. N Engl J Med. 2004;351(13):1296–305.
10. Herzog CA, Shroff GR. Atherosclerotic versus nonatherosclerotic evaluation: the Yin and Yang of cardiovascular imaging in advanced chronic kidney disease. JACC Cardiovasc Imaging. 2014;7(7):729–32.
11. Charytan D, Kuntz RE. The exclusion of patients with chronic kidney disease from clinical trials in coronary artery disease. Kidney Int. 2006;70(11):2021–30.
12. Reddan DN, Szczech LA, Tuttle RH, Shaw LK, Jones RH, Schwab SJ, et al. Chronic kidney disease, mortality, and treatment

strategies among patients with clinically significant coronary artery disease. J Am Soc Nephrol. 2003;14(9):2373–80.
13. Keeley EC, McCullough PA. Coronary revascularization in patients with coronary artery disease and chronic kidney disease. Adv Chronic Kidney Dis. 2004;11(3):254–60.
14. Best PJ, Lennon R, Ting HH, Bell MR, Rihal CS, Holmes DR, et al. The impact of renal insufficiency on clinical outcomes in patients undergoing percutaneous coronary interventions. J Am Coll Cardiol. 2002;39(7):1113–9.
15. Ziada KM. Coronary revascularization in end-stage renal disease. Curr Cardiol Rep. 2007;9(5):389–95.
16. Kannan A, Poongkunran C, Medina R, Ramanujam V, Poongkunran M, Balamuthusamy S. Coronary revascularization in chronic and end-stage renal disease: a systematic review and meta-analysis. Am J Ther. 2016;23(1):e16–28.
17. Tsai TT, Messenger JC, Brennan JM, Patel UD, Dai D, Piana RN, et al. Safety and efficacy of drug-eluting stents in older patients with chronic kidney disease: a report from the linked CathPCI Registry-CMS claims database. J Am Coll Cardiol. 2011;58(18):1859–69.
18. Bangalore S, Kumar S, Fusaro M, Amoroso N, Attubato MJ, Feit F, et al. Short-and long-term outcomes with drug-eluting and bare-metal coronary stents: a mixed-treatment comparison analysis of 117,762 patient-years of follow-up from randomized trials. Circulation. 2012;125(23):2873–91.
19. Bangalore S, Toklu B, Amoroso N, Fusaro M, Kumar S, Hannan EL, et al. Bare metal stents, durable polymer drug eluting stents, and biodegradable polymer drug eluting stents for coronary artery disease: mixed treatment comparison meta-analysis. BMJ. 2013;347:f6625.
20. Lentine KL, Costa SP, Weir MR, Robb JF, Fleisher LA, Kasiske BL, et al. Cardiac disease evaluation and management among kidney and liver transplantation candidates: a scientific statement from the American Heart Association and the American College of Cardiology Foundation. J Am Coll Cardiol. 2012;60(5):434–80.
21. Valgimigli M, Patialiakas A, Thury A, McFadden E, Colangelo S, Campo G, et al. Zotarolimus-eluting versus bare-metal stents in uncertain drug-eluting stent candidates. J Am Coll Cardiol. 2015;65(8):805–15.
22. El-Hayek G, Messerli F, Bangalore S, Hong MK, Herzog E, Benjo A, et al. Meta-analysis of randomized clinical trials comparing short-term versus long-term dual antiplatelet therapy following drug-eluting stents. Am J Cardiol. 2014;114(2):236–42.
23. Task Force M, Montalescot G, Sechtem U, Achenbach S, Andreotti F, Arden C, et al. ESC guidelines on the management of stable coronary artery disease: the Task Force on the management of stable coronary artery disease of the European Society of Cardiology. Eur Heart J. 2013;34(38):2949–3003.
24. Bangalore S, Silbaugh TS, Normand SL, Lovett AF, Welt FG, Resnic FS. Drug-eluting stents versus bare metal stents prior to noncardiac surgery. Catheter Cardiovasc Interv. 2015;85(4):533–41.
25. Miao Y, Yu-Jie Z, Zhi-Jian W, Dong-Mei S, Yu-Yang L, Ying-Xin Z, et al. Chronic kidney disease and the risk of stent thrombosis after percutaneous coronary intervention with drug-eluting stents. Catheter Cardiovasc Interv. 2012;80(3):361–7.
26. Toutouzas K, Patsa C, Synetos A, Karanasos A, Karampelas J, Tsiamis E, et al. The impact of new generation drug-eluting stent implantation on patients with chronic kidney disease and a single lesion in the proximal segment of the left anterior descending artery. HJC. 2011;52(2):103–10.
27. Chang TI, Leong TK, Boothroyd DB, Hlatky MA, Go AS. Acute kidney injury after CABG versus PCI: an observational study using 2 cohorts. J Am Coll Cardiol. 2014;64(10):985–94.
28. Anderson RJ, O'Brien M, MaWhinney S, VillaNueva CB, Moritz TE, Sethi GK, et al. Renal failure predisposes patients to adverse outcome after coronary artery bypass surgery. VA Cooperative Study #5. Kidney Int. 1999;55(3):1057–62.
29. Cooper WA, O'Brien SM, Thourani VH, Guyton RA, Bridges CR, Szczech LA, et al. Impact of renal dysfunction on outcomes of coronary artery bypass surgery: results from the Society of Thoracic Surgeons National Adult Cardiac Database. Circulation. 2006;113(8):1063–70.
30. Liu JY, Birkmeyer NJ, Sanders JH, Morton JR, Henriques HF, Lahey SJ, et al. Risks of morbidity and mortality in dialysis patients undergoing coronary artery bypass surgery. Northern New England Cardiovascular Disease Study Group. Circulation. 2000;102(24):2973–7.
31. Szczech LA, Best PJ, Crowley E, Brooks MM, Berger PB, Bittner V, et al. Outcomes of patients with chronic renal insufficiency in the bypass angioplasty revascularization investigation. Circulation. 2002;105(19):2253–8.
32. Mehta RH, Hafley GE, Gibson CM, Harrington RA, Peterson ED, Mack MJ, et al. Influence of preoperative renal dysfunction on one-year bypass graft patency and two-year outcomes in patients undergoing coronary artery bypass surgery. J Thorac Cardiovasc Surg. 2008;136(5):1149–55.
33. Hillis LD, Smith PK, Anderson JL, Bittl JA, Bridges CR, Byrne JG, et al. 2011 ACCF/AHA guideline for coronary artery bypass graft surgery: executive summary: a report of the American College of Cardiology Foundation/American Heart Association Task Force on Practice Guidelines. J Thorac Cardiovasc Surg. 2012;143(1):4–34.
34. Authors/Task Force m, Windecker S, Kolh P, Alfonso F, Collet JP, Cremer J, et al. ESC/EACTS Guidelines on myocardial revascularization: The Task Force on Myocardial Revascularization of the European Society of Cardiology (ESC) and the European Association for Cardio-Thoracic Surgery (EACTS)Developed with the special contribution of the European Association of Percutaneous Cardiovascular Interventions (EAPCI). Eur Heart J. 2014;35(37):2541–619.
35. Ahmed WH, Shubrooks SJ, Gibson CM, Baim DS, Bittl JA. Complications and long-term outcome after percutaneous coronary angioplasty in chronic hemodialysis patients. Am Heart J. 1994;128(2):252–5.
36. Herzog CA, Ma JZ, Collins AJ. Long-term outcome of dialysis patients in the United States with coronary revascularization procedures. Kidney Int. 1999;56(1):324–32.
37. Ix JH, Mercado N, Shlipak MG, Lemos PA, Boersma E, Lindeboom W, et al. Association of chronic kidney disease with clinical outcomes after coronary revascularization: the Arterial Revascularization Therapies Study (ARTS). Am Heart J. 2005;149(3):512–9.
38. Chen YY, Wang JF, Zhang YJ, Xie SL, Nie RQ. Optimal strategy of coronary revascularization in chronic kidney disease patients: a meta-analysis. Eur J Int Med. 2013;24(4):354–61.
39. Farkouh ME, Domanski M, Sleeper LA, Siami FS, Dangas G, Mack M, et al. Strategies for multivessel revascularization in patients with diabetes. N Engl J Med. 2012;367(25):2375–84.
40. Bangalore S, Guo Y, Samadashvili Z, Blecker S, Xu J, Hannan EL. Revascularization in patients with multivessel coronary artery disease and chronic kidney disease: everolimus–Eluting stents versus coronary artery bypass graft surgery. J Am Coll Cardiol. 2015;66(11):1209–20.
41. Holmes DR, Mohr FW, Serruys PW, Mack MJ, Vermeersch P, Van Cauwelaert P, Virtanen K, Harjula AL, Leadley K, Dawkins KD. The impact of renal insufficiency of 2-year outcomes following PCI or CABG in the SYNTAX Trial. J Am Coll Cardiol. 2010;55(A184):E1724.

42. Kappetein AP, Feldman TE, Mack MJ, Morice MC, Holmes DR, Stahle E, et al. Comparison of coronary bypass surgery with drug-eluting stenting for the treatment of left main and/or three-vessel disease: 3-year follow-up of the SYNTAX trial. Eur Heart J. 2011;32(17):2125–34.
43. Sellke FW, DiMaio JM, Caplan LR, Ferguson TB, Gardner TJ, Hiratzka LF, et al. Comparing on-pump and off-pump coronary artery bypass grafting: numerous studies but few conclusions—a scientific statement from the American Heart Association council on cardiovascular surgery and anesthesia in collaboration with the interdisciplinary working group on quality of care and outcomes research. Circulation. 2005;111(21):2858–64.
44. Ashrith G, Elayda MA, Wilson JM. Revascularization options in patients with chronic kidney disease. Tex Heart Inst J. 2010;37(1):9–18.
45. Burfeind WR Jr, Glower DD, Wechsler AS, Tuttle RH, Shaw LK, Harrell FE Jr, et al. Single versus multiple internal mammary artery grafting for coronary artery bypass: 15-year follow-up of a clinical practice trial. Circulation. 2004;110(11 Suppl 1):II27–35.

Revascularization Strategies in CKD: Antiplatelet Therapy, Stent Type, Timing, and Complications of PCI

31

Marwan Y. Qattan and Somjot S. Brar

Antiplatelet Therapy Post-PCI in CKD

Dual antiplatelet therapy (DAPT) remains the mainstay of treatment post-PCI. This includes treatment with aspirin and one additional antiplatelet agent. Nowadays there are multiple antiplatelet agents available that have shown to be effective when administered with aspirin for the prevention of ischemic events post-PCI. The impact of these antiplatelet therapies in patients with CKD and which is the preferred antiplatelet agent are in debate.

Clopidogrel

Clopidogrel is a thienopyridine that via an active metabolite, selectively inhibits the binding of adenosine diphosphate to platelet P2Y12 receptor and the subsequent activation of the glycoprotein IIb/IIIa complex and platelet aggregation. Clopidogrel use was associated with favorable cardiovascular outcomes in the Clopidogrel in Unstable Angina to Prevent Recurrent Events (CURE) Trial for unstable angina and non-ST segment elevation myocardial infarction [1] and the Clopidogrel for the Reduction of Events during Observation (CREDO) trial for stable angina [2].

In the CURE trial, the efficacy and safety of clopidogrel was studied in 12,245 patients with non-ST segment elevation myocardial infarction in three strata of GFR (low: GFR < 60 ml/min/1.73 m^2; intermediate: GFR 64–81.2 ml/min/1.73 m^2; and normal or near normal: GFR > 81.3 ml/min/1.73 m^2). Patients were randomized to placebo or clopidogrel (clopidogrel 300 mg loading dose followed by 75 mg daily) and followed for 3–12 months (mean duration 9 months). The efficacy of clopidogrel on reducing the primary composite of cardiovascular death, nonfatal myocardial infarction (MI) or stroke was observed in all three strata: lower GFR (RR 0.89; 95% CI 0.76–1.05), medium GFR (RR 0.68, 95% CI 0.56–0.84), and near normal GFR (RR 0.74; 95% CI 0.60–0.93; *P* for heterogeneity = 0.11). Moreover, the event rate of the primary composite endpoint was higher as the GFR declined in the clopidogrel and placebo groups. The absolute bleeding risk was higher in patients with CKD, however, the relative increase of bleeding was similar. This study suggested adding clopidogrel to standard non-ST segment elevation myocardial infarction treatment is beneficial and safe in patients with CKD [3].

The Clopidogrel for the Reduction of Events During Observation (CREDO) trial assessed the efficacy and safety of clopidogrel in elective PCI for stable angina in 2002 patients, including with CKD. Patients were treated with clopidogrel 300 mg or placebo loading dose followed by 75 mg daily for 12-months in the clopiogrel group and with clopidogrel for 28 days in the placebo group. All patients were treated with aspirin. Outcomes were analyzed in three strata of renal function: normal (GFR > 90 ml/min/1.73 m^2, n = 999], mild CKD (GFR of 60–89 ml/min/1.73 m^2, n = 672) and moderate CKD (GFR < 60 ml/min/1.73 m^2, n = 331). Patients with normal renal function in the clopidogrel group had a marked reduction in the primary composite endpoint of death, myocardial infarction, or stroke compared with the placebo group (10.4 vs. 4.4%, $P < 0.001$), but patients with mild or moderate CKD had no significant difference in the primary composite outcome (mild: 12.8 vs. 10.3%, P = 0.30; moderate: 13.1 vs. 17.8%, P = 0.24). Clopidogrel use was associated with more major or minor bleeding, but it was not different based on renal function [4]. This study suggested that clopidogrel may not be as

M.Y. Qattan
Department of Cardiology, Kaiser Permanente, Los Angeles Medical Center, 1526 Edgemont St, Second Floor, Cardiology, Los Angeles, CA 90027, USA
e-mail: marwan.qattan@kp.org

S.S. Brar (✉)
Department of Cardiology and Regional Cardiac Cath Lab, Kaiser Permanente, Los Angeles Medical Center, 4867 Sunset Blvd, 3rd Floor, Rm 3755, Los Angeles, CA 90027, USA
e-mail: SBrar@cvri.org

J. Rangaswami et al. (eds.), *Cardio-Nephrology*,
DOI 10.1007/978-3-319-56042-7_31

beneficial in patients with stable angina and CKD undergoing PCI as it is in patients with normal renal function.

Ticagrelor

Ticagrelor is a reversibly binding oral P2Y12 receptor antagonist that blocks ADP-induced platelet aggregation. In the Platelet Inhibition and Patient Outcomes (PLATO) trial, tricagrelor showed clinical and biochemical superiority to clopidogrel in patient with ACS [5] impact of tricagelor by renal function (GFR > 60 ml/min/1.73 m^2 vs. GFR < 60 ml/min/1.73 m^2) was studied in 18,624 patients with acute coronary syndrome (ST and non-ST elevation myocardial infarctions) from the PLATO trial. Ticagrelor significantly reduced the primary composite endpoint of cardiovascular death, MI and stroke [17.3 vs. 22.0%; hazard ratio (HR), 0.77; 95% CI 0.65–0.90]. All-cause death was reduced in the tricagelor group with GFR < 60 ml/min/1.73 m^2 (10.0 vs. 14.0%; HR 0.72; 95% CI 0.58–0.89). Major bleeding (15.1 vs. 14.3%; HR 1.07; 95% CI 0.88–1.30), fatal bleeding (0.34 vs. 0.77%; HR 0.48; 95% CI 0.15–1.54), and non-coronary bypass related major bleeding (8.5 vs. 7.3%; HR 1.28; 95% CI 0.97–1.68) were not significantly different between the two groups [6].

Prasugrel

Prasugrel is a thienopyridine with potent and selective P2Y12 receptor blockade that exhibits dose-dependent inhibition of platelet aggregation. In the Trial to Assess Improvement in Therapeutic Outcomes by Optimizing Platelet Inhibition with Prasugrel–Thrombolysis In Myocardial Infarction 38 (TRITON-TIMI 38) trial, prasugrel significantly reduced primary ischemic outcomes in patients with ACS compared to clopidogrel (9.9% versus 12.1%, HR 0.81;95% CI 0.73–0.9) and in the subgroup with creatinine clearance of < 60 ml/min/1.73 m^2 [7]. In a substudy from the TRITON-TIMI 38 trial, prasugrel significantly reduced cardiovascular death, nonfatal myocardial infarction, or nonfatal stroke among patients with and without DM. Renal function was an independent factor for this outcome [8]. These data support the effectiveness of prasugrel in patients with CKD.

Dual Antiplatelet Therapy Duration in CKD

According to the 2016 ACC/AHA updated guidelines on the duration of dual antiplatelet therapy (DAPT) after PCI, patients with stable ischemic heart disease (SIHD) should be given DAPT for a minimum of 1 month in BMS and 6 months in DES (class I) and the guideline suggests that it may be reasonable to continue for longer than 1 month in BMS and longer than 6 months in DES (class IIB) in patient who tolerate DAPT without a bleeding complication and are not at high bleeding risk (e.g., prior bleeding on DAPT, coagulopathy, or oral anticoagulant use). On the contrary, patients with SIDH and DES who develop a high risk of bleeding (e.g., treatment with oral anticoagulant therapy), are at high risk of severe bleeding complication (e.g., major intracranial surgery), or develop significant overt bleeding, it is reasonable to discontinue P2Y12 inhibitor therapy after 3 months (class IIB). In patients with acute coronary syndrome (ACS) who are treated with PCI (DES or BMS) the recommended duration of DAPT in the 2016 ACC/AHA updated guideline has not changed from at least 12 months of therapy (class I). However, for patients with a high risk of bleeding (e.g., treatment with oral anticoagulant therapy), or those who develop significant overt bleeding, it is reasonable to stop P2Y12 inhibitor therapy after 6 months (class IIB). A longer DAPT duration (>12 months) may be reasonable in patients with ACS treated with PCI who have completed 12 months of DAPT without a bleeding complication and are not at high bleeding risk (e.g., prior bleeding on DAPT, coagulopathy, oral anticoagulant use), especially in patients with a high DAPT score (≥ 2) who have favorable ischemic to bleeding risk ratio (class IIB).

The duration of DAPT in patients with CKD is controversial. The 2016 ACC/AHA updated DAPT guideline included CKD as a factor associated with increased ischemic events implying longer DAPT duration may be of benefit. Patients with CKD have delayed arterial healing and neoinitimal coverage of coronary stents [9]; thus the proper duration of dual antiplatelet therapy may be longer. In a retrospective cohort study of 23,042 patients with and without CKD (defined as GFR < 60 ml/min/1.73 m^2) who received BMS or first-generation DES, clopidogrel therapy for more than 12 months reduced death or MI (18 vs. 24%, HR 0.74; 95% CI 0.58–0.95), and death (15 vs 23%, HR 0.61; 95% CI 0.47–0.80) in patients with CKD and DES compared to 12 months or less. Such benefit was not significant in patients with GFR > 60 ml/min/1.73 m^2 or with BMS. In this study, longer clopidogrel therapy was not associated with increase bleeding in patients with CKD [10]. However, CKD is also included as factor associated with increased bleeding risk. Thus, appropriate risk stratification and patient selection are important factors in determining the optimal duration of DAPT in patients with CKD.

PCI in CKD

Coronary Artery Lesions Characteristics in CKD

In an autopsy study of coronary artery plaques, end-stage kidney disease (ESKD) was associated with significantly more calcification than coronary artery disease with normal renal function, where plaques are mostly fibro-atheromatous. Also the luminal area was significantly lower in patients with ESKD [11].

An intravascular ultrasound (IVUS) study of coronary plaque in patients with ESKD on hemodialysis and evidence of myocardial ischemia, showed smaller cross-sectional area (4.2 ± 1.6 vs. 5.2 ± 1.8 mm^2; $P < 0.02$), and calcification in the deeper arterial layer (69 vs. 9%; $P < 0.004$) compared to patients with normal renal function, suggesting a greater remodeling effect in response to a more aggressive atherosclerotic process in the medial portion of the artery [12].

An optical coherence tomography (OCT) study [13] of coronary plaques characteristics in non-culprit vessels in patient with CKD compared to patients without CKD, showed larger lipid index (mean lipid arc × lipid length, 1248.4 ± 782.8 versus 1716.1 ± 1116.2 mm; $P = 0.003$), calcification (50.8 vs. 34.8%; $P = 0.041$), cholesterol crystals (23.0 vs. 11.2%; $P = 0.048$), and plaque disruption (13.1 vs 5.5%; $P = 0.049$) in patient with CKD. However, fibrous cap thickness was not significantly different between the two groups [13].

PCI Versus Fibrinolytic Therapy in CKD and STEMI

To date, few randomized trials have reported on the comparative effectiveness of reperfusion strategies in patients with an acute myocardial infarction and CKD. In a retrospective analysis of reperfusion therapy strategy (fibrinolytic therapy or primary PCI) among patients with or without CKD (GFR < 60 ml/min) and STEMI, primary PCI was associated with lower 30-day unadjusted mortality compared to fibrinolytic therapy (17.9 vs 29.4%, $P < 0.05$, in CKD group and 3.1 vs 5.4%, $P < 0.05$, in the normal renal function group), but the adjusted mortality favored primary PCI in the normal renal function group (OR 0.41; 95% CI 0.19–0.89, $P = 0.02$) but not in the impaired renal function group (OR 0.70; 95% CI 0.31–1.60, $P = 0.4$) [14].

Early Invasive Versus Conservative PCI Strategy in CKD and NSTEMI

Among patients with high-risk non-ST elevation myocardial infarction, an early invasive strategy improves long-term survival and reduces late myocardial infarction and hospitalization [15]. The benefit of early invasive strategy in patients with CKD was explored in a meta-analysis of 5 randomized trials ($n = 1453$) [16]. There was a significantly lower risk for hospitalization and a trend toward lower risk for death and re-infarction. Patients with CKD stage 4 were under represented, ($n < 300$) and patients with CKD stage 5 were not included in this study.

A retrospective study from Sweden evaluated the 1-year mortality benefit of an early invasive therapy vs. medical therapy across renal function stages in 23,262 patients with non-ST segment elevation myocardial infarction. The percentage of patients treated invasively were significantly lower as GFR declined ($P < 0.001$): 62% (>90 ml/min/1.73 m^2), 55% (89–60 ml/min/1.73 m^2), 36% (59–30 ml/min/1.73 m^2), 14% (29–15 ml/min/1.73 m^2) and 15% (<15 ml/min/1.73 m^2). The overall 1-year mortality was 36% lower with an invasive strategy (HR 0.64; 95% CI 0.56–0.73; $P < 0.001$). However, this benefit declined with lower levels of renal function and no difference in mortality was observed in patients with stage 5 CKD (GFR < 15 ml/min/1.73 m^2) or receiving dialysis (HR 1.61; 95% CI 0.84–3.09; $P = 0.15$) [17].

Coronary Stent Type in CKD

Coronary restenosis is major limitation of PCI therapy, particularly in patients with CKD. The restenosis rate is higher with worsening renal function and among patients on hemodialysis [18, 19]. In a study of 1184 patients treated with PCI for NSTEMI or unstable angina, the incidence of restenosis at 1 month was 4.6% with normal renal function, 5.3% in CKD stage 1 and 2, 6.8% in CKD stage 3, 7.3% in CKD stage 4 and 9.6% in CKD stage 5 ($P = 0.001$), and at 6 months was 11.2% with normal renal function, 13.5% in CKD stage 1 and 2, 15.7% in CKD stage 3, 16.4% in CKD stage 4 and 19.7% in CKD stage 5 ($P = 0.001$) [19]. The increased restenosis rate in CKD may be explained, in part, by older age and greater number and severity of comorbidities [20], accelerated atherosclerosis rate, stent under expansion caused by higher CAD complexity and plaque calcification [11, 12, 21–24], and underuse of medical therapy [25, 26].

Drug-Eluting Stents Versus Bare-Metal Stents in CKD

The risk of restenosis is reduced with the use of DES, including in subjects with CKD [18]. Studies have shown that using DES in CAD revascularization is associated with lower risk of in-stent restenosis and need for repeat revascularization compared to BMS. In patients with CKD this benefit is attenuated as they have higher risk of in-stent restenosis after PCI compared to patients with normal renal function. In a prospective registry study of 436 patients with CKD (GFR < 60 ml/min/1.73 m^2), multivariable analyses with propensity adjustment, at 3 years of follow-up, DES use was an independent predictor of lower rates of all-cause death (HR 0.48; 95% CI 0.25–0.92), target vessel revascularization (HR 0.50; 95% CI 0.27–0.94) and major adverse cardiac events (MACE) (HR 0.62; 95% CI 0.41–0.94) compared to BMS [27]. DES use was not associated with an increased risk of myocardial infarction or stent thrombosis; however, the patients who received DES in this study had more stable coronary artery disease. A prospective registry study for long-term outcomes (7 years) of DES in patients with CKD (<60 ml/min/1.73 m^2) showed no reduction in mortality (HR 0.85; 95% CI 0.69–1.05; $P = 0.1$) but reduced rate of revascularization (HR 0.68; 95% CI 0.53–0.88; $P = 0.004$) and MACE (HR 0.81; 95% CI 0.69–0.95; $P = 0.011$) [28]. Similarly, a study of 504 patients showed that the target lesion revascularization rates were similar after PCI with DES in patients with normal renal function or CKD: 5.6 versus 4.8%, respectively ($P = 0.7$) [29]. In the BASKET-PROVE trial, patients with CKD (GFR < 60 ml/min/1.73 m^2) who needed large vessel coronary stenting ($\geq$3.0 mm) had a lower major adverse cardiac event rate with DES than with BMS (4.9 vs. 15.2%; HR 0.29; 95% CI 0.10–0.80; $P = 0.017$) [30].

In a study of PCI in elderly patients (65 years and older), placement of a DES compared to BMS was associated with lower rates of MI and mortality in all CKD subgroups, except for MI in long-term dialysis patients, where decreased rates of revascularization did not extend to any subgroup of patients with CKD [31]. In a study from US Renal Data System database, restenosis was associated with higher mortality in dialysis patients [32]. In contrast, in the Prevention of Restenosis with Tranilast and its Outcomes (PRESTO) trial, the higher mortality in patients with CKD after PCI (2.2, 1.2, 0.8% in GFR <60, 60–89, >89 ml/min/1.73 m^2, respectively; $P < 0.001$) was not associated with restenosis [33].

Drug-Eluting Versus Bare-Metal Stent in Dialysis Patients

In a study of patients on chronic dialysis, use of DES was associated with a significant reduction in target vessel revascularization (OR 0.07; 95% CI 0.01–0.84; $P = 0.036$) and composite of death, myocardial infarction and target vessel revascularization (OR 0.11; 95% CI 0.02–0.51; $P = 0.005$) compared to BMS [34]. Also, in another study of patients on dialysis, DES use was independently associated with freedom from the composite major adverse cardiac events (HR 0.24; 95% CI 0.10–0.60; $P = 0.002$) and with a trend to lower all-cause mortality (HR 0.40; 95% CI 0.15–1.05; $P = 0.06$) at 1 year compared to BMS [35].

However, not all studies show a beneficial effect of DES in patients on dialysis. In a study of 54 dialysis patients with 69 lesions treated with DES compared to 54 dialysis patients with 58 lesions treated with BMS, the angiographic and clinical follow-ups at 9 months showed lower in-stent restenosis rate in lesions treated with DES than BMS (22 vs. 40%, $P = 0.048$); however, there were no difference between in-segment restenosis (31 vs. 43%, $P = 0.3$), incidence of death, myocardial infarction, or target lesion revascularization (TLR) (14 vs. 21%, $P = 0.4$) [36]. Another study compared 88 patients on hemodialysis with 121 lesions treated with sirolimus-eluting stents, to 78 patients on hemodialysis with 95 lesions treated with BMS [18]. In this study, the rates of restenosis did not differ at 1 year (22.2% in the DES vs. 24.4% in the BMS, $P = 0.73$) [18]. In another study of 42 patients on hemodialysis who underwent PCI with DES for 46 de novo lesions compared with 74 patients with 78 de novo lesions that were treated with BMS, the restenosis (34 vs. 43%) and target lesion revascularization (25 vs. 36%) rates were similar by stent type. Major adverse cardiac events, a composite of death, myocardial infarction, and target vessel revascularization were also similar between groups [37].

Drug-Eluting Stent in Dialysis Versus Non-Dialysis Patients

Drug-eluting stents in hemodialysis patients have poorer clinical outcomes compared to non-hemodialysis patients. The incidence of clinical event is significantly higher in the hemodialysis patient (50.0 vs. 12.5%, $P < 0.0001$) as is the rate of target lesion revascularization (33.3 vs. 4.6%, $P < 0.0001$). Hemodialysis status was an explanatory factor for cardiac events (HR 2.70, $P = 0.03$), target lesion revascularization (HR 6.92, $P = 0.0004$), and in-stent restenosis (HR 3.32, $P = 0.03$) [38].

A study investigated the clinical outcomes of patients with CAD treated with DES who were grouped to GFR $\geq$ 60 ml/min/1.73 m^2, <60 ml/min/1.73 m^2, or hemodialysis and showed that the late lumen loss at 8 months was significantly different among the 3 groups: GFR $\geq$ 60 ml/min/1.73 m^2, 0.16 ± 0.46 mm; GFR < 60 ml/min/1.73 m^2, 0.44 ± 0.62 mm; hemodialysis, 0.81 ± 0.88 mm ($P < 0.0001$). Major adverse cardiac events were 10.8% with GFR $\geq$ 60 ml/min/1.73 m^2, 18.8% with GFR < 60 ml/min/1.73 m^2, and 38.7% in the hemodialysis group ($P = 0.0002$) [39]. In contrast, in a study of 3,442 patients who underwent PCI with DES implantation, the restenosis rate was low and comparable between dialysis and non-dialysis patients at 6 months but mortality occurred more often in dialysis patients (16 vs. 3.8%; $P < 0.001$). Multivariate analysis showed cardiogenic shock to be an independent predictor of mortality ($P = 0.04$) [40]

Access Site: Femoral Versus Radial in CKD

The femoral artery is the traditional vascular access to the heart; however, in the past decade the radial artery has become increasingly popular as it is associated with lower risk of bleeding, earlier ambulation and is easily accessible. The radial artery approach limits the use of large-size catheters and some interventional devices due to its smaller caliber. Spasm of the radial artery can be a challenge in patients with severe vasculopathy, which is more common with CKD. Radial access is associated with increased risk of radiation and contrast exposure in less-experienced operators.

A large cohort study from the British Columbia Cardiac Registry showed cardiac catheterization, including PCI, via the radial approach was associated with lower risk of CKD progression. Six months post-PCI there were less new dialysis events (0.2 vs. 0.4%, $P < 0.0001$), fewer CKD stage 4 or 5 cases (0.1 vs. 0.4, $P < 0.0001$) or new CKD (0.2% vs. 1.2%, $P = <0.0001$) with the radial compared to femoral approach. This low risk for CKD was attributed to lower use of contrast, and possibly lower risk of cholesterol embolization by avoiding catheter contact with the descending thoracic and abdominal aorta. Radial access was also associated with reduced access site bleeding and blood transfusion requirements, which have been shown in other studies to be independent predictors of worsening renal function [41].

PCI Complications in CKD

Stent Thrombosis

Stent thrombosis is associated with premature discontinuation of DAPT, long stents, bifurcation lesions, stent under expansion, and acute coronary syndrome at time of PCI [42]. In a retrospective study aimed to investigate the 1-year incidence of stent thrombosis after elective DES PCI in patients with CKD (GFR < 60 ml/min/1.73 m^2), the incidence of probable or definite stent thrombosis was significantly higher in patients with CKD compared to patients with normal renal function (1.8 vs. 0.6%, $P = 0.014$) [43]. CKD was an independent predictor of stent thrombosis after adjustment for clinical and biochemical covariates.

A study by Lakovou et al. evaluated predictors of stent thrombosis in DES. Renal failure was found to have a significant hazard for stent thrombosis at 9-month follow-up, second only to premature discontinuation of dual antiplatelet therapy [44]. Similarly, Machecourt et al. [45] showed in the EVASTENT matched-cohort registry, that chronic kidney disease is an important predictor for stent thrombosis in patients with DES. In a study by Choi et al. [46] the rate of stent thrombosis was significantly higher in the lowest GFR quartile compared with the highest GFR quartile and high levels of high-sensitivity C-reactive protein. The increased incidence of stent thrombosis in patients with CKD could be explained by the delayed arterial healing and incomplete neoinitimal coverage [9], which may be associated with atheromatous changes, remodeling and stiffness of the arterial wall in patients with CKD [47] and higher risk of clopidogrel resistance in patients with CKD [48–50].

Vascular Access Complications

Vascular complications including hematoma, retroperitoneal bleeding, pseudoaneurysm, arteriovenous fistula, occlusion, dissection, embolization, femoral neuropathy, and infection are well-known complications of PCI and associated with increased morbidity, mortality, and length of stay in the hospital.

Patients with CKD (GFR < 60 ml/min/1.73 m^2) experience higher rates of major vascular complications after PCI via the femoral access compared to patients without normal renal function (8.4 vs. 4.2%; $P = 0.045$) [51]. In a retrospective analysis of the combined incidence of pseudoaneurysm, retroperitoneal hematoma, femoral artery thrombosis, surgical vascular repair, and groin infection after PCI in patients with different levels of renal functions, renal function was the strongest independent predictor for the primary outcome (OR 1.032; 95% CI 1.019–1.046; $P < 0.0001$), driven by higher infection ($P < 0.0001$), thrombosis ($P = 0.003$) and hematoma ($P = 0.007$). There was an inverse relationship between the vascular access site complication rate and GFR, such that lower GFR levels were a predictor of vascular access complications ($P < 0.001$) [52].

Vascular Closure Devices

Vascular closure devices after femoral access have shown to improve patient comfort, free medical staff resources, and shorten the time needed for hemostasis, ambulation, and discharge. However, the role of these devices in decreasing vascular complications remains controversial. In a study comparing vascular access complications among patients with CKD who received a vascular closure device or manual compression after PCI via the femoral access, complications were significantly lower in the vascular closure device group

(4.7 vs. 21.6%; P = 0.003) a vascular closure device was independently associated with a decreased risk of major vascular complications in patients with CKD (OR 0.11; 95% CI 0.03–0.41; P =0.001) [51].

Conclusions

Patients with CKD continue to experience inferior outcomes after PCI owing to a complex interplay of factors. Optimal strategies for duration and type of antiplatelet therapy and stent choice remain understudied areas that deserve attention, toward the goal of optimizing post interventional outcomes in this high-risk group of patients.

References

1. Yusuf S, Zhao F, Mehta SR, Chrolavicius S, Tognoni G, Fox KK. Effects of clopidogrel in addition to aspirin in patients with acute coronary syndromes without ST-segment elevation. N Engl J Med. 2001;345(7):494–502.
2. Steinhubl SR, Berger PB, Mann JT 3rd, Fry ET, DeLago A, Wilmer C, et al. Early and sustained dual oral antiplatelet therapy following percutaneous coronary intervention: a randomized controlled trial. JAMA. 2002;288(19):2411–20.
3. Keltai M, Tonelli M, Mann JF, Sitkei E, Lewis BS, Hawken S, et al. Renal function and outcomes in acute coronary syndrome: impact of clopidogrel. Eur J Cardiovasc Prev Rehabil. 2007;14(2): 312–8.
4. Best PJ, Steinhubl SR, Berger PB, Dasgupta A, Brennan DM, Szczech LA, et al. The efficacy and safety of short- and long-term dual antiplatelet therapy in patients with mild or moderate chronic kidney disease: results from the Clopidogrel for the Reduction of Events During Observation (CREDO) trial. Am Heart J. 2008; 155(4):687–93.
5. Wallentin L, Becker RC, Budaj A, Cannon CP, Emanuelsson H, Held C, et al. Ticagrelor versus clopidogrel in patients with acute coronary syndromes. N Engl J Med. 2009;361(11):1045–57.
6. James S, Budaj A, Aylward P, Buck KK, Cannon CP, Cornel JH, et al. Ticagrelor versus clopidogrel in acute coronary syndromes in relation to renal function: results from the Platelet Inhibition and Patient Outcomes (PLATO) trial. Circulation. 2010;122(11): 1056–67.
7. Wiviott SD, Braunwald E, McCabe CH, Montalescot G, Ruzyllo W, Gottlieb S, et al. Prasugrel versus clopidogrel in patients with acute coronary syndromes. N Engl J Med. 2007; 357(20):2001–15.
8. Wiviott SD, Braunwald E, Angiolillo DJ, Meisel S, Dalby AJ, Verheugt FW, et al. Greater clinical benefit of more intensive oral antiplatelet therapy with prasugrel in patients with diabetes mellitus in the trial to assess improvement in therapeutic outcomes by optimizing platelet inhibition with Prasugrel-Thrombolysis in Myocardial Infarction 38. Circulation. 2008;118(16):1626–36.
9. Kotani J, Awata M, Nanto S, Uematsu M, Oshima F, Minamiguchi H, et al. Incomplete neointimal coverage of sirolimus-eluting stents: angioscopic findings. J Am Coll Cardiol. 2006;47(10):2108–11.
10. Siddiqi OK, Smoot KJ, Dufour AB, Cho K, Young M, Gagnon DR, et al. Outcomes with prolonged clopidogrel therapy after coronary stenting in patients with chronic kidney disease. Heart. 2015;101(19):1569–76.
11. Schwarz U, Buzello M, Ritz E, Stein G, Raabe G, Wiest G, et al. Morphology of coronary atherosclerotic lesions in patients with end-stage renal failure. Nephrol Dial Transpl. 2000;15(2):218–23.
12. Varela AM, Taniguchi E, Stadler N, Faria-Neto JR, Pecoits-Filho R. Use of intravascular ultrasonography for the characterization of coronary artery disease in patients with chronic kidney disease. J Bras Nefrol. 2011;33(4):413–21.
13. Kato K, Yonetsu T, Jia H, Abtahian F, Vergallo R, Hu S, et al. Nonculprit coronary plaque characteristics of chronic kidney disease. Circ Cardiovasc Imaging. 2013;6(3):448–56.
14. Chan MY, Becker RC, Sim LL, Tan V, Lee CH, Low AF, et al. Reperfusion strategy and mortality in ST-elevation myocardial infarction among patients with and without impaired renal function. Ann Acad Med Singap. 2010;39(3):179–84.
15. Bavry AA, Kumbhani DJ, Rassi AN, Bhatt DL, Askari AT. Benefit of early invasive therapy in acute coronary syndromes: a meta-analysis of contemporary randomized clinical trials. J Am Coll Cardiol. 2006;48(7):1319–25.
16. Charytan DM, Wallentin L, Lagerqvist B, Spacek R, De Winter RJ, Stern NM, et al. Early angiography in patients with chronic kidney disease: a collaborative systematic review. Clin J Am Soc Nephrol. 2009;4(6):1032–43.
17. Szummer K, Lundman P, Jacobson SH, Schon S, Lindback J, Stenestrand U, et al. Influence of renal function on the effects of early revascularization in non-ST-elevation myocardial infarction: data from the Swedish Web-System for Enhancement and Development of Evidence-Based Care in Heart Disease Evaluated According to Recommended Therapies (SWEDEHEART). Circulation. 2009;120(10):851–8.
18. Aoyama T, Ishii H, Toriyama T, Takahashi H, Kasuga H, Murakami R, et al. Sirolimus-eluting stents vs bare metal stents for coronary intervention in Japanese patients with renal failure on hemodialysis. Circ J. 2008;72(1):56–60.
19. Attallah N, Yassine L, Fisher K, Yee J. Risk of bleeding and restenosis among chronic kidney disease patients undergoing percutaneous coronary intervention. Clin Nephrol. 2005;64(6): 412–8.
20. Rubenstein MH, Harrell LC, Sheynberg BV, Schunkert H, Bazari H, Palacios IF. Are patients with renal failure good candidates for percutaneous coronary revascularization in the new device era? Circulation. 2000;102(24):2966–72.
21. Charytan DM, Garg P, Varma M, Garshick MS, Jeon C, Mauri L. Angiographic characteristics of coronary arterial segments progressing to myocardial infarction in patients with and without chronic kidney disease. Clin Exp Nephrol. 2013;17(2):232–9.
22. Chonchol M, Whittle J, Desbien A, Orner MB, Petersen LA, Kressin NR. Chronic kidney disease is associated with angiographic coronary artery disease. Am J Nephrol. 2008;28(2): 354–60.
23. Coskun U, Orta Kilickesmez K, Abaci O, Kocas C, Bostan C, Yildiz A, et al. The relationship between chronic kidney disease and SYNTAX score. Angiology. 2011;62(6):504–8.
24. Kono K, Fujii H, Miyoshi N, Kawamori H, Shite J, Hirata K, et al. Coronary plaque morphology using virtual histology-intravascular ultrasound analysis in hemodialysis patients. Ther Apher Dial. 2011;15(1):44–50.
25. Berger AK, Duval S, Krumholz HM. Aspirin, beta-blocker, and angiotensin-converting enzyme inhibitor therapy in patients with end-stage renal disease and an acute myocardial infarction. J Am Coll Cardiol. 2003;42(2):201–8.
26. Latif F, Kleiman NS, Cohen DJ, Pencina MJ, Yen CH, Cutlip DE, et al. In-hospital and 1-year outcomes among percutaneous coronary intervention patients with chronic kidney disease in the

era of drug-eluting stents: a report from the EVENT (Evaluation of Drug Eluting Stents and Ischemic Events) registry. JACC Cardiovasc Interv. 2009;2(1):37–45.
27. Shenoy C, Boura J, Orshaw P, Harjai KJ. Drug-eluting stents in patients with chronic kidney disease: a prospective registry study. PLoS ONE. 2010;5(11):e15070.
28. Appleby CE, Ivanov J, Lavi S, Mackie K, Horlick EM, Ing D, et al. The adverse long-term impact of renal impairment in patients undergoing percutaneous coronary intervention in the drug-eluting stent era. Circ Cardiovasc Interv. 2009;2(4):309–16.
29. Osorio Gomes V, Blaya P, Lasevitch R, Oliveira D, Hickmann P, Smidt L, et al. Impact of chronic kidney disease on the efficacy of drug-eluting stents: long-term follow-up study. Arq Bras Cardiol. 2011;96(5):346–51.
30. Wanitschek M, Pfisterer M, Hvelplund A, De Servi S, Bertel O, Jeger R, et al. Long-term benefits and risks of drug-eluting compared to bare-metal stents in patients with versus without chronic kidney disease. Int J Cardiol. 2013;168(3):2381–8.
31. Tsai TT, Messenger JC, Brennan JM, Patel UD, Dai D, Piana RN, et al. Safety and efficacy of drug-eluting stents in older patients with chronic kidney disease: a report from the linked CathPCI Registry-CMS claims database. J Am Coll Cardiol. 2011;58(18): 1859–69.
32. Herzog CA, Ma JZ, Collins AJ. Comparative survival of dialysis patients in the United States after coronary angioplasty, coronary artery stenting, and coronary artery bypass surgery and impact of diabetes. Circulation. 2002;106(17):2207–11.
33. Best PJ, Berger PB, Davis BR, Grines CL, Sadeghi HM, Williams BA, et al. Impact of mild or moderate chronic kidney disease on the frequency of restenosis: results from the PRESTO trial. J Am Coll Cardiol. 2004;44(9):1786–91.
34. Das P, Moliterno DJ, Charnigo R, Mukherjee D, Steinhubl SR, Sneed JD, et al. Impact of drug-eluting stents on outcomes of patients with end-stage renal disease undergoing percutaneous coronary revascularization. J Invasive Cardiol. 2006;18(9):405–8.
35. Halkin A, Selzer F, Marroquin O, Laskey W, Detre K, Cohen H. Clinical outcomes following percutaneous coronary intervention with drug-eluting vs. bare-metal stents in dialysis patients. J Invasive Cardiol. 2006;18(12):577–83.
36. Ishio N, Kobayashi Y, Takebayashi H, Iijima Y, Kanda J, Nakayama T, et al. Impact of drug-eluting stents on clinical and angiographic outcomes in dialysis patients. Circ J. 2007;71 (10):1525–9.
37. Suzuki K, Inoue N, Matsuo A, Shiono Y, Nakanishi N, Otsuki Y, et al. Limitation on efficacy of sirolimus-eluting stent implantation in patients on hemodialysis. J Cardiol. 2007;49(6):331–6.
38. Sasao H, Hotta D, Maeda T, Saito N, Takagi S, Shimamoto K. Comparison of long-term clinical outcome after sirolimus-eluting stent implantation in patients with and without hemodialysis. Int Heart J. 2007;48(6):689–700.
39. Nakazawa G, Tanabe K, Aoki J, Yamamoto H, Higashikuni Y, Onuma Y, et al. Impact of renal insufficiency on clinical and angiographic outcomes following percutaneous coronary intervention with sirolimus-eluting stents. Catheter Cardiovasc Interv. 2007;69(6):808–14.
40. Hassani SE, Chu WW, Wolfram RM, Kuchulakanti PK, Xue Z, Gevorkian N, et al. Clinical outcomes after percutaneous coronary intervention with drug-eluting stents in dialysis patients. J Invasive Cardiol. 2006;18(6):273–7.
41. Vuurmans T, Byrne J, Fretz E, Janssen C, Hilton JD, Klinke WP, et al. Chronic kidney injury in patients after cardiac catheterisation or percutaneous coronary intervention: a comparison of radial and femoral approaches (from the British Columbia Cardiac and Renal Registries). Heart. 2010;96(19):1538–42.
42. de la Torre-Hernandez JM, Alfonso F, Hernandez F, Elizaga J, Sanmartin M, Pinar E, et al. Drug-eluting stent thrombosis: results from the multicenter Spanish registry ESTROFA (Estudio ESpanol sobre TROmbosis de stents FArmacoactivos). J Am Coll Cardiol. 2008;51(10):986–90.
43. Miao Y, Yu-Jie Z, Zhi-Jian W, Dong-Mei S, Yu-Yang L, Ying-Xin Z, et al. Chronic kidney disease and the risk of stent thrombosis after percutaneous coronary intervention with drug-eluting stents. Catheter Cardiovasc Interv. 2012;80(3):361–7.
44. Iakovou I, Schmidt T, Bonizzoni E, Ge L, Sangiorgi GM, Stankovic G, et al. Incidence, predictors, and outcome of thrombosis after successful implantation of drug-eluting stents. JAMA. 2005;293(17):2126–30.
45. Machecourt J, Danchin N, Lablanche JM, Fauvel JM, Bonnet JL, Marliere S, et al. Risk factors for stent thrombosis after implantation of sirolimus-eluting stents in diabetic and nondiabetic patients: the EVASTENT Matched-Cohort Registry. J Am Coll Cardiol. 2007;50(6):501–8.
46. Choi DH, Park KW, Yang HM, Lee HY, Park JS, Kang HJ, et al. Renal dysfunction and high levels of hsCRP are additively associated with hard endpoints after percutaneous coronary intervention with drug eluting stents. Int J Cardiol. 2011;149(2): 174–81.
47. Krasniak A, Drozdz M, Pasowicz M, Chmiel G, Michalek M, Szumilak D, et al. Factors involved in vascular calcification and atherosclerosis in maintenance haemodialysis patients. Nephrol Dial Transpl. 2007;22(2):515–21.
48. Cuisset T, Frere C, Moro PJ, Quilici J, Pons C, Gaborit B, et al. Lack of effect of chronic kidney disease on clopidogrel response with high loading and maintenance doses of clopidogrel after Acute Coronary Syndrome. Thromb Res. 2010;126(5):e400–2.
49. Htun P, Fateh-Moghadam S, Bischofs C, Banya W, Muller K, Bigalke B, et al. Low responsiveness to clopidogrel increases risk among CKD patients undergoing coronary intervention. J Am Soc Nephrol. 2011;22(4):627–33.
50. Park SH, Kim W, Park CS, Kang WY, Hwang SH, Kim W. A comparison of clopidogrel responsiveness in patients with versus without chronic renal failure. Am J Cardiol. 2009;104(9): 1292–5.
51. Prada-Delgado O, Estevez-Loureiro R, Calvino-Santos R, Barge-Caballero E, Salgado-Fernandez J, Pinon-Esteban P, et al. Renal insufficiency and vascular complications after primary angioplasty via femoral route Impact of vascular closure devices use. Rev Esp Cardiol (Engl Ed). 2012;65(3):258–64.
52. Aziz EF, Pulimi S, Coleman C, Florita C, Musat D, Tormey D, et al. Increased vascular access complications in patients with renal dysfunction undergoing percutaneous coronary procedures using arteriotomy closure devices. J Invasive Cardiol. 2010;22(1):8–13.

Peripheral Arterial Disease in CKD: Disease Burden, Outcomes and Interventional Strategies

32

Bhalaghuru Chokkalingam Mani and Nicholas J. Ruggiero II

Disease Burden

Peripheral arterial disease (PAD) has been described as the "global pandemic" of our time [1]. In comparison to the 30 million individuals living with HIV, peripheral arterial disease far outnumbers many other chronic diseases. Studies comparing the trend of peripheral arterial disease prevalence have revealed that approximately 200 million individuals were living with peripheral arterial disease in the year 2010. This indicates a dramatic rise in prevalence, with an additional 40 million individuals compared to the year 2000 when the prevalence was estimated to be around 160 million [2]. In the United States, conservative estimates place the figure in the range of at least 8–10 million individuals suffering from peripheral arterial disease [3, 4].

The reasons for increasing prevalence of peripheral arterial disease can be explained by the alarming rise of other conditions such as hypertension, diabetes and hypercholesterolemia [2]. Peripheral arterial disease was traditionally believed to be more common in men when compared to women. However, recent studies show that the prevalence of PAD in men and women is almost equal in the high income regions of the world, and the prevalence is higher in women compared to men in the low and mid income regions [2]. Other studies have showed a similar prevalence between men and women in the US [5]. The prevalence of peripheral arterial disease also rises with increasing age. While the prevalence is roughly around 4% for individuals older than 40 years, it sharply increases to 15% for individuals over 70 years of age [6]. The American College of Cardiology and the American Heart Association recommends the use of an Ankle brachial index (ABI) as the diagnostic test of choice for evaluating lower extremity peripheral arterial disease. An ABI of 1 is considered normal and an ABI of less than 0.9 is considered abnormal. When the ABI is abnormally high (greater than 1.4) (such as in CKD) it is recommended to use the Toe Brachial index (TBI) to establish the diagnosis in individuals with high clinical suspicion [7].

Chronic kidney disease (CKD) is defined by the National Kidney Foundation as a glomerular filtration rate (GFR) of less than 60 ml/min per 1.73 m^2 for greater than 3 months. CKD is listed by the Centers for Disease Control (CDC) as one of the most prevalent chronic illnesses, with one in seven adults living in the United States with some degree of CKD [8, 9]. CKD is closely intertwined with PAD, with individuals with kidney disease being twice as likely to have peripheral arterial disease compared with those preserved kidney function. In addition, there is a linear relationship between the severity of CKD and the severity of peripheral arterial disease. The National Health and Nutrition Examination survey estimates at least 1 million individuals above the age of 40 with even mild to moderate CKD suffer from peripheral arterial disease defined as Ankle Brachial Index (ABI) less than 0.9 [10]. CKD is also associated with abnormally high ABIs, in particular ABIs greater than 1.4 which inherently is a marker for arterial stiffening and or calcification [11]. When the ABI is abnormally high (greater than 1.4), it is recommended to use the Toe Brachial index (TBI) to establish the diagnosis in individuals with high clinical suspicion [12]. In those individuals who have end stage kidney disease (ESKD), as many as 20–30% have coexistent peripheral arterial disease [13]. The other risk factors strongly associated with peripheral arterial disease include the traditional cardiovascular risk factors namely hypertension, smoking, hypercholesterolemia and diabetes [6].

B.C. Mani
Jefferson Heart and Vascular Institute, Thomas Jefferson University Hospital, Sidney Kimmel College of Medicine, 925 Chestnut Street, Mezzanine Level, Philadelphia, PA 19107, USA
e-mail: bhalaghuru.chokkalingammani@jefferson.edu

N.J. Ruggiero II (✉)
Jefferson Angioplasty Center, Thomas Jefferson University Hospital, 111 South 11th Street, Suite 6210, Philadelphia, PA 19107, USA
e-mail: Nicholas.ruggiero@jefferson.edu

J. Rangaswami et al. (eds.), *Cardio-Nephrology*,
DOI 10.1007/978-3-319-56042-7_32

The disease burden estimated for peripheral arterial disease, albeit staggering, may still not represent the true prevalence, since many of the studies did not utilize toe brachial index or duplex ultrasound in addition to ABI to detect peripheral arterial disease [1]. In addition many other forms of peripheral arterial disease go misdiagnosed or remain under diagnosed. The prevalence of renal artery disease ranges from 20 to 60% in individuals diagnosed with PAD, whereas literature on mesenteric artery disease is largely lacking [8]. The prevalence of abdominal aortic aneurysms ≥ 3 cm in diameter is approximately 3–4% [14].

Impact of PAD and CKD

Peripheral arterial disease is associated independently with increased mortality [15–17]. Patients with peripheral arterial disease have increased risk of cardiac events during the course of their life [18–20]. There is also a trend towards increased occurrence of stroke and cerebrovascular events in the PAD patient population [21]. Patients with PAD are plagued by lower quality of life and limited mobility [22]. Similarly, CKD currently ranks among the top 10 causes of mortality in the United States and is an important cause of disability and years lost to life [23].

From a health care economic perspective, analysis of Medicare data in the United States reveals that roughly 7% of the beneficiaries were treated for PAD. The average spending per person with PAD was close to $2000 dollars per year. The overall cost of managing PAD based on just the Medicare data from 2001 was roughly around 4.4 billion dollars [24]. This compounds the fact that the expenditure for management of all forms of CKD including ESKD was an astounding 87 billion dollars in 2012 [25].

Clinical Presentation and Management of PAD

Aorto Iliac Disease

Clinical Presentation

Aortoiliac disease can result in buttock claudication, infra-inguinal claudication symptoms of thighs and or calves and vasculogenic erectile dysfunction. Aortoiliac disease can worsen other coexisting lower extremity arterial disease by decreasing arterial inflow.

Non-interventional Management

Smoking cessation is universally recommended. Control of risk factors like hypertension and diabetes along with exercise forms the cornerstone of non-interventional management [26]. Interestingly supervised exercise has been shown to be superior to medical therapy alone [27].

Once symptomatic aorto iliac peripheral arterial disease is identified, medical therapy with low dose aspirin should be initiated [24]. In addition, symptomatic peripheral arterial disease of any bed would be considered as clinically significant atherosclerotic cardiovascular disease. Hence dyslipidemia in this setting should be managed with high dose statin therapy according to the most recent American College of Cardiology cholesterol guidelines [28]. In cases of aspirin intolerance, clopidogrel 75 mg a day is an alternative [24].

Interventional Management

The Trans-Atlantic Inter Society consensus (TASC) group categorizes aorto-iliac and femoral popliteal lesions into A, B, C and D based on anatomy and lesion complexity [24]. (Table 32.1)

For TASC A aorto iliac lesions, endovascular therapy is the treatment of choice. For type B and C lesions endovascular therapy is the preferred option. Surgery can be an alternative in a suitable risk patient [24]. In patients with TASC D lesions, surgery has been the gold standard but percutaneous strategies are now equivalent [29].

Surgical techniques for aorto-iliac disease include aorto-iliac thromboendarterectomy, aorto bifemoral bypass surgery and extra anatomic bypass surgery. Extra anatomic bypass surgery includes axillo-femoral and femorofemoral techniques. Extra anatomic bypass has the advantage of avoiding an open abdominal procedure and thereby the morbidity associated with it however long term patency rates are lower compared with the other approaches [27].

Endovascular therapy with angioplasty and stents has comparable outcomes to surgical techniques with less morbidity and mortality. Stents for aorto-iliac lesions can be self-expandable, balloon expandable or covered stents (stents that are covered with materials such as polytetrafluoroethylene PTFE, Goretex etc.). Calcified focal lesions commonly seen in CKD requiring higher radial force are better managed by balloon expandable stents whereas larger diameter lesions are better served with self-expandable stents. For aorto-iliac disease in general, covered stents are used in situations where rupture of the vessel is likely (neocarinal formation, calcified lesions and aneurysmal lesions). Primary patency rates for stents in the aortoiliac location are very promising with 1 and 4 year rates approaching 100 and 80% respectively. Also, covered stenting of the iliac artery has specifically shown to decrease the need for repeat interventions. For bifurcation aortic disease involving aorta and the iliacs, the preferred technique is by way of "aorto-iliac" kissing stents [26].

Intravascular ultrasound (IVUS) has been used as an alternative to contrast angiography in endovascular aortic repair with comparable outcomes without the risk of compromising renal function [30, 31]. More recently intracardiac

Table 32.1 Trans-Atlantic Inter Societal Consensus (TASC) classification of aorto-iliac and femoral popliteal lesions

	Aorto-iliac lesions	Femoral popliteal
TASC A	Unilateral or bilateral stenoses of CIA Unilateral or bilateral single short (≤ 3 cm) stenosis of EIA	Single stenosis ≤ 10 cm in length Single occlusion ≤ 5 cm in length
TASC B	Short (≤ 3 cm) stenosis of infrarenal aorta Unilateral CIA occlusion Single or multiple stenosis totaling 3–10 cm involving the EIA not extending into the CFA Unilateral EIA occlusion not involving the origins of internal iliac or CFA	Multiple lesions (stenoses or occlusions) each ≤ 5 cm Single stenosis or occlusion ≤ 15 cm not involving the infra geniculate popliteal artery Single or multiple lesions in the absence of continuous tibial vessels to improve inflow for a distal bypass Heavily calcified occlusion ≤ 5 cm in length Single popliteal stenosis
TASC C	Bilateral CIA occlusions Bilateral EIA stenoses 3–10 cm long not extending into the CFA Unilateral EIA stenosis extending into the CFA Unilateral EIA occlusion that involves the origins of internal iliac and/or CFA Heavily calcified unilateral EIA occlusion with or without involvement of origins of internal iliac and/or CFA	Multiple stenoses or occlusions totaling ≥ 15 cm with or without heavy calcification Recurrent stenoses or occlusions that need treatment after two endovascular interventions
TASC D	Infra-renal aortoiliac occlusion Diffuse disease involving the aorta and both iliac arteries requiring treatment Diffuse multiple stenoses involving the unilateral CIA, EIA and CFA Unilateral occlusions of both CIA and EIA Bilateral occlusions of EIA Iliac stenoses in patients with AAA requiring treatment and not amenable to endograft placement or other lesions requiring open aortic or iliac surgery	Chronic total occlusions of CFA or SFA (≥ 20 cm, involving the popliteal artery) Chronic total occlusion of popliteal artery and proximal trifurcation vessels

CIA Common Iliac Artery, *EIA* External Iliac Artery, *CFA* Common Femoral Artery, *AAA* Abdominal Aortic Aneurysm, *SFA* Superficial Femoral Artery

echocardiography (ICE) catheter which is used for intracardiac imaging has been used similar to IVUS in endovascular repair of abdominal aortic aneurysm. ICE catheter use is associated with minimal or no use of contrast in the patients who underwent the procedure [32]. Whether used solely or in conjunction with contrast angiography these are valuable tools in reducing the need for iodinated contrast in patients with CKD or those who are intolerant to iodinated contrast media.

Infrainguinal Peripheral Arterial Disease

Clinical Presentation

Symptomatic infra inguinal peripheral arterial disease manifests as claudication of the thighs, calves, non-healing ulcers of lower leg following trauma and critical limb ischemia. Critical limb ischemia is defined as chronic rest pain, ulcers, gangrene that is attributable to arterial occlusive disease.

Non Interventional Management

For both asymptomatic and symptomatic lower extremity PAD, smoking cessation is universally recommended. Supervised exercise programs consisting of at least 30 min of walking, at least 3 times a week lasting at least for 12 weeks is a Class I recommendation for patients with claudication symptoms. For those individuals who are unable to participate in a supervised program, a home based program can be a suitable alternative. For symptomatic PAD, low dose aspirin and statin therapy in addition to aggressive management of risk factors like hypertension, diabetes, dyslipidemia is recommended [26].

In situations where aspirin is not tolerated, clopidogrel 75 mg once a day is an alternative [33]. For patients with intermittent claudication and without any contraindications, a trial of oral cilostazol 100 mg twice daily is recommended. In those patients who cannot tolerate cilostazol, a trial of oral pentoxifylline 400 mg three times daily is recommended [26].

Interventional Management

For individuals with ongoing lifestyle limiting symptomatic lower extremity peripheral arterial disease who have failed all non-interventional measures, surgical revascularization or endovascular therapy is recommended [26].

For TASC A femoral popliteal lesions, endovascular therapy is the treatment of choice. For TASC B and C lesions, endovascular therapy is the preferred modality with surgery being an option if the surgical risk is good [24]. For TASC D lesions surgery has historically been the treatment of choice, but with improved equipment and procedural technique, this is more equivocal [27]. Endovascular strategy includes plain balloon angioplasty, bare metal stents, PTFE covered stents and drug-coated stents [27]. Finally drug coated balloons are emerging as a superior alternative to plain balloon angioplasty [34].

For infrapopliteal disease, revascularization is recommended primarily where there is critical limb ischemia. Surgical techniques are available with autologous venous conduits from femoral or popliteal to the pedal or tibial arteries. Synthetic grafts are only a second choice if autologous veins are not available since veins offer higher patency rates compared with synthetic material [26]. Endovascular therapy for infra popliteal lesions primarily involves use of balloon angioplasty with bare metal stents being used as bailout if necessary. Paclitaxel coated balloon angioplasty has showed promise in infra popliteal disease by significantly decreasing rates of restenosis and amputation [35, 36]. Small series of drug coated coronary stents have also showed promise, but would require more robust studies to validate. Notably, limb salvage rates for endovascular therapy and surgery for infra popliteal disease are comparable (80–85%) [37].

For patients with infra inguinal peripheral arterial disease and CKD requiring percutaneous interventions, carbon dioxide angiography is an alternative to iodinated contrast angiography [38]. The use of carbon dioxide has been studied as a sole agent or supplementary agent along with iodinated contrast in individuals with CKD. Carbon dioxide angiography has proven to reduce the amount of contrast exposure, radiation time while preserving renal function [39, 40].

Extra Cranial Carotid Artery Disease

Clinical Presentation

Extracranial carotid artery disease is responsible for 15% of ischemic strokes. Symptomatic or clinically significant carotid artery disease is defined as focal disease associated with stroke, transient ischemic attacks (TIA) or transient mono-ocular blindness (amaurosis fugax) [28].

Non Interventional Management

Medical therapy for symptomatic extracranial carotid artery disease is similar to management of PAD in other arterial beds and involves management of risk factors namely, hypertension, diabetes, smoking cessation, statin therapy. Aspirin, clopidogrel or the combination of aspirin-dipyridamole is recommended for individuals who have symptomatic disease [28].

Interventional Management

Carotid artery endarterectomy is recommended in individuals with extra cranial carotid artery stenosis greater than 70% by non-invasive imaging or greater than 50% by catheter angiography who have experienced non disabling stroke, TIA or amaurosis fugax and who are at low to average risk for surgical complications. Similarly, carotid artery stenting can be considered in the above situation if the risk of stenting is low to average [28]. In patients with stroke or a TIA carotid artery revascularization with either stenting or surgery can be performed within 2 weeks of the index clinical event [28].

In the asymptomatic individual with carotid artery stenosis greater than 70%, recent data from ACT-1 [41] and CREST [42] showed that outside the peri-operative period, there was no difference in the rate of ipsilateral late stroke after endarterectomy or stenting. This however does not help resolve the vexing question of how best to treat the asymptomatic patient, especially in centers with less angiographer experience. It is hoped that with Carotid Revascularization and Medical Management for Asymptomatic Carotid Stenosis Trial (CREST-2), data will emerge on outcomes with both interventions as well as optimal medical management.

Carotid artery revascularization is not recommended when the stenosis is less than 50% or if the artery is known to be chronically occluded [28].

Vertebral Artery Disease

Clinical Presentation

Vertebral artery disease results in symptoms related to the posterior circulation (dizziness, vertigo, diplopia, perioral numbness, blurred vision, tinnitus, ataxia, bilateral sensory deficits, and syncope). Vertebral artery disease is estimated to be responsible for roughly 20% of posterior circulation strokes [28].

Non Interventional Management

Non interventional management is similar to extracranial carotid artery disease which involves management of vascular risk factors, anti-platelet therapy and statin.

Interventional Management

Asymptomatic vertebral artery disease does not require any interventions. Even when vertebral artery disease is identified, interventions are not commonly done due to the presence of 2 vertebral arteries and most patients remain asymptomatic and unrecognized [43]. Compounding the above factors is the paucity on data on the subject. Surgical correction of vertebral artery disease or angioplasty is rarely performed. There is also a paucity of data on the subject [44].

Peripheral Arterial Disease Outcomes in the CKD Population

As mentioned previously, PAD is associated with an increased risk of future major adverse cardiac events and mortality (Fig. 32.1) [13–19].

Even in asymptomatic individuals with abnormal ABIs, the relative risk of 10-year all-cause mortality has been shown to be twice as high and cardiac mortality, four times as high compared with individuals with normal ABIs [45]. Patients with stable peripheral arterial disease also have a high incidence of acute limb ischemia and acute visceral ischemia defined as arterial events of less than 2-week duration resulting in symptoms. The prognosis after acute peripheral vascular events is very poor with significantly high disability and mortality (about 70%) at 1 and (90%) at 5 years [46]. Individuals with CKD frequently have more severe grades of peripheral arterial disease. CKD as a risk factor on its own increases the chance of future cardiovascular outcomes and worse mortality. There is a linear relationship between the severity of CKD measured by decline in GFR and the risk of death or cardiovascular event [47]. This is shown in Table 32.2.

CKD also doubles the lower extremity amputation rate in PAD patients compared to those without it. Co existent CKD tends to increase the propensity for hospital acquired infections and patients with CKD and PAD are twice as likely to have sepsis [48]. Chronic kidney disease greatly affects outcomes in peripheral arterial disease (Table 32.3). In patients with lower extremity arterial disease, death rates are roughly 3–5 times higher compared with people with normal renal function [51]. The presence of both CKD and PAD increases mortality to a greater degree than the presence of either one alone (Fig. 32.2) [52].

Repair and treatment of peripheral arterial disease is also complicated by the presence of CKD. In the case of peripheral lower extremity interventions, the presence of CKD increased the likelihood of requiring interventions for multiple vessels. The presence of severe CKD increased the likelihood of death or amputation at 30 days by three times. Also severe CKD increased the risk of requiring repeat intervention in infra inguinal arteries with previous angioplasty [53]. In individuals undergoing aorto iliac stenting however, there has not been conclusive data to show that CKD decreases stent patency or increases repeat

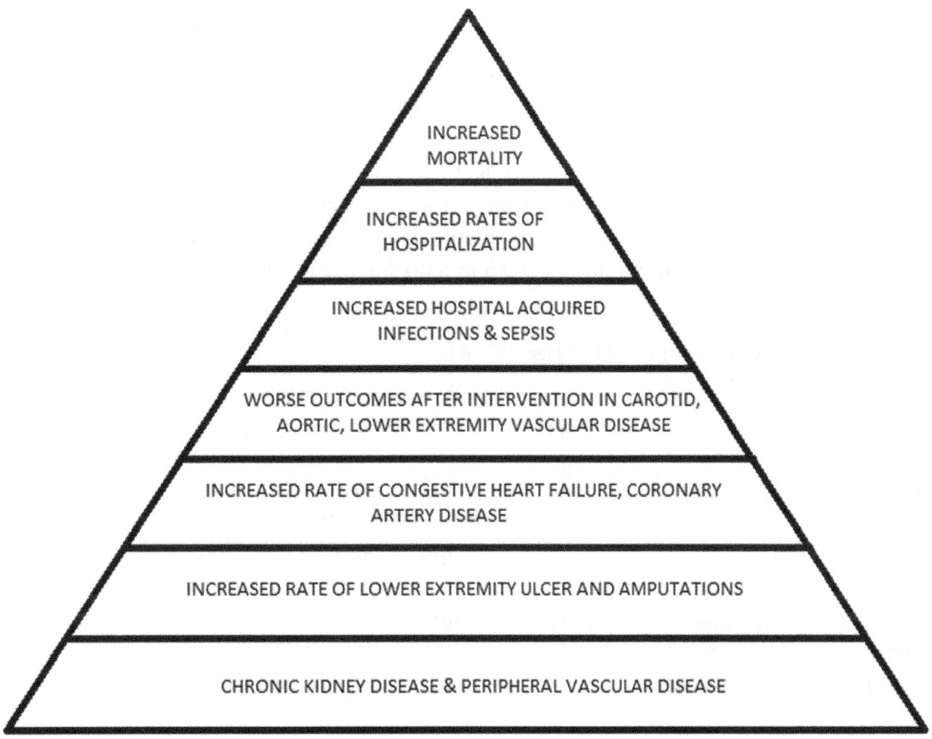

Fig. 32.1 Association of adverse outcomes with the presence of both chronic kidney disease and peripheral vascular disease

Table 32.2 Showing adjusted hazard ratio for any cardiovascular even and all cause mortality among 1,120,295 ambulatory adults stratified by estimated GFR

Estimated GFR in ml/min/1.73 m^2	Cardiovascular event	All cause mortality
≥ 60	1.00	1.00
45–59	1.4	1.2
30–44	2.0	1.8
15—29	2.8	3.2
<15	3.4	5.9

The group with GFR $\geq$ 60 served as the reference group
Adapted with permission from Ref. [47]

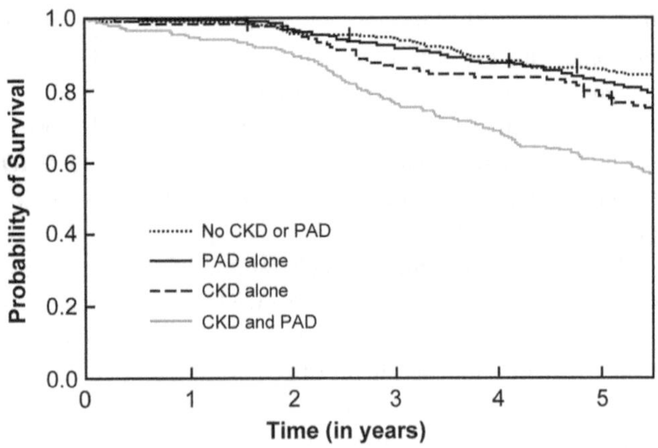

Fig. 32.2 Kaplan–Meier plot of survival probability over time stratified by presence or absence of CKD and PAD. *CKD* Chronic Kidney disease, *PAD* Peripheral arterial disease. Log-rank test for overall difference $P < 0.0001$ (With permission from Ref. [52])

interventions [54]. In individuals undergoing lower extremity bypass surgery as a means of revascularization, severe CKD worsens mortality and amputation free survival [55].

In the case of abdominal aortic aneurysms, the risk of complications and cardiovascular events associated with open or endovascular repair rise in proportion to the severity of CKD. (Refer to Table 32.4) The 30-day mortality is twice as high in individuals with severe CKD (6 vs. 3%; $P = 0.0081$) compared with milder disease [56, 57] and patients with severe CKD who underwent open repair of AAA had a 30-day mortality rate of 10% and a 40% rate of any complication [43]. While it is clear that acutely there is an increased association of morbidity and mortality in individuals undergoing surgical repair of abdominal and infra inguinal arterial disease, data specifically on graft patency rates in this population is still unclear.

Similar to other peripheral disease in other arterial beds, carotid artery disease in conjunction with CKD appears to fare worse (Table 32.5). The impact of CKD on patients undergoing carotid interventions has been examined. In more than 20,000 patients undergoing carotid endarterectomy, moderate CKD (GFR 30–60 ml/min/1.73 m^2) increased the risk of cardiac events (1.7 vs. 0.9% for controls, $P < 0.001$) and pulmonary complications (2.1 vs. 1.3% control; $P < 0.001$) without an increase in mortality. However, severe CKD (GFR less than 30 ml/min/1.73 m^2) had a significantly increased mortality (3.1 vs. 1.0% control, $P < 0.001$) [59]. GFR less than 60 ml/min/1.73 m^2 has also been identified as a risk factor for poor 5-year survival in individuals undergoing carotid endarterectomy for asymptomatic carotid artery disease [60]. The trend appears to be the same in patients undergoing carotid artery stenting. There does not appear to be a significant difference in mortality in individuals with moderate CKD (GFR 30–60 ml/min/1.73 m^2) compared with those having GFR greater than 60 ml/min/1.73 m^2. However, once GFR declines to the range of severe CKD, the 30-day mortality climbs up to roughly 5 times. (0.66% normal renal function, 1.15% moderate renal insufficiency, and 5.45% severe renal insufficiency; $P = 0.005$) [61]

Table 32.3 Pad outcomes stratified by stages of CKD

Study	Outcome	GFR estimation	CKD stratification				Length of follow up	*P* value
			eGFR > 90	eGFR 60–89	eGFR 30–59	eGFR < 30		
Lacroix et al. [49]	Amputation	MDRD	53/219 (24.2%)	80/344 (23.3%)	98/325 (30.1%)	52/122 (42.6%)	1 year	0.0003
Lacroix et al. [48]	Mortality	MDRD	35/219 (16.0%)	62/344 (18.0%)	103/325 (31.7%)	54 (44.3%)	1 year	<0.0001
Otte et al. [50]	Foot ulceration rate per 1000 patients per year	MDRD			29	98		0.02

MDRD Modified Diet and Renal Disease, *eGFR* estimated Glomerular Filtration Rate

Table 32.4 AAA outcomes stratified by stages of CKD

Study	Outcome	GFR estimation	CKD stratification				Length of follow up	*P* value
			eGFR > 90	eGFR 60–89	eGFR 30–59	eGFR < 30		
Patel VI et al. [43]	Mortality after EVAR	MDRD		2.6% (*n* = 746)		5.7% (*n* = 370)	30 days	0.0081
Patel VI et al. [43]	Mortality after open AAA repair	MDRD		4.1 (*n* = 367)		9.9 (*n* = 202)	30 days	0.0057
Saratzis et al. [43]	Non fatal MI after EVAR	CKD EPI	0.5% (1/173)	3% (3/110)	5% (5/80)	30% (6/20)	34+/ 12 months	<0.001
Saratzis et al. [44]	Non fatal stroke after EVAR	CKD EPI	0% (0/173)	0% (0/110)	10% (8/80)	5% (1/20)	34+/ 12 months	<0.001
Saratzis et al. [44]	Mortality after EVAR	CKD EPI	0.5% (1/173)	2% (2/110)	12% (10/80)	35% (7/20)	34+/ 12 months	<0.001

CKD EPI Chronic Kidney Disease Epidemiology Collaboration formula, *EVAR* Endovascular Abdominal Aortic Aneurysm Repair, *AAA* Abdominal Aortic Aneurysm

Table 32.5 Carotid artery disease outcomes stratified by stages of CKD

Study	Outcome	GFR estimation	CKD stratification			Length of follow up	*P* value
			eGFR > 60	eGFR 30-59	eGFR < 30		
Sidawy AN et al. [45]	Mortality following CEA	MDRD	% (*n* = 13,965)	1.4% (*n* = 6423)	3.1% (*n* = 511)	30 days	<0.05
Protack CD et al. [47]	Mortality following CAS	MDRD	1.02% (*n* = 604)	3.33% (*n* = 262)	15.39 (*n* = 55)	30 days	0.02
Protack CD et al. [47]	Stroke following CAS	MDRD	4.08% (*n* = 604)	3.33% (*n* = 262)	23.08% (*n* = 55)	30 days	0.01
Avgerinos et al. [58]		MDRD	5/868 0.6%	5/414 1.2%	2/60 3.3%	30 days	<0.05

CEA Carotid Endarterectomy, *CAS* Carotid Artery Stenting, *MI* Myocardial Infarction

Conclusion

The management of PAD and CKD both independently and together is an arduous task. CKD increases the chance of adverse cardiovascular and cerebrovascular outcomes. It also increases the risk of interventional strategies currently available. Clinicians need to be cognizant of this so as to provide optimal management strategies to patients and also to avoid the burden of cost that these two conditions impale on the healthcare system. Hence management of these conditions requires a thorough understanding of their pathophysiology and relationship. Management of these complex conditions will require a multi-disciplinary team approach involving cardiologists, nephrologists, vascular surgeons, podiatrists, and wound care experts to integrate all aspects of care in these complex patients.

References

1. Hirsch AT, Duval S. The global pandemic of peripheral artery disease. Lancet. 2013;382(9901):1312–4.
2. Fowkes FG, Rudan D, Rudan I, Aboyans V, Denenberg JO, McDermott MM, et al. Comparison of global estimates of prevalence and risk factors for peripheral artery disease in 2000 and 2010: a systematic review and analysis. Lancet. 2013;382 (9901):1329–40.
3. Hirsch AT, Hartman L, Town RJ, Virnig BA. National health care costs of peripheral arterial disease in the medicare population. Vasc Med. 2008;13(3):209–15.
4. Roger VL, Go AS, Lloyd-Jones DM, Adams RJ, Berry JD, Brown TM, et al. Heart disease and stroke statistics—2011 update: a report from the American Heart Association. Circulation. 2011;123(4):e18–209.
5. McDermott MM, Liu K, Criqui MH, Ruth K, Goff D, Saad MF, et al. Ankle-brachial index and subclinical cardiac and carotid

disease: the multi-ethnic study of atherosclerosis. Am J Epidemiol. 2005;162(1):33–41.
6. Selvin E, Erlinger TP. Prevalence of and risk factors for peripheral arterial disease in the United States: results from the National Health and Nutrition Examination Survey, 1999–2000. Circulation. 2004;110(6):738–43.
7. Hirsch AT, Haskal ZJ, Hertzer NR, Bakal CW, Creager MA, Halperin JL, et al. ACC/AHA 2005 Practice Guidelines for the Management of Patients With Peripheral Arterial Disease (Lower Extremity, Renal, Mesenteric, and Abdominal Aortic): A Collaborative Report from the American Association for Vascular Surgery/Society for Vascular Surgery,* Society for Cardiovascular Angiography and Interventions, Society for Vascular Medicine and Biology, Society of Interventional Radiology, and the ACC/AHA Task Force on Practice Guidelines (Writing Committee to Develop Guidelines for the Management of Patients With Peripheral Arterial Disease): Endorsed by the American Association of Cardiovascular and Pulmonary Rehabilitation; National Heart, Lung, and Blood Institute; Society for Vascular Nursing; TransAtlantic Inter-Society Consensus; and Vascular Disease Foundation. Circulation. 2006;113(11):e463–654.
8. Hoerger TJ, Simpson SA, Yarnoff BO, Pavkov ME, Rios Burrows N, Saydah SH, et al. The future burden of CKD in the United States: a simulation model for the CDC CKD Initiative. Am J Kidney Dis. 2015;65(3):403–11.
9. Hirsch AT, Haskal ZJ, Hertzer NR, Bakal CW, Creager MA, Halperin JL, et al. ACC/AHA 2005 Practice Guidelines for the Management of Patients With Peripheral Arterial Disease (Lower Extremity, Renal, Mesenteric, and Abdominal Aortic): A Collaborative Report from the American Association for Vascular Surgery/Society for Vascular Surgery,* Society for Cardiovascular Angiography and Interventions, Society for Vascular Medicine and Biology, Society of Interventional Radiology, and the ACC/AHA Task Force on Practice Guidelines (Writing Committee to Develop Guidelines for the Management of Patients With Peripheral Arterial Disease): Endorsed by the American Association of Cardiovascular and Pulmonary Rehabilitation; National Heart, Lung, and Blood Institute; Society for Vascular Nursing; TransAtlantic Inter-Society Consensus; and Vascular Disease Foundation. Circulation. 2006;113(11): e463–654.
10. O'Hare AM, Glidden DV, Fox CS, Hsu CY. High prevalence of peripheral arterial disease in persons with renal insufficiency: results from the National Health and Nutrition Examination Survey 1999–2000. Circulation. 2004;109(3):320–3.
11. Ix JH, Katz R, De Boer IH, Kestenbaum BR, Allison MA, Siscovick DS, et al. Association of chronic kidney disease with the spectrum of ankle brachial index the CHS (Cardiovascular Health Study). J Am Coll Cardiol. 2009;54(13):1176–84.
12. Hirsch AT, Haskal ZJ, Hertzer NR, Bakal CW, Creager MA, Halperin JL, et al. ACC/AHA 2005 Practice Guidelines for the Management of Patients With Peripheral Arterial Disease (Lower Extremity, Renal, Mesenteric, and Abdominal Aortic): A Collaborative Report from the American Association for Vascular Surgery/Society for Vascular Surgery,* Society for Cardiovascular Angiography and Interventions, Society for Vascular Medicine and Biology, Society of Interventional Radiology, and the ACC/AHA Task Force on Practice Guidelines (Writing Committee to Develop Guidelines for the Management of Patients With Peripheral Arterial Disease): Endorsed by the American Association of Cardiovascular and Pulmonary Rehabilitation; National Heart, Lung, and Blood Institute; Society for Vascular Nursing; TransAtlantic Inter-Society Consensus; and Vascular Disease Foundation. Circulation. 2006;113(11): e463–654.
13. Stack AG. Coronary artery disease and peripheral vascular disease in chronic kidney disease: an epidemiological perspective. Cardiol Clin. 2005;23(3):285–98.
14. Lederle FA, Johnson GR, Wilson SE, Chute EP, Hye RJ, Makaroun MS, et al. The aneurysm detection and management study screening program: validation cohort and final results. Aneurysm Detection and Management Veterans Affairs Cooperative Study Investigators. Arch Intern Med. 2000;160(10):1425–30.
15. Criqui MH, Langer RD, Fronek A, Feigelson HS, Klauber MR, McCann TJ, et al. Mortality over a period of 10 years in patients with peripheral arterial disease. N Engl J Med. 1992;326(6):381–6.
16. Newman AB, Sutton-Tyrrell K, Vogt MT, Kuller LH. Morbidity and mortality in hypertensive adults with a low ankle/arm blood pressure index. JAMA. 1993;270(4):487–9.
17. Vogt MT, Cauley JA, Newman AB, Kuller LH, Hulley SB. Decreased ankle/arm blood pressure index and mortality in elderly women. JAMA. 1993;270(4):465–9.
18. Criqui MH, McClelland RL, McDermott MM, Allison MA, Blumenthal RS, Aboyans V, et al. The ankle-brachial index and incident cardiovascular events in the MESA (Multi-Ethnic Study of Atherosclerosis). J Am Coll Cardiol. 2010;56(18):1506–12.
19. Lee AJ, Price JF, Russell MJ, Smith FB, van Wijk MC, Fowkes FG. Improved prediction of fatal myocardial infarction using the ankle brachial index in addition to conventional risk factors: the Edinburgh Artery Study. Circulation. 2004;110 (19):3075–80.
20. Resnick HE, Lindsay RS, McDermott MM, Devereux RB, Jones KL, Fabsitz RR, et al. Relationship of high and low ankle brachial index to all-cause and cardiovascular disease mortality: the Strong Heart Study. Circulation. 2004;109(6):733–9.
21. Tsai AW, Folsom AR, Rosamond WD, Jones DW. Ankle-brachial index and 7-year ischemic stroke incidence: the ARIC study. Stroke. 2001;32(8):1721–4.
22. Regensteiner JG, Hiatt WR, Coll JR, Criqui MH, Treat-Jacobson D, McDermott MM, et al. The impact of peripheral arterial disease on health-related quality of life in the Peripheral Arterial Disease Awareness, Risk, and Treatment: New Resources for Survival (PARTNERS) Program. Vasc Med. 2008;13(1):15–24.
23. GBD 2013 Mortality and Causes of Death Collaborators. Global, regional, and national age-sex specific all-cause and cause-specific mortality for 240 causes of death, 1990–2013: a systematic analysis for the Global Burden of Disease Study 2013. Lancet. 2015;385(9963):117–71.
24. Hirsch AT, Hartman L, Town RJ, Virnig BA. National health care costs of peripheral arterial disease in the Medicare population. Vasc Med. 2008;13(3):209–15.
25. Saran R, Li Y, Robinson B, Ayanian J, Balkrishnan R, Bragg-Gresham J, et al. US Renal Data System 2014 Annual Data Report: Epidemiology of Kidney Disease in the United States. Am J Kidney Dis. 2015;66(1 Suppl 1):Svii, S1-305.
26. Norgren L, Hiatt WR, Dormandy JA, Nehler MR, Harris KA, Fowkes FG, et al. Inter-society consensus for the management of peripheral arterial disease (TASC II). Eur J Vasc Endovasc Surg. 2007;33(Suppl 1):S1–75.
27. Murphy TP, Cutlip DE, Regensteiner JG, Mohler ER III, Cohen DJ, Reynolds MR, et al. Supervised exercise, stent revascularization, or medical therapy for claudication due to aortoiliac peripheral artery disease: the CLEVER study. J Am Coll Cardiol. 2015;65(10):999–1009.
28. Society for Vascular Surgery Lower Extremity Guidelines Writing Group, Conte MS, Pomposelli FB, Clair DG, Geraghty PJ, McKinsey JF, et al. Society for Vascular Surgery practice guidelines for atherosclerotic occlusive disease of the lower extremities: management of asymptomatic disease and claudication. J Vasc Surg. 2015;61(3 Suppl):2S–41S.

29. Ruggiero NJ II, Jaff MR. The current management of aortic, common iliac, and external iliac artery disease: basic data underlying clinical decision making. Ann Vasc Surg. 2011;25 (7):990–1003.
30. von Segesser LK, Marty B, Ruchat P, Bogen M, Gallino A. Routine use of intravascular ultrasound for endovascular aneurysm repair: angiography is not necessary. Eur J Vasc Endovasc Surg. 2002;23(6):537–42.
31. Hoshina K, Kato M, Miyahara T, Mikuriya A, Ohkubo N, Miyata T. A retrospective study of intravascular ultrasound use in patients undergoing endovascular aneurysm repair: its usefulness and a description of the procedure. Eur J Vasc Endovasc Surg. 2010;40(5):559–63.
32. Belenky A, Atar E, Orron DE, Litvin S, Knizhnik M, Almog M, et al. Endovascular abdominal aortic aneurysm repair using transvenous intravascular US catheter guidance in patients with chronic renal failure. J Vasc Interv Radiol. 2014;25(5):702–6.
33. Brott TG, Halperin JL, Abbara S, Bacharach JM, Barr JD, Bush RL, et al. 2011 ASA/ACCF/AHA/AANN/AANS/ACR/ASNR/CNS/SAIP/SCAI/SIR/SNIS/SVM/SVS guideline on the management of patients with extracranial carotid and vertebral artery disease: a report of the American College of Cardiology Foundation/American Heart Association Task Force on Practice Guidelines, and the American Stroke Association, American Association of Neuroscience Nurses, American Association of Neurological Surgeons, American College of Radiology, American Society of Neuroradiology, Congress of Neurological Surgeons, Society of Atherosclerosis Imaging and Prevention, Society for Cardiovascular Angiography and Interventions, Society of Interventional Radiology, Society of NeuroInterventional Surgery, Society for Vascular Medicine, and Society for Vascular Surgery. J Am Coll Cardiol. 2011;57(8):e16–94.
34. Rosenfield K, Jaff MR, White CJ, Rocha-Singh K, Mena-Hurtado C, Metzger DC, et al. Trial of a Paclitaxel-coated balloon for femoropopliteal artery disease. N Engl J Med. 2015;373(2):145–53.
35. Fanelli F, Cannavale A, Corona M, Lucatelli P, Wlderk A, Salvatori FM. The "DEBELLUM"—lower limb multilevel treatment with drug eluting balloon—randomized trial: 1-year results. J Cardiovasc Surg (Torino). 2014;55(2):207–16.
36. Liistro F, Porto I, Angioli P, Grotti S, Ricci L, Ducci K, et al. Drug-eluting balloon in peripheral intervention for below the knee angioplasty evaluation (DEBATE-BTK): a randomized trial in diabetic patients with critical limb ischemia. Circulation. 2013;128 (6):615–21.
37. Steering Committee TASC, Jaff MR, White CJ, Hiatt WR, Fowkes GR, Dormandy J, et al. An update on methods for revascularization and expansion of the TASC lesion classification to include below-the-knee arteries: a supplement to the Inter-Society Consensus for the Management of Peripheral Arterial Disease (TASC II). Vasc Med. 2015;20(5):465–78.
38. Scalise F, Novelli E, Auguadro C, Casali V, Manfredi M, Zannoli R. Automated carbon dioxide digital angiography for lower-limb arterial disease evaluation: safety assessment and comparison with standard iodinated contrast media angiography. J Invasive Cardiol. 2015;27(1):20–6.
39. Palena LM, Diaz-Sandoval LJ, Candeo A, Brigato C, Sultato E, Manzi M. Automated carbon dioxide angiography for the evaluation and endovascular treatment of diabetic patients with critical limb ischemia. J Endovasc Ther. 2016;23(1):40–8.
40. Stegemann E, Tegtmeier C, Bimpong-Buta NY, Sansone R, Uhlenbruch M, Richter A, et al. Carbondioxide-aided angiography decreases contrast volume and preserves kidney function in peripheral vascular interventions. Angiology. 2016;67(9):875–81.
41. Rosenfield K, Matsumura JS, Chaturvedi S, Riles T, Ansel GM, Metzger DC, et al. Randomized trial of stent versus surgery for asymptomatic carotid stenosis. N Engl J Med. 2016;374(11): 1011–20.
42. Brott TG, Howard G, Roubin GS, Meschia JF, Mackey A, Brooks W, et al. Long-term results of stenting versus endarterectomy for carotid-artery stenosis. N Engl J Med. 2016;374 (11):1021–31.
43. European Association for Cardiovascular Prevention & Rehabilitation, Reiner Z, Catapano AL, De Backer G, Graham I, Taskinen MR, et al. ESC/EAS Guidelines for the management of dyslipidaemias: the Task Force for the management of dyslipidaemias of the European Society of Cardiology (ESC) and the European Atherosclerosis Society (EAS). Eur Heart J. 2011;32(14):1769–818.
44. Coward LJ, McCabe DJ, Ederle J, Featherstone RL, Clifton A, Brown MM, et al. Long-term outcome after angioplasty and stenting for symptomatic vertebral artery stenosis compared with medical treatment in the Carotid And Vertebral Artery Transluminal Angioplasty Study (CAVATAS): a randomized trial. Stroke. 2007;38(5):1526–30.
45. Kornitzer M, Dramaix M, Sobolski J, Degre S, De Backer G. Ankle/arm pressure index in asymptomatic middle-aged males: an independent predictor of ten-year coronary heart disease mortality. Angiology. 1995;46(3):211–9.
46. Howard DP, Banerjee A, Fairhead JF, Hands L, Silver LE, Rothwell PM, et al. Population-based study of incidence, risk factors, outcome, and prognosis of ischemic peripheral arterial events: implications for prevention. Circulation. 2015;132 (19):1805–15.
47. Go AS, Chertow GM, Fan D, McCulloch CE, Hsu C. Chronic kidney disease and the risks of death, cardiovascular events, and hospitalization. N Engl J Med 2004 09/23; 2016/01; 351 (13):1296–1305.
48. Luders F, Bunzemeier H, Engelbertz C, Malyar NM, Meyborg M, Roeder N, et al. CKD and acute and long-term outcome of patients with peripheral artery disease and critical limb ischemia. Clin J Am Soc Nephrol. 2016;11(2):216–22.
49. Lacroix P, Aboyans V, Desormais I, Kowalsky T, Cambou JP, Constans J, et al. Chronic kidney disease and the short-term risk of mortality and amputation in patients hospitalized for peripheral artery disease. J Vasc Surg. 2013;58(4):966–71.
50. Otte J, van Netten JJ, Woittiez AJ. The association of chronic kidney disease and dialysis treatment with foot ulceration and major amputation. J Vasc Surg. 2015;62(2):406–11.
51. Pasqualini L, Schillaci G, Pirro M, Vaudo G, Siepi D, Innocente S, et al. Renal dysfunction predicts long-term mortality in patients with lower extremity arterial disease. J Intern Med. 2007;262 (6):668–77.
52. Liew YP, Bartholomew JR, Demirjian S, Michaels J, Schreiber MJ Jr. Combined effect of chronic kidney disease and peripheral arterial disease on all-cause mortality in a high-risk population. Clin J Am Soc Nephrol. 2008;3(4):1084–9.
53. Patel VI, Mukhopadhyay S, Guest JM, Conrad MF, Watkins MT, Kwolek CJ, et al. Impact of severe chronic kidney disease on outcomes of infrainguinal peripheral arterial intervention. J Vasc Surg. 2014;59(2):368–75.
54. Aihara H, Soga Y, Iida O, Suzuki K, Tazaki J, Shintani Y, et al. Long-term outcomes of endovascular therapy for aortoiliac bifurcation lesions in the real-AI registry. J Endovasc Ther. 2014;21(1):25–33.
55. Owens CD, Ho KJ, Kim S, Schanzer A, Lin J, Matros E, et al. Refinement of survival prediction in patients undergoing lower

extremity bypass surgery: stratification by chronic kidney disease classification. J Vasc Surg. 2007;45(5):944–52.

56. Patel VI, Lancaster RT, Mukhopadhyay S, Aranson NJ, Conrad MF, LaMuraglia GM, et al. Impact of chronic kidney disease on outcomes after abdominal aortic aneurysm repair. J Vasc Surg. 2012;56(5):1206–13.
57. Saratzis A, Sarafidis P, Melas N, Saratzis N, Kitas G. Impaired renal function is associated with mortality and morbidity after endovascular abdominal aortic aneurysm repair. J Vasc Surg. 2013;58(4):879–85.
58. Avgerinos ED, Go C, Ling J, Makaroun MS, Chaer RA. Survival and long-term cardiovascular outcomes after carotid endarterectomy in patients with chronic renal insufficiency. Ann Vasc Surg. 2015;29(1):15–21.
59. Sidawy AN, Aidinian G, Johnson ON III, White PW, DeZee KJ, Henderson WG. Effect of chronic renal insufficiency on outcomes of carotid endarterectomy. J Vasc Surg. 2008;48(6):1423–30.
60. Wallaert JB, Cronenwett JL, Bertges DJ, Schanzer A, Nolan BW, De Martino R, et al. Optimal selection of asymptomatic patients for carotid endarterectomy based on predicted 5-year survival. J Vasc Surg. 2013;58(1):112–8.
61. Protack CD, Bakken AM, Saad WE, Davies MG. Influence of chronic renal insufficiency on outcomes following carotid revascularization. Arch Surg. 2011;146(10):1135–41.

Contrast Induced Nephropathy

33

Jatinder Kohli, Akash N. Sethi, and Michael R. Rudnick

Introduction

Contrast Induced Nephropathy (CIN) is a generally reversible, non-oliguric cause of acute kidney injury (AKI) that usually occurs within 48–72 h after intravascular contrast administration. However, AKI after contrast administration cannot be automatically attributed to the contrast agent. The KDIGO AKI guidelines recommend evaluation of other possible causes of AKI in all such cases [1].

Clinical Significance

CIN is associated with significant morbidity and mortality. Multiple studies have reported its relationship with prolonged hospitalization, as well as other clinically significant adverse outcomes including early and late cardiovascular events [2]. McCullough et al. [3] evaluated the relationship between renal outcomes and in-hospital mortality after coronary intervention. The adjusted odds ratios were reported to be 6.56 [95% Confidence interval (CI) 3.34–12.62; $P < 0.00001$] for CIN of any severity and 13.54 (95% CI 3.92–46.8; $P < 0.00001$) for CIN requiring dialysis. The 2-year survival rate for patients with CIN requiring dialysis was only 18.8%.

Although CIN is usually a reversible form of AKI, reports in literature have shown higher incidence of chronic kidney disease (CKD) in patients who develop CIN after coronary angiography. Nemoto et al. [4] reported CIN as an independent risk factor for continuous deterioration of renal function at 6–8 months after percutaenous coronary intervention (PCI) following acute coronary syndrome (ACS). Thus, a careful long-term follow up of renal function is needed following episodes of CIN.

Pathogenesis

The primary pathways by which contrast agents cause nephropathy are by renal ischemia (by increasing oxygen demand or decreasing blood flow), and tubular injury via Reactive Oxygen Species (ROS) or direct cytotoxic effects (Fig. 33.1).

The renal medulla is poorly oxygenated at baseline, making it susceptible to hypoxic injury. Reasons for poor oxygenation even under normal conditions are countercurrent exchange of oxygen between vasa recta, and oxygen use by active transport of sodium in ascending limb of loop of henle [5].

After contrast is injected there is a transient increase in renal blood flow followed by variable duration of decreased blood flow resulting in renal ischemia. Hyperosmolar contrast agents by inducing osmotic diuresis can increase oxygen demand due to increased work of active transporters. Furthermore, the release of vasoconstrictive mediators like endothelin and adenosine, as well as blockade of vasodilator compounds such as nitric oxide and prostaglandins appear to exacerbate medullary hypoxic injury [6].

ROS formed as a result of post ischemic oxidative stress can cause tubular injury via their effects on renal endothelial cells. In vitro cell culture studies as well as some animal data

M.R. Rudnick (✉)
Department of Medicine, Penn Presbyterian Medical Center, Perelman School of Medicine of the University of Pennsylvania, 39th and Market Streets, MOB Suite 240, Philadelphia, PA 19104, USA
e-mail: rudnickm@uphs.upenn.edu

J. Kohli
Renal, Electrolyte and Hypertension Division, Department of Medicine, Hospital of University of Pennsylvania, 3400 Spruce Street, Founders 1, Philadelphia, PA 19104, USA
e-mail: Jatinder.kohli@uphs.upenn.edu

A.N. Sethi
Renal, Electrolytes and Hypertension, Hospital of University of Pennsylvania, 3400 Spruce Stree, Philadelphia, PA 19104, USA
e-mail: asethi87@gmail.com

J. Rangaswami et al. (eds.), *Cardio-Nephrology*,
DOI 10.1007/978-3-319-56042-7_33

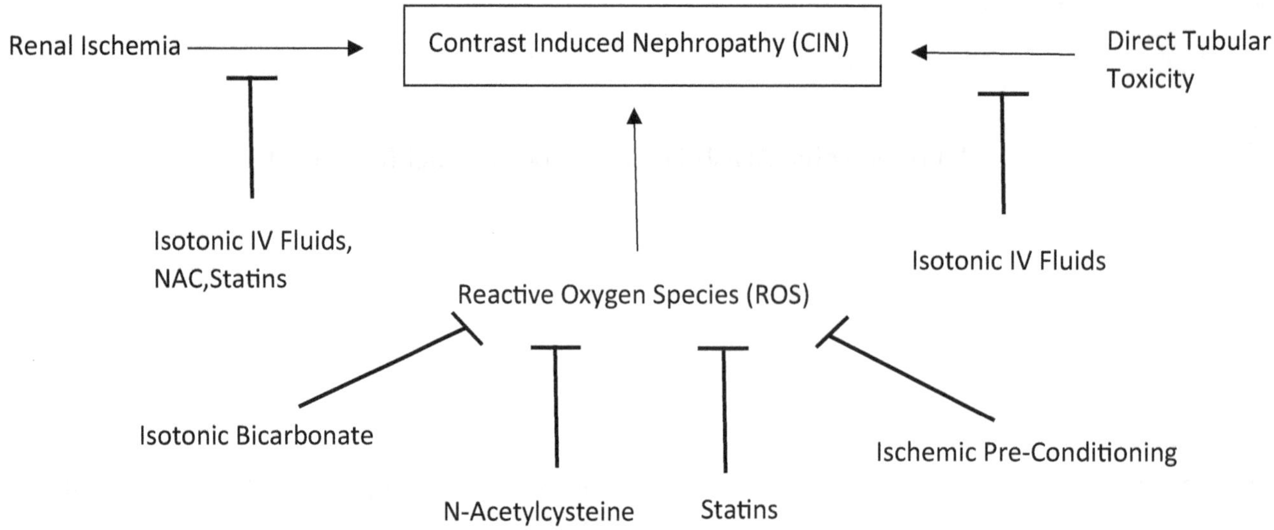

Fig. 33.1 Pathogenic mechanisms and preventive strategies for CIN

have shown contrast mediated activation of various pro-inflammatory and pro-apoptotic molecules such as JNK kinases, p38transcription factor NF-Kb and caspases, as well as deactivation of pro-proliferative kinases such as ERK1/2 and Akt [7].

Direct toxicity of contrast agents to renal epithelial cells has also been suggested to contribute to the pathogenesis of CIN.

Risk Factors

There are several risk factors for the development of CIN, of which the following dominate in terms of relative risk of injury:

- CKD: Pre-existing renal insufficiency is the single most important risk factor for CIN, and the risk increases with increase in severity of baseline renal dysfunction. A clinical significant risk is usually thought to be associated with eGFR below 60 mL/min/1.73 m^2 although this threshold may be different between intravenous and intra-arterial contrast administration.
- Diabetes Mellitus: Although diabetes is often considered to be a risk factor for CIN, the risk is likely related to the co-existing renal insufficiency rather than diabetes itself. In diabetic patients with normal renal function the incidence of CIN is similar to non-diabetic patients with normal renal function. On the other hand, the risk of CIN is higher in patients with diabetes and pre-existing renal insufficiency compared to non-diabetic patients with similar levels of pre-existing renal insufficiency.
- Contrast agent characteristics: The type (hyperosmolar vs. lowosmolar vs. or iso-osmolar), volume as well as route of administration (intra-arterial vs. intravenous) are all related to the risk of CIN.

The earlier generation contrast agents which were ionic and hyperosmolar (around 2000 mosm/L) are more nephrotoxic compared to newer agents i.e., low-osmolar (600–900 mosm/L) and iso-osmolar agents (300 mOsm/L). However, iso-osmolar agents have not been shown to be less nephrotoxic compared to low-osmolar agents. This may possibly be related to the increased viscosity of iso-osmolar agents [8].

Although low doses have been variably defined in literature (from <30 to 125 mL), the lower doses are considered to be less nephrotoxic compared to higher doses. In general, it is recommended to use the lowest possible doses of contrast, particularly in patients at higher risk for CIN.

Other risk factors for CIN include advancing age, co-existing volume depletion, congestive heart failure (CHF), hemodynamic instability, hyperglycemia (independent of diabetes mellitus) and concurrent use of nephrotoxic medications. Multiple myeloma, use of angiotensin converting enzyme inhibitors/angiotensin receptor blockers (ACEI-/ARB), renal transplant and cirrhosis are considered to be synergizing risk factors, with controversial evidence.

Validated risk prediction models have been developed to assess the risk of CIN in patients undergoing PCI. An example of one such prediction model based on patient and procedure characteristics developed by Mehran et al. [9] is shown in Fig. 33.2. While such prediction models would not alter the ultimate decisions to perform coronary procedures in any individual patient, they do help risk stratify patients pre procedure, and help draw attention to optimizing co-existing risk factors for CIN to the extent feasible.

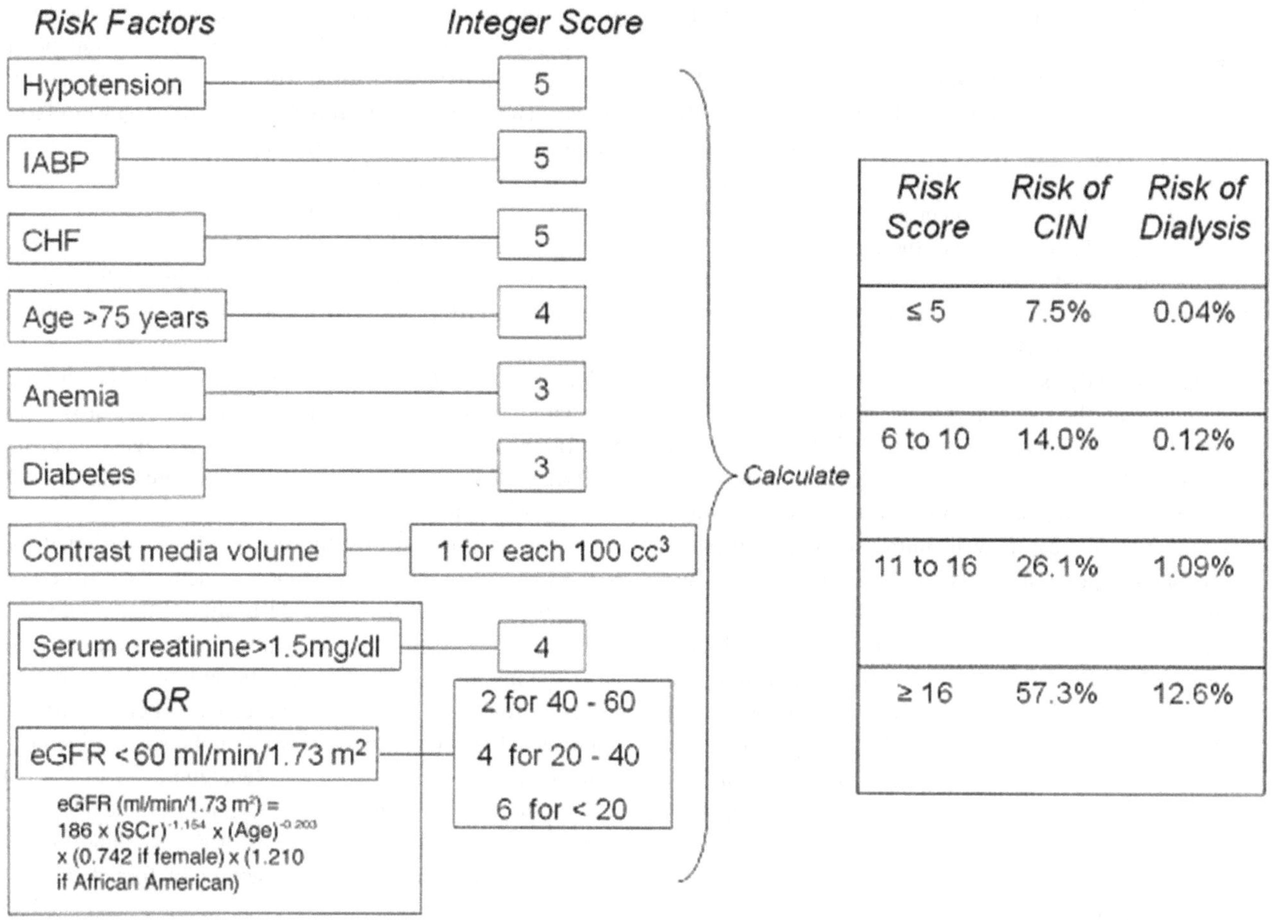

Fig. 33. 2 CIN risk scoring model for percutaneous coronary intervention (PCI); *CHF* congestive heart failure, *egfr* estimated glomerular filtration rate, *IABP* intra-aortic balloon pump

Clinical Features/Diagnosis

CIN is typically characterized by an AKI developing within 24–48 h of contrast media exposure, with the rise in serum creatinine reaching its peak at 3–5 days, followed by return to baseline in 7–10 days. AKI from CIN is usually non oliguric although severe AKI requiring hemodialysis can occur particularly in patients with underlying significant CKD.

The urinalysis is helpful in excluding other causes of AKI and is usually characterized by findings of acute tubular necrosis (ATN), including muddy brown casts and tubular epithelial cells. However, absence of these findings does not exclude the diagnosis. Proteinuria is usually absent or mild, when present. Though AKI is mediated via tubular injury, fractional excretion of sodium (FeNa) has been reported to be <1% reflective of the significant renal arteriolar hypoperfusion that is typical of the post contrast sequelae. Other causes of AKI that should be considered in patients post cardiac catheterization include atheroembolic disease, cardiorenal syndrome and any procedure related hypoperfusion causing ischemic ATN independent of contrast media.

Prevention

Currently, there is no treatment to reverse or ameliorate CIN once it has occurred. Preventive strategies are the best option for patients at risk of developing CIN. Many preventive strategies have been tried that may interfere with one or more of the currently accepted pathogenic mechanisms (Fig. 33.1). The strategies shown to have definite value in CIN prevention include parenteral hydration, the use of low-osmolar and iso-osmolar contrast media as well as a low volume of contrast media. The major CIN preventive strategies will be discussed here.

Intravenous Fluids

Theoretically, extracellular volume expansion helps by counteracting different mechanisms involved in the pathogenesis of CIN. These include decreasing the direct tubular toxicity by dilution of contrast media as well as preventing the renal medullary ischemia via inhibition of renin angiotensin system (RAS) as well as vasopressin.

Isotonic saline has been shown to be more protective than equivalent volumes of hypotonic saline [10], likely because isotonic fluids are better volume expanders. It has been postulated that isotonic bicarbonate, by altering tubular fluid pH may protect against free radical mediated injury and thus may be superior to isotonic saline. However, the role of isotonic bicarbonate remains uncertain as multiple trials and systemic reviews have shown conflicting results [11]. A recent meta-analysis evaluated the data from 22 randomized controlled trials (RCT's) and concluded that sodium bicarbonate is not superior to isotonic saline in preventing CIN, the need for dialysis or mortality [11]. In addition to uncertain benefit, the risk of formulation errors with isotonic bicarbonate should be considered as well. KDIGO recommends that either fluid can be used for CIN prevention.

The data regarding optimal rate, timing and duration of fluids remain equivocal as well. Intravenous (IV) hydration 12 h before and after the cardiac catheterization has been shown to have better outcomes compared to IV hydration only during the procedure [12]. In the absence of large, prospective, randomized trials to guide the timing and duration of IV hydration, it is a common practice to administer 1 mL/kg/h for 6–12 h' pre-procedure, intra-procedure and for 6–12 h' post-procedure for inpatients scheduled for a contrast procedure. For outpatients with high risk to develop CIN, isotonic fluids starting 1 h prior and continuing up to 4–6 h post contrast administration is a common practice.

It has been suggested that optimal hydration should be defined according to pre-defined clinical markers. Markers which been shown to decrease the incidence of CIN compared to standard hydration include left ventricular end diastolic pressure (LVEDP) [13], urine flow rate [14], and central venous pressure (CVP) [15]. The beneficial effects hydration protocols are perhaps related to the ability to administer higher mean volume compared to standard hydration groups. As an example, Brar et al. [13] evaluated the fluid replacement protocol guided by LVEDP. In this trial, 396 patients with CKD (egfr < 60 mL/min/1.73 m^2) and various other risk factors for CIN, including age >75 years, diabetes mellitus and history of congestive heart failure were randomized to LVEDP guided fluid management (n = 196) or standard hydration group (n = 200). All patients received intravenous isotonic saline (3 mL/kg) 1 h prior to the cardiac catheterization. In addition, LVEDP guided group patients received 5 mL/kg/h if LVEDP was lower than 13 mmHg, 3 mL/Kg/h if LVEDP was between 13 and 18 mmHg, and 1.5 mL/Kg/h if LVEDP was greater than 18 mmHg. In comparison, the control group received 1.5 mL/kg/h. Both groups received intravenous fluid throughout and for 4 h following the procedure. CIN (defined as >0.5 mg/dL or >25% increase in serum creatinine between 1 and 4 days after the procedure) occurred less frequently in the LVEDP group compared with control [6.7 vs. 16.3%, respectively (RR 0.41, 95% CI 0.22–0.79)]. There was no statistically significant difference in the adverse events among the two groups. These findings need further confirmation from larger multicenter trials before this approach can be recommended as a standard hydration protocol.

Oral hydration is currently not recommended as an effective strategy for prevention of CIN. The use of diuretics is currently not recommended unless required for volume overload. In a RCT (n = 78) of CKD (mean serum creatinine 2.1 mg/dL) patients undergoing cardiac catheterization Solomon et al. [16] showed IV hydration to be better when compared to IV hydration plus mannitol or furosemide. Several other small trials have also reported higher incidence of AKI with the use of diuretics for CIN prevention, likely related to volume depletion.

However, subsequently Stevens et al. [14] reported that irrespective of baseline renal function, achieving urine flow rates above 150 mL/h in first 24 h after contrast exposure with forced diuresis while attempting to hold the intravascular volume in a constant state with replacement of urinary losses provides a modest protective benefit against contrast-induced renal injury. Based on the same principle, a fluid management system called Renalguard^{TM} (PLC Medical system, Inc. Franklin, MA, USA) has been developed. It is designed to guide fluid replacement by matching volume repletion to the urine output in setting of forced diuresis. Two small randomized trials have reported its beneficial effects on reducing the incidence of CIN [17, 18]. The potential benefit that it offers is likely from higher urine output per hour without the concerns for volume depletion. For example, the target urine output in both these trials was at least 300 mL/h for up to 4 h after the contrast procedure. Though these results in absence of any significant adverse events look promising but its efficacy, safety and cost effectiveness still needs to be evaluated by additional large, randomized control trials.

N-acetylcysteine (NAC)

NAC is thought to have a role in prevention of CIN due to its antioxidant and vasodilatory effects. The largest RCT (n = 2308) that evaluated the role of NAC in CIN prevention concluded that acetylcysteine does not reduce the risk of contrast-induced acute kidney injury or other clinically relevant outcomes in at-risk patients undergoing coronary and peripheral vascular angiography [19]. However, it should be noted that this study was likely underpowered to exclude a benefit from NAC in high-risk patients (i.e., patients with severe CKD) as majority of the patients included in this study had rather mild degree of renal dysfunction (eGFR 45–60 mL/min/1.73 m^2) and thus represented patients at lower

Table 33.1 Novel-technique proposed by Nayak et al to minimize contrast volume during angiography or intervention

Key elements of the ultra-low contrast technique
1. Use small diameter catheters (i.e., 5–6 French) without side-holes
2. All contrast injections require simultaneous cine angiogram, i.e., "no dye without the cine's eye"
3. Limit the volume of contrast injected from the catheter to 1–2 cm^3 per injection using a 3-cm^3 syringe
4. During PCI, prior to exchange of devices such as balloon catheters, remove contrast from the guide catheter by back bleeding contrast out of the "Y" connector
5. If available, display previous angiographic images (including angiography from past procedures) alongside active fluoroscopy screen as a reference to use as guidance during guide wire, balloon, stent and ultrasound passage
6. Absolutely no contrast "puffing" during the procedure
7. Use IVUS liberally for pre-PCI assessment of the lesion, selection of therapeutic modalities, and post-PCI result assessment

risk of CIN. Several other trials as well meta-analyses have produced conflicting results, but given its safety profile and cost it continues to be commonly used for CIN prevention. KDIGO suggests the use of oral NAC together with intravenous crystalloids in patients at high risk for CIN. The preferred dose is 1200 mg twice daily starting a day prior to and on the day of the procedure.

Contrast Volume

Contrast volume increases the risk of CIN in a dose dependent fashion. Table 33.1 highlights a novel approach to minimize the contrast volume during coronary procedures described by Nayak et al. [20]. Among other strategies, this approach suggested the use of intravascular ultrasound (IVUS). IVUS has now been shown to significantly reduce the contrast volume during diagnostic and therapeutic coronary procedures. Mariani Jr. et al. [21] evaluated to the impact of using IVUS on final contrast volume in patients undergoing PCI, the median total contrast volume in IVUS group was found to be 20 mL (minimum 3 mL; maximum 54 mL) compared to median total volume of 64.5 mL (minimum 19 mL; maximum 170 mL) in angiography guided group ($P < 0.001$). Thus, the use of IVUS should be strongly considered, particularly for high-risk patients undergoing coronary angiography.

Statins

The role of statins in prevention of CIN is currently controversial as well. Given their pleotropic effects including their anti-inflammatory profile, low cost and favorable side effect profile there has been much interest in evaluating the role of statins in the prevention of CIN. Statins are thought to modulate kidney hypoperfusion after contrast administration by downregulation of angiotensin receptors and decreased synthesis of endothelin-1, while at the same time increasing nitric oxide production (a potent vasodilator) which in turn decreases ischemic injury. In addition, statins have also have been thought to decrease the toxic damage and inflammation on the tubular cells by scavenging oxygen-free radicals and down regulating the pro-inflammatory cytokines, which in turn inhibits tissue factor expression by macrophages and prevent the activation of nuclear factor-kB.

However, multiple RCT's as well as meta-analyses have reported conflicting results. A meta-analysis by Zhang et al. [22] evaluated 6 RCT's and concluded that the data on statins and CIN risk reduction were inconclusive, due to the inherent limitations of included studies. Another recent meta-analysis [23] which included the data from 9 RCT's supported the use of pre-procedure statin to decrease the risk of CIN. Given the conflicting results as well as difficulty in interpreting the results of various meta-analyses due to heterogeneous data, there is no consensus on the use of statins in the prevention of CIN. This uncertainty merits further randomized trials in high-risk patients to evaluate the role of statins in CIN prevention. However, in patients who would need statins anyways (e.g. patients with acute myocardial infarctions), it seems a reasonable approach to start or maintain statin therapy prior to the coronary angiography.

Remote Ischemic Preconditioning

Remote ischemic preconditioning (RIPC) is a technique which inducing brief periods of non-injurious ischemia and reperfusion that is thought to reduce kidney ischemic-reperfusion injury. The technique either involves using sphygmomanometer and inflating above systolic pressure or using a stent balloon to transiently occlude blood flow. The proposed mechanism of action for RIPC involves neuronal pathways, which releases adenosine, bradykinin, endogenous peptides and possibly some other unidentified humoral factors that mediate protection of remote organs via their anti-inflammatory and antioxidant properties. Over past few years, several small observational and randomized trials reported reduced incidence of CIN as well as AKI post cardiac surgery with RIPC. However, a recent large, randomized trial (n = 1612) in patients undergoing cardiac surgery by Hausenloy et al. [24] did not show any improvement in clinical outcomes (including death from cardiovascular causes, nonfatal myocardial infarction, coronary revascularization, acute kidney injury, or stroke) with the use of RIPC. This trial also speculated the possible risks associated with RIPC including release of various pro-inflammatory stimuli. In conclusion, this seems to be an exciting prospect whose efficacy as well as safety still needs to examined before it can be routinely recommended as a preventive measure for CIN or AKI post cardiac surgeries.

Renin Angiotensin Aldosterone System (RAAS) Blockade

Angiotensin converting enzyme (ACE) inhibitors and aldosterone receptor blockers (ARBs) are one of the most commonly used agents in patients with cardiovascular risk factors. The effect of withholding these agents on the incidence of CIN in patients undergoing contrast procedure remains controversial [25]. Given the insufficient data as well as the theoretical benefits of RAAS blockade including prevention of renal vasoconstriction and angiotensin II mediated generation of ROS, there are currently no standardized recommendations for or against their cessation pre procedure, except in the volume depleted patient.

Summary

CIN remains one of the major complications of coronary and vascular angiography, with significant morbidity and mortality burden. It is imperative to risk stratify patients at high risk for CIN based on eGFR, diabetes, volume status and concomitant nephrotoxins before dye exposure. Using judicious and individualized peri-procedural fluid management and minimizing tubulotoxic pathways are the mainstay of reducing the burden of this entity. Novel strategies targeted at the inflammatory response to tubular ischemia hold promise in being able to reduce nephron loss after contrast media exposure, in the future.

References

1. KDIGO AKI. Work Group: KDIGO clinical practice guideline for acute kidney injury. Kidney Int Suppl. 2012;2:1–138.
2. Rudnick M, Feldman H. Contrast induced nephropathy: what are the true clinical consequences? Clin J Am Soc Nephrol. 2008;3: 263–72.
3. McCullough PA, Wolyn R, Rocher LL, Levin RN, O'Neill WW. Acute renal failure after coronary intervention: incidence, risk factors, and relationship to mortality. Am J Med. 1997;103: 368–75.
4. Nemoto N, Iwasaki M, Nakanishi M, Araki T, Utsunomiya M, Hori M, et al. Impact of continuous deterioration of kidney function 6–8 months after percutaneous coronary intervention for acute coronary syndrome. Am J Cardiol. 2014;113:1647–51.
5. Heyman SN, Rosen S, Brezis M. Radiocontrast nephropathy: a paradigm for the synergism between toxic and hypoxic insults in the kidney. Exp Nephrol. 1994;2:153–7.
6. Rudnick, et al. Contrast-induced nephropathy: How it develops, how to prevent it. Cleve Clin J Med. 2006;73:75–87.
7. Michael A, Faga T, Pisani A, et al. Molecular mechanisms of renal cellular nephrotoxicity due to radiocontrast media. BioMed Res Int. 2014;2014:10.
8. Sterling KA, Tehrani T, Rudnick MR. Clinical significance and preventive strategies for contrast-induced nephropathy. Curr Opin Nephrol Hypertens. 2008;17:616–23.
9. Mehran R, Aymong ED, Nikolsky E, et al. A simple risk score for prediction of contrast-induced nephropathy after percutaneous coronary intervention: development and initial validation. J Am Coll Cardiol. 2004;44:1393–9.
10. Mueller C, Buerkle G, Buettner HJ, et al. Prevention of contrast media associated nephropathy: randomized comparison of 2 hydration regimens in 1620 patients undergoing coronary angioplasty. Arch Intern Med. 2002;162:329–36.
11. Zapata-Chica CA, Bello Marquez D, Serna-Hiquita LM, et al. Sodium bicarbonate vs. isotonic saline solution to prevent Contrast-induced nephropathy: a systematic review and meta-analysis. Colomb Med (Cali). 2015;46(3):90–103.
12. Bader BD, Berger ED, Heede MB, et al. What is the best hydration regimen to prevent contrast media-induced nephrotoxicity? Clin Nephrol. 2004;62(1):1–7.
13. Brar SS, Aharonian V, Mansukhani P, et al. Haemodynamic-guided fluid administration for the prevention of contrast-induced acute kidney injury: the POSEIDON randomized controlled trial. Lancet. 2014;383:1814–23.
14. Stevens MA, McCullough PA, Tobin KJ, et al. A prospective randomized trial of prevention measures in patients at high risk for contrast nephropathy: results of the P.R.I.N.c.e. study. Prevention of radiocontrast induced nephropathy clinical evaluation. J Am Coll Cardiol. 1999;33:403–11.
15. Qian Geng, Zhenhong Fu, Guo Jun, et al. Prevention of contrast-induced nephropathy by central venous pressure-guided fluid administration in chronic kidney disease and congestive heart failure patients. J Am Coll Cardiol Interv. 2017;9(1):89–96.
16. Solomon R, Werner C, Mann D, et al. Effects of saline, mannitol and furosemide to prevent acute decreases in renal function induced by radiocontrast agents. N Engl J Med. 1994;331:1416.
17. Briguori C, Visconti G, Focaccio A, et al. Renal insufficiency after contrast media administration trial II (REMEDIAL II): renal guard system in high-risk patients for contrast-induced acute kidney injury. Circulation. 2011;124:1260–9.
18. Marenzi G, Ferrari C, Marana I, et al. Prevention of contrast nephropathy by furosemide with matched hydration: the MYTHOS (Induced diuresis with matched hydration compared to standard hydration for contrast induced nephropathy prevention) trial. JACC Cardiovasc Interv. 2012;5:90–7.
19. Investigators ACT. Acetylcysteine for prevention of renal outcomes in patients undergoing coronary and peripheral vascular angiography: main results from the randomized acetylcysteine for contrast-induced nephropathy trial (ACT). Circulation. 2011;124:1250.
20. Nayak KR, Mehta HS, Price MJ, et al. A novel technique for ultra-low contrast administration during angiography or intervention. Catheter Cardiovasc Interv. 2010;75:1076–83.
21. Mariani J Jr, Guedes C, Soares P, et al. Intravascular ultrasound guidance to minimize the use of iodine contrast in percutaneous coronary intervention: the MOZART (minimizing contrast utilization with IVUS guidance in coronary angioplasty) randomized controlled trial. JACC Cariovasc Interv. 2014;7(11):1287–93.

22. Zhang T, Shen LH, Hu LH, He B. Statins for the prevention of contrast-induced nephropathy: a systematic review and meta-analysis. Am J Nephrol. 2011;33(4):344–51.
23. Liu YH, Liu Y, Duan CY, et al. Statins for the Prevention of contrast-induced nephropathy after coronary angiography/percutaneous interventions: a meta-analysis of randomized controlled trials. J Cardiovasc Pharmacol Ther. 2015;20(2):181–92.
24. Hausenloy DJ, Candilio L, Evans R, et al. Remote ischemic preconditioning and outcomes of cardiac surgery. N Engl J Med. 2015;373(15):1408–17.
25. Balta S, Aparci M. The relation between renin-angiotensin-aldosterone system blockade and contrast-induced nephropathy: an unresolved issue. Cardiology. 2015;130(1):1–3.

Acute Kidney Injury After Cardiac Surgery

34

Andrea Perrotti, Benoit Barrucand, and Sidney Chocron

Abbreviations and Acronyms Dictionary

ACE inhibitor	Angiotensin-converting enzyme inhibitors
AKI	Acute kidney injury
AKIN	Acute kidney injury network
ATP	Adenosine triphosphate
CABG	Coronary artery bypass graft
CPB	Cardiopulmonary bypass
CSA-AKI	Cardiac surgery associated acute kidney injury
eGFR	Estimated glomerular filtration rate
GFR	Glomerular filtration rate
L-FABP	L-type fatty acid-binding protein
MECC	Mini-extracorporeal circulation
NAG	*N*-acetyl-B-d-glucosaminidase
NGAL	Neutrophil gelatinase-associated lipocalin
RAA	Renin-angiotensin-aldosterone
RBC	Red blood cells
RIFLE	Risk, injury, failure, loss, and end-stage renal disease
RTT	Renal replacement therapy
SCr	Serum creatinine
SRI	Simplified renal index
UO	Urine output

Incidence and Prognosis of Acute Kidney Injury After Cardiac Surgery

Cardiac surgery remains one of the most common high-risk surgeries in the world. Every year, over 2 million operations are performed worldwide. Acute kidney injury (AKI) is one of the most frequent and serious complications to occur following cardiac surgery [1]. Depending on the specific definition of AKI and the preoperative renal status of the patient, it has been reported that the incidence of postoperative AKI in cardiac surgery ranges from 5 to 40% [2, 3]. The incidence of AKI depends on the type of surgery; for example, isolated CABG has the lowest incidence of AKI, while valvular surgery and combined CABG plus valvular

A. Perrotti (✉) · S. Chocron
Department of Thoracic and Cardio-Vascular Surgery, University Hospital Jean Minjoz, EA3920, University of Franche-Comté, 3 Boulevard Fleming, 25030 Besançon, France
e-mail: a.perrotti@hotmail.it

S. Chocron
e-mail: sidney.chocron@univ-fcomte.fr

B. Barrucand
Department of Anesthesiology and Surgical Critical Care Medicine, University Hospital Jean Minjoz, 3 Boulevard Fleming, 25000 Besançon, France
e-mail: bbarrucand@chu-besancon.fr

J. Rangaswami et al. (eds.), *Cardio-Nephrology*,
DOI 10.1007/978-3-319-56042-7_34

surgery are associated with a higher incidence [4]. Postoperative AKI is associated with high mortality, more complicated hospital course, and a higher risk of infectious complications [5]. Although postoperative AKI requiring dialysis (AKI-D) is rare (1.2–3.0%), it is independently associated with mortality. Indeed, among patients who require dialysis, the risk of mortality is high, averaging around 60–70% [6]. Moreover, the majority of patients who develop AKI-D remain dialysis-dependent, leading to significant long-term morbidity and mortality [7]. In fact, Hobson et al. reported that up to 45% of patients who required dialysis after cardiac surgery may remain dialysis-dependent, 33% may have a partial renal recovery and only 21% may achieve complete renal recovery at the time of hospital discharge [8]. Even slight rises in serum creatinine (sCr) may increase postoperative mortality significantly. Lassnigg et al. [9] demonstrated that a minimal increase (0.3–0.5 mg/dL) in sCr after cardiac surgery was associated with a nearly threefold increase in 30-day mortality and a >0.5 mg/dL rise in sCr was associated with an 18.64-fold increase in 30-day mortality.

The link between postoperative AKI and mortality is driven by several factors, including some that are directly related to hemodialysis, such as catheter-related infections, visceral ischemia, platelet dysfunction, and immunodeficiency. Thakar et al. reported that the infection rate is higher in patients with postoperative AKI, regardless of baseline renal function, and that postoperative mortality in patients with serious infection was 31.7% [10]. In a prospective, multicenter, community-based study, Liano and Pascual reported that infections were the cause of death in 40% of patients with AKI [11]. For these reasons, it is important to improve our understanding of the pathophysiology of AKI associated with cardiac surgery, and implement specific therapies based on this knowledge.

Definition of Acute Kidney Injury

Historically, the lack of a consensual definition of AKI has posed a major problem that has substantially complicated research in this field. The use of several, different, and arbitrary definitions by various authors made it difficult to determine the true incidence and risk factors of AKI or to draw comparisons between different studies. In 2004, the Acute Dialysis Quality Initiative Group introduced the RIFLE classification in order to provide a uniform definition of AKI and facilitate early detection and grading for patients suffering from renal failure [12]. RIFLE stands for "Risk, Injury, Failure, Loss of kidney function and End stage kidney disease," and is based on two criteria, namely: serum creatinine levels (sCr) and urine output (UO), using a 7-day time window. Another version of the RIFLE classification was proposed by the Acute Kidney Injury Network (AKIN) in 2007. The AKIN group suggested four important changes in the new classification as compared with the original RIFLE, namely: omission of glomerular filtration rate (GFR), considering creatinine changes as low as 0.3 mg/dL as AKI; the use of a 48 h time window; and the removal of the last two levels of AKI (loss of function and end-stage kidney disease) [13] (Table 34.1). Data have shown that the AKIN score applied in cardiac surgery patients without correction of sCr for fluid balance may lead to overdiagnosis of AKI (poor positive predictive value), while modification of RIFLE by staging all patients with dialysis in the failure class "F" may improve the predictive value. In view of the limitations of both these AKI definitions, the use of the RIFLE criteria in patients undergoing cardiac surgery seems to be preferable [14].

Pathogenesis of AKI

The pathogenesis of AKI in cardiac surgery is complex and multifactorial. We can identify some of the mechanisms that cause the injury during the preoperative, intraoperative, and postoperative phases. Several processes in cardiac surgery can lead to cellular ischemia in the kidney, explaining tubular epithelial and vascular endothelial injury [15]. Autoregulation of kidney perfusion normally preserves a stable GFR despite changes in systemic blood pressure (ranging from 80 to 180 mmHg). However, often, during cardiac surgery, the mean pressure can fall below the limits of autoregulation, especially in the event of hemodynamic instability. Moreover, in many cardiac surgery patients, autoregulation does not work, due to several factors such as advanced age, chronic hypertension, or chronic use of drugs that may impact kidney autoregulation (e.g., angiotensin receptor blockers, ACE inhibitors, nonsteroidal antiinflammatory drugs, and radiocontrast agents). In these patients, renal function may worsen, even when the mean arterial blood pressure is within normal limits [16]. Another pathophysiologic mechanism that leads to ischemic kidney injury is the strong systemic inflammatory response [5]. CPB-associated systemic inflammatory response syndrome is triggered, first of all, by direct contact between blood components and the artificial surface of the bypass circuit; and this exposure to the CPB circuit initiates several types of cascades that can cause kidney injury, such as complement activation, free radical formation, and inflammatory cytokine production. Concurrently, exogenous and endogenous toxins, ischemia-reperfusion injury, and operative trauma all play a central role in the development of inflammation [17]. Moreover, the kidney may be affected by microemboli composed of platelet aggregates, fibrin, lipids, atheromatous plaques, and air. In fact, emboli smaller than 40 μm are not

Table 34.1 Definition and classification for acute kidney injury

	RIFLE classification		AKIN classification	
	Serum creatinine/GFR criteria	Urine output criteria	Serum creatinine/GFR criteria	Urine output criteria
Definition	SCr rise ≥ 1.5 times baseline or GFR decrease >25% within 7 d		SCr rise ≥ 1.5 times baseline or ≥ 0.3 mg/dL within 48 h	
Staging	R (Risk) SCr rise up to 2 times baseline or GFR decrease >25%	<0.5 mL/kg/h for ≥ 6 h	Stage 1 SCr rise up to 2 times baseline or ≥ 0.3 mg/dL	<0.5 mL/kg/h for ≥ 6 h
	I (Injury) SCr rise up to 3 times baseline or GFR decrease >50%	<0.5 mL/kg/h for ≥ 12 h	Stage 2 SCr rise up to 3 times baseline	<0.5 mL/kg/h for ≥ 12 h
	F (Failure) SCr rise 3 times baseline or more or GFR decrease >75% or absolute SCr ≥ 4 mg/dL with acute rise ≥ 0.5 mg/dL	<0.5 mL/kg/h for ≥ 24 h or anuria ≥ 12 h	Stage 3 SCr rise 3 times baseline or more or absolute SCr ≥ 4 mg/dL with acute rise ≥ 0.5 mg/dL with acute rise ≥ 0.5 mg/dL or need for RRT	<0.3 mL/kg/h for ≥ 24 h or anuria ≥ 12 h
	L (loss) persistent AKI >4 wk, need for RRT			
	E (ESRD) persistent loss >3 mo, need for dialysis			

RIFLE risk, injury, failure, loss and end-stage renal disease, *AKIN* acute kidney injury network, *GFR* glomerular filtration rate, *SCr* serum creatinine, *h* hours, *d* days, *AKI* acute kidney injury, *RRT* renal replacement therapy, *ESRD* end-stage renal disease, *mo* months

effectively filtered by CPB systems, with the risk of damaging renal capillaries directly [17]. Lastly, another important cause of kidney injury during CPB is haemolysis and release of free hemoglobin. Increased levels of free red blood cell constituents, together with exhaustion of their scavengers, transferrin, and haptoglobin, result in a variety of serious clinical sequelae including increased systemic vascular resistance, altered coagulation activity, platelet dysfunction, and renal tubular damage [18]. The combination of all these factors explains the considerable risk of renal tubular injury in patients undergoing cardiac surgery.

Diagnosis of Cardiac Surgery Associated Acute Kidney Injury: The Role of Biomarkers

Serum creatinine is still the most important biomarker routinely used to identify kidney injury since, to date, there is no substitute that is equally as feasible and inexpensive. On the other hand, the detective ability of serum creatinine is low, and its response to renal insult is slow and late. In fact, circulating levels of creatinine vary with age, gender, ethnicity, muscle mass, diet, vigorous exercise, and medication. Creatinine levels start to rise only when 50% of renal function has already been lost. Therefore, it may take up to 24 h for AKI to be diagnosed owing to the slow increase in creatinine levels [19]. This delay, which may prevent early and effective intervention, highlights the need for immediate markers of AKI. The ability to detect the initiation or early phases of AKI could improve monitoring, facilitate care, and achieve better outcomes. Ideally, such a biomarker would identify injury as it occurs intraoperatively or at least within a few hours after surgery. Recent research efforts have identified multiple proteins that may be the starting point for early diagnosis of AKI. Neutrophil gelatinase-associated lipocalin (Ngal) is a protein that normally binds to small iron-carrying molecules. Ngal is significantly overexpressed in response to acute renal injury, and has been investigated in both serum and urine for the early diagnosis of ischaemic renal injury. It has been highlighted that in pediatric surgery, Ngal is a powerful immediate biomarker with a significantly earlier rise following injury as compared to creatinine [20, 21]. While Ngal has shown good sensitivity and specificity in pediatric surgery populations, its reliability is still controversial in adult cardiac patients due to the various comorbidities affecting this population. In the study by Wagener et al., urinary NGAL was shown to be a reliable biomarker for postoperative AKI, with concentrations continuing to increase and remaining significantly higher at 3 and 18 h after cardiac surgery [22]. Conversely, McIlroy et al. [23] reported that urine NGAL may have diminished ability to detect AKI in patients with preexisting renal disease, but performs better in those with baseline eGFR > 60 mL/min. Equally controversial are the results obtained with plasma Ngal. Perry et al. [24] reported that Ngal had a limited predictive value at 2 h post-surgery in contrast with Haase, who reported a significant predictive value at 6 h [25]. Finally, we previously reported that plasma Ngal is a useful marker of AKI in patients with chronic renal failure prior to surgery [26].

Several other biomarkers such as cystatin C, IL-18, L-type fatty acid-binding protein (L-FABP), and *N*-acetyl-B-d-glucosaminidase (NAG) have been identified. However, the results of studies investigating IL-18 continue to be conflicting. An important study reported that urinary IL-18 was an early predictor of AKI after cardiac surgery, as demonstrated by an area under the receiver operating characteristic curve for diagnosis of AKI at 4, 12, and 24 h after CPB of 61, 75, and 73%, respectively [27]. Conversely, a study by Haase et al. asserted that 24 h after surgery, urinary IL-18 did not appear to be reliable in identifying patients who go on to develop AKI after cardiac surgery, but rather, represents a nonspecific marker of CPB-associated systemic inflammation [28]. Likewise, cystatin C appears to be a biomarker that is not influenced by age, sex, or muscle mass. However, due to conflicting results, its precise value in the diagnosis and prognosis of CSA-AKI remains unclear [29]. Moreover, a recent meta-analysis of 28 studies reporting intraoperative and/or early postoperative measurement of current biomarkers found that known biomarkers have poor, and at best moderate, discrimination for AKI when measured within the first 24 h after cardiac surgery in adults [30]. The problem is that the pathogenesis of CSA-AKI is multifactorial, and thus, a single biomarker cannot capture sufficient information to be highly accurate in the diagnosis of AKI. Combining different biomarkers improves the sensitivity of early detection of CSA-AKI as compared with individual biomarkers [31]. A large multicenter prospective study involving 1219 patients showed that plasma NGAL and IL-18 peaking 6 h after surgery were significantly linked to AKI, mortality, and longer hospital stay after cardiac surgery [32]. Another observational study by Koyner et al. evaluated the interest of simultaneous use of IL-18, plasma and urinary NGAL, and urinary albumin-to-creatinine ratio (ACR). The authors showed that biomarkers measured on the day of AKI diagnosis improved risk stratification and identified patients at higher risk of progression of AKI and worse outcomes [33]. Nevertheless, clinicians unfortunately cannot yet avail themselves of these new biomarkers in everyday practice, because diagnostic features have been found to vary widely, and also because the identification of confounders of biomarkers is still in progress. In summary, considerable research is still warranted into AKI biomarkers to optimize these tools before they can be used to guide risk stratification, therapeutic intervention, and prognostication of CSA-AKI.

Risk Factors for CSA-AKI

Several risk factors associated with the development of CSA-AKI have been identified. There are two main groups of risk factors, namely preoperative and intraoperative factors. Most preoperative risk factors are patient-related, while most intraoperative factors depend on the surgical procedure (Table 34.2).

Preoperative Risk Factors for AKI

The most frequently reported preoperative risk factors for the occurrence of AKI post-surgery include female gender, reduced left ventricular function or the presence of congestive heart failure, advanced age, diabetes mellitus, peripheral vascular disease, preoperative use of an intra-aortic balloon pump, chronic obstructive pulmonary disease, emergency surgery, redo surgery, and preoperative renal impairment [estimated glomerular filtration rate (eGRF) < 60 mL/min creatinine >2.1 mg/dL] [2, 5, 34]. Moreover, a multicenter study by Perez-Valdivieso et al. suggested that preoperative diuretic use was an independent risk factor for CSA-AKI [35]. In addition, surgery performed too early after contrast angiography may be a major risk factor affecting postoperative AKI according to a multivariate analysis by Medalion et al. of patients after CABG surgery. In fact, these authors identified surgery within 24 h of contrast administration and a contrast dose over >1.4 mL/kg as being risk factors for CSA-AKI if surgery took place within 5 days of angiography [36]. Equally, Kramer et al. underline the fact that cardiac catheterization and cardiac surgery should not be performed together in the same hospitalization, to allow renal cell recovery, prior to the new insults to renal cells from the surgery itself, with a view to decreasing the risk of postoperative AKI [37]. Furthermore, administering some medications such as nonsteroidal antiinflammatory drugs and angiotensin receptor blockers may be an additional risk factor, because it impairs the autoregulation of renal blood flow in patients already suffering from major renal insults following chronic or acute cardiac disease [38].

During the perioperative period, the volume status of the patients is of importance, especially in case of low cardiac output. This condition leads to hyperactivity of the sympathetic nervous system, with the corresponding activation of the renin-angiotensin aldosterone (RAA) system, increasing renal vasoconstriction, and it is directly related to AKI risk [39]. Finally, genetic predisposition to AKI has been

Table 34.2 Risk factors for cardiac surgery associated acute kidney injury

Preoperative	Intraoperative	Postoperative
Female gender	Anemia	Hemodynamic instability
Reduced LV function or the presence of CHF	Hemodilution	Operative trauma
Advanced age	Off-pump vs on-pump CABG	Anemia
Diabetes mellitus	Hemodynamic alterations	Blood transfusion
Peripheral vascular disease	Hypothermia	Surgical reexploration
Preoperative use of IABP	Embolism	
Chronic obstructive pulmonary disease	Duration of CPB	
Emergency surgery		
Redo surgery and preoperative renal impairment		
Adequate hydration and avoid loop diuretics		
Surgery after 5 days of coronary angiography		
Chronic obstructive pulmonary disease		

LV left ventricular, *CHF* congestive heart failure, *CABG* coronary artery bypass graft, *IABP* intra-aortic balloon pump, *CPB* cardiopulmonary bypass

described in one study from Duke University, reporting that patients with the inherited apolipoprotein epsilon-4 allele are less likely to develop AKI compared to patients with other forms of this allele [40].

Several research groups have developed risk stratification models that help to predict the risk of CSA-AKI. Identification and categorization of high-risk patients allows for the adoption of optimal strategies aimed at better management and efficient application of prophylactic and therapeutic measures. Risk prediction models can also be used as research tools to select high-risk patients for studies on AKI, and to facilitate more detailed informed consent. Chertow et al. in 1997 published the first risk score using a large population database [2]. Three additional predictive risk models, the Cleveland Clinic score, the Mehta score, and the Simplified Renal Index (SRI) score [41–43], have since been developed to predict the need for dialysis as an outcome. Published by Thakar et al. in 2005, the Cleveland Clinic score is the most validated model for its high level of precision and the best discriminatory power, resulting from an analysis of a population of 33,217 patients. It is derived from 13 preoperative factors, and the overall score ranges from 0 to 17. In the lowest risk group (score 0–2), the risk of AKI was 0.4%, while patients with the highest score [9–13] had a risk of 21.5% [41]. In 2006, Mehta et al. developed a predictive model for postoperative AKI-D, including a bedside tool to calculate the additive risk score, based on the analysis of a multicenter dataset of more than 600 hospitals [42]. Wijeysundera et al. subsequently proposed the SRI model in 2007, a "simplified renal index" using only eight factors to predict postoperative AKI-D [43]. Finally, two validation studies concluded that the Cleveland Clinic score has the best discriminatory capacity for postoperative AKI-D [44, 45]. In another publication from the Cleveland Clinic, new predictive risk models integrating intraoperative factors have been published, and these seem to represent an advance over previous predictive scores [46]. Other models have been suggested to predict AKI not requiring dialysis. However, the use of varying definitions of AKI may impact the general clinical utilization of these risk models. Furthermore, urine IL-18 and plasma NGAL when added to the risk model improved risk prediction by 25 and 18% respectively [32]. A universally accepted definition of AKI, together with the use of new biomarkers, should pave the way for the development of a complete and final score for the prediction of early stages of AKI.

Intraoperative Events

The intraoperative period is a critical time when patients are exposed to anesthesia and cardiopulmonary bypass (CPB). As already mentioned above, these events plays a critical role in causing hemodynamic alterations, and in inducing activation of both innate and adaptive immune responses leading to CSA-AKI. Loss of pulsatile flow, hemodilution, hypothermia, and embolism are all postulated to be contributing factors. At this stage; the surgeon has a wide range of choices concerning the best procedures to achieve a successful outcome of the patient.

Events Associated with CPB

The main aim of CPB is to maintain adequate regional perfusion at a level that allows optimal cellular and organ function. Thus, any inadequate change in flow rate or in perfusion pressure, depending on its duration and importance, may lead to renal injury [47]. In general, CPB flow rates of 1.8–2.21/min/m^2 along with a mean perfusion pressure of 50–70 mmHg [48] are advised. The loss of pulsatile flow during CPB may cause an increase in peripheral vascular resistance, interstitial oedema and subsequently, have a negative impact on the microcirculation [49]. While there has much investigation into the feasibility of reproducing the pulsatile flow during CPB, the practical advantages of its application have never yet been universally accepted. In fact, a recent meta-analysis carried out by Sievert et al. [50] among 1185 patients demonstrated that the pulsatile flow protects renal function in patients undergoing cardiac surgery, but Baraki et al., in their study involving 1959 patients, concluded that keeping the pulsatile flow during surgery had no positive impact on either mortality or renal function, and only shortened hospitalization [51]. During CPB, uncontrolled hemodilution is to be avoided, as it decreases the oxygen-carrying capacity of the blood. Renal function may be affected both by a reduction in regional blood flow and by decreased oxygen transport [5, 38]. In a retrospective study of 1760 patients, Habib et al. showed that intraoperative hematocrits below 24% were significantly associated with increased risk of postoperative AKI [52]. A more recent prospective study [53] reported that patients with low haematocrit (<24%) who present with a lactate rise signaling tissue hypoxemia are more prone to renal damage.

Several factors linked to CPB seem to explain red blood cell (RBC) destruction that is the basis of hemolysis. The mechanisms responsible for RBC damage may be shear stress, blood temperature control if the pump is not properly set, a mismatch between patient size and the diameter of cannulae or poor positioning, the air–fluid interface in the reservoir, and more especially, cardiotomy suction, due to the traumatic contact when blood is concurrently suctioned with air [54]. Replacing cardiotomy suction with the use of red blood cell salvage reduces haemolysis, thereby avoiding mechanical damage. In this process, only RBCs are retained during blood processing, while plasma, platelets, heparin, plasma-free hemoglobin, and inflammatory mediators are discarded with the wash solution. The consequent RBCs are finally suspended at a hematocrit of 50–70% in normal saline and reinfused [54]. Macroscopic and microscopic emboli, both gaseous and particulate, are often generated during CPB. These emboli are closely related to some intraoperative manipulations such as aortic cannulation, cross clamp placement and release [54]. In a retrospective review, Sreeram et al. found a significant correlation between the total number of transcranial Doppler-detected emboli and postoperative changes in serum creatinine [55]. Epiaortic echocardiography has become a valuable tool to choose an optimal site for cannulation and clamping in patients likely to have aortic atherosclerosis. In the presence of extensive aortic disease, the surgeon may apply peripheral cannulation. Arterial perfusion through the axillary artery provides adequate antegrade aortic flow with fewer atheroembolic complications. A further alternative is femoral cannulation, which exposes the patient to the risk of a retrograde flow. An attractive device to avoid damage caused by emboli is the use of intra-aortic filtration (e.g., the EMBOL-X System, Edwards Lifesciences, Irvine, CA, USA), a cannula with an expandable filtration trap incorporated, that is able to capture emboli in the ascending aorta during surgical manipulation, after aortic cross-clamping and before aortic declamping. Considering the damage caused by CPB, it is natural to wonder whether CSA-AKI is related to the duration of CPB. A recent meta-analysis of 12,466 patients found a significant link between the duration of CPB and cross-clamp time and incidence of CSA-AKI [56]. Individual patient characteristics together with CPB duration are responsible for the renal damage. This makes it difficult to define an average "safe time" cutoff beyond which AKI may occur. However, in a study by Salis et al. including over 5000 patients, a mean cutoff of 115 min was identified as the limit beyond which the risk of AKI increased [57]. Depending on the type of intervention, different levels of hypothermia may be required, ranging from quasi-normothermia to deep hypothermia at 18 °C. The role of hypothermia in the occurrence of CSA-AKI remains debate [58, 59]. Beyond the degree of hypothermia, it has been purported that the rewarming technique may be implicated in the occurrence of postoperative AKI [60].

On-Pump Versus off-Pump

Avoiding CPB may decrease systemic inflammatory response syndrome, but the act of splitting the sternum and entering the mediastinal cavity is, by itself, already a major biological aggression. While off-pump coronary artery bypass avoids many CPB-related complications and aortic manipulation, it may nonetheless be responsible for low cardiac output, due to contortion of the heart, and this is liable to cause AKI. In 2009, Nigwekar et al. [61] published a meta-analysis of 22 studies including a total of 27,000 patients evaluating the results of on-pump versus off-pump surgery. They reported a significant reduction in overall AKI and in AKI-D in patients operated on using the off-pump technique, compared with those in whom the on-pump technique was used. Conversely, according to the large randomized controlled ROOBY [62] and CORONARY [63] trials, there were no significant differences between the on-pump and off-pump techniques when AKI-D was taken as the primary endpoint. To date, there have been no randomized clinical trials proving the superiority of one technique over the other in reducing CSA-AKI. For this reason, it is up to each surgeon, according to their clinical judgement and experience, to choose the technique that they deem most likely to produce the best results in light of the patient's condition.

Blood Transfusion

While preoperative and intraoperative anemia may contribute to kidney injury by reducing renal oxygen delivery and worsening oxidative stress [34, 64], there is also evidence to suggest that transfusion of RBCs is strongly associated with CSA-AKI [34, 35]. Stored RBCs become less deformable, undergo ATP and 2,3-diphosphoglycerate depletion, lose their ability to generate nitric oxide, have increased adhesiveness to vascular endothelium, release procoagulant phospholipids, and accumulate proinflammatory molecules, as well as free iron and hemoglobin [65, 66]. As a result, transfusion of stored RBCs promotes an inflammatory state, intensifies tissue oxidative stress and activates the coagulation cascade [34, 65, 66]. In cardiac surgery patients, these events can lead to kidney dysfunction. Karkouti et al. reported that it is not the absolute level of hemoglobin that is important, but rather, its relative change from the baseline [67]. They found that the risk of AKI was significantly increased when hemoglobin decreased by more than 50% below baseline levels [67]. In light of these data, blood sparing techniques are of fundamental utility, such as the use of mini-extracorporeal circulation (MECC) with retro-priming using the patient's blood, intraoperative blood salvage using CellSaver® autotransfusion system, hemostatic glue, cryoprecipitate, and factor VII to minimize the need for transfusion.

Surgical Reexploration

The preoperative use of antiplatelet agents, or surgery requiring a long duration of CBP, and/or hypothermia, can make it difficult to control hemostasis, causing delayed chest closure or surgical reexploration. Surgical reexploration after cardiac surgery is strongly linked to AKI, owing to many factors such ensuing haemodynamic instability, operative trauma, anemia, and blood transfusion [68]. Therefore, it is advisable to proceed as follows: the use of platelet antiaggregants or other medications that lower blood coagulation should be discontinued preoperatively, where possible. While surgery is in progress, blood transfusion, platelets, and blood coagulating drugs should be administered in a timely manner. Lastly, meticulous hemostasis by the surgeon and close monitoring of the patient, especially in the early postoperative period, are of prime importance.

Pharmacological Renal Protection

Preoperative

Before cardiac surgery, it is important to preserve, and even optimize the patient's renal function. Among the various risk factors that have been identified for AKI after surgery, some of them can be targeted for specific measures. Several approaches have been proposed for protecting renal function.

Improving renal perfusion by optimizing preoperative volemia has shown promise for the improvement of postoperative renal status. In a prospective study in a tertiary centre, it was shown that preoperative intravenous infusion of half-isotonic saline was associated with a reduction in the rate of postoperative acute renal failure in patients with moderate-to-severe CKD prior to surgery [69]. To confirm these results, further studies with larger populations are warranted to identify the impact of optimizing volemia prior to surgery in patients with normal preoperative renal function. Indeed, preoperative hydration is likely not a suitable strategy in patients with congestive heart disease, in whom vascular filling is not tolerated.

In general, patients admitted to undergo cardiac surgery mostly benefit from cardiovascular treatments that may have repercussions on renal function. Statins have been reported to have a protective effect. Welten et al. reported that statin use was associated with an increased odds of complete kidney function recovery in patients who developed AKI after vascular surgery [70]. Similarly, Billings et al. showed that early postoperative statin use was associated with a lower incidence of AKI [71]. In another recent study, the use of statins was associated with a lower risk of elevation of certain biomarkers of AKI [72].

Regarding ACE inhibitors and angiotensin-II receptor blockers, results of studies to date have been conflicting as regards the potential benefits on renal function [73–75].

Taken together, these results regarding the effects of cardiovascular on renal function do not make it possible to identify a single therapeutic strategy as being the most beneficial. However, treatment of congestive heart disease should be pursued if it is deemed to be useful in order to maintain hemodynamic status.

Perioperative

Several different molecules have been proposed for renal protection in the context of cardiac surgery.

Fenoldopam is a selective inhibitor of dopaminergic receptors. It is synthetically derived from dopamine, and increases renal output. In a meta-analysis of 13 studies including a total of 1059 patients, fenoldopam was shown to confer significant benefits in preventing renal replacement therapy and reducing mortality in patients undergoing cardiovascular surgery [76]. A further meta-analysis of randomized, placebo-controlled studies suggested that fenoldopam reduced the incidence of postoperative AKI [77]. Conversely, Bove et al., in a prospective, randomized study among patients with AKI after cardiac surgery and reported that fenoldopam did not reduce the need for renal replacement therapy or risk of 30-day mortality, and was associated with an increased rate of hypotension [78].

Nesiritide is another drug that has been tested in this context. In a multicentre randomized, placebo-controlled trial, Mentzer et al. showed that nesiritide in perioperative nesiritide in patients with impaired left ventricular function undergoing CABG was associated with improved postoperative renal function [79], and the findings were especially pronounced in the subgroup of patients with preoperative renal failure. However, further prospective studies in larger sample sizes are necessary to reach consensus on the utility of this drug in improving renal outcomes post-cardiac surgery.

Acidity is known to worsen tubular lesions, and therefore, bicarbonate has been proposed to prevent postoperative AKI in cardiac surgery. However, recent data do not plead in favor of the use of bicarbonate, with reports of deleterious effects and an increase in renal failure in treated patients [80, 81]. However, studies of this approach were heterogeneous, and did not use the same doses or endpoints [82].

Mannitol acts as a diuretic by inducing osmotic dieresis. It increases intravascular volume, thereby contributing to increasing cardiac preload, and increasing cardiac output. This in turn leads to increased renal blood flow and urine output by enhancing tubular output. However, recent studies failed to find any benefit of mannitol on renal function after CABG surgery in patients with established renal dysfunction [83] or in those with normal preoperative kidney function [84].

Lastly, dopamine is a neurotransmitter that has a dose-dependent action on adrenergic alpha and beta1 receptors. In experimental conditions, it stimulates renal dopamine receptors, thereby increasing renal blood flow and filtration. However, results of its application in clinical practice have been disappointing, and based on studies investigating its potential clinical effects, dopamine cannot be recommended for use in routine practice.

Postoperative

Once AKI has been diagnosed post-surgery, it is mandatory to rapidly initiate measures to correct the causative mechanism(s), if they are amenable to therapy. Late diagnosis can lead to worsening of renal damage.

The appropriate therapy must be chosen based on clinical analysis of each case. Blood and urine tests should help to orient the diagnosis toward either an organic lesion, or a pre-renal cause. The presence of a functional component is difficult to identify, but is of paramount importance, as treatment will take effect most rapidly on the functional component, if any.

1. The quality of renal perfusion depends on what the level of effective renal perfusion pressure is. Evaluating effective renal perfusion pressure should take into account the patient's baseline pressure (hypertensive or elderly patient). Once the level of effective renal perfusion pressure has been achieved, it is necessary to check that the pressure being created is not stemming mainly from substantial vascular resistance. Renal perfusion tests are not performed in routine practice. There have been reports in the literature investigating the renal resistive index, which was shown to be associated with the postoperative AKI [85, 86]. In clinical practice, measuring cardiac output and vascular resistance can yield an estimation of the quality of renal perfusion.
2. Renal tissue oxygenation also depends on perfusion pressure, as well as on renal blood flow and the rate of hemoglobin, which transports oxygen. Analysis of overall oxygen consumption as a function of oxygen transport is an interesting parameter. Indeed, analysis of the patient's SV02 levels can contribute to this analysis. However, it should be noted that SV02 only reflects the macrocirculation.
3. Venous hypertension has deleterious effects on renal perfusion. Therefore, measures of venous pressure showing extreme values (central venous pressure >15 mmHg) indicate a compelling need to reduce the fluid overload rapidly. In critically ill patients with renal failure, fluid accumulation and fluid overload are associated with a reduced capacity to recover renal function [87].

4. Strict glycemic control during the perioperative period has been shown to reduce the incidence of acute renal failure requiring dialysis [88].
5. In case of occurrence of AKI post-surgery, rapid initiation of renal replacement therapy improves prognosis and survival [89, 90].

Conclusion

AKI remains a common complication after cardiac surgery and is associated with poorer patient outcomes. Early identification of AKI after surgery should prompt rapid initiation of corrective therapies, and physicians should be attentive to early signs of AKI after surgery. Preventive measures before and during surgery may help to lessen the risk of post-surgical AKI. Nonetheless, further studies into the mechanisms, predictors, and risk factors for AKI are necessary to identify targets for prevention and therapy, and to prevent this deleterious complication in the context of cardiac surgery.

References

1. Stafford-Smith M, Shaw A, Swaminathan M. Cardiac surgery and acute kidney injury: emerging concepts. Curr Opin Crit Care. 2009;15(6):498–502.
2. Chertow GM, Lazarus JM, Christiansen CL, Cook EF, Hammermeister KE, Grover F, Daley J. Preoperative renal risk stratification. Circulation. 1997;95(4):878–84.
3. Mao H, Katz N, Ariyanon W, Blanca-Martos L, Adybelli Z, Giuliani A, Danesi TH, Kim JC, Nayak A, Neri M, Virzi GM, Brocca A, Scalzotto E, Salvador L, Ronco C. Cardiac surgery-associated acute kidney injury. Cardiorenal Med. 2013;3(3):178–99.
4. Grayson AD, Khater M, Jackson M, Fox MA. Valvular heart operation is an independent risk factor for acute renal failure. Ann Thorac Surg. 2003;75(6):1829–35.
5. Rosner MH, Okusa MD. Acute kidney injury associated with cardiac surgery. Clin J Am Soc Nephrol. 2006;1(1):19–32.
6. Chertow GM, Levy EM, Hammermeister KE, Grover F, Daley J. Independent association between acute renal failure and mortality following cardiac surgery. Am J Med. 1998;104(4):343–8.
7. Leacche M, Rawn JD, Mihaljevic T, Lin J, Karavas AN, Paul S, Byrne JG. Outcomes in patients with normal serum creatinine and with artificial renal support for acute renal failure developing after coronary artery bypass grafting. Am J Cardiol. 2004;93(3):353–6.
8. Hobson CE, Yavas S, Segal MS, Schold JD, Tribble CG, Layon AJ, Bihorac A. Acute kidney injury is associated with increased long-term mortality after cardiothoracic surgery. Circulation. 2009;119(18):2444–53.
9. Lassnigg A, Schmidlin D, Mouhieddine M, Bachmann LM, Druml W, Bauer P, Hiesmayr M. Minimal changes of serum creatinine predict prognosis in patients after cardiothoracic surgery: a prospective cohort study. J Am Soc Nephrol. 2004;15(6):1597–605.
10. Thakar CV, Yared JP, Worley S, Cotman K, Paganini EP. Renal dysfunction and serious infections after open-heart surgery. Kidney Int. 2003;64(1):239–46.
11. Liano F, Pascual J. Epidemiology of acute renal failure: a prospective, multicenter, community-based study. Madrid Acute Renal Failure Study Group. Kidney Int. 1996;50(3):811–8.
12. Bellomo R, Ronco C, Kellum JA, Mehta RL, Palevsky P. Acute renal failure—definition, outcome measures, animal models, fluid therapy and information technology needs: the second international consensus conference of the acute dialysis quality initiative (ADQI) Group. Crit Care. 2004;8(4):R204–12.
13. Mehta RL, Kellum JA, Shah SV, Molitoris BA, Ronco C, Warnock DG, Levin A. Acute kidney injury network: report of an initiative to improve outcomes in acute kidney injury. Crit Care. 2007;11(2):R31.
14. Englberger L, Suri RM, Li Z, Casey ET, Daly RC, Dearani JA, Schaff HV. Clinical accuracy of RIFLE and Acute Kidney Injury Network (AKIN) criteria for acute kidney injury in patients undergoing cardiac surgery. Crit Care. 2011;15(1):R16.
15. Sutton TA, Fisher CJ, Molitoris BA. Microvascular endothelial injury and dysfunction during ischemic acute renal failure. Kidney Int. 2002;62(5):1539–49.
16. Abuelo JG. Normotensive ischemic acute renal failure. N Engl J Med. 2007;357(8):797–805.
17. Okusa MD. The inflammatory cascade in acute ischemic renal failure. Nephron. 2002;90(2):133–8.
18. Vercaemst L. Hemolysis in cardiac surgery patients undergoing cardiopulmonary bypass: a review in search of a treatment algorithm. J Extra Corpor Technol. 2008;40(4):257–67.
19. Bagshaw SM, Gibney RT. Conventional markers of kidney function. Crit Care Med. 2008;36(4 Suppl):S152–8.
20. Mishra J, Dent C, Tarabishi R, Mitsnefes MM, Ma Q, Kelly C, Ruff SM, Zahedi K, Shao M, Bean J, Mori K, Barasch J, Devarajan P. Neutrophil gelatinase-associated lipocalin (NGAL) as a biomarker for acute renal injury after cardiac surgery. Lancet. 2005;365(9466):1231–8.
21. Dent CL, Ma Q, Dastrala S, Bennett M, Mitsnefes MM, Barasch J, Devarajan P. Plasma neutrophil gelatinase-associated lipocalin predicts acute kidney injury, morbidity and mortality after pediatric cardiac surgery: a prospective uncontrolled cohort study. Crit Care. 2007;11(6):R127.
22. Wagener G, Jan M, Kim M, Mori K, Barasch JM, Sladen RN, Lee HT. Association between increases in urinary neutrophil gelatinase-associated lipocalin and acute renal dysfunction after adult cardiac surgery. Anesthesiology. 2006;105(3):485–91.
23. McIlroy DR, Wagener G, Lee HT. Neutrophil gelatinase-associated lipocalin and acute kidney injury after cardiac surgery: the effect of baseline renal function on diagnostic performance. Clin J Am Soc Nephrol. 2010;5(2):211–9.
24. Perry TE, Muehlschlegel JD, Liu KY, Fox AA, Collard CD, Shernan SK, Body SC. Plasma neutrophil gelatinase-associated lipocalin and acute postoperative kidney injury in adult cardiac surgical patients. Anesth Analg. 2010;110(6):1541–7.
25. Haase M, Bellomo R, Devarajan P, Ma Q, Bennett MR, Mockel M, Matalanis G, Dragun D, Haase-Fielitz A. Novel biomarkers early predict the severity of acute kidney injury after cardiac surgery in adults. Ann Thorac Surg. 2009;88(1):124–30.
26. Perrotti A, Miltgen G, Chevet-Noel A, Durst C, Vernerey D, Bardonnet K, Davani S, Chocron S. Neutrophil gelatinase-associated lipocalin as early predictor of acute kidney injury after cardiac surgery in adults with chronic kidney failure. Ann Thorac Surg. 2015;99(3):864–9.
27. Parikh CR, Mishra J, Thiessen-Philbrook H, Dursun B, Ma Q, Kelly C, Dent C, Devarajan P, Edelstein CL. Urinary IL-18 is an

early predictive biomarker of acute kidney injury after cardiac surgery. Kidney Int. 2006;70(1):199–203.
28. Haase M, Bellomo R, Story D, Davenport P, Haase-Fielitz A. Urinary interleukin-18 does not predict acute kidney injury after adult cardiac surgery: a prospective observational cohort study. Crit Care. 2008;12(4):R96.
29. McIlroy DR, Wagener G, Lee HT. Biomarkers of acute kidney injury: an evolving domain. Anesthesiology. 2010;112(4):998–1004.
30. Ho J, Tangri N, Komenda P, Kaushal A, Sood M, Brar R, Gill K, Walker S, MacDonald K, Hiebert BM, Arora RC, Rigatto C. Urinary, plasma, and serum biomarkers' utility for predicting acute kidney injury associated with cardiac surgery in adults: a meta-analysis. Am J Kidney Dis. 2015;66(6):993–1005.
31. Han WK, Wagener G, Zhu Y, Wang S, Lee HT. Urinary biomarkers in the early detection of acute kidney injury after cardiac surgery. Clin J Am Soc Nephrol. 2009;4(5):873–82.
32. Parikh CR, Coca SG, Thiessen-Philbrook H, Shlipak MG, Koyner JL, Wang Z, Edelstein CL, Devarajan P, Patel UD, Zappitelli M, Krawczeski CD, Passik CS, Swaminathan M, Garg AX. Postoperative biomarkers predict acute kidney injury and poor outcomes after adult cardiac surgery. J Am Soc Nephrol. 2011;22(9):1748–57.
33. Koyner JL, Garg AX, Coca SG, Sint K, Thiessen-Philbrook H, Patel UD, Shlipak MG, Parikh CR. Biomarkers predict progression of acute kidney injury after cardiac surgery. J Am Soc Nephrol. 2012;23(5):905–14.
34. Karkouti K, Wijeysundera DN, Yau TM, Callum JL, Cheng DC, Crowther M, Dupuis JY, Fremes SE, Kent B, Laflamme C, Lamy A, Legare JF, Mazer CD, McCluskey SA, Rubens FD, Sawchuk C, Beattie WS. Acute kidney injury after cardiac surgery: focus on modifiable risk factors. Circulation. 2009;119(4):495–502.
35. Perez-Valdivieso JR, Monedero P, Vives M, Garcia-Fernandez N, Bes-Rastrollo M. Cardiac-surgery associated acute kidney injury requiring renal replacement therapy. A Spanish retrospective case-cohort study. BMC Nephrol. 2009;10:27.
36. Medalion B, Cohen H, Assali A, Vaknin Assa H, Farkash A, Snir E, Sharoni E, Biderman P, Milo G, Battler A, Kornowski R, Porat E. The effect of cardiac angiography timing, contrast media dose, and preoperative renal function on acute renal failure after coronary artery bypass grafting. J Thorac Cardiovasc Surg. 2010;139(6):1539–44.
37. Kramer RS, Quinn RD, Groom RC, Braxton JH, Malenka DJ, Kellett MA, Brown JR. Same admission cardiac catheterization and cardiac surgery: is there an increased incidence of acute kidney injury? Ann Thorac Surg. 2010;90(5):1418–23 (discussion 23–4).
38. Rosner MH, Portilla D, Okusa MD. Cardiac surgery as a cause of acute kidney injury: pathogenesis and potential therapies. J Intensive Care Med. 2008;23(1):3–18.
39. Bellomo R, Auriemma S, Fabbri A, D'Onofrio A, Katz N, McCullough PA, Ricci Z, Shaw A, Ronco C. The pathophysiology of cardiac surgery-associated acute kidney injury (CSA-AKI). Int J Artif Organs. 2008;31(2):166–78.
40. Chew ST, Newman MF, White WD, Conlon PJ, Saunders AM, Strittmatter WJ, Landolfo K, Grocott HP, Stafford-Smith M. Preliminary report on the association of apolipoprotein E polymorphisms, with postoperative peak serum creatinine concentrations in cardiac surgical patients. Anesthesiology. 2000;93(2):325–31.
41. Thakar CV, Arrigain S, Worley S, Yared JP, Paganini EP. A clinical score to predict acute renal failure after cardiac surgery. J Am Soc Nephrol. 2005;16(1):162–8.
42. Mehta RH, Grab JD, O'Brien SM, Bridges CR, Gammie JS, Haan CK, Ferguson TB, Peterson ED. Bedside tool for predicting the risk of postoperative dialysis in patients undergoing cardiac surgery. Circulation. 2006;114(21):2208–16 (quiz).
43. Wijeysundera DN, Karkouti K, Dupuis JY, Rao V, Chan CT, Granton JT, Beattie WS. Derivation and validation of a simplified predictive index for renal replacement therapy after cardiac surgery. JAMA. 2007;297(16):1801–9.
44. Candela-Toha A, Elias-Martin E, Abraira V, Tenorio MT, Parise D, de Pablo A, Centella T, Liano F. Predicting acute renal failure after cardiac surgery: external validation of two new clinical scores. Clin J Am Soc Nephrol. 2008;3(5):1260–5.
45. Englberger L, Suri RM, Li Z, Dearani JA, Park SJ, Sundt TM III, Schaff HV. Validation of clinical scores predicting severe acute kidney injury after cardiac surgery. Am J Kidney Dis. 2010;56(4):623–31.
46. Demirjian S, Schold JD, Navia J, Mastracci TM, Paganini EP, Yared JP, Bashour CA. Predictive models for acute kidney injury following cardiac surgery. Am J Kidney Dis. 2012;59(3):382–9.
47. Urzua J, Troncoso S, Bugedo G, Canessa R, Munoz H, Lema G, Valdivieso A, Irarrazaval M, Moran S, Meneses G. Renal function and cardiopulmonary bypass: effect of perfusion pressure. J Cardiothorac Vasc Anesth. 1992;6(3):299–303.
48. Parolari A, Alamanni F, Gherli T, Bertera A, Dainese L, Costa C, Schena M, Sisillo E, Spirito R, Porqueddu M, Rona P, Biglioli P. Cardiopulmonary bypass and oxygen consumption: oxygen delivery and hemodynamics. Ann Thorac Surg. 1999;67(5):1320–7.
49. Poswal P, Mehta Y, Juneja R, Khanna S, Meharwal ZS, Trehan N. Comparative study of pulsatile and nonpulsatile flow during cardio-pulmonary bypass. Ann Card Anaesth. 2004;7(1):44–50.
50. Sievert A, Sistino J. A meta-analysis of renal benefits to pulsatile perfusion in cardiac surgery. J Extra Corpor Technol. 2012;44(1):10–4.
51. Baraki H, Gohrbandt B, Del Bagno B, Haverich A, Boethig D, Kutschka I. Does pulsatile perfusion improve outcome after cardiac surgery? A propensity-matched analysis of 1959 patients. Perfusion. 2012;27(3):166–74.
52. Habib RH, Zacharias A, Schwann TA, Riordan CJ, Engoren M, Durham SJ, Shah A. Role of hemodilutional anemia and transfusion during cardiopulmonary bypass in renal injury after coronary revascularization: implications on operative outcome. Crit Care Med. 2005;33(8):1749–56.
53. Huybregts RA, de Vroege R, Jansen EK, van Schijndel AW, Christiaans HM, van Oeveren W. The association of hemodilution and transfusion of red blood cells with biochemical markers of splanchnic and renal injury during cardiopulmonary bypass. Anesth Analg. 2009;109(2):331–9.
54. Lau K, Shah H, Kelleher A, Moat N. Coronary artery surgery: cardiotomy suction or cell salvage? J Cardiothorac Surg. 2007;2:46.
55. Sreeram GM, Grocott HP, White WD, Newman MF, Stafford-Smith M. Transcranial Doppler emboli count predicts rise in creatinine after coronary artery bypass graft surgery. J Cardiothorac Vasc Anesth. 2004;18(5):548–51.
56. Kumar AB, Suneja M, Bayman EO, Weide GD, Tarasi M. Association between postoperative acute kidney injury and duration of cardiopulmonary bypass: a meta-analysis. J Cardiothorac Vasc Anesth. 2012;26(1):64–9.
57. Salis S, Mazzanti VV, Merli G, Salvi L, Tedesco CC, Veglia F, Sisillo E. Cardiopulmonary bypass duration is an independent predictor of morbidity and mortality after cardiac surgery. J Cardiothorac Vasc Anesth. 2008;22(6):814–22.
58. Algarni KD, Yanagawa B, Rao V, Yau TM. Profound hypothermia compared with moderate hypothermia in repair of acute type A aortic dissection. J Thorac Cardiovasc Surg. 2014;148(6):2888–94.

59. Tsai JY, Pan W, Lemaire SA, Pisklak P, Lee VV, Bracey AW, Elayda MA, Preventza O, Price MD, Collard CD, Coselli JS. Moderate hypothermia during aortic arch surgery is associated with reduced risk of early mortality. J Thorac Cardiovasc Surg. 2013;146(3):662–7.
60. Boodhwani M, Rubens FD, Wozny D, Nathan HJ. Effects of mild hypothermia and rewarming on renal function after coronary artery bypass grafting. Ann Thorac Surg. 2009;87(2):489–95.
61. Nigwekar SU, Kandula P, Hix JK, Thakar CV. Off-pump coronary artery bypass surgery and acute kidney injury: a meta-analysis of randomized and observational studies. Am J Kidney Dis. 2009;54 (3):413–23.
62. Shroyer AL, Grover FL, Hattler B, Collins JF, McDonald GO, Kozora E, Lucke JC, Baltz JH, Novitzky D. On-pump versus off-pump coronary-artery bypass surgery. N Engl J Med. 2009;361 (19):1827–37.
63. Lamy A, Devereaux PJ, Prabhakaran D, Taggart DP, Hu S, Paolasso E, Straka Z, Piegas LS, Akar AR, Jain AR, Noiseux N, Padmanabhan C, Bahamondes JC, Novick RJ, Vaijyanath P, Reddy S, Tao L, Olavegogeascoechea PA, Airan B, Sulling TA, Whitlock RP, Ou Y, Ng J, Chrolavicius S, Yusuf S. Off-pump or on-pump coronary-artery bypass grafting at 30 days. N Engl J Med. 2012;366(16):1489–97.
64. Karkouti K, Wijeysundera DN, Beattie WS. Risk associated with preoperative anemia in cardiac surgery: a multicenter cohort study. Circulation. 2008;117(4):478–84.
65. Almac E, Ince C. The impact of storage on red cell function in blood transfusion. Best Pract Res Clin Anaesthesiol. 2007;21 (2):195–208.
66. Cardo LJ, Hmel P, Wilder D. Stored packed red blood cells contain a procoagulant phospholipid reducible by leukodepletion filters and washing. Transfus Apher Sci. 2008;38(2):141–7.
67. Karkouti K, Wijeysundera DN, Yau TM, McCluskey SA, van Rensburg A, Beattie WS. The influence of baseline hemoglobin concentration on tolerance of anemia in cardiac surgery. Transfusion. 2008;48(4):666–72.
68. Moulton MJ, Creswell LL, Mackey ME, Cox JL, Rosenbloom M. Reexploration for bleeding is a risk factor for adverse outcomes after cardiac operations. J Thorac Cardiovasc Surg. 1996;111 (5):1037–46.
69. Marathias KP, Vassili M, Robola A, Alivizatos PA, Palatianos GM, Geroulanos S, Vlahakos DV. Preoperative intravenous hydration confers renoprotection in patients with chronic kidney disease undergoing cardiac surgery. Artif Organs. 2006;30(8):615–21.
70. Welten GM, Chonchol M, Schouten O, Hoeks S, Bax JJ, van Domburg RT, van Sambeek M, Poldermans D. Statin use is associated with early recovery of kidney injury after vascular surgery and improved long-term outcome. Nephrol Dial Transplant. 2008;23(12):3867–73.
71. Billings FT, Pretorius M, Siew ED, Yu C, Brown NJ. Early postoperative statin therapy is associated with a lower incidence of acute kidney injury after cardiac surgery. J Cardiothorac Vasc Anesth. 2010;24(6):913–20.
72. Molnar AO, Parikh CR, Coca SG, Thiessen-Philbrook H, Koyner JL, Shlipak MG, Myers ML, Garg AX. Association between preoperative statin use and acute kidney injury biomarkers in cardiac surgical procedures. Ann Thorac Surg. 2014;97 (6):2081–7.
73. Arora P, Rajagopalam S, Ranjan R, Kolli H, Singh M, Venuto R, Lohr J. Preoperative use of angiotensin-converting enzyme inhibitors/angiotensin receptor blockers is associated with increased risk for acute kidney injury after cardiovascular surgery. Clin J Am Soc Nephrol. 2008;3(5):1266–73.
74. Cittanova ML, Zubicki A, Savu C, Montalvan C, Nefaa N, Zaier K, Riou B, Coriat P. The chronic inhibition of angiotensin-converting enzyme impairs postoperative renal function. Anesth Analg. 2001;93(5):1111–5.
75. Ouzounian M, Buth KJ, Valeeva L, Morton CC, Hassan A, Ali IS. Impact of preoperative angiotensin-converting enzyme inhibitor use on clinical outcomes after cardiac surgery. Ann Thorac Surg. 2012;93(2):559–64.
76. Landoni G, Biondi-Zoccai GG, Marino G, Bove T, Fochi O, Maj G, Calabro MG, Sheiban I, Tumlin JA, Ranucci M, Zangrillo A. Fenoldopam reduces the need for renal replacement therapy and in-hospital death in cardiovascular surgery: a meta-analysis. J Cardiothorac Vasc Anesth. 2008;22(1):27–33.
77. Zangrillo A, Biondi-Zoccai GG, Frati E, Covello RD, Cabrini L, Guarracino F, Ruggeri L, Bove T, Bignami E, Landoni G. Fenoldopam and acute renal failure in cardiac surgery: a meta-analysis of randomized placebo-controlled trials. J Cardiothorac Vasc Anesth. 2012;26(3):407–13.
78. Bove T, Zangrillo A, Guarracino F, Alvaro G, Persi B, Maglioni E, Galdieri N, Comis M, Caramelli F, Pasero DC, Pala G, Renzini M, Conte M, Paternoster G, Martinez B, Pinelli F, Frontini M, Zucchetti MC, Pappalardo F, Amantea B, Camata A, Pisano A, Verdecchia C, Dal Checco E, Cariello C, Faita L, Baldassarri R, Scandroglio AM, Saleh O, Lembo R, Calabro MG, Bellomo R, Landoni G. Effect of fenoldopam on use of renal replacement therapy among patients with acute kidney injury after cardiac surgery: a randomized clinical trial. JAMA. 2014;312(21):2244–53.
79. Mentzer RM Jr, Oz MC, Sladen RN, Graeve AH, Hebeler RF Jr, Luber JM Jr, Smedira NG. Effects of perioperative nesiritide in patients with left ventricular dysfunction undergoing cardiac surgery: the NAPA trial. J Am Coll Cardiol. 2007;49(6):716–26.
80. Haase M, Haase-Fielitz A, Plass M, Kuppe H, Hetzer R, Hannon C, Murray PT, Bailey MJ, Bellomo R, Bagshaw SM. Prophylactic perioperative sodium bicarbonate to prevent acute kidney injury following open heart surgery: a multicenter double-blinded randomized controlled trial. PLoS Med. 2013;10(4):e1001426.
81. Heringlake M, Heinze H, Schubert M, Nowak Y, Guder J, Kleinebrahm M, Paarmann H, Hanke T, Schon J. A perioperative infusion of sodium bicarbonate does not improve renal function in cardiac surgery patients: a prospective observational cohort study. Crit Care. 2012;16(4):R156.
82. Kristeller JL, Zavorsky GS, Prior JE, Keating DA, Brady MA, Romaldini TA, Hickman TL, Stahl RF. Lack of effectiveness of sodium bicarbonate in preventing kidney injury in patients undergoing cardiac surgery: a randomized controlled trial. Pharmacotherapy. 2013;33(7):710–7.
83. Smith MN, Best D, Sheppard SV, Smith DC. The effect of mannitol on renal function after cardiopulmonary bypass in patients with established renal dysfunction. Anaesthesia. 2008;63 (7):701–4.
84. Yallop KG, Sheppard SV, Smith DC. The effect of mannitol on renal function following cardio-pulmonary bypass in patients with normal pre-operative creatinine. Anaesthesia. 2008;63(6):576–82.
85. Guinot PG, Bernard E, Abou Arab O, Badoux L, Diouf M, Zogheib E, Dupont H. Doppler-based renal resistive index can assess progression of acute kidney injury in patients undergoing cardiac surgery. J Cardiothorac Vasc Anesth. 2013;27(5):890–6.
86. Bossard G, Bourgoin P, Corbeau JJ, Huntzinger J, Beydon L. Early detection of postoperative acute kidney injury by Doppler renal resistive index in cardiac surgery with cardiopulmonary bypass. Br J Anaesth. 2011;107(6):891–8.
87. Bouchard J, Mehta RL. Fluid accumulation and acute kidney injury: consequence or cause. Curr Opin Crit Care. 2009;15 (6):509–13.
88. van den Berghe G, Wouters P, Weekers F, Verwaest C, Bruyninckx F, Schetz M, Vlasselaers D, Ferdinande P, Lauwers P,

Bouillon R. Intensive insulin therapy in critically ill patients. N Engl J Med. 2001;345(19):1359–67.
89. Elahi MM, Lim MY, Joseph RN, Dhannapuneni RR, Spyt TJ. Early hemofiltration improves survival in post-cardiotomy patients with acute renal failure. Eur J Cardiothorac Surg. 2004;26(5):1027–31.
90. Garcia-Fernandez N, Perez-Valdivieso JR, Bes-Rastrollo M, Vives M, Lavilla J, Herreros J, Monedero P. Timing of renal replacement therapy after cardiac surgery: a retrospective multicenter Spanish cohort study. Blood Purif. 2011;32(2):104–11.

Part VII

The Cardiorenometabolic Spectrum

35 Dyslipidemias in CKD and ESKD: Outcomes and Management

David Carruthers and Anand Rohatgi

Introduction

Cardiovascular disease (CVD) is the leading cause of death in the United States, with an estimated 375,000 deaths attributed to heart disease per year. Both dyslipidemia and chronic kidney disease (CKD) are major risk factors for CVD [1], and are linked via multiple derangements, including oxidative stress, inflammation, physical inactivity, anemia, hypertension, vascular calcification, endothelial dysfunction, depressed nitric oxide availability, and dyslipidemia [2–9].

In this chapter, we discuss the variation in the lipid profile across a spectrum of kidney disease, including chronic kidney disease, nephrotic syndrome, end-stage kidney disease on dialysis, and kidney transplantation. We also review the trials 4D, AURORA, SHARP, ALERT, and meta-analyses which form the basis of the current KDIGO recommendations for medical management of dyslipidemia in patients with CKD.

Dyslipidemias and Chronic Kidney Disease

CKD is associated with multiple lipid abnormalities, including consistently elevated triglycerides (>200 mg/dL in over half of patients with CKD), and varying low-density lipoprotein cholesterol (LDL-C) levels (decreased, increased, or unchanged). The severe lipid perturbations observed in CKD is termed "uremic dyslipidemia" [10, 11].

The hypertriglyceridemia seen in CKD is thought to be related to the concomitant hyperparathyroid state. In essence, hepatic and lipoprotein lipase activity are blunted by elevated parathyroid levels, leading to decreased clearance of triglyceride-rich lipoproteins such as very low-density lipoprotein (VLDL), intermediate-density lipoprotein (IDL), and chylomicron remnants. Parathyroidectomy partially reverses these lipase-mediated perturbations but does not fully reverse the decreased receptor-mediated clearance of triglyceride-rich lipoproteins that is observed in CKD [12].

CKD decreases enzymatic activity necessary for high-density lipoprotein (HDL) maturation (LCAT and CETP) [13], preventing efficient movement of cholesterol through the reverse cholesterol transport pathway. This impairment leads to dysfunctional triglyceride exchange from LDL and VLDL particles to HDL particles [10, 14]. The triglyceride-enriched LDL particles, also described as small dense LDL, are more prone to penetrate vessel walls and undergo oxidation, promoting increased atherosclerosis in patients with CKD [15].

The uremic dyslipidemia profile of small atherogenic LDL, decreased mature HDL, and increased serum triglycerides is also seen in patients with insulin resistance syndromes such as type 2 diabetes mellitus. CKD has been linked to worsening insulin resistance, which is thought to play a role in decreasing enzymatic activity leading to uremic dyslipidemia [16, 17].

As CKD progresses to nephrotic-range proteinuria, the lipid profile changes to a phenotype of increased LDL-C as well as increased triglycerides. In nephrotic syndrome, HMG CoA reductase (the rate-limiting enzyme for hepatic cholesterol synthesis) is upregulated and cholesterol 7α[alpha]-hydroxylase is downregulated [18, 19], resulting in increased production of LDL particles. In addition, LDL catabolism is decreased as LDL receptor activity diminishes, leading to higher circulating LDL-C levels.

D. Carruthers · A. Rohatgi (✉)
Department of Cardiology, University of Texas Southwestern, 5323 Harry Hines Blvd, Dallas, TX 75390-8830, USA
e-mail: anand.rohatgi@utsouthwestern.edu

D. Carruthers
e-mail: David.carruthers@parkland.org

J. Rangaswami et al. (eds.), *Cardio-Nephrology*,
DOI 10.1007/978-3-319-56042-7_35

End-Stage Kidney Disease (ESKD)

Peritoneal Dialysis (PD)

Patients on peritoneal dialysis continue to lose protein across the peritoneal membrane (5–15 g/day) and, therefore, exhibit a cholesterol profile similar to those with nephrotic syndrome [20]. Moreover, the glucose absorbed during PD serves as a substrate for lipoprotein synthesis [21]. In one study, patients on PD had decreased cholesterol levels when icodextrin substrate dialysis replaced glucose [22].

Hemodialysis

In patients on hemodialysis, the lipid profile remains largely similar to that seen in earlier stages of CKD: elevated triglycerides and decreased HDL cholesterol. However, long-term hemodialysis can lead to changes distinct from the typical uremic dyslipidemia. In contrast to use of unfractionated heparin, repeated exposure to low molecular weight heparin during hemodialysis releases lipoprotein lipase, which hydrolyzes circulating triglyceride content and results in moderate reductions of triglyceride levels [21]. Sevelemar hydrochloride, which is often given to patients on HD to treat hyperphosphatemia, has a cholestyramine-like ability to bind bile acids, phosphate, and cholesterol in the intestines, mildly decreasing cholesterol levels [21].

Kidney Transplantation

Patients receiving kidney transplants typically have increased triglyceride and LDL cholesterol levels. In 1999, it was reported that 90–97% of patients who received kidney transplants had LDL levels over 100 mg/dL [23], yet these numbers have decreased in recent years with newer immunosuppressant therapy and concomitant statin treatment [24]. This profile of elevated LDL cholesterol is thought to be due to a combination of underlying CKD and nephrotic syndrome. In addition, the effects of immunosuppressive agents such as steroid treatment, calcineurin inhibitors, and rapamycin exacerbate the dyslipidemia. In order to prevent allograft failure, dyslipidemia due to immunosuppressive medications can be tolerated, but certain adjustments of immunosuppressive therapy, such as replacing cyclosporine with tacrolimus, can improve the lipid profile of transplant patients [25–28].

Treating Dyslipidemia in CKD: The Evidence and Recommendations

Lowering LDL cholesterol is a proven treatment strategy in reducing atherosclerotic cardiovascular events including myocardial infarction and stroke. As such, the 2013 ACC/AHA cholesterol guidelines suggest using a moderate-intensity therapy statin (goal to lower LDL by 30–50%) or high-intensity statin (lowering LDL by approximately >50%) in order to reduce atherosclerotic cardiovascular disease (ASCVD). The 2013 ACC/AHA guidelines have identified fourmajor groups that would benefit from statin therapy:

- Clinical ASCVD (high-intensity statin if age <75, moderate intensity if age >75)
- Primary elevations of LDL-C greater than 190 mg/dL (high-intensity statin)
- Diabetes aged 40–75 with LDL-C 70 to 189 mg/dL and without clinical ASCVD (moderate-intensity statin, high intensity if estimated 10-year ASCVD risk >7.5%)
- Without clinical ASCVD or diabetes with LDL-C 70–189 mg/dL and estimated 10-year ASCVD risk >7.5% (moderate–high-intensity statin)

However, trials forming the basis of the 2013 ACC/AHA recommendations excluded patients with CKD and ESKD from their cohorts. Studies that directly tested the efficacy of statin therapy in patients with CKD are reviewed below, including the 4D trial, the AURORA trial, and the SHARP trial (Table 35.1) [29].

4D

The first large, randomized placebo-controlled trial evaluating statins in ESKD was the 4D trial (Deutsche Diabetes Dialyse Studie), published in 2005 [30]. The study enrolled 1255 patients (619 to atorvastatin, 636 to placebo) age 18–80 in Germany with type 2 diabetes mellitus, and who were on hemodialysis for <2 years. Exclusion factors included LDL-C <80 mg/dL or >190 mg/dL, triglycerides >1000 mg/dL, liver enzymes over three times the normal limits, hematopoietic disease, systemic disease unrelated to ESKD, vascular intervention, congestive heart failure, or myocardial infarction within three months of enrollment, unsuccessful kidney transplantation, and resistant hypertension (systolic blood pressure >200 mmHg, diastolic >110 mmHg).

Table 35.1 Randomized controlled trials of statins in patients with CKD/ESRD

Trial	Intervention	N/CKD stage	Follow-up (years)	LDL-C reduction (%)	Primary outcome	Results
4D [30]	Atorvastatin 20 mg	1255/HD	4	42	Death from cardiac cause, nonfatal MI, and stroke	HR 0.92 (0.77–1.10)
Aurora [31]	Rosuvastatin 10 mg	2776/HD	3.2	43	Nonfatal MI, nonfatal stroke, or death from cardiovascular causes	HR 0.96 (0.84–1.11)
Sharp [32]	Simvastatin 20 mg + ezetimibe 10 mg	9270/All stages	4.9	68	Nonfatal MI, coronary death, non-hemorrhagic stroke, or revascularization	RR 0.83 (0.74–0.94)
Alert [33]	Fluvastatin 40 or 80 mg	2102/Transplant	5.1	32	Major cardiovascular events ($p = 0.139$)	RR 0.72 (0.6–1.06)

The trial randomized participants to atorvastatin 20 mg once daily versus placebo. If LDL-C fell below 50 mg/dL, the dose of atorvastatin was reduced to 10 mg/day. At randomization, median LDL-C was 121 mg/dL in the atorvastatin group, and 125 mg/dL in the placebo arm. At 4 weeks, those randomized to atorvastatin had a median level of 72 mg/dL versus unchanged in placebo.

There was no benefit associated with atorvastatin versus placebo for the composite primary endpoint (243 vs. 226 $p = 0.37$). Analysis by component end points of the primary end point included death from cardiac causes (20% in atorvastatin vs. 23% placebo $p = 0.08$), fatal stroke (4% atorvastatin vs, 2% placebo $p = 0.04$) nonfatal myocardial infarction (20% atorvastatin vs. 23% placebo $p = 0.08$), or nonfatal stroke (5% atorvastatin vs. 5% placebo, $p = 0.89$).

Randomization to atorvastatin had inconsistent associations with secondary end points, including death from all causes (45% in atorvastatin group vs. 50% in placebo $p = 0.33$), all cardiac events combined (33% in atorvastatin group vs. 39% in placebo $p = 0.03$), all cerebrovascular events combined (13% atorvastatin vs. 11% placebo $p = 0.49$), death from any cause other than cardiac disease or cerebrovascular disease (24% in atorvastatin vs. 25% placebo, $p = 0.62$).

In summary, among patients with ESKD on HD and diabetes, atorvastatin 20 mg daily lowered LDL cholesterol by 42% to 72 mg per deciliter but failed to improve cardiovascular outcomes.

AURORA

The AURORA study [31], published four years later in 2009, was a double-blind, randomized, multicenter study evaluating the effects of rosuvastatin 10 mg daily versus placebo in 2776 hemodialysis patients over a mean follow-up period of 3.2 years. This study differed from the 4D trial in that it enrolled both patients with ($n = 731$) and without diabetes ($n = 1545$). The primary endpoint was time to a major cardiovascular event (cardiovascular death, nonfatal myocardial infarction or nonfatal stroke).

Baseline LDL-C levels in AURORA were 100 mg/dL. Randomization to rosuvastatin led to a reduction in LDL-C by 43% at 3 months. There was no benefit of rosuvastatin for the primary end point (28.5% in rosuvastatin vs. 29.5% in placebo; p value 0.59). In sub-analysis, there was no significant difference in death from cardiovascular cause ($p = 0.97$), nonfatal myocardial infarction ($p = 0.23$), or nonfatal stroke ($p = 0.42$). The lack of significance in stroke is notable, as this differs from the prior 4D trial, in which there was a greater incidence of stroke in the treatment arm.

Within the secondary endpoints, there was no difference in death from any cause ($p = 0.51$), death from non-cardiovascular cause ($p = 0.34$), vascular access procedures ($p = 0.19$), atherosclerotic cardiac events ($p = 0.64$), or revascularization ($p = 0.88$).

Lastly, it was shown that statin therapy was safe in hemodialysis patients, with no increase in muscle-related adverse events, rhabdomyolysis, or liver disease.

Notably, Aurora did not include patients who were on statin therapy prior to initiating hemodialysis, so it was still unclear what the benefit of continuing treatment in this group would be. Also, the yearly event rate for the primary end point was lower than expected, suggesting a possible selection bias toward a healthier dialysis cohort. Lastly, there were a high proportion of patients who discontinued the study medication due to a high rate of hospitalization for coexisting illness, adverse events, and renal transplantation.

SHARP

The last major randomized, double-blind placebo-controlled trial of statins in patients with CKD was the SHARP trial, published in 2011 [32]. This study was the largest to date, enrolling 9438 patients randomized to simvastatin

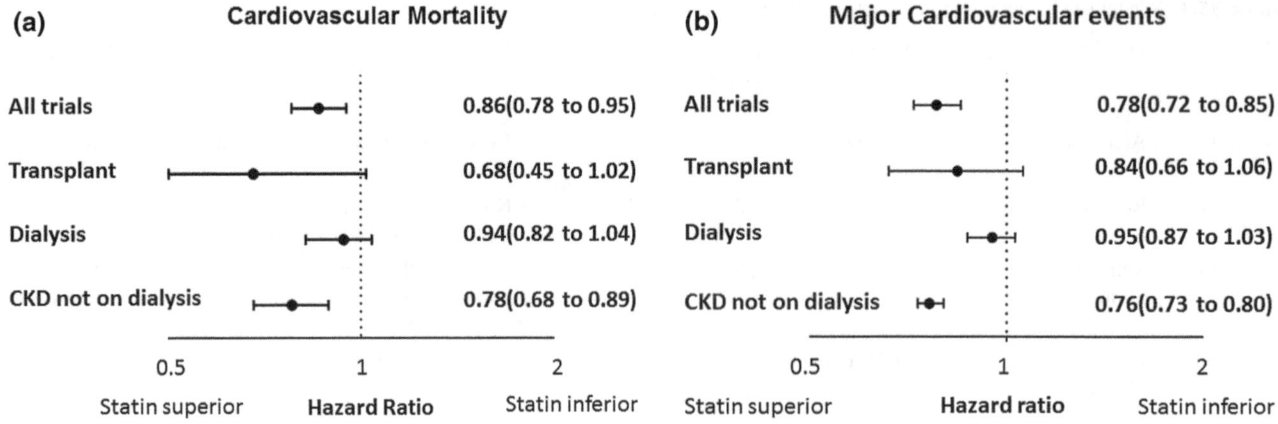

Fig. 35.1 Meta-analysis of statin trials in patients with various stages of CKD. **a** CV mortality, **b** MACE. [35]

20 mg + ezetimibe 10 mg versus simvastatin 20 mg versus placebo. After the first year, no safety concerns were identified with the addition of ezetimibe 10 mg, so the simvastatin alone arm was re-randomized to either simvastatin + ezetimibe or to placebo. In the study, 33% of the patients were on maintenance dialysis at randomization. Among patients not on dialysis, 35% had CKD stage 3 (eGFR 30–59 mL/min/1.73 m^2), 43% had stage 4 disease (eGFR 15–29 mL/min/1.73 m^2), and 20% had stage 5 CKD (eGFR < 15 mL/min/1.73 m^2). The mean follow-up time was 4.9 years. The primary end point in the trial included nonfatal MI, coronary death, non-hemorrhagic stroke, or arterial revascularization.

Randomization to simvastatin + ezetimibe was associated with a significant reduction in the primary end point, with an 11.3% event rate in the treatment group versus 13.4% in placebo ($p = 0.002$). In sub-analyses, the simvastatin + ezetimibe group had significantly lower non-hemorrhagic stroke ($p = 0.01$) and number of arterial revascularizations ($p = 0.0036$). There was no significant difference in cardiac deaths ($p = 0.38$), or in death from any cause ($p = 0.87$), with the majority of the benefit driven by decreased revascularization in the treatment group. Simvastatin + ezetimibe did not result in increased risk of elevated creatinine kinase, myopathy (0.2% in simvastatin + ezetimibe vs. 0.1% in placebo), or rhabdomyolysis (0.1 vs. 0%). SHARP also showed no difference between subgroups based on individual CKD staging, though the study was not powered adequately to study individual CKD stages.

Statin Therapy in CKD: Reviews and Meta-Analysis

In addition to the evidence in SHARP in favor of treating patients with CKD not on hemodialysis with cholesterol-lowering therapy, several reviews and meta-analyses have been published, further supporting treatment. A 2014 Cochrane review on statin use for CKD patients not on dialysis evaluated 50 studies ($n = 45{,}285$), showing the benefit of statin therapy in improving cardiovascular events (RR 0.72, 95% CI 0.66–0.79), all-cause mortality (RR 0.79, 95% CI 0.69–0.91), cardiovascular death (RR 0.79, 95% CI 0.69–0.87), and MI (RR 0.55, 95% CI 0.42–0.72), with uncertain effects on fatal and nonfatal strokes (RR 0.62, 95% CI 0.35–1.12) [34]. This data further supports what was seen in the SHARP trial, and supports cholesterol-lowering therapy with statin (or statin + ezetimibe) for all patients with CKD not on hemodialysis.

A separate 2012 review and meta-analysis analyzed data for statin use on CKD including patients with end-stage renal disease on hemodialysis and renal transplant patients. The study group reviewed 80 randomized trials ($n = 51{,}099$), comparing the effects of statins against placebo or no treatment. The results of this review are summarized in Fig. 35.1: statin treatment was associated with significant reductions in all-cause mortality, cardiovascular mortality, major cardiovascular events, fatal or nonfatal myocardial infarction, and fatal or nonfatal stroke among patients with CKD not on dialysis. Patients already with end-stage renal disease on hemodialysis did not see benefits from statin therapy, and those with kidney transplants had a trend towards benefit from statin therapy [35].

Other Treatments

Due to the increased prevalence of hypertriglyceridemia among patients with CKD (over 50% of CKD patients have triglyceride level >200 mg/dL), several studies have evaluated fibrates in this population [11]. A sub-analysis of The Veterans Affairs High-Density Lipoprotein Intervention

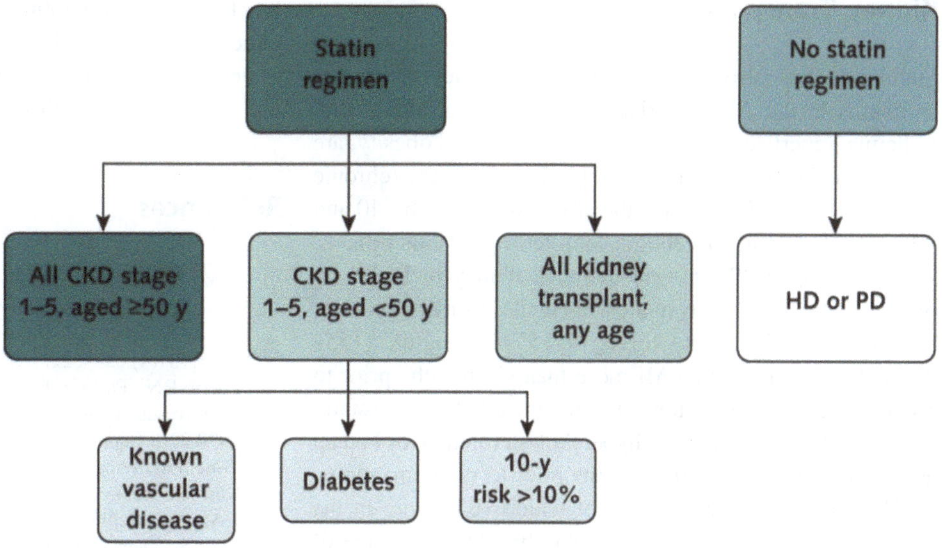

Fig. 35.2 Flow chart for statin treatment in CKD [40]

Trial (VA-HIT) looked at 1046 men with kidney insufficiency, defined by creatinine clearance <75 mL/min using the Cockcroft-Gault equation. Within this subgroup, the primary outcome of coronary death or nonfatal myocardial infarction was lower in the gemfibrozil treatment group ($p = 0.02$), but no total mortality benefit was observed with treatment ($p = 0.85$). Patients in the gemfibrozil arm did have significantly worsened kidney function compared to placebo measured by an increase in serum creatinine (5.9 vs. 2.8%, $p = 0.02$). Given the increased risks of gemfibrozil to kidney function, no mortality benefit seen with treatment, and increased risk of myopathy when fibrates are combined with statin therapy [36], it is not recommended to treat patients with CKD with fibrate therapy [37]. Patients with fasting triglyceride levels >500 mg/dL should attempt lifestyle modifications with diet, weight loss, exercise, decreased alcohol, and hyperglycemia treatment first but may require additional treatment if the risk of pancreatitis remains elevated.

KDIGO Recommendations

Although patients with chronic kidney disease are at greater risk for coronary disease, the association between absolute LDL-C level and cardiovascular outcomes is weaker than in patients without CKD. As such, cholesterol-lowering therapy may be less effective in chronic kidney disease compared to the general population [38]. The etiology of cardiovascular events in patients with kidney disease is multifactorial, and non-atherosclerotic etiologies such as sudden cardiac death, arrhythmia and heart failure, likely caused by increased oxidative stress, inflammation, physical inactivity, anemia, hypertension, vascular calcification, endothelial dysfunction, and depressed nitric oxide availability [5–9], prevail. Specifically in hemodialysis patients, cardiovascular events may be more related to increased prevalence of left ventricular hypertrophy, rapid volume changes, and electrolyte abnormalities [39]. As the correlation between absolute LDL-C levels and cardiac death are not strong in kidney disease, KDIGO advises treatment based on absolute risks factors, rather than LDL-C levels. Notably, all patients with a decreased eGFR (not on dialysis) over the age of 50 should be treated with cholesterol-lowering therapy with a statin or statin + ezetimibe. This is because all patients with chronic kidney disease over age 50 are at an increased risk for cardiovascular disease, with a 10-year risk for coronary death or nonfatal MI to be >10%. Patients who are under age 50, but who have prior cardiovascular disease, diabetes mellitus, or calculated ASCVD risk score >10% are also recommended to be on cholesterol-lowering therapy.

However, there is no evidence for beginning statin therapy in patients with ESKD on dialysis [30, 31, 35]. In the above-mentioned trials, patients who were taking statins and progressed to ESKD were not evaluated, and therefore it is a weak recommendation to continue therapy in this subgroup. In SHARP, 2141 patients without kidney failure at baseline commenced dialysis during the trial, and there was a benefit within this group [32]. Yet the study was not powered for this or analyzed as its own separate subgroup, and studies are needed to further evaluate this subgroup (Fig. 35.2) [40].

Kidney Transplant

Statin use has also been evaluated in kidney transplant recipients in the ALERT trial. Hyperlipidemia, along with ischemia–reperfusion damage, hypertension, and obesity, are risk factors leading to chronic allograft nephropathy (chronic rejection). ALERT evaluated the effects of fluvastatin 40 and 80 mg daily versus placebo on long-term graft function.

Patients aged 30–75 were included if they had a transplant for greater than 6 months at randomization and had baseline total cholesterol levels of 155–348 mg/dL (155–270 if the patient had an MI more than six months prior to randomization). Exclusion criteria included prior statin therapy, a history of familial hypercholesterolemia, or had an acute rejection in the three months prior to randomization.

2102 patients were enrolled, of which 1050 were in the treatment arm and 1052 were in placebo. At an average of 2.8 years, the dose of the study medication was doubled in 65% of the patients. The major cause of renal failure in patients enrolled were glomerulonephritis and polycystic kidney disease, and all patients in the study were on cyclosporine, 81% on steroids, 65% received azathioprine, and 16% received mycophenolate mofetil.

In the study, fluvastatin treatment lowered LDL cholesterol by a mean of 32%, but there was no significant difference between the treatment and placebo arms in the primary endpoint of major adverse cardiac events, cardiac death, nonfatal MI, or coronary intervention procedure ($p = 0.139$). There was also no significant difference in renal endpoints, namely graft losses, doubling of serum creatinine, or patient death. However, within subgroup analysis, there was a significant reduction in cardiac death and nonfatal MI ($p = 0.005$) among the treatment arm, leading to a 2B recommendation by KDIGO to treat all renal transplant patients with statin therapy [33, 40].

Conclusion

Uremic dyslipidemia is a unique lipid profile seen in CKD, caused by changes in lipid enzymatic activity, increased PTH levels, and increased insulin resistance. Although lowering LDL-C levels is correlated to lowering CVD risk in the general population, the correlation is not as strong in CKD. Several landmark trials, including 4D, AURORA, SHARP, and ALERT, have driven the current recommendations by the KDIGO committee for treating patients with CKD not on hemodialysis with statin or statin + ezetimibe, but not initiating statins in those already on hemodialysis [40]. Although hypertriglyceridemia is a key component of uremic dyslipidemia, fibrates are not recommended in CKD, due to little significant benefits and worsening renal function. Areas for future research include whether to continue patients with CKD on statin therapy as they transition to hemodialysis, and whether high-intensity statin treatment will be associated with benefit [30–33].

References

1. Mozaffarian D, Benjamin EJ, Go AS, Arnett DK, Blaha MJ, Cushman M, et al. Heart disease and stroke statistics—2015 update: a report from the American Heart Association. Circulation. 2015;131(4):e29–322.
2. Foley RN, Parfrey PS, Sarnak MJ. Clinical epidemiology of cardiovascular disease in chronic renal disease. Am J Kidney Dis. 1998;32(5 Suppl 3):S112–9.
3. Tonelli M, Wiebe N, Culleton B, House A, Rabbat C, Fok M, et al. Chronic kidney disease and mortality risk: a systematic review. J Am Soc Nephrol. 2006;17(7):2034–47.
4. Go AS, Chertow GM, Fan D, McCulloch CE, Hsu CY. Chronic kidney disease and the risks of death, cardiovascular events, and hospitalization. N Engl J Med. 2004;351(13):1296–305.
5. Himmelfarb J, Stenvinkel P, Ikizler TA, Hakim RM. The elephant in uremia: oxidant stress as a unifying concept of cardiovascular disease in uremia. Kidney Int. 2002;62(5):1524–38.
6. McCullough PA. Why is chronic kidney disease the "spoiler" for cardiovascular outcomes? J Am Coll Cardiol. 2003;41(5):725–8.
7. Stenvinkel P, Alvestrand A. Inflammation in end-stage renal disease: sources, consequences, and therapy. Semin Dial. 2002;15(5):329–37.
8. Vaziri ND, Ni Z, Wang XQ, Oveisi F, Zhou XJ. Downregulation of nitric oxide synthase in chronic renal insufficiency: role of excess PTH. Am J Physiol. 1998;274(4 Pt 2):F642–9.
9. Vaziri ND. Effect of chronic renal failure on nitric oxide metabolism. Am J Kidney Dis. 2001;38(4 Suppl 1):S74–9.
10. Vaziri ND. Dyslipidemia of chronic renal failure: the nature, mechanisms, and potential consequences. Am J Physiol Renal Physiol. 2006;290(2):F262–72.
11. Weiner DE, Sarnak MJ. Managing dyslipidemia in chronic kidney disease. J Gen Intern Med. 2004;19(10):1045–52.
12. Liang K, Oveisi F, Vaziri ND. Role of secondary hyperparathyroidism in the genesis of hypertriglyceridemia and VLDL receptor deficiency in chronic renal failure. Kidney Int. 1998;53(3):626–30.
13. Guarnieri GF, Moracchiello M, Campanacci L, Ursini F, Ferri L, Valente M, et al. Lecithin-cholesterol acyltransferase (LCAT) activity in chronic uremia. Kidney Int Suppl. 1978;8:S26–30.
14. Attman PO, Samuelsson O, Alaupovic P. Lipoprotein metabolism and renal failure. Am J Kidney Dis. 1993;21(6):573–92.
15. Deighan CJ, Caslake MJ, McConnell M, Boulton-Jones JM, Packard CJ. Atherogenic lipoprotein phenotype in end-stage renal failure: origin and extent of small dense low-density lipoprotein formation. Am J Kidney Dis. 2000;35(5):852–62.
16. Kaysen GA. Hyperlipidemia in chronic kidney disease. Int J Artif Organs. 2007;30(11):987–92.
17. Charlesworth JA, Kriketos AD, Jones JE, Erlich JH, Campbell LV, Peake PW. Insulin resistance and postprandial triglyceride levels in primary renal disease. Metab Clin Exp. 2005;54(6):821–8.
18. Liang K, Vaziri ND. Gene expression of LDL receptor, HMG-CoA reductase, and cholesterol-7 alpha-hydroxylase in chronic renal failure. Nephrol Dial Transplant. 1997;12(7):1381–6.
19. Vaziri ND. Molecular mechanisms of lipid disorders in nephrotic syndrome. Kidney Int. 2003;63(5):1964–76.

20. Prinsen BH, de Sain-van der Velden MG, de Koning EJ, Koomans HA, Berger R, Rabelink TJ. Hypertriglyceridemia in patients with chronic renal failure: possible mechanisms. Kidney Int Suppl. 2003;84:S121–4.
21. Attman PO, Samuelsson O, Johansson AC, Moberly JB, Alaupovic P. Dialysis modalities and dyslipidemia. Kidney Int Suppl. 2003;84:S110–2.
22. Bredie SJ, Bosch FH, Demacker PN, Stalenhoef AF, van Leusen R. Effects of peritoneal dialysis with an overnight icodextrin dwell on parameters of glucose and lipid metabolism. Perit Dial Int. 2001;21(3):275–81.
23. Moore R, Thomas D, Morgan E, Wheeler D, Griffin P, Salaman J, et al. Abnormal lipid and lipoprotein profiles following renal transplantation. Transpl Proc. 1993;25(1 Pt 2):1060–1.
24. Gaston RS, Kasiske BL, Fieberg AM, Leduc R, Cosio FC, Gourishankar S, et al. Use of cardioprotective medications in kidney transplant recipients. Am J Transplant. 2009;9(8):1811–5.
25. Vanrenterghem Y, Lebranchu Y, Hene R, Oppenheimer F, Ekberg H. Double-blind comparison of two corticosteroid regimens plus mycophenolate mofetil and cyclosporine for prevention of acute renal allograft rejection. Transplantation. 2000;70(9):1352–9.
26. Kuster GM, Drexel H, Bleisch JA, Rentsch K, Pei P, Binswanger U, et al. Relation of cyclosporine blood levels to adverse effects on lipoproteins. Transplantation. 1994;57(10):1479–83.
27. Artz MA, Boots JM, Ligtenberg G, Roodnat JI, Christiaans MH, Vos PF, et al. Improved cardiovascular risk profile and renal function in renal transplant patients after randomized conversion from cyclosporine to tacrolimus. J Am Soc Nephrol. 2003;14 (7):1880–8.
28. Groth CG, Backman L, Morales JM, Calne R, Kreis H, Lang P, et al. Sirolimus (rapamycin)-based therapy in human renal transplantation: similar efficacy and different toxicity compared with cyclosporine. Sirolimus European Renal Transplant Study Group. Transplantation. 1999;67(7):1036–42.
29. Robinson JG, Stone NJ. The 2013 ACC/AHA guideline on the treatment of blood cholesterol to reduce atherosclerotic cardiovascular disease risk: a new paradigm supported by more evidence. Eur Heart J. 2015;36(31):2110–8.
30. Wanner C, Krane V, Marz W, Olschewski M, Mann JF, Ruf G, et al. Atorvastatin in patients with type 2 diabetes mellitus undergoing hemodialysis. New Engl J Med. 2005;353(3):238–48.
31. Fellstrom BC, Jardine AG, Schmieder RE, Holdaas H, Bannister K, Beutler J, et al. Rosuvastatin and cardiovascular events in patients undergoing hemodialysis. New Engl J Med. 2009;360(14):1395–407.
32. Baigent C, Landray MJ, Reith C, Emberson J, Wheeler DC, Tomson C, et al. The effects of lowering LDL cholesterol with simvastatin plus ezetimibe in patients with chronic kidney disease (study of heart and renal protection): a randomised placebo-controlled trial. Lancet. 2011;377(9784):2181–92.
33. Holdaas H, Fellstrom B, Jardine AG, Holme I, Nyberg G, Fauchald P, et al. Effect of fluvastatin on cardiac outcomes in renal transplant recipients: a multicentre, randomised, placebo-controlled trial. Lancet. 2003;361(9374):2024–31.
34. Palmer SC, Navaneethan SD, Craig JC, Johnson DW, Perkovic V, Hegbrant J, et al. HMG CoA reductase inhibitors (statins) for people with chronic kidney disease not requiring dialysis. Cochrane Database Syst Rev. 2014;5:CD007784.
35. Palmer SC, Craig JC, Navaneethan SD, Tonelli M, Pellegrini F, Strippoli GF. Benefits and harms of statin therapy for persons with chronic kidney disease: a systematic review and meta-analysis. Ann Intern Med. 2012;157(4):263–75.
36. Sarnak MJ, Bloom R, Muntner P, Rahman M, Saland JM, Wilson PW, et al. KDOQI US commentary on the 2013 KDIGO clinical practice guideline for lipid management in CKD. Am J Kidney Dis. 2015;65(3):354–66.
37. Tonelli M, Collins D, Robins S, Bloomfield H, Curhan GC. Veterans' affairs high-density lipoprotein intervention trial I. Gemfibrozil for secondary prevention of cardiovascular events in mild to moderate chronic renal insufficiency. Kidney Int. 2004;66 (3):1123–30.
38. Tonelli M, Muntner P, Lloyd A, Manns B, Klarenbach S, Pannu N, et al. Association between LDL-C and risk of myocardial infarction in CKD. J Am Soc Nephrol. 2013;24(6):979–86.
39. Green D, Roberts PR, New DI, Kalra PA. Sudden cardiac death in hemodialysis patients: an in-depth review. Am J Kidney Dis. 2011;57(6):921–9.
40. Wanner C, Tonelli M. Kidney disease: Improving Global Outcomes Lipid Guideline Development Work Group M. KDIGO clinical practice guideline for lipid management in CKD: summary of recommendation statements and clinical approach to the patient. Kidney Int. 2014;85(6):1303–9.

The Cardiac Impact of Atherosclerotic Renovascular Disease (ARVD)

36

Diana Vassallo, Darren Green, and Philip A. Kalra

Introduction

The prevalence of atherosclerotic renovascular disease (ARVD) seems to be ever increasing due to the combination of an increasingly ageing population, rising atherosclerotic burden and easier access to noninvasive imaging of the renal arteries. Although ARVD is asymptomatic in the large majority of patients, the presence of this disease has important implications; it is associated with a threefold increased risk of death and up to fourfold increased risk of adverse cardiovascular events [1, 2]. A small proportion of patients with ARVD can present with overt clinical manifestations such as recurrent episodes of acute heart failure, severe hypertension or rapidly deteriorating renal function. Prognosis in this 'high-risk' subgroup of patients is even worse. In this review, we shall focus on the close relationship between ARVD and the heart, focusing on epidemiology, pathophysiology, and recommendations for treatment.

Epidemiology

Typical risk factors for ARVD are older age, diabetes, smoking, dyslipidemia, and pre-existing systemic atherosclerosis, hence it is not surprising that these patients are at a significantly increased risk of cardiovascular disease as these are the main risk factors for heart disease. Renal artery stenosis (RAS) of at least 50% was found in 15% of 1235 patients who underwent abdominal aortography in conjunction with coronary catheterization and a similar study showed that 11.7% of 843 patients had RAS of at least 75%. Conversely, atherosclerotic heart disease is found in at least two-thirds of patients with ARVD [2].

Symptomatic heart failure as defined by the Framingham criteria has been reported in around one third of the ARVD population [2] while more than half of outpatients with chronic heart failure and left ventricular ejection fraction <40% may have RAS >50% [3]. Around 10% of patients with ARVD, typically those with bilateral severe ARVD, can present with acute decompensated heart failure, sometimes referred to as 'flash pulmonary edema' (FPE) [4].

Prognosis

Patients with concomitant ARVD and coronary artery disease (CAD) have a worse prognosis than those without coexisting ARVD; 4-year survival in patients with both CAD and ARVD is 65% compared to 86% in patients without ARVD and the risk increases with increasing severity of RAS [1]. Similarly, patients with both chronic heart failure and ARVD have a significantly increased risk of vascular events, prolonged hospitalizations, progression to end-stage kidney disease, and indeed a threefold increased risk of mortality compared to patients without chronic heart failure [5]. Other studies have not been able to show that ARVD is an independent predictor of mortality probably because such patients characteristically have multiple comorbidities and many competing risks for death. Flash pulmonary edema has been shown to be associated with a two-to-threefold increased risk of death and cardiovascular events [6].

D. Vassallo (✉) · D. Green · P.A. Kalra
Department of Renal Medicine, Salford Royal NHS Foundation Trust, Stott Lane, Salford, M6 8HD, UK
e-mail: vassallodi@gmail.com

D. Green
e-mail: darrengreen@doctors.org.uk

P.A. Kalra
e-mail: philip.kalra@srft.nhs.uk

J. Rangaswami et al. (eds.), *Cardio-Nephrology*,
DOI 10.1007/978-3-319-56042-7_36

Pathophysiology of Cardiac Disease in ARVD

Cardiac Remodeling

Although hypertension is the commonest cause of cardiovascular disease and heart failure in the general population, hypertension does not appear to be the sole contributing factor to cardiac dysfunction in the ARVD population and neurohormonal activation appears to play a major role. The point at which the degree of RAS becomes clinically significant is difficult to judge from simple cross-sectional renal angiography as this does not take into account flow hemodynamics, vessel geometry, or the degree of irreversible intraparenchymal injury downstream to the stenosis. Nevertheless, experimental evidence supports expert consensus which states that angiographic stenosis $\geq 70\%$ can be considered hemodynamically significant. Renal artery stenosis of 50–70% can be considered significant if on catheter angiography and physiologic testing there is a resting translesional mean pressure gradient of >10 mmHg, a hyperemic peak systolic pressure gradient of >20 mmHg or renal fractional flow reserve ≤ 0.8 [7].

Hemodynamically significant RAS leads to renin–angiotensin–aldosterone system (RAAS) activation, which in turn causes an increase in renin secretion and production of angiotensin II. This induces hypertension both through its potent vasoconstrictive effects and by increasing sodium and water retention. Angiotensin II is also known to stimulate myocardial fibrosis through production of fibroblast growth factor-23 (FGF-23), platelet-derived growth factor (PDGF) and transforming growth factor-beta (TGF-ß) whilst the ischemic kidney can itself activate the sympathetic nervous system with resulting secretion of noradrenaline [8, 9]. All these pathways serve to augment the risk of both coronary artery disease and cardiac structural abnormalities in patients with ARVD.

Detailed echocardiographic studies have characterized the different myocardial remodeling patterns that occur in response to increased cardiac afterload in ARVD. Concentric remodeling is an early stage of ventricular remodeling characterized by the absence of left ventricular hypertrophy (LVH) but with an increase in wall thickness. This can then progress to either concentric hypertrophy or eccentric hypertrophy and left ventricular dilatation, which are typically associated with pressure and volume overload, respectively [10]. A cross-sectional study comparing echocardiographic characteristics between 79 patients with ARVD and 50 control patients with a similar degree of hypertension and renal impairment showed that only 5% of ARVD patients had a structurally normal heart [11]. Concentric hypertrophy is found in almost half of patients with ARVD patients; the majority of these patients have a normal ejection fraction but are at risk of developing diastolic heart failure. Conversely, a quarter of patients have eccentric hypertrophy; decreased ejection fraction is more common in these patients [10].

A longitudinal echocardiographic study has shown that with time, patients with ARVD develop progressive left ventricular dilatation; a low estimated glomerular filtration rate (eGFR) at baseline can predispose to this [12]. Impaired renal function is associated with a worse prognosis in patients with ARVD and chronic heart failure due to a variety of reasons: decreased use of vasculoprotective therapy such as renin–angiotensin blockade, fluid overload, electrolyte disturbances leading to arrhythmias, vascular calcification, and uremic cardiomyopathy.

Flash Pulmonary Edema

FPE is the presenting feature in 5–10% of patients with ARVD. It was first described in 1988 by Pickering et al. who observed episodes of acute decompensated heart failure in patients with renovascular hypertension and azotemia [4]. FPE tends to occur more frequently in patients with severe bilateral ARVD. Although there is no formal definition of FPE, it is characterized by an acute increase in end-diastolic left ventricular pressure in patients with stiff, hypertrophied ventricles and preserved ejection fraction, leading to rapid fluid accumulation in the pulmonary interstitial and alveolar spaces. Neurohormonal activation can facilitate development of FPE by increasing pulmonary capillary permeability. Patients with bilateral ARVD are especially at risk of FPE as they have impaired pressure natriuresis; however, this condition can also occur in patients with coronary artery disease and myocardial ischemia, and in those with valvular pathology [13].

Unstable Angina

Unstable angina is caused by myocardial ischemia and is defined as severe chest pain with recent onset, or with increasing frequency or severity. It is typically caused by atherosclerotic plaque rupture with partial thrombosis of a coronary artery. ARVD can however worsen unstable angina by causing an increase in cardiac afterload and left ventricular oxygen demands, exacerbating myocardial ischemia.

Treatment

Medical

Patients with ARVD typically have a high cardiovascular risk burden and hence smoking cessation advice together with adequate diabetic and weight control, should be coupled with multi-targeted vascular protective therapy, consisting of renin–angiotensin blockade, statins and aspirin. They usually also require diuretics to control symptoms of fluid overload.

Although the use of renin–angiotensin blockade has not been studied in patients with concomitant ARVD and chronic heart failure, separate studies have shown that this treatment can improve survival in patients with ARVD and in those with chronic heart failure [8, 14]. More specifically, angiotensin-receptor blockers (ARB) have been shown to reduce left ventricular mass in patients with hypertensive diastolic dysfunction [15]. The main concern with renin–angiotensin blockade is the risk of acute kidney injury due to reduced renal efferent arteriolar pressure and impaired autoregulation in patients with hemodynamically significant RAS, especially as these patients are usually also on concurrent diuretic therapy. Patients on renin–angiotensin blockade require frequent monitoring of their renal function; if following initiation of an angiotensin converting enzyme inhibitor (ACEI) or ARB, serum creatinine concentration increases by more than 30% or eGFR declines by more than 25%, and there is no other precipitating cause of acute kidney injury (AKI) such as dehydration or concurrent nephrotoxic medication (e.g., nonsteroidal anti-inflammatory agents), the dose of the ACEI or ARB may need to be reduced to a previously tolerated level or stopped altogether. In the event of an intercurrent illness which can cause hypotension, such as diarrhea, vomiting or sepsis, it is recommended that the ACEI or ARB should be temporarily stopped until the patient has recovered from the hypovolemic illness [8, 16]. As discussed below, revascularization may be considered to permit the use of renin–angiotensin blockade for optimization of cardiac status.

While beta-blockers can improve outcomes in patients with heart failure and reduced ejection fraction, and there is some evidence that they can improve survival and reduce the incidence of nonfatal cardiovascular events in patients with ARVD [17], their role in patients with diastolic heart failure and normal resting heart rates is unclear. It is thought that beta-blockers can worsen exercise intolerance due to their negative chronotropic effects and they have not been shown to improve survival or reduce hospitalizations in this population of patients [15].

Revascularization

Randomized Controlled Studies

Contemporary renal revascularization techniques involve percutaneous transluminal angioplasty with stenting (PTRAS) as opposed to the more hazardous open surgical reconstruction techniques used in the past. To date, six randomized controlled trials (RCTs) have not shown that PTRAS confers any added benefit to optimal medical therapy in terms of blood pressure control, improvement in renal function, cardiovascular events or mortality [18–23]. Predefined clinical end points for the first four trials involved renal function and blood pressure control; the numbers of patients recruited into these earlier studies were relatively small hence these studies were underpowered to investigate the effect of revascularization on cardiac end points. On the other hand, the two more recent multicenter trials, Angioplasty and Stent for Renal Artery Lesions Trial (ASTRAL) and the Cardiovascular Outcomes for Renal Atherosclerotic Lesions Trial (CORAL), recruited large numbers of patients [22, 23]. However, they were criticized because patients with 'high-risk' features such as unstable cardiac status, deteriorating renal function, or uncontrolled hypertension were usually excluded from participation in these studies by their managing clinician, hence it is argued that the results cannot be extrapolated to higher risk patients typically encountered in clinical practice.

The ASTRAL trial randomized 806 patients with ARVD to receive either medical therapy alone or renal revascularization. Around 50% of patients in both groups had coronary artery disease and mean eGFR was around 40 ml/min. The primary outcome measure was change in renal function from baseline while secondary outcomes included blood pressure control, renal outcomes, cardiovascular events and death; there was no difference in any of these parameters between patients who underwent revascularization and those treated with medical therapy alone. Over a median follow-up period of 33.6 months, 35% suffered a cardiovascular event in both arms. The results of a cardiac magnetic resonance sub-study performed in 44 patients originally recruited into ASTRAL have recently been published. Over a 12-month period, there was nonsignificant improvement in left ventricular structural parameters in both arms, which could reflect the effect of appropriate medical therapy. Revascularization was again not shown to confer any added benefit, possibly because patients with acute heart failure were not recruited into this study, but also because the study population was unselected, with many having relatively modest RAS [24].

These findings are in keeping with the results of the Stenting of Renal Artery Stenosis in Coronary Artery Disease (RAS-CAD) trial, which looked at the effect of revascularization on left ventricular mass index (LVMI) in 84 patients with both ARVD and underlying coronary artery disease over a 12-month period. Medical therapy led to improved LVMI, however revascularization had no added effect. Again, patients with severe ARVD and a high-risk profile were excluded from this study [25].

The more recent CORAL study looked at the effect of revascularization in 947 patients randomized to intervention or medical therapy on the composite clinical end point consisting of death from cardiovascular or renal causes,

Table 36.1 Observational studies describing the effect of renal revascularization in patient with chronic or acute heart failure

Authors and year of publication	Number of patients	Type of heart failure presentation	Coronary artery disease	Left ventricular systolic dysfunction	ACEI use	RAS degree	Intervention	Heart failure end points
Pickering et al. [4]	11	Acute	Yes 5/11	No	Yes 8/11 showed WRF	7 bilateral, 2 unilateral to SFK, 2 unilateral	8 PTRA, 3 surgery	10/11 no further FPE
Meissner et al. [32]	6	Chronic	Yes	Yes	Yes with WRF	Severe bilateral or unilateral to SFK	4 PTRA, 1 surgery, one none	Undefined clinical improvement
Messina et al. [33]	17	Acute	Yes 11/17	Yes 6/17	Unknown	Severe bilateral	1 PTRA, 16 surgery	No FPE over mean follow-up of 2.4 years
Khosla et al. [26]	28	Chronic	Yes 24/28	Yes 22/28	Unknown	>70% stenosis, 8 unilateral, 20 bilateral	28 PTRA with stent	16/28 improvement in NYHA class
Bloch et al. [34]	25	19 acute 6 chronic	Yes 15/25	Yes 4/25	Unknown	22 Bilateral, 3 Unilateral	25 PTRAS	18/25 no recurrent, 3 with FPE, 4 with CHF at 1 year
Missouris et al. [35]	6	Chronic	Unknown	Unknown	Yes with WRF	4 severe bilateral, 5 severe unilateral	8 PTRA, 1 surgery	Unspecified improvement
Gray et al. [36]	39	Chronic and Acute	Unknown	Unknown	Yes 6/39	18/39 severe bilateral, 21/39 severe unilateral to SFK	26 PTRAS	Reduction in hospitalization for heart failure

Adapted from De Silva [8]
ACEI angiotensin converting enzyme inhibitor, *CHF* chronic heart failure, *FPE* flash pulmonary edema, *PTRA* percutaneous transluminal angioplasty, *PTRAS* percutaneous transluminal angioplasty with stenting, *RAS* renal artery stenosis, *SFK* single functioning kidney, *WRF* worsening renal function

myocardial infarction, stroke, hospitalization from congestive heart failure, progressive renal impairment, or need for renal replacement therapy. Only 12–15% of patients had a documented history of heart failure whereas 26–30% had had a prior myocardial infarction; the mean eGFR was higher than in ASTRAL at around 58 ml/min. In comparison to ASTRAL, around 6% of patients in each arm suffered a myocardial infarction and a similar proportion required hospitalization for congestive heart failure over a median follow-up period of 43 months. These results could reflect the low-risk cardiac and renal status of patients recruited into this trial.

Retrospective Studies, Case Series and Case Reports

A number of uncontrolled case series and case reports suggest that revascularization can confer benefit to specific patients who present with 'cardiac destabilization syndromes' such as flash pulmonary edema or unstable angina (see Table 36.1). This was first described by Pickering in a case series of 11 patients with acute pulmonary edema who underwent revascularization; 10 patients had no further episodes over a mean follow-up period of 28 months, although mortality data was not reported. A similar benefit has been reported in 20 patients presenting with unstable angina who all underwent renal revascularization with or without coronary intervention. There was an improvement in the mean Canadian Cardiovascular Society angina classification from 3.1 to 1.4 up to 8 months post-intervention which was independent of whether patients received coronary intervention [26]. A recent retrospective single-center study has shown that revascularization was associated with reduced risk of death (HR 0.4, $p = 0.01$) in patients presenting with flash pulmonary edema, and reduced risk of death (HR 0.15, $p = 0.04$) and cardiovascular events (HR 0.23, $p = 0.02$) in patients with combined uncontrolled hypertension and rapidly deteriorating renal function [6].

Revascularization may also optimize outcomes in patients with chronic heart failure although this has been less well described. Kane et al. performed a retrospective study looking specifically at the effect of revascularization in 163 patients with ARVD, 50 of whom had predominantly chronic diastolic heart failure as defined by clinical and echocardiographic criteria. Outcomes for 50 patients who underwent revascularization were compared with 50 matched patients, also with underlying ARVD and chronic heart

Table 36.2 Recommendations for renal revascularization

High-risk clinical presentation	Recommendation classification	Level of evidence
Cardiac disturbance		
Haemodynamically significant RAS[c] with: Recurrent unexplained CHF or Sudden unexplained pulmonary edema	Class I	B
RAS and unstable angina	Class IIa	B
Resistant hypertension[a]		
RAS with Accelerated, Resistant or malignant hypertension Hypertension with unilateral small kidney Hypertension with medication intolerance	Class IIa	B
Ischemic nephropathy[b]		
RAS and chronic renal insufficiency with: Bilateral RAS or RAS to a solitary functioning kidney	Class IIa	B
RAS and chronic renal insufficiency with unilateral RAS (2 kidneys present)	Class IIb	C
Asymptomatic bilateral or solitary viable kidney with haemodynamically significant RAS	Class IIb	C
Asymptomatic unilateral haemodynamically significant RAS in a viable kidney	Class IIb	C

Adapted from Parikh et al. [7]
RAS renal artery stenosis
[a]Defined as uncontrolled hypertension despite use of maximally tolerated doses of at least three antihypertensive agents, one of which is a diuretic, or intolerance to medication
[b]Defined as chronic kidney disease with eGFR <45 ml/min in the context of atheroscerlotic renovascular disease (ARVD) usually with potential global renal ischemia (unilateral RAS with a solitary functioning kidney or bilateral significant RAS)
[c]Defined as angiographic stenosis ≥ 70 or 50–70% with a resting translesional mean pressure gradient >10 mmHg, hyperemic mean systolic pressure gradient >20 mmHg or renal fractional flow reserve ≤ 0.8

failure, who were treated exclusively medically. Results showed that more patients with chronic heart failure who underwent revascularization were receiving renin–angiotensin blockade at follow-up, which was thought to partly explain the better systolic blood pressure control, fivefold reduction in hospitalizations and reduced New York Heart Association (NYHA) class (1.9 vs. 2.6) noted in this group. However, overall mortality was not different between the two groups, possibly as a result of the significant cardiovascular risk of these patients and other confounding factors [5].

Three observational studies to date have described changes in cardiac morphology following renal artery revascularization. Zeller et al. showed a decrease in LVMI of 10 g/m^2 at a mean follow-up of 24 months in 102 ARVD patients following revascularization and this was independent of the reduction in blood pressure also noted in this group. In contrast, LVMI was seen to increase by 9 g/m^2 in 101 contemporaneous patients with chronic kidney disease and essential hypertension who were managed medically; blood pressure in this group was noted to increase during follow-up. However, this retrospective study is limited by inherent differences between these two groups of patients. Patients in the ARVD group had better renal function and lower blood pressure at baseline, although a higher proportion of these patients were diabetic and had coronary artery disease, hence the pathophysiology of cardiac structural changes in the two groups is likely to be different [27].

Corriere et al. performed echocardiography at baseline and at a mean of 7.7 months following revascularization in 20 ARVD patients; there was a statistically significant improvement in LVMI but no difference in ejection fraction [28]. A very similar study performed by Rzeznik et al. looked at echocardiographic parameters at baseline and 3 and 12 months post-revascularization in 84 patients with ARVD. There was an improvement in left ventricular mass (LVM) and LVMI independent of blood pressure change. However, there was no corresponding improvement in diastolic function parameters [29]. The latter two studies were uncontrolled hence it is not possible to deduce whether these changes occurred independently of medical therapy. In addition, only a very small proportion of these patients had overt symptoms of heart failure.

An individual case report looked at echocardiographic parameters before and after revascularization in a patient with bilateral ARVD and recurrent episodes of flash pulmonary edema. Post-revascularization, the patient experienced improvement in NYHA classification, better blood pressure control, and renal function. There was marked improvement in echocardiographic morphology and function at 4 months (left ventricular mass decreased from 161 to 116 g and ejection fraction improved from 39 to 65%) and these changes were sustained at 1-year of follow-up. There was an accompanying increase in vascular endothelial growth factor (VEGF) and, as expected, a decrease in angiotensin II levels following revascularization. All these changes may have been augmented by the use of concomitant antihypertensive and cardioprotective medication [30].

Recommendations and Future Directions

Despite the neutral results of RCTs and the lack of robust evidence, the American College of Cardiology/American Heart Association strongly recommend revascularization for patients with hemodynamically significant ARVD and recurrent episodes of chronic heart failure or acute, unexplained pulmonary edema [31] (see Table 36.2).

More research is required to help understand the close relationship between heart and kidney pathophysiology in ARVD. It is hoped that advanced imaging techniques such as speckle-track echocardiography, detailed cardiac MRI studies, and the application of novel biomarkers can help identify ARVD patients who have potentially reversible myocardial changes, so that they can benefit from timely referral for revascularization.

Conclusion

There is a high prevalence of cardiac morbidity and mortality in patients with ARVD both due to shared atherosclerotic risk factors leading to coronary artery disease, and due to adverse cardiac structural remodeling secondary to a combination of neurohormonal activation, renal impairment, and hypertension. Intensive vascular protective therapy, in particular the use of renin–angiotensin blockade, is essential to mitigate the high risk of adverse cardiovascular events in these patients. There is evidence that the use of revascularization in combination with optimal medical therapy may be of benefit in a small subgroup of patients who present with cardiac destabilization syndromes such as acute flash pulmonary edema or unstable angina. Further research is required to help identify these patients accurately and to ensure timely referral for revascularization.

References

1. Conlon PJ, Athirakul K, Kovalik E, Schwab SJ, Crowley J, Stack R, et al. Survival in renal vascular disease. J Am Soc Nephrol [Internet]. 1998;9(2):252–6. http://www.ncbi.nlm.nih.gov/pubmed/19352127.
2. Kalra PA, Guo H, Kausz AT, Gilbertson DT, Liu J, Chen S-C, et al. Atherosclerotic renovascular disease in United States patients aged 67 years or older: risk factors, revascularization, and prognosis. Kidney Int. 2005;68(1):293–301.
3. de Silva R, Loh H, Rigby AS, Nikitin NP, Witte KKA, Goode K, et al. Epidemiology, associated factors, and prognostic outcomes of renal artery stenosis in chronic heart failure assessed by magnetic resonance angiography. Am J Cardiol [Internet]. 2007 Jul 15 [cited 2014 Dec 5];100(2):273–9. http://www.ncbi.nlm.nih.gov/pubmed/17631082.
4. Pickering TG, Herman L, Devereux RB, Sotelo JE, James GD, Sos TA, et al. Recurrent pulmonary oedema in hypertension due to bilateral renal artery stenosis: treatment by angioplasty or surgical revascularisation. Lancet. 1988;2(8610):551–2.
5. Kane GC, Xu N, Mistrik E, Roubicek T, Stanson AW, Garovic VD. Renal artery revascularization improves heart failure control in patients with atherosclerotic renal artery stenosis. Nephrol Dial Transplant. 2010;25:813–20.
6. Ritchie J, Green D, Chrysochou C, Chalmers N, Foley RN, Kalra PA. High-risk clinical presentations in atherosclerotic renovascular disease: prognosis and response to renal artery revascularization. Am J Kidney Dis. 2014;63(2):186–97.
7. Parikh SA, Shishehbor MH, Gray BH, White CJ, Jaff MR. SCAI expert consensus statement for renal artery stenting appropriate use. Catheter Cardiovasc Interv. 2014;84(7):1163–71.
8. De Silva R, Nikitin NP, Bhandari S, Nicholson A, Clark AL, Cleland JGF. Atherosclerotic renovascular disease in chronic heart failure: should we intervene? Eur Heart J. 2005;26(16):1596–605.
9. De Mello WC, Danser AH. Angiotensin II and the heart: on the intracrine renin-angiotensin system. Hypertension [Internet]. 2000;35(6):1183–8. doi:10.1080/09585199200000155.
10. Khan AR, Sheikh M, Kaw D, Cooper CJ, Khouri SJ. Prevalence and factors associated with left ventricular remodeling in renal artery stenosis. J Am Soc Hypertens [Internet]. 2014;1–8. http://www.ncbi.nlm.nih.gov/pubmed/24582873.
11. Wright JR, Shurrab AE, Cooper A, Kalra PR, Foley RN, Kalra PA. Left ventricular morphology and function in patients with atherosclerotic renovascular disease. J Am Soc Nephrol [Internet]. 2005;16(9):2746–53. http://jasn.asnjournals.org/cgi/content/abstract/16/9/2746.
12. Wright JR, Shurrab AE, Cooper A, Kalra PR, Foley RN, Kalra PA. Progression of cardiac dysfunction in patients with atherosclerotic renovascular disease. QJM [Internet]. 2009;102(10):695–704. http://qjmed.oxfordjournals.org/content/102/10/695.abstract.
13. Rimoldi SF, Yuzefpolskaya M, Allemann Y, Messerli F. Flash pulmonary edema. Prog Cardiovasc Dis [Internet]. 2009;52(3):249–59. doi:10.1016/j.pcad.2009.10.002.
14. Chrysochou C, Foley RN, Young JF, Khavandi K, Cheung CM, Kalra PA. Dispelling the myth: the use of renin-angiotensin blockade in atheromatous renovascular disease. Nephrol Dial Transplant [Internet]. 2012 Apr [cited 2014 Aug 27];27(4):1403–9. http://www.ncbi.nlm.nih.gov/pubmed/21993376.
15. From AM, Borlaug BA. Heart failure with preserved ejection fraction: pathophysiology and emerging therapies. Cardiovasc Ther. 2011;29(4):6–21.
16. National Institute for Health and Care Excellence. Acute Kidney Injury [Internet]. 2013. https://www.nice.org.uk/guidance/cg169.
17. Ritchie J, Green D, Alderson H V., Chrysochou C, Vassallo D, Sinha S, et al. Associations of antiplatelet therapy and beta

blockade with patient outcomes in atherosclerotic renovascular disease. J Am Soc Hypertens [Internet]. 2015;1–10. http://linkinghub.elsevier.com/retrieve/pii/S1933171115008025.

18. Plouin P-F, Chatellier G, Darné B, Raynaud A, Study G for the EMM vs A (EMMA). Blood pressure outcome of angioplasty in atherosclerotic renal artery stenosis: a randomized trial. Hypertension. 1998;31(3):823–9.
19. Webster J, Marshall F, Abdalla M, Dominiczak A, Edwards R, Isles CG, et al. Randomised comparison of percutaneous angioplasty vs continued medical therapy for hypertensive patients with atheromatous renal artery stenosis. Scottish and Newcastle Renal Artery Stenosis Collaborative Group. J Hum Hypertens. 1998;12:329–35.
20. Van Jaarsveld BC, Krijnen P, Pieterman H, Derkx F, Deinum J, Postma CT, et al. The effect of balloon angioplasty on hypertension. N Engl J Med. 2000;342(14):1007–14.
21. Bax L, Woittiez A, Kouwenberg H, Mali W, Buskens E, Beek F, et al. Stent placement in patients with atherosclerotic renal artery stenosis and impaired renal function. Ann Intern Med. 2010;150 (12):840–8.
22. Wheatley K, Ives N, Gray R, Kalra PA, Moss JG, Baigent C, et al. Revascularization versus medical therapy for renal-artery stenosis. N Engl J Med. 2009;361(20):1953–62.
23. Cooper CJ, Murphy TP, Cutlip DE, Jamerson K, Henrich W, Reid DM, et al. Stenting and medical therapy for atherosclerotic renal-artery stenosis. N Engl J Med. 2014;370(1):13–22.
24. Ritchie J, Green D, Chrysochou T, Hegarty J, Handley K, Ives N, et al. Effect of renal artery revascularization upon cardiac structure and function in atherosclerotic renal artery stenosis: cardiac magnetic resonance sub-study of the ASTRAL trial. Nephrol Dial Transplant [Internet]. 2016;gfw107. doi:10.1093/ndt/gfw107.
25. Marcantoni C, Zanoli L, Rastelli S. Effect of renal artery stenting on left ventricular mass: a randomised clinical trial. Am J Kidney Dis. 2012;60(1):39–46.
26. Khosla S, White CJ, Collins TJ, Jenkins JS, Shaw D, Ramee SR. Effects of renal artery stent implantation in patients with renovascular hypertension presenting with unstable angina or congestive heart failure. Am J Cardiol [Internet]. 1997;80(3):363–6. http://www.ncbi.nlm.nih.gov/pubmed/9264441.
27. Zeller T, Rastan A, Schwarzwalder U, Muller C, Frank U, Burgelin K, et al. Regression of left ventricular hypertrophy following stenting of renal artery stenosis. J Endovasc Ther [Internet]. 2007;14(2):189–97. http://www.ncbi.nlm.nih.gov/pubmed/17488176.
28. Corriere M, Hoyle J, Craven T, D'Agostino RJ, Edwards M, Moore P, et al. Changes in left ventricular structure and function following renal artery revascularization. Ann Vasc Surg. 2010;24 (1):80–4.
29. Rzeznik D, Przewlocki T, Kablak-Ziembicka A, Kozanecki A, Roslawiecka A, Lach J, et al. Effect of renal artery revascularization on left ventricular hypertrophy, diastolic function, blood pressure, and the one-year outcome. J Vasc Surg Off Publ Soc Vasc Surg [and] Int Soc Cardiovasc Surgery, North Am Chapter [Internet]. 2011;53(3):692–7. doi:10.1016/j.jvs.2010.09.054.
30. Chrysochou C, Schmitt M, Siddals K, Hudson J, Fitchet A, Kalra PA. Reverse cardiac remodelling and renal functional improvement following bilateral renal artery stenting for flash pulmonary oedema. Nephrol Dial Transplant. 2013;28(2):479–83.
31. Hirsch AT, Haskal ZJ, Hertzer NR, Bakal CW, Creager MA, Halperin JL, et al. ACC/AHA 2005 practice guidelines for the management of patients with peripheral arterial disease (lower extremity, renal, mesenteric, and abdominal aortic). Circulation. 2006;113(11):e463–5.
32. Meissner M, Wilson A, Jessup M. Renal artery stenosis in heart failure. Am J Cardiol. 1988;62(17):1307–8.
33. Messina LM, Zelenock GB, Yao KA, Stanley JC, Mich AA. Renal revascularization for recurrent pulmonary edema in patients with poorly controlled hypertension and renal insufficiency: a distinct subgroup of patients with arteriosclerotic renal artery occlusive disease. J Vasc Surg. 1992;15(1):73–82. doi:10.1016/0741-5214 (92)70015-D.
34. Bloch M, Trost D, Pickering T, Sos T, August P. Prevention of recurrent pulmonary oedema in patients with bilateral renovascular disease through renal artery stent placement. Am J Hypertens. 1999;12(1):1–7.
35. Missouris CG, Belli AM, MacGregor GA. "Apparent" heart failure: a syndrome caused by renal artery stenoses. Heart [Internet]. 2000;83(2):152–5. http://www.pubmedcentral.nih.gov/articlerender.fcgi?artid=1729312&tool=pmcentrez&rendertype=abstract.
36. Gray BH, Olin JW, Childs MB, Sullivan TM, Bacharach JM. Clinical benefit of renal artery angioplasty with stenting for the control of recurrent and refractory congestive heart failure. Vasc Med. 2002;7(4):275–9.

Preeclampsia: A Mirror into Future Cardiovascular and Renal Health

37

Scott Blumhof and Janani Rangaswami

Introduction

Preeclampsia, a leading cause of morbidity and mortality in pregnancy, complicates up to 5% of pregnancies worldwide [1]. The spectrum of hypertensive disorders during pregnancy comes in four varieties: gestational hypertension, preeclampsia and eclampsia syndrome, chronic hypertension, and preeclampsia superimposed on chronic hypertension [2]. Gestational hypertension is the development of elevated blood pressure of greater than 140/90 mmHg in previously normotensive women after 20 weeks of gestation. Proteinuria does not develop, and the elevated blood pressures resolve by 12 weeks postpartum. Preeclampsia is gestational hypertension with the presence of proteinuria and/or signs of end organ damage. The progression of the preeclampsia syndrome to eclampsia is signified by the onset of worsening hypertension and generalized tonic-clonic seizures. Preeclampsia and eclampsia are both definitively treated by delivery of the placenta, resulting in resolution of the acute syndrome. However, it has been shown that women who suffer from preeclampsia have a higher lifetime risk of cardiovascular disease (CVD), chronic kidney disease (CKD), cerebrovascular disease, and metabolic derangements including insulin resistance, overt diabetes mellitus, hyperlipidemia, and the metabolic syndrome. In this chapter, we will focus on preeclampsia, its diagnosis, and characteristics as a syndrome, risk factors for its development, the current understanding of the molecular mechanisms behind this disorder, and finally will discuss the implications of preeclampsia as they pertain to the long-term risk for development of CVD, CKD, cerebrovascular disease, and insulin resistance.

Definition and Epidemiology

According to the American College of Obstetrics and Gynecology, preeclampsia is defined as either a maternal blood pressure >140/90 mmHg on two occasions at least 4 h apart after 20 weeks gestation in a woman with previously measured normal blood pressure, or a single blood pressure reading of >160/110 mmHg combined with proteinuria, $\geq$ 300 mg per 24 h urine collection. In severe disease, other manifestations include renal insufficiency defined as serum creatinine concentrations above 1.1 mg/dL or a doubling of the serum creatinine in the absence of preexisting renal disease, pulmonary edema, and cerebral or visual symptoms [2].

The incidence of preeclampsia is higher in women with baseline hypertension, affecting 15–25% of pregnancies in these women and further increasing maternal and fetal risks [3]. When preeclampsia is superimposed upon chronic hypertension this subset of patients develops the disease earlier in the pregnancy and have more severe disease than in women without an underlying diagnosis of hypertension. While 16% of maternal deaths are due to the hypertensive disorders as a group [4], 10–12.3% are due to preeclampsia itself [5, 6].

Risk factors for preeclampsia include preexisting vascular conditions such as hypertension, obesity, chronic renal disease, diabetes mellitus, and thrombophilia [7], nulliparity [8], a change in paternity [9], a history of preeclampsia [10], extremes of age [11], race [12], socioeconomic status, and altitude [11, 13, 14]. Conditions that result in an increase in placental mass, for example, multiple gestations and molar

S. Blumhof (✉)
Department of Pulmonary, Allergy, and Critical Care Medicine, UAB, 1900 University Blvd, Tinsley Harrison Tower, Suite 422, Birmingham, AL, USA
e-mail: sblumhof@gmail.com

J. Rangaswami
Department of Medicine, Einstein Medical Center, 5401 Old York Road, Suite 363, Philadelphia, PA 19141, USA
e-mail: rangaswj@einstein.edu

J. Rangaswami
Sidney Kimmel College, Thomas Jefferson University, Philadelphia, PA, USA

J. Rangaswami et al. (eds.), *Cardio-Nephrology*,
DOI 10.1007/978-3-319-56042-7_37

pregnancies, have also been shown to make it more likely that preeclampsia will complicate that particular pregnancy [11]. This observation strongly implicates a placental trigger in the pathogenesis of this syndrome. Interestingly, active tobacco use has actually been associated with a decreased risk for preeclampsia though the mechanism is not fully understood [15]. Despite this, the risks of smoking during pregnancy far outweigh this one benefit.

Although no single gene has been implicated, several studies have suggested that genetic elements have a role in the incidence and development of preeclampsia. Polymorphisms in genes coding for renin, angiotensinogen, endothelial nitric oxide synthase, prothrombin, factor V Leiden, and methyltetrahydrofolate reductase showed promise in initial small trials [16–19], but could not be confirmed in larger studies [20–24]. However, a study of families in Iceland looking for potential preeclampsia genes revealed a significant locus on chromosome 2p13 [25] and this locus was confirmed in a similar study of patients from New Zealand and Australia [26]. Despite discovery of this locus, the exact mechanism through which it predisposes a woman to preeclampsia remains unknown. Another potential culprit could be a locus on chromosome 13, as it has been observed that mothers of fetuses with trisomy 13 have a higher incidence of preeclampsia than mothers pregnant with normal fetuses, but again its exact role remains elusive [27].

Pathogenesis

Placental Factors

The placenta is requisite for preeclampsia to appear, not the fetus. This is demonstrated by the fact that molar pregnancies, which harbor no viable fetus, have been shown to have increased incidence of preeclampsia [11]. Placentae from preeclamptic women, when examined pathologically, classically reveal numerous infarcts, sclerotic narrowing of arteries and arterioles, and fibrin deposition and thrombosis [28]. In normal placentation, the cytotrophoblasts alter the uterine vasculature so that it can supply the placenta and fetus with the necessary amounts of blood and nutrients needed to sustain a normal pregnancy. These invading cells also modulate the production of vascular endothelial growth factor (VEGF) ligands and receptors, being able to, at certain points in the pregnancy, express every mammalian member of this family of proteins. The end result is transformation of these vessels from small resistance vessels to flaccid, high-caliber capacitance vessels able to perfuse the placenta [29–33].

In preeclampsia the normal placentation process is disrupted as evidenced by insufficient endovascular invasion by cytotrophoblasts and failure of uterine artery remodeling [29]. When the cytotrophoblast cells invade the uterine spiral arteries they adopt a cell profile more akin to endothelial cells than their epithelial origin. In the preeclamptic patient, not only do the cells not invade as deep into the uterine tissue as they need to, they also fail to undergo this process of "pseudovasculogenesis," which involves switching of cell surface integrins and adhesion molecules to resemble endothelial cells [34–36]. This suggests that faulty differentiation eventually leads to ischemia and tissue hypoxia characteristic of the preeclamptic placenta. However, the cause of this failure is unknown. It has been suggested by some that initial hypoxia causes this aberrant invasion and differentiation [37]. It is interesting that hypoxia would both lead to the syndrome and then contribute to its development. Another hypothesis is that a decrease in soluble antiangiogenic factors is possibly involved in the faulty remodeling [38]. This diminished perfusion and hypoxic environment eventually leads to the release of placental debris, microparticles, and factors into the maternal circulation that lead to the systemic inflammatory response and the second stage of the syndrome (Fig. 37.1) [39, 40].

Angiogenic Factors

It is evident by 21 days post conception that placental vasculogensis has begun. Involved in this process are numerous pro- and antiangiogenic substances, of which the best studied are the VEGF and angiopoietin families. It is hypothesized that the hypoxic environment that is created as previously described results in angiogenic imbalance, and the overproduction of antiangiogenic factors. It has been shown that in preeclamptic women, the placenta

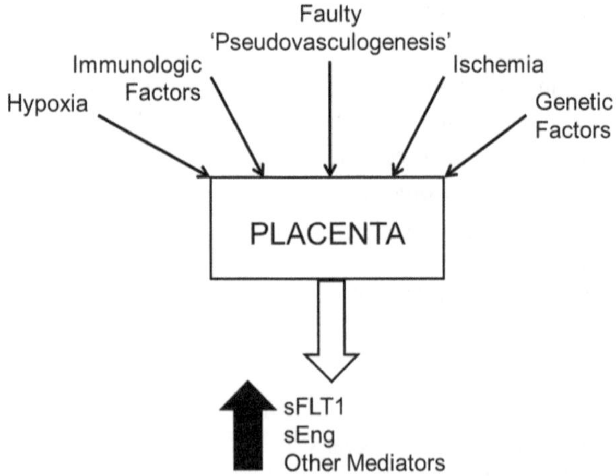

Fig. 37.1 The placental factors that lead to the release of antiangiogenic molecules and contribute to the antiangiogenic milieu of preeclampsia (*sFlt-1* soluble Fms-like tyrosine kinase 1, *sEng* soluble endoglin)

overproduces at least two antiangiogenic peptides that enter the maternal circulation: soluble Fms-like tyrosine kinase 1 (sFlt-1) and soluble endoglin (sEng) [41]. Before we discuss the roles of these molecules in the development of the maternal syndrome, we will first review their role in vascular homeostasis.

VEGF are secreted proteins that are responsible for regulating vasculogenesis, the formation of blood vessels in embryonic life, and angiogenesis, the process of forming new blood vessels. The important members of this family for our discussions are VEGF-A (VEGF) and placental growth factor (PlGF). VEGF is proangiogenic which promotes the proliferation and survival of endothelial cells [42, 43] and PlGF is a homolog released by the placenta with similar activity [44]. The family of VEGF receptors present on vascular endothelial cells is large, but those apropos to our discussion include Flt-1 (VEFGR-1) and KDR (VEGFR-2). VEGF binds to both Flt-1 and KDR, while PlGF binds only to Flt-1 [45]. When Flt-1 is absent in a mouse model, the mice die in embryonic life due to overgrowth of endothelial cells and blood vessel disarray [46] which implies that the function of Flt-1 is as a negative regulator of angiogenesis [47]. Recent work also suggests that the role of the Flt-1 gene is to express sFlt-1 which acts as a soluble VEGF signaling inhibitor and regulates and guides emerging vessel sprouts through control of local VEGF concentrations [48]. Aside from being involved in embryonic vasculogenesis and angiogenesis, the VEGF family of proteins plays a role in the survival of endothelial cells and vascular homeostasis in mature vessels. It is especially important in differentiation and survival of fenestrated endothelium in the choroid plexus, renal podocytes, and hepatocytes [49]. Inhibition of VEGF has been seen in vivo to lead to pathology in many of those organs. In the mouse, kidney knockout of VEGF has been shown to result in the classic kidney lesions of preeclampsia [50]. In fact, the role of VEGF in vascular homeostasis was best noted in humans during testing of anti-VEGF chemotherapies for the treatment of cancer the common side effects were headaches, hypertension, proteinuria, glomerular endothelial damage, coagulopathy, and rarely the reversible posterior leukoencephalopathy syndrome [51–54].

As early as 1989 Roberts and Taylor et al. hypothesized that preeclampsia results from the release of circulating factors by the placenta which lead to widespread maternal endothelial dysfunction [55, 56]. In fact, to this day, evidence continues to support this early hypothesis. For one, the most well-known manifestations of preeclampsia occur in organs that contain fenestrated endothelial cells and involve the vasculature of those organs. In addition, there is also evidence that establishes the presence of factors released by the injured endothelium in the circulation of women with clinical preeclampsia including, to name a few, endothelin-1 [57], fibronectin [58–60], von Willebrand factor [58, 61], thrombomodulin [62, 63], markers of oxidative stress [64], and inflammatory cytokines [65]. To further support the theory that a circulating factor results in endothelial dysfunction, serum from preeclamptic women induces endothelial injury in vitro [56, 64, 66].

Efforts to identify this circulating factor resulted in the observation by Karumanchi et al. that sFlt-1 mRNA is upregulated in preeclamptic women [67]. SFlt-1 is a soluble form of the VEGF/PlGF receptor Flt-1 produced by alternative splicing, and is a potent inhibitor of both VEGF and PlGF activity [68]. In support of sFlt-1 as the causative agent of the endothelial dysfunction rampant in preeclampsia, administration of sFlt-1 to pregnant rats induced a syndrome of hypertension, preoteinuria, and glomerular endotheliosis almost identical to preeclampsia [67]. However, absent from this syndrome was the liver dysfunction and cerebral changes notable in severe preeclampsia. It was then discovered by gene expression that sEng was noted to be present at fourfold greater concentrations in preeclamptic pregnancy than in normal pregnancy [47]. sEng was seen to combine with sFlt-1 to induce the features of severe preeclampsia not caused by sFlt-1 inhibition of VEGF alone [49, 69]. The proposed mechanism is that sEng reduces binding of transforming growth factor beta (TGF-B1) and blocks TGF-B1 induced vasodilation of vessels in rats, likely through the downregulation of nitric oxide synthetase [69]. It was also shown that sEng could induce increased capillary permeability in mouse lung, liver, and kidney. The most important observation came when pregnant rats were injected with both sFlt-1 and sEng and subsequently develop a syndrome reminiscent of severe preeclampsia with hypertension, nephrotic range proteinuria, low platelet count, elevated liver enzymes, and reduced fetal weight [69]. Thus, it can be seen that most, if not all of the symptoms of the preeclampsia syndrome can be explained by the actions of these antiangiogenic molecules.

Epidemiological studies have revealed that sFlt-1 levels are elevated in preeclamptic women beginning at least 5 weeks before the onset of the syndrome and remain elevated when compared with unaffected women [70–72]. In fact, levels of sFlt-1 correlate with the severity of the syndrome [72]. Low levels of PlGF in the first trimester are a risk for subsequent preeclampsia, and levels of PlGF in the urine of women prior to 25 weeks gestation are lower in women with preeclampsia than in those with normotensive pregnancies [72]. The degree of suppression correlates with the severity of the syndrome [73]. However, the ratio of sFlt-1 to PlGF has proven to be a better marker of preeclampsia than either alone, implying that it is the balance of the angiogenic and antiangiogenic factors or not their absolute levels that leads to preeclampsia [72, 74, 75]. In support of this, it has most recently been reported that a serum ratio of sFlt-1 to PlGF less than 38 could be used to predict the absence of preeclampsia in women with suspected preeclampsia after 24 weeks gestation [76]. Levels of sEng are also elevated in the serum of women who develop preeclampsia when compared with women who do not [77]. Recent work has also associated alterations in sFlt-1, PlGF, and sEng concentrations with maternal vascular dysfunction and impaired nitric oxide formation [78]. From all this evidence, it can easily be seen how these three molecules are possible causative agents of the syndrome of preeclampsia.

Immune Factors

Loss of maternal immune tolerance to paternally derived placental and fetal antigens is another possible pathway to the development of the preeclampsia syndrome [79]. This loss of immune tolerance for fetal antigen can be observed during pathologic examination of preeclampatic placentas which reveals increased dendritic cell and macrophage infiltration and signs of inflammation similar to acute graft rejection [80–82].

Clinical Manifestations

The cardinal features of the preeclamptic syndrome are elevated blood pressure, proteinuria, and edema. As the syndrome becomes more severe neurologic abnormalities, coagulopathy, liver dysfunction, and eclampsia, heralded by the onset of seizures, occur.

In a normal pregnancy, peripheral vascular resistance and blood pressure typically decrease, but in preeclampsia the opposite occurs. This increase in peripheral vascular resistance is likely accomplished by an increase in sympathetic activation [83], increased concentrations of circulating catecholamine [84], and an exaggerated response to angiotensin II and other hypertensive stimuli when compared to normotensive pregnant controls [41]. Also contributing to elevated blood pressure is an increased effective circulating volume which would effectively result in a rise in blood pressure resulting in the observed suppressed levels of rennin and aldosterone in preeclamptic patients [85]. Generalized vascular constriction is also evident when compared with normal controls, which is likely due to dysfunction of the maternal endothelium caused by the circulating antiangiogenic factors discussed earlier as evinced by alterations in levels of markers of endothelial activation [86].

Proteinuria in preeclampsia results due to a loss of both size and charge selectivity of the glomerular barrier, and either accompanies or follows the development of hypertension [87]. The glomerular lesion characteristic of preeclampsia is called "glomerular capillary endotheliosis." Light microscopy of renal biopsies of preeclamptic patients reveals enlarged glomeruli and the glomerular capillary lumen appears to be bloodless due to endothelial and mesangial swelling and hypertrophy, and the glomerular podocytes are swollen and contain periodic acid-Schiff positive hyaline droplets. On electron microscopy, endothelial cells demonstrate a loss of fenestrations with cytoplasmic swelling owing to fluid and lipid accumulation and capillary occlusion [88]. This loss of fenestrations points to the decreased action of VEGF as an important part of the pathophysiology underlying preeclampsia as one of its important roles in homeostasis is to maintain fenestrated endothelium.

Preeclampsia is also complicated by neurologic symptoms that range from headache, blurred vision, temporary loss of vision, and seizures (eclampsia). These neurologic symptoms have been attributed to cerebral edema and vasoconstriction likely due to disruption of the blood brain barrier due to do endothelial damage [89]. As mentioned earlier, one of the specific cell types the VEGF is involved in maintaining are the ependymal cells of the CNS, the foot processes of which form the blood brain barrier.

Implications for Future Vascular Disease

The signs and symptoms of preeclampsia resolve in the several weeks following removal of the placenta, however women who develop the syndrome are affected by it for the rest of their lives.

Women with preeclampsia have been shown to have a future risk of hypertension that is three to four times higher than that of their non-preeclamptic counterparts [90–96]. This risk of future hypertension is dose dependent and increases with severity of the preeclampsia [92] and also with early onset of preeclampsia [97]. Studies have also shown that women diagnosed with a hypertensive complication of pregnancy have a twofold increased risk of future ischemic heart disease as well as stroke [90, 92, 96, 98–103]. It is not just the risk of cardiovascular disease that is increased, but the risk of death from a cardiovascular event is increased as well [98]. The dose-dependent relationship is again seen, as one study associated a twofold increased risk of CVD with mild preeclampsia but a fivefold increase in risk in severe disease [104]. These women are also at a fivefold increased risk of development of chronic kidney disease and progression to end stage renal disease, which increases with each subsequent pregnancy complicated by preeclampsia [105]. There has also been an association between preeclampsia and the future development of diabetes mellitus to the tune of a threefold increase in risk [92]. Preeclampsia has also been associated with the development of unfavorable lipid profiles [106], hypothyroidism [107], depression [108], and venous thromboembolic disease [90].

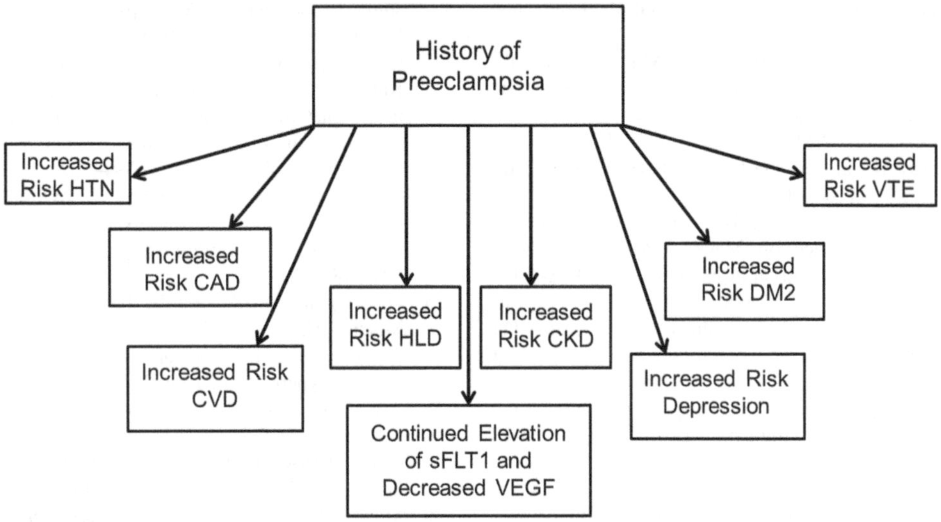

Fig. 37.2 Patients with a history of preeclampsia remain at increased risk of many diseases after the syndrome has resolved (*HTN* hypertension, *CAD* coronary artery disease, *CVD* cerebrovascular disease, *HLD* hyperlipidemia, *sFlt-1* soluble FMs-like tyrosine kinase 1, *VEGF* vascular endothelial growth factor, *CKD* chronic kidney disease, *DM2* type 2 diabetes mellitus, *VTE* venous thromboembolism)

The exact reason why these women are at such an increased risk of future disease has not yet been described. However, theories abound that again return to the antiangiogenic milieu that exists in preeclampsia and the potential for permanent vascular damage from inflammatory stress, coagulation dysregulation, and endothelial damage secondary to the preeclamptic episode. Studies have shown that preeclampsia induces long-term changes in the proteome of animal models associated with cardiovascular disease [109]. Although the levels of sFlt-1 have been shown to decrease after delivery of the placenta, studies have shown that levels remain higher in women who have suffered from preeclampsia as compared to those who have not [110]. These elevated levels of sFlt-1 have been shown to be correlated with exacerbations of congestive heart failure [111] and also with hospitalization for the same [112]. This persistent milieu of endothelial dysfunction increases risk for cardiovascular, metabolic and renal disease when taking into account the fact that lower levels of VEGF have been implicated in heart failure [113], ischemic heart disease in diabetic and insulin resistant patients [114], and several forms of kidney disease (Fig. 37.2) [115].

Conclusion

Preeclampsia is a two-stage disease that begins with abnormal placentation and ends with maternal endothelial dysfunction which leads to the classic symptoms of hypertension, edema, and proteinuria, as well as to the symptoms of more severe disease such as renal failure, HELLP syndrome, neurologic symptoms, and the seizures of eclampsia. While parts of its pathophysiology remain unclear, the role of a soluble antiangiogenic molecule, sFlt-1, and its effects on levels of angiogenic molecules such as VEGF and PlGF is paramount to the development of the maternal syndrome. Most important though is that once a woman is diagnosed with preeclampsia she becomes a patient who is at high risk for the development of a host of cardiorenal disease including hypertension, CAD, and CKD that is likely to progress to ESRD. Despite the overwhelming evidence of these increased risks, no studies have been done or guidelines developed about how to treat these patients to effectively reduce their risk of future morbidity and mortality. In fact, a previous diagnosis of preeclampsia, let alone an obstetric history is not part of any cardiovascular disease risk score These women should be treated as 'high-risk' for CVD with aggressive risk reduction, and that internists, cardiologists, and nephrologists should be aware of preeclampsia and the impact they have on the cardiovascular risk profile of their patients.

References

1. Abalos E, Cuesta C, Grosso AL, Chou D, Say L. Global and regional estimates of preeclampsia and eclampsia: a systematic review. Eur J Obstet Gynecol Reprod Biol. 2013;170(1):1–7.
2. American College of O, Gynecologists, Task Force on Hypertension in P. Hypertension in pregnancy. Report of the American College of Obstetricians and Gynecologists' Task Force on hypertension in pregnancy. Obstet Gynecol. 2013;122(5): 1122–31.
3. Caritis S, Sibai B, Hauth J, Lindheimer MD, Klebanoff M, Thom E, et al. Low-dose aspirin to prevent preeclampsia in women at high risk. National Institute of Child Health and

Human Development Network of Maternal-Fetal Medicine Units. N Engl J Med. 1998;338(11):701–5.
4. Khan KS, Wojdyla D, Say L, Gulmezoglu AM, Van Look PF. WHO analysis of causes of maternal death: a systematic review. Lancet. 2006;367(9516):1066–74.
5. Berg CJ, Callaghan WM, Syverson C, Henderson Z. Pregnancy-related mortality in the United States, 1998 to 2005. Obstet Gynecol. 2010;116(6):1302–9.
6. Saucedo M, Deneux-Tharaux C, Bouvier-Colle MH, French National Experts Committee on Maternal M. Ten years of confidential inquiries into maternal deaths in France, 1998–2007. Obstet Gynecol. 2013;122(4):752–60.
7. Karumanchi SA, Maynard SE, Stillman IE, Epstein FH, Sukhatme VP. Preeclampsia: a renal perspective. Kidney Int. 2005;67(6):2101–13.
8. Trupin LS, Simon LP, Eskenazi B. Change in paternity: a risk factor for preeclampsia in multiparas. Epidemiology. 1996;7 (3):240–4.
9. Robillard PY, Hulsey TC, Alexander GR, Keenan A, de Caunes F, Papiernik E. Paternity patterns and risk of preeclampsia in the last pregnancy in multiparae. J Reprod Immunol. 1993;24(1):1–12.
10. Lachmeijer AM, Dekker GA, Pals G, Aarnoudse JG, ten Kate LP, Arngrimsson R. Searching for preeclampsia genes: the current position. Eur J Obstet Gynecol Reprod Biol. 2002;105(2): 94–113.
11. Chesley LC. History and epidemiology of preeclampsia-eclampsia. Clin Obstet Gynecol. 1984;27(4):801–20.
12. Myatt L, Clifton RG, Roberts JM, Spong CY, Hauth JC, Varner MW, et al. First-trimester prediction of preeclampsia in nulliparous women at low risk. Obstet Gynecol. 2012;119 (6):1234–42.
13. Lawlor DA, Morton SM, Nitsch D, Leon DA. Association between childhood and adulthood socioeconomic position and pregnancy induced hypertension: results from the Aberdeen children of the 1950s cohort study. J Epidemiol Community Health. 2005;59(1):49–55.
14. Palmer SK, Moore LG, Young D, Cregger B, Berman JC, Zamudio S. Altered blood pressure course during normal pregnancy and increased preeclampsia at high altitude (3100 meters) in Colorado. Am J Obstet Gynecol. 1999;180(5):1161–8.
15. Bainbridge SA, Sidle EH, Smith GN. Direct placental effects of cigarette smoke protect women from pre-eclampsia: the specific roles of carbon monoxide and antioxidant systems in the placenta. Med Hypotheses. 2005;64(1):17–27.
16. Arngrimsson R, Hayward C, Nadaud S, Baldursdottir A, Walker JJ, Liston WA, et al. Evidence for a familial pregnancy-induced hypertension locus in the eNOS-gene region. Am J Hum Genet. 1997;61(2):354–62.
17. Dizon-Townson DS, Nelson LM, Easton K, Ward K. The factor V Leiden mutation may predispose women to severe preeclampsia. Am J Obstet Gynecol. 1996;175(4 Pt 1):902–5.
18. Sohda S, Arinami T, Hamada H, Yamada N, Hamaguchi H, Kubo T. Methylenetetrahydrofolate reductase polymorphism and pre-eclampsia. J Med Genet. 1997;34(6):525–6.
19. Ward K, Hata A, Jeunemaitre X, Helin C, Nelson L, Namikawa C, et al. A molecular variant of angiotensinogen associated with preeclampsia. Nat Genet. 1993;4(1):59–61.
20. Arngrimsson R, Geirsson RT, Cooke A, Connor M, Bjornsson S, Walker JJ. Renin gene restriction fragment length polymorphisms do not show linkage with preeclampsia and eclampsia. Acta Obstet Gynecol Scand. 1994;73(1):10–3.
21. Guo G, Wilton AN, Fu Y, Qiu H, Brennecke SP, Cooper DW. Angiotensinogen gene variation in a population case-control study of preeclampsia/eclampsia in Australians and Chinese. Electrophoresis. 1997;18(9):1646–9.
22. Lachmeijer AM, Arngrimsson R, Bastiaans EJ, Pals G, ten Kate LP, de Vries JI, et al. Mutations in the gene for methylenetetrahydrofolate reductase, homocysteine levels, and vitamin status in women with a history of preeclampsia. Am J Obstet Gynecol. 2001;184(3):394–402.
23. Lade JA, Moses EK, Guo G, Wilton AN, Grehan M, Cooper DW, et al. The eNOS gene: a candidate for the preeclampsia susceptibility locus? Hypertens Pregnancy. 1999;18(1):81–93.
24. O'Shaughnessy KM, Fu B, Ferraro F, Lewis I, Downing S, Morris NH. Factor V Leiden and thermolabile methylenetetrahydrofolate reductase gene variants in an East Anglian preeclampsia cohort. Hypertension. 1999;33(6):1338–41.
25. Arngrimsson R, Siguroardottir S, Frigge ML, Bjarnadottir RI, Jonsson T, Stefansson H, et al. A genome-wide scan reveals a maternal susceptibility locus for pre-eclampsia on chromosome 2p13. Hum Mol Genet. 1999;8(9):1799–805.
26. Moses EK, Lade JA, Guo G, Wilton AN, Grehan M, Freed K, et al. A genome scan in families from Australia and New Zealand confirms the presence of a maternal susceptibility locus for pre-eclampsia, on chromosome 2. Am J Hum Genet. 2000;67 (6):1581–5.
27. Tuohy JF, James DK. Pre-eclampsia and trisomy 13. Br J Obstet Gynaecol. 1992;99(11):891–4.
28. Salafia CM, Pezzullo JC, Lopez-Zeno JA, Simmens S, Minior VK, Vintzileos AM. Placental pathologic features of preterm preeclampsia. Am J Obstet Gynecol. 1995;173(4):1097–105.
29. Brosens IA, Robertson WB, Dixon HG. The role of the spiral arteries in the pathogenesis of preeclampsia. Obstet Gynecol Annu. 1972;1:177–91.
30. Fisher SJ. Why is placentation abnormal in preeclampsia? Am J Obstet Gynecol. 2015;213(4 Suppl):S115–22.
31. Librach CL, Werb Z, Fitzgerald ML, Chiu K, Corwin NM, Esteves RA, et al. 92-kD type IV collagenase mediates invasion of human cytotrophoblasts. J Cell Biol. 1991;113(2):437–49.
32. Wewer UM, Faber M, Liotta LA, Albrechtsen R. Immunochemical and ultrastructural assessment of the nature of the pericellular basement membrane of human decidual cells. Lab Invest. 1985;53(6):624–33.
33. Zhou Y, Genbacev O, Fisher SJ. The human placenta remodels the uterus by using a combination of molecules that govern vasculogenesis or leukocyte extravasation. Ann N Y Acad Sci. 2003;995:73–83.
34. Zhou Y, Damsky CH, Chiu K, Roberts JM, Fisher SJ. Preeclampsia is associated with abnormal expression of adhesion molecules by invasive cytotrophoblasts. J Clin Invest. 1993;91(3):950–60.
35. Zhou Y, Damsky CH, Fisher SJ. Preeclampsia is associated with failure of human cytotrophoblasts to mimic a vascular adhesion phenotype. One cause of defective endovascular invasion in this syndrome? J Clin Invest. 1997;99(9):2152–64.
36. Zhou Y, Fisher SJ, Janatpour M, Genbacev O, Dejana E, Wheelock M, et al. Human cytotrophoblasts adopt a vascular phenotype as they differentiate. A strategy for successful endovascular invasion? J Clin Invest. 1997;99(9):2139–51.
37. Genbacev O, Joslin R, Damsky CH, Polliotti BM, Fisher SJ. Hypoxia alters early gestation human cytotrophoblast differentiation/invasion in vitro and models the placental defects that occur in preeclampsia. J Clin Invest. 1996;97(2):540–50.
38. McMahon K, Karumanchi SA, Stillman IE, Cummings P, Patton D, Easterling T. Does soluble fms-like tyrosine kinase-1 regulate placental invasion? Insight from the invasive placenta. Am J Obstet Gynecol. 2014;210(1):68e1–4.

39. Lee SM, Romero R, Lee YJ, Park IS, Park CW, Yoon BH. Systemic inflammatory stimulation by microparticles derived from hypoxic trophoblast as a model for inflammatory response in preeclampsia. Am J Obstet Gynecol. 2012;207(4):337e1–8.
40. Redman CW, Tannetta DS, Dragovic RA, Gardiner C, Southcombe JH, Collett GP, et al. Review: Does size matter? Placental debris and the pathophysiology of pre-eclampsia. Placenta. 2012;33(Suppl):S48–54.
41. Karumanchi SARS, Taylor RN. Angiogensis and preeclampsia. In: Taylor RNRJ, Cunningham FG, editors. Chesley's hypertensive disorders of pregnancy. 4th ed. Amsterdam: Academic Press; 2014.
42. Keck PJ, Hauser SD, Krivi G, Sanzo K, Warren T, Feder J, et al. Vascular permeability factor, an endothelial cell mitogen related to PDGF. Science. 1989;246(4935):1309–12.
43. Leung DW, Cachianes G, Kuang WJ, Goeddel DV, Ferrara N. Vascular endothelial growth factor is a secreted angiogenic mitogen. Science. 1989;246(4935):1306–9.
44. Maglione D, Guerriero V, Viglietto G, Delli-Bovi P, Persico MG. Isolation of a human placenta cDNA coding for a protein related to the vascular permeability factor. Proc Natl Acad Sci USA. 1991;88(20):9267–71.
45. Park JE, Chen HH, Winer J, Houck KA, Ferrara N. Placenta growth factor. Potentiation of vascular endothelial growth factor bioactivity, in vitro and in vivo, and high affinity binding to Flt-1 but not to Flk-1/KDR. J Biol Chem. 1994;269(41):25646–54.
46. Shalaby F, Rossant J, Yamaguchi TP, Gertsenstein M, Wu XF, Breitman ML, et al. Failure of blood-island formation and vasculogenesis in Flk-1-deficient mice. Nature. 1995;376(6535):62–6.
47. Powe CE, Levine RJ, Karumanchi SA. Preeclampsia, a disease of the maternal endothelium: the role of antiangiogenic factors and implications for later cardiovascular disease. Circulation. 2011;123(24):2856–69.
48. Chappell JC, Taylor SM, Ferrara N, Bautch VL. Local guidance of emerging vessel sprouts requires soluble Flt-1. Dev Cell. 2009;17(3):377–86.
49. Maharaj AS, Saint-Geniez M, Maldonado AE, D'Amore PA. Vascular endothelial growth factor localization in the adult. Am J Pathol. 2006;168(2):639–48.
50. Eremina V, Sood M, Haigh J, Nagy A, Lajoie G, Ferrara N, et al. Glomerular-specific alterations of VEGF-A expression lead to distinct congenital and acquired renal diseases. J Clin Invest. 2003;111(5):707–16.
51. Glusker P, Recht L, Lane B. Reversible posterior leukoencephalopathy syndrome and bevacizumab. N Engl J Med. 2006;354(9):980–2 (discussion –2).
52. Kabbinavar F, Hurwitz HI, Fehrenbacher L, Meropol NJ, Novotny WF, Lieberman G, et al. Phase II, randomized trial comparing bevacizumab plus fluorouracil (FU)/leucovorin (LV) with FU/LV alone in patients with metastatic colorectal cancer. J Clin Oncol. 2003;21(1):60–5.
53. Kuenen BC, Levi M, Meijers JC, Kakkar AK, van Hinsbergh VW, Kostense PJ, et al. Analysis of coagulation cascade and endothelial cell activation during inhibition of vascular endothelial growth factor/vascular endothelial growth factor receptor pathway in cancer patients. Arterioscler Thromb Vasc Biol. 2002;22(9):1500–5.
54. Yang JC, Haworth L, Sherry RM, Hwu P, Schwartzentruber DJ, Topalian SL, et al. A randomized trial of bevacizumab, an anti-vascular endothelial growth factor antibody, for metastatic renal cancer. N Engl J Med. 2003;349(5):427–34.
55. Roberts JM, Taylor RN, Musci TJ, Rodgers GM, Hubel CA, McLaughlin MK. Preeclampsia: an endothelial cell disorder. Am J Obstet Gynecol. 1989;161(5):1200–4.
56. Rodgers GM, Taylor RN, Roberts JM. Preeclampsia is associated with a serum factor cytotoxic to human endothelial cells. Am J Obstet Gynecol. 1988;159(4):908–14.
57. Nova A, Sibai BM, Barton JR, Mercer BM, Mitchell MD. Maternal plasma level of endothelin is increased in preeclampsia. Am J Obstet Gynecol. 1991;165(3):724–7.
58. Deng L, Bremme K, Hansson LO, Blomback M. Plasma levels of von Willebrand factor and fibronectin as markers of persisting endothelial damage in preeclampsia. Obstet Gynecol. 1994;84(6):941–5.
59. Stubbs TM, Lazarchick J, Horger EO III. Plasma fibronectin levels in preeclampsia: a possible biochemical marker for vascular endothelial damage. Am J Obstet Gynecol. 1984;150(7):885–7.
60. Taylor RN, Crombleholme WR, Friedman SA, Jones LA, Casal DC, Roberts JM. High plasma cellular fibronectin levels correlate with biochemical and clinical features of preeclampsia but cannot be attributed to hypertension alone. Am J Obstet Gynecol. 1991;165(4 Pt 1):895–901.
61. Thorp JM Jr, White GC II, Moake JL, Bowes WA Jr. von Willebrand factor multimeric levels and patterns in patients with severe preeclampsia. Obstet Gynecol. 1990;75(2):163–7.
62. Hsu CD, Iriye B, Johnson TR, Witter FR, Hong SF, Chan DW. Elevated circulating thrombomodulin in severe preeclampsia. Am J Obstet Gynecol. 1993;169(1):148–9.
63. Minakami H, Takahashi T, Izumi A, Tamada T. Increased levels of plasma thrombomodulin in preeclampsia. Gynecol Obstet Invest. 1993;36(4):208–10.
64. Musci TJ, Roberts JM, Rodgers GM, Taylor RN. Mitogenic activity is increased in the sera of preeclamptic women before delivery. Am J Obstet Gynecol. 1988;159(6):1446–51.
65. Cackovic M, Buhimschi CS, Zhao G, Funai EF, Norwitz ER, Kuczynski E, et al. Fractional excretion of tumor necrosis factor-alpha in women with severe preeclampsia. Obstet Gynecol. 2008;112(1):93–100.
66. Myers J, Mires G, Macleod M, Baker P. In preeclampsia, the circulating factors capable of altering in vitro endothelial function precede clinical disease. Hypertension. 2005;45(2):258–63.
67. Maynard SE, Min JY, Merchan J, Lim KH, Li J, Mondal S, et al. Excess placental soluble fms-like tyrosine kinase 1 (sFlt1) may contribute to endothelial dysfunction, hypertension, and proteinuria in preeclampsia. J Clin Invest. 2003;111(5):649–58.
68. Kendall RL, Thomas KA. Inhibition of vascular endothelial cell growth factor activity by an endogenously encoded soluble receptor. Proc Natl Acad Sci USA. 1993;90(22):10705–9.
69. Venkatesha S, Toporsian M, Lam C, Hanai J, Mammoto T, Kim YM, et al. Soluble endoglin contributes to the pathogenesis of preeclampsia. Nat Med. 2006;12(6):642–9.
70. Chaiworapongsa T, Romero R, Espinoza J, Bujold E, Mee Kim Y, Goncalves LF, et al. Evidence supporting a role for blockade of the vascular endothelial growth factor system in the pathophysiology of preeclampsia. Young Investigator Award. Am J Obstet Gynecol. 2004;190(6):1541–7 (discussion 7–50).
71. Hertig A, Berkane N, Lefevre G, Toumi K, Marti HP, Capeau J, et al. Maternal serum sFlt1 concentration is an early and reliable predictive marker of preeclampsia. Clin Chem. 2004;50(9):1702–3.
72. Levine RJ, Maynard SE, Qian C, Lim KH, England LJ, Yu KF, et al. Circulating angiogenic factors and the risk of preeclampsia. N Engl J Med. 2004;350(7):672–83.
73. Levine RJ, Thadhani R, Qian C, Lam C, Lim KH, Yu KF, et al. Urinary placental growth factor and risk of preeclampsia. JAMA. 2005;293(1):77–85.
74. Buhimschi CS, Norwitz ER, Funai E, Richman S, Guller S, Lockwood CJ, et al. Urinary angiogenic factors cluster

hypertensive disorders and identify women with severe preeclampsia. Am J Obstet Gynecol. 2005;192(3):734–41.
75. Verlohren S, Galindo A, Schlembach D, Zeisler H, Herraiz I, Moertl MG, et al. An automated method for the determination of the sFlt-1/PIGF ratio in the assessment of preeclampsia. Am J Obstet Gynecol. 2010;202(2):161 e1–e11.
76. Zeisler H, Llurba E, Chantraine F, Vatish M, Staff AC, Sennstrom M, et al. Predictive value of the sFlt-1:PlGF Ratio in women with suspected preeclampsia. N Engl J Med. 2016;374 (1):13–22.
77. Levine RJ, Lam C, Qian C, Yu KF, Maynard SE, Sachs BP, et al. Soluble endoglin and other circulating antiangiogenic factors in preeclampsia. N Engl J Med. 2006;355(10):992–1005.
78. Sandrim VC, Palei AC, Metzger IF, Gomes VA, Cavalli RC, Tanus-Santos JE. Nitric oxide formation is inversely related to serum levels of antiangiogenic factors soluble fms-like tyrosine kinase-1 and soluble endogline in preeclampsia. Hypertension. 2008;52(2):402–7.
79. Erlebacher A. Mechanisms of T cell tolerance towards the allogeneic fetus. Nat Rev Immunol. 2013;13(1):23–33.
80. Hiby SE, Walker JJ, O'Shaughnessy KM, Redman CW, Carrington M, Trowsdale J, et al. Combinations of maternal KIR and fetal HLA-C genes influence the risk of preeclampsia and reproductive success. J Exp Med. 2004;200(8):957–65.
81. Huang SJ, Chen CP, Schatz F, Rahman M, Abrahams VM, Lockwood CJ. Pre-eclampsia is associated with dendritic cell recruitment into the uterine decidua. J Pathol. 2008;214(3): 328–36.
82. Lockwood CJ, Matta P, Krikun G, Koopman LA, Masch R, Toti P, et al. Regulation of monocyte chemoattractant protein-1 expression by tumor necrosis factor-alpha and interleukin-1beta in first trimester human decidual cells: implications for preeclampsia. Am J Pathol. 2006;168(2):445–52.
83. Schobel HP, Fischer T, Heuszer K, Geiger H, Schmieder RE. Preeclampsia—a state of sympathetic overactivity. N Engl J Med. 1996;335(20):1480–5.
84. Manyonda IT, Slater DM, Fenske C, Hole D, Choy MY, Wilson C. A role for noradrenaline in pre-eclampsia: towards a unifying hypothesis for the pathophysiology. Br J Obstet Gynaecol. 1998;105(6):641–8.
85. Tapia HR, Johnson CE, Strong CG. Renin-angiotensin system in normal and in hypertensive disease of pregnancy. Lancet. 1972;2 (7782):847–50.
86. Agatisa PK, Ness RB, Roberts JM, Costantino JP, Kuller LH, McLaughlin MK. Impairment of endothelial function in women with a history of preeclampsia: an indicator of cardiovascular risk. Am J Physiol Heart Circ Physiol. 2004;286(4):H1389–93.
87. Moran P, Baylis PH, Lindheimer MD, Davison JM. Glomerular ultrafiltration in normal and preeclamptic pregnancy. J Am Soc Nephrol. 2003;14(3):648–52.
88. Stillman IE, Karumanchi SA. The glomerular injury of preeclampsia. J Am Soc Nephrol. 2007;18(8):2281–4.
89. Schwartz RB, Feske SK, Polak JF, DeGirolami U, Iaia A, Beckner KM, et al. Preeclampsia-eclampsia: clinical and neuroradiographic correlates and insights into the pathogenesis of hypertensive encephalopathy. Radiology. 2000;217(2):371–6.
90. Bellamy L, Casas JP, Hingorani AD, Williams DJ. Pre-eclampsia and risk of cardiovascular disease and cancer in later life: systematic review and meta-analysis. BMJ. 2007;335(7627):974.
91. Hannaford P, Ferry S, Hirsch S. Cardiovascular sequelae of toxaemia of pregnancy. Heart. 1997;77(2):154–8.
92. Lykke JA, Langhoff-Roos J, Sibai BM, Funai EF, Triche EW, Paidas MJ. Hypertensive pregnancy disorders and subsequent cardiovascular morbidity and type 2 diabetes mellitus in the mother. Hypertension. 2009;53(6):944–51.
93. Magnussen EB, Vatten LJ, Smith GD, Romundstad PR. Hypertensive disorders in pregnancy and subsequently measured cardiovascular risk factors. Obstet Gynecol. 2009;114(5):961–70.
94. Marin R, Gorostidi M, Portal CG, Sanchez M, Sanchez E, Alvarez J. Long-term prognosis of hypertension in pregnancy. Hypertens Pregnancy. 2000;19(2):199–209.
95. Wang IK, Muo CH, Chang YC, Liang CC, Chang CT, Lin SY, et al. Association between hypertensive disorders during pregnancy and end-stage renal disease: a population-based study. CMAJ. 2013;185(3):207–13.
96. Wilson BJ, Watson MS, Prescott GJ, Sunderland S, Campbell DM, Hannaford P, et al. Hypertensive diseases of pregnancy and risk of hypertension and stroke in later life: results from cohort study. BMJ. 2003;326(7394):845.
97. Lazdam M, de la Horra A, Diesch J, Kenworthy Y, Davis E, Lewandowski AJ, et al. Unique blood pressure characteristics in mother and offspring after early onset preeclampsia. Hypertension. 2012;60(5):1338–45.
98. Irgens HU, Reisaeter L, Irgens LM, Lie RT. Long term mortality of mothers and fathers after pre-eclampsia: population based cohort study. BMJ. 2001;323(7323):1213–7.
99. Kestenbaum B, Seliger SL, Easterling TR, Gillen DL, Critchlow CW, Stehman-Breen CO, et al. Cardiovascular and thromboembolic events following hypertensive pregnancy. Am J Kidney Dis. 2003;42(5):982–9.
100. Lin YS, Tang CH, Yang CY, Wu LS, Hung ST, Hwa HL, et al. Effect of pre-eclampsia-eclampsia on major cardiovascular events among peripartum women in Taiwan. Am J Cardiol. 2011;107 (2):325–30.
101. Mongraw-Chaffin ML, Cirillo PM, Cohn BA. Preeclampsia and cardiovascular disease death: prospective evidence from the child health and development studies cohort. Hypertension. 2010;56 (1):166–71.
102. Pell JP, Smith GC, Walsh D. Pregnancy complications and subsequent maternal cerebrovascular events: a retrospective cohort study of 119,668 births. Am J Epidemiol. 2004;159 (4):336–42.
103. Smith GC, Pell JP, Walsh D. Pregnancy complications and maternal risk of ischaemic heart disease: a retrospective cohort study of 129,290 births. Lancet. 2001;357(9273):2002–6.
104. McDonald SD, Malinowski A, Zhou Q, Yusuf S, Devereaux PJ. Cardiovascular sequelae of preeclampsia/eclampsia: a systematic review and meta-analyses. Am Heart J. 2008;156 (5):918–30.
105. Vikse BE, Irgens LM, Leivestad T, Skjaerven R, Iversen BM. Preeclampsia and the risk of end-stage renal disease. N Engl J Med. 2008;359(8):800–9.
106. Hubel CA, Snaedal S, Ness RB, Weissfeld LA, Geirsson RT, Roberts JM, et al. Dyslipoproteinaemia in postmenopausal women with a history of eclampsia. BJOG. 2000;107(6): 776–84.
107. Levine RJ, Vatten LJ, Horowitz GL, Qian C, Romundstad PR, Yu KF, et al. Pre-eclampsia, soluble fms-like tyrosine kinase 1, and the risk of reduced thyroid function: nested case–control and population based study. BMJ. 2009;339:b4336.
108. Delahaije DH, Dirksen CD, Peeters LL, Smits LJ. Anxiety and depression following preeclampsia or hemolysis, elevated liver enzymes, and low platelets syndrome. A systematic review. Acta Obstet Gynecol Scand. 2013;92(7):746–61.
109. Bytautiene E, Bulayeva N, Bhat G, Li L, Rosenblatt KP, Saade GR. Long-term alterations in maternal plasma proteome after sFlt1-induced preeclampsia in mice. Am J Obstet Gynecol. 2013;208(5):388 e1–e10.
110. Wolf M, Hubel CA, Lam C, Sampson M, Ecker JL, Ness RB, et al. Preeclampsia and future cardiovascular disease: potential

role of altered angiogenesis and insulin resistance. J Clin Endocrinol Metab. 2004;89(12):6239–43.
111. Seno ATY, Matsui M, Nakada Y, Ueda T, Okuda A, Jonckx B, Nakagawa H, Onoue K, Watanabe M, Kawata H. Soluble Flt-1 deficiency plays a significant role in the exacerbation of cardiac hypertrophy and heart failure. Circulation. 2014;130(Suppl 2): A17078.
112. Vorovich E, French B, Ky B, Goldberg L, Fang JC, Sweitzer NK, et al. Biomarker predictors of cardiac hospitalization in chronic heart failure: a recurrent event analysis. J Card Fail. 2014;20 (8):569–76.
113. Taimeh Z, Loughran J, Birks EJ, Bolli R. Vascular endothelial growth factor in heart failure. Nat Rev Cardiol. 2013;10(9):519–30.
114. Chou E, Suzuma I, Way KJ, Opland D, Clermont AC, Naruse K, et al. Decreased cardiac expression of vascular endothelial growth factor and its receptors in insulin-resistant and diabetic States: a possible explanation for impaired collateral formation in cardiac tissue. Circulation. 2002;105(3):373–9.
115. Schrijvers BF, Flyvbjerg A, De Vriese AS. The role of vascular endothelial growth factor (VEGF) in renal pathophysiology. Kidney Int. 2004;65(6):2003–17.

Obstructive Sleep Apnea: A Unifying Link Between Cardiovascular and Renal Disease

38

Parasuram Melarcode Krishnamoorthy, Virend K. Somers, and Abel Romero-Corral

Introduction

Obstructive sleep apnea (OSA) is an important and common comorbidity, especially in patients with obesity. It is characterized by transient, repetitive partial (hypopnea) or complete (apnea) upper airway obstruction during sleep causing $\geq$ 10 s pause in respiration [1]. It is usually associated with sleep disturbance, snoring, daytime fatigue, and chronic intermittent hypoxia. Although it is estimated that one in five Americans may have OSA as defined by an apnea–hypopnea index score of ≥ 5 [2], approximately 80% of individuals have not been diagnosed [3], and common conditions such as age, male sex, and obesity are important risk factors for its development [4]. Screening for common risk factors for, and associations with OSA, has been recommended as a part of routine health examination as per the recent adult Obstructive Sleep Apnea Task Force of the American Academy of Sleep Medicine guidelines [5]. OSA may be an independent predictor of all-cause mortality [6], hypertension [7–9], coronary artery disease [10], heart failure [11, 12], and stroke [13]. In addition, patients with OSA are at increased risk of sudden death from cardiac causes during sleep [14], and also shown to be an independent predictor of sudden cardiac death in a cohort of 10,701 patients referred for their first polysomnogram [15]. Patients likely to have OSA usually also have risk factors in common with chronic cardiovascular and kidney diseases, such as obesity, hypertension and diabetes mellitus, suggestive of a possible link between these conditions [16].

P.M. Krishnamoorthy · A. Romero-Corral (✉)
Department of Cardiology, Einstein Medical Center, 5501 Old York Road, Philadelphia, PA 19141, USA
e-mail: romeroab@einstein.edu

P.M. Krishnamoorthy
e-mail: parasumk@yahoo.com

V.K. Somers
Department of Cardiovascular Diseases, Mayo Clinic, 200 First Street SW, Rochester, MN 55905, USA
e-mail: somers.virend@mayo.edu

J. Rangaswami et al. (eds.), *Cardio-Nephrology*,
DOI 10.1007/978-3-319-56042-7_38

Prevalence of OSA in CKD

OSA is an important clinical comorbidity with significant impact in patients with CKD [17]. The reported prevalence of OSA in this population has ranged from 27 to 54%, which is considerably higher than the general population [18]. Male gender was found to be the single strongest predictor of OSA in CKD. Although OSA is increasingly common in patients with CKD, it may not be clinically apparent. Patients may not have the typical constellation of symptoms, and hence will need low threshold for objective screening for OSA. Okubo et al. studied the cost effectiveness of OSA screening in all middle-aged male outpatients with CKD and diabetes. The authors recommended routine screening for OSA in middle-aged patients between the ages of 35–65 years with CKD. It was cost effective and may have also helped reduce primary and secondary CVD risk [19]. Sleep disordered breathing and daytime sleepiness have been well studied in patients with end stage kidney disease (ESKD) on dialysis [20, 21] and even in CKD patients with stable creatinine clearance and not on dialysis [22, 23]. Roumelioti et al. [20] studied 89 patients with CKD and 75 patients on hemodialysis (HD) comparing them to 224 controls. Sleep disordered breathing was more common in patients with advanced CKD both not on HD (OR 2.19, 95% confidence interval [CI] 1.22–3.92) and on HD (OR 4.14, 95% CI 2.26–7.60) compared to controls, and nocturnal hypoxemia was significantly elevated in patients on HD compared to controls and to CKD not on HD (OR 2.12, 95% CI 1.05–4.23, $p = 0.04$). In another study by Sakaguchi et al. [23] of 100 patients, multivariate regression showed that a 10-ml/min/1.73 m^2 decrease in eGFR was associated with a 42% increased odds of OSA even after adjusting for multiple confounding risk factors including age, gender, and BMI. Patients with an estimated GFR of less than 90 ml/min/1.73 m^2 were at an increased risk of developing OSA compared to patients with normal renal function with an odds ratio of 1.22 to 1.42 for each 15 ml/min decrease in the GFR [24]. In the next paragraphs we will attempt to describe the pathophysiology associated with these findings and a summary of these studies are listed in Table 38.1.

Pathophysiology of OSA in CKD

Different mechanisms have been proposed to explain the pathophysiological link between OSA and CKD [6, 17, 25] (Figs. 38.1 and 38.2). OSA is associated with sleep fragmentation and hypoxemia re-oxygenation episodes which activate central sympathetic outflow to the kidney and other vascular beds, resulting in elevations in blood pressure both transiently during airway obstruction, and chronically in the awake state, which has been linked to the progression of CKD [26, 27]. Multiple studies have shown direct relationships between apnea–hypopnea index (AHI) and hypertension [7, 28]. In a large community based study of 6132 healthy middle aged and older patients by Nieto et al. [7], high AHI scores or sleep time below 90% oxygen saturation were associated with greater odds of hypertension, even after adjusting for common confounding factors including age, gender, BMI, smoking, and alcohol use. Hass et al. [29] aimed to study the relation between AHI and hypertension phenotype (systolic/diastolic hypertension vs isolated systolic hypertension) in 6120 participants from the Sleep Heart Health Study. Interestingly, sleep disordered breathing was associated with systolic/diastolic hypertension only in patients younger than 60 years. Also, isolated systolic hypertension was not associated with sleep disordered breathing in any age group. Although the authors did not comment on kidney function or prevalence of chronic kidney disease in this patient population, there were two important conclusions from this study; (1) OSA is a significant cause for secondary hypertension in the young; and (2) It is important to identify type of hypertension, namely systolic/diastolic hypertension versus isolated systolic hypertension, when considering OSA as a contributing factor for hypertension.

Sympathetic activation also results in upregulation of the renin–angiotensin–aldosterone system (RAAS), altering cardiovascular hemodynamics, causing increased salt and water retention. Increased renin-angiotensin activity also results in endothelial dysfunction mediated by free radical oxidative stress and inflammation [30]. OSA patients also have elevated levels of aldosterone, which has been linked to fibrosis and accelerated progression of CKD. Animal models have shown that increased aldosterone may result in glomerular sclerosis [31], which can be reversed by

Table 38.1 Summary of studies involving CKD patients with OSA

Study name	Study group	Study *N*	Study type	Study aim	Findings
Nicholl et al. [18]	CKD with and without OSA vs OSA without CKD	119 (CKD) vs 230 (no CKD)	Case control study	Clinical presentation of OSA in patients with CKD	1. Male gender was strongest predictor of OSA in CKD 2. Prevalence of OSA in CKD was unlikely to be clinically apparent
Roumelioti et al. [20]	CKD not on HD, on HD and no CKD	85 (not on HD) vs 74 (HD) vs 224 (no CKD)	Case control study	Sleep disordered breathing and excessive day time sleepiness in patients with CKD	1. SDS and EDS are common among patients with CKD 2. Modest correlation of EDS with SDB in HD group
Unruh et al. [21]	HD vs no CKD	46 (HD) vs 137 (no CKD)	Case control study	SDB and sleep cycle in patients on HD vs controls	1. HD had a higher odds of SDB and more severe nocturnal hypoxemia 2. HD group demonstrated shorter sleep time and greater sleep fragmentation
Markou et al. [22]	CKD not on HD	35	Cohort study	SDB in non-dialyzed CKD patients	1. Prevalence of SDB and RLS is high in dialysis-independent CRF 2. SDB weakly correlates with indices of kidney function and this association becomes stronger in nondiabetics
Sakaguchi et al. [23]	CKD not on HD	100	Cohort study	Prevalence of OSA and association with renal function in CKD patients not on HD	1. Increased prevalence of OSA (65%) among patients with CKD not on HD in Japan 2. Decreased GFR was a significant predictor of OSA. 10-ml/min per 1.73 m^2 BSA decrease in eGFR was associated with a 42% increased odds of OSA
Sim et al. [24]	Early stages of CKD	1,102,089	Cross sectional study	Prevalence of OSA in early stages of CKD	1. Increased risk of OSA in patients with early CKD

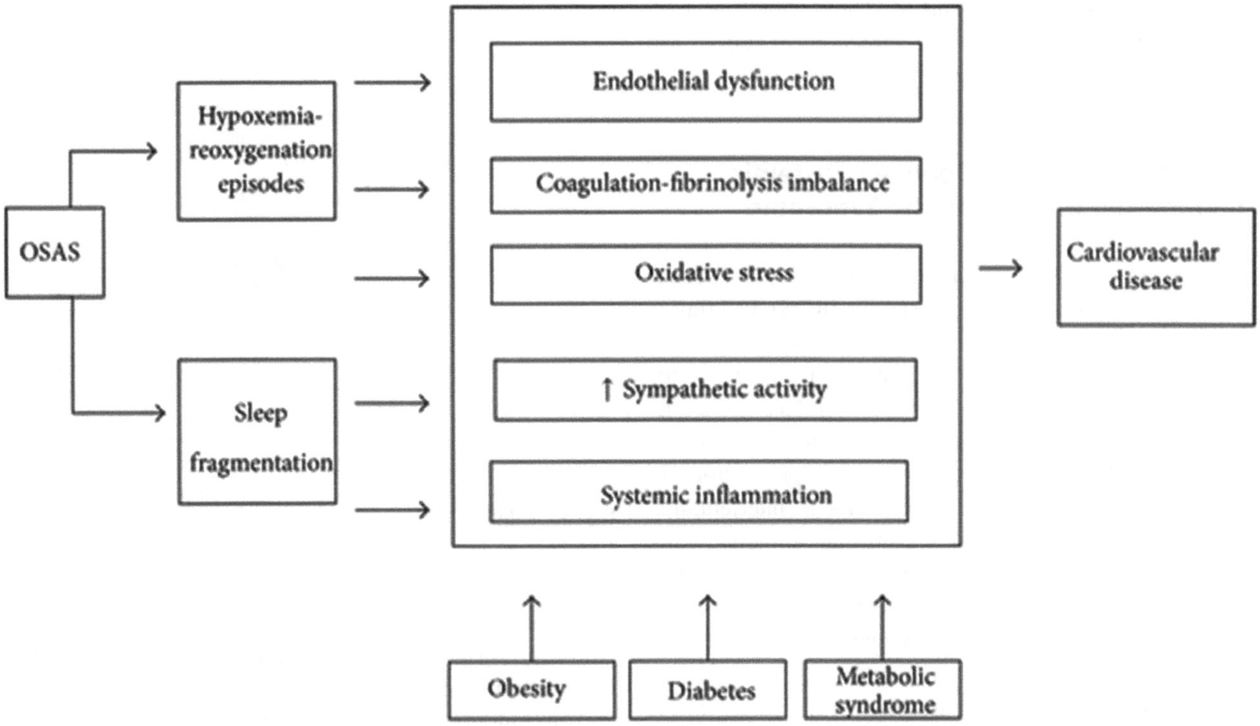

Fig. 38.1 A schematic summary of the proposed sequence of events in obstructive sleep apnea syndrome starting from episodic hypoxia and sleep fragmentation. Adapted from Zamarrón et al. [25]

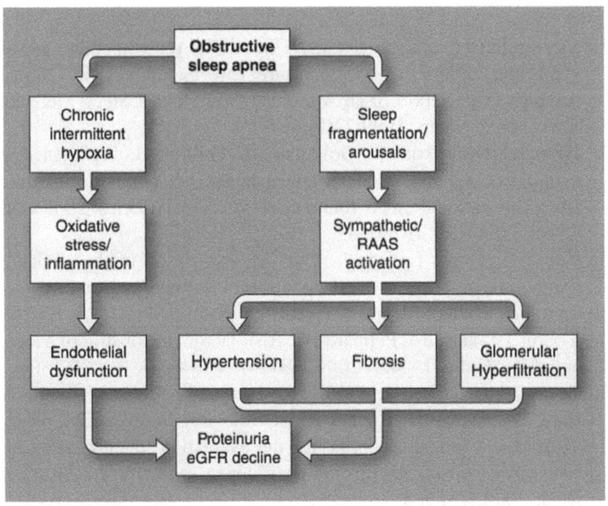

Fig. 38.2 Pathophysiologic links between obstructive sleep apnea (OSA) and chronic kidney disease (CKD). Adapted from Adeseun and Rosas [17]

aldosterone blockade [32]. OSA has also been linked to glomerular hyperfiltration in a study where continuous positive airway pressure (CPAP) use was associated with decreased hyperfiltration and significant increases in renal plasma flow without significant change in GFR after treatment with CPAP [33]. Kinebuchi et al. [33] studied glomeruli in 27 patients with OSA compared it to 32 healthy controls and demonstrated that patients with OSA have hyperfiltrating glomeruli as estimated by increased in filtration fraction (EF) in OSA compared to controls (0.26 ± 0.04 vs 0.21 ± 0.03; $p < 0.01$). There was a significant decrease in FF in patients with OSA on CPAP treatment (0.26 ± 0.04 to 0.23 ± 0.03; $p < 0.01$) who did not receive ACEI/ARB at baseline ($n = 21$). In six patients who received ACEI/ARB, there was no significant change in FF after CPAP treatment. The direct consequences of glomerular hyperfiltration are glomerular enlargement and glomerular sclerosis, which are both characteristics of focal segmental glomerulosclerosis. Plausible mechanisms include high sympathetic activity in patients with OSA, and hormones like atrial natriuretic peptide promoting glomerular hyperfiltration. The role of OSA causing proteinuria resulting in progression of CKD is controversial, due to the interplay of underlying common factors such as obesity [34]. Obesity in itself can cause hyperfiltration, glomerulomegaly, and focal glomerulosclerosis, eventually resulting in proteinuria [35]. Two small trials showed that OSA therapy resulted in decreases in proteinuria [36, 37]. In a study of 34 patients with OSA compared to 34 controls, Chaudhary et al. [36] observed regression of proteinuria after 3 years of follow up in 4 patients treated for OSA. In another study by Sklar et al. [37], two patients with severe OSA and high-grade proteinuria were studied. The authors observed remissions in proteinuria with correction of OSA and improvement in nocturnal hypoxemia.

OSA: A Potential Link Between Systemic Inflammation and Metabolic Syndrome

OSA-induced chronic intermittent hypoxemia can produce free radicals and reactive oxygen species (ROS) resulting in oxidative stress [17]. These free radicals generated by both NADPH and xanthine oxidase pathways are pro-inflammatory and are thought to produce ischemic-reperfusion injury. There is an upregulation of the inflammatory cascade resulting in increased production of cytokines including tumor necrosis factor-α, interleukin-6, interleukin-8, and monocyte chemoattractant protein-1 [38]. In addition, OSA also causes increases in platelet aggregation, insulin resistance, and metabolic dysregulation, which are the same factors involved in initiation and progression of CKD (Fig. 38.3). Supporting these findings, CPAP therapy in OSA improves endothelial function [39], attenuates the abnormally high levels of circulating apoptotic endothelial cells [40], reduces free radical production from neutrophils [41], decreases inflammatory mediators [42], increases vasodilator levels [43], and mediates a decline in vasoconstrictor levels in patients with sleep apnea [44]. In a study of 10 newly diagnosed untreated moderate-to-severe patients with OSA by Lattimore et al. [39], treatment with CPAP improved baseline endothelial nitric oxide release, stimulating endothelium dependent vaso-relaxation in the systemic circulation. Yokoe et al. [42] measured levels of CRP and IL-6 produced by monocytes in patients with OSA and found them significantly elevated compared to obese controls. The levels of CRP were directly associated with BMI and IL-6 was associated with apnea–hypopnea index and BMI. The authors also studied the effect of CPAP and noted that the levels of inflammatory biomarkers, including CRP and IL-6, decreased with treatment of OSA and improved sleep architecture. Whether OSA therapy with CPAP could delay the progression or help prevent the development of CKD remains unknown [42].

In summary, we conclude that OSA may be a unifying process between chronic kidney disease and cardiovascular disease, as they share common etiologies including hypertension, diabetes mellitus, and obesity. Possible pathophysiologic mechanisms underlying this relationship include (1) increased oxidative stress leading to insulin resistance and metabolic syndrome; (2) endothelial dysfunction from systemic inflammation; and (3) increased sympathetic system/RAAS activation leading to hypertension and fibrosis.

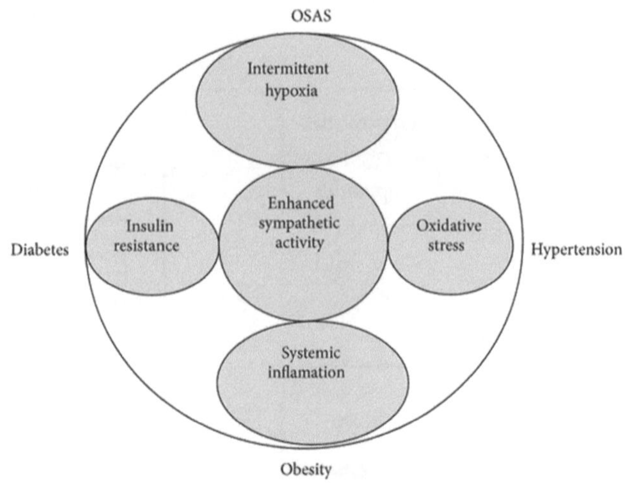

Fig. 38.3 OSAS and metabolic syndrome. Adapted from Zamarrón et al. [25]

There needs to be an increasing awareness among practicing clinicians regarding OSA as a multisystem pathophysiologic entity, warranting early diagnosis and prompt treatment to prevent long-term morbidity and mortality.

References

1. Sleep-related breathing disorders in adults: recommendations for syndrome definition and measurement techniques in clinical research. The Report of an American Academy of Sleep Medicine Task Force. Sleep. 1999;22(5):667–89.
2. Hiestand DM, Britz P, Goldman M, Phillips B. Prevalence of symptoms and risk of sleep apnea in the US population: results from the national sleep foundation sleep in America 2005 poll. Chest. 2006;130(3):780–6.
3. Young T, Evans L, Finn L, Palta M. Estimation of the clinically diagnosed proportion of sleep apnea syndrome in middle-aged men and women. Sleep. 1997;20(9):705–6.
4. Young T, Skatrud J, Peppard PE. Risk factors for obstructive sleep apnea in adults. JAMA. 2004;291(16):2013–6.
5. Epstein LJ, Kristo D, Strollo PJ Jr, Friedman N, Malhotra A, Patil SP, Ramar K, Rogers R, Schwab RJ, Weaver EM, Weinstein MD. Clinical guideline for the evaluation, management and long-term care of obstructive sleep apnea in adults. J Clin Sleep Med. 2009;5(3):263–76.
6. He J, Kryger MH, Zorick FJ, Conway W, Roth T. Mortality and apnea index in obstructive sleep apnea. Experience in 385 male patients. Chest. 1988;94(1):9–14.
7. Nieto FJ, Young TB, Lind BK, Shahar E, Samet JM, Redline S, D'Agostino RB, Newman AB, Lebowitz MD, Pickering TG. Association of sleep-disordered breathing, sleep apnea, and hypertension in a large community-based study. Sleep Heart Health Study. JAMA. 2000;283(14):1829–36.
8. Drager LF, Genta PR, Pedrosa RP, Nerbass FB, Gonzaga CC, Krieger EM, Lorenzi-Filho G. Characteristics and predictors of obstructive sleep apnea in patients with systemic hypertension. Am J Cardiol. 2010;105(8):1135–9.

9. Gus M, Goncalves SC, Martinez D, de Abreu Silva EO, Moreira LB, Fuchs SC, Fuchs FD. Risk for obstructive sleep apnea by Berlin Questionnaire, but not daytime sleepiness, is associated with resistant hypertension: a case–control study. Am J Hypertens. 2008;21(7):832–5.
10. Peker Y, Kraiczi H, Hedner J, Loth S, Johansson A, Bende M. An independent association between obstructive sleep apnoea and coronary artery disease. Eur Respir J. 1999;14(1):179–84.
11. Devulapally K, Pongonis R Jr, Khayat R. OSA: the new cardiovascular disease: part II: Overview of cardiovascular diseases associated with obstructive sleep apnea. Heart Fail Rev. 2009;14(3):155–64.
12. Shahar E, Whitney CW, Redline S, Lee ET, Newman AB, Nieto FJ, O'Connor GT, Boland LL, Schwartz JE, Samet JM. Sleep-disordered breathing and cardiovascular disease: cross-sectional results of the Sleep Heart Health Study. Am J Respir Crit Care Med. 2001;163(1):19–25.
13. Yaggi HK, Concato J, Kernan WN, Lichtman JH, Brass LM, Mohsenin V. Obstructive sleep apnea as a risk factor for stroke and death. N Engl J Med. 2005;353(19):2034–41.
14. Gami AS, Howard DE, Olson EJ, Somers VK. Day-night pattern of sudden death in obstructive sleep apnea. N Engl J Med. 2005;352(12):1206–14.
15. Gami AS, Olson EJ, Shen WK, Wright RS, Ballman KV, Hodge DO, Herges RM, Howard DE, Somers VK. Obstructive sleep apnea and the risk of sudden cardiac death: a longitudinal study of 10,701 adults. J Am Coll Cardiol. 2013;62(7):610–6.
16. Rosas SE. Sleep apnea in individuals with chronic kidney disease: a wake-up call. Clin J Am Soc Nephrol. 2011;6(5):954–6.
17. Adeseun GA, Rosas SE. The impact of obstructive sleep apnea on chronic kidney disease. Curr Hypertens Rep. 2010;12(5):378–83.
18. Nicholl DD, Ahmed SB, Loewen AH, Hemmelgarn BR, Sola DY, Beecroft JM, Turin TC, Hanly PJ. Clinical presentation of obstructive sleep apnea in patients with chronic kidney disease. J Clin Sleep Med. 2012;8(4):381–7.
19. Okubo R, Kondo M, Hoshi S. Cost-effectiveness of obstructive sleep apnea screening for patients with diabetes or chronic kidney disease. Sleep Breath. 2015;19:1081–92.
20. Roumelioti ME, Buysse DJ, Sanders MH, Strollo P, Newman AB, Unruh ML. Sleep-disordered breathing and excessive daytime sleepiness in chronic kidney disease and hemodialysis. Clin J Am Soc Nephrol. 2011;6(5):986–94.
21. Unruh ML, Sanders MH, Redline S, Piraino BM, Umans JG, Hammond TC, Sharief I, Punjabi NM, Newman AB. Sleep apnea in patients on conventional thrice-weekly hemodialysis: comparison with matched controls from the Sleep Heart Health Study. J Am Soc Nephrol. 2006;17(2):3503–9.
22. Markou N, Kanakaki M, Myrianthefs P, Hadjiyanakos D, Vlassopoulos D, Damianos A, Siamopoulos K, Vasiliou M, Konstantopoulos S. Sleep-disordered breathing in nondialyzed patients with chronic renal failure. Lung. 2006;184(1):43–9.
23. Sakaguchi Y, Shoji T, Kawabata H, Niihata K, Suzuki A, Kaneko T, Okada N, Isaka Y, Rakugi H, Tsubakihara Y. High prevalence of obstructive sleep apnea and its association with renal function among nondialysis chronic kidney disease patients in Japan: a cross-sectional study. Clin J Am Soc Nephrol. 2011;6(5):995–1000.
24. Sim JJ, Rasgon SA, Kujubu DA, Kumar VA, Liu IL, Shi JM, Pham TT, Derose SF. Sleep apnea in early and advanced chronic kidney disease: Kaiser Permanente Southern California cohort. Chest. 2009;135(3):710–6.
25. Zamarrón C, Valdés Cuadrado L, Alvarez-Sala R. Pathophysiologic mechanisms of cardiovascular disease in obstructive sleep apnea syndrome. Pulm Med. 2013;2013:521087.
26. Foley RN, Parfrey PS, Sarnak MJ. Clinical epidemiology of cardiovascular disease in chronic renal disease. Am J Kidney Dis. 1998;32(5 Suppl 3):S112–9.
27. Schohn D, Weidmann P, Jahn H, Beretta-Piccoli C. Norepinephrine-related mechanism in hypertension accompanying renal failure. Kidney Int. 1985;28(5):814–22.
28. Bixler EO, Vgontzas AN, Lin HM, Ten Have T, Leiby BE, Vela-Bueno A, Kales A. Association of hypertension and sleep-disordered breathing. Arch Intern Med. 2000;160(15):2289–95.
29. Haas DC, Foster GL, Nieto FJ, Redline S, Resnick HE, Robbins JA, Young T, Pickering TG. Age-dependent associations between sleep-disordered breathing and hypertension: importance of discriminating between systolic/diastolic hypertension and isolated systolic hypertension in the Sleep Heart Health Study. Circulation. 2005;111(5):614–21.
30. Budhiraja R, Parthasarathy S, Quan SF. Endothelial dysfunction in obstructive sleep apnea. J Clin Sleep Med. 2007;3(4):409–15.
31. Greene EL, Kren S, Hostetter TH. Role of aldosterone in the remnant kidney model in the rat. J Clin Invest. 1996;98(4):1063–8.
32. Aldigier JC, Kanjanbuch T, Ma LJ, Brown NJ, Fogo AB. Regression of existing glomerulosclerosis by inhibition of aldosterone. J Am Soc Nephrol. 2005;16(11):3306–14.
33. Kinebuchi S, Kazama JJ, Satoh M, Sakai K, Nakayama H, Yoshizawa H, Narita I, Suzuki E, Gejyo F. Short-term use of continuous positive airway pressure ameliorates glomerular hyperfiltration in patients with obstructive sleep apnoea syndrome. Clin Sci (Lond). 2004;107(3):317–22.
34. Casserly LF, Chow N, Ali S, Gottlieb DJ, Epstein LJ, Kaufman JS. Proteinuria in obstructive sleep apnea. Kidney Int. 2001;60(4):1484–9.
35. Serra A, Romero R, Lopez D, Navarro M, Esteve A, Perez N, Alastrue A, Ariza A. Renal injury in the extremely obese patients with normal renal function. Kidney Int. 2008;73(8):947–55.
36. Chaudhary BA, Sklar AH, Chaudhary TK, Kolbeck RC, Speir WA Jr. Sleep apnea, proteinuria, and nephrotic syndrome. Sleep. 1988;11(1):69–74.
37. Sklar AH, Chaudhary BA. Reversible proteinuria in obstructive sleep apnea syndrome. Arch Intern Med. 1988;148(1):87–9.
38. Quercioli A, Mach F, Montecucco F. Inflammation accelerates atherosclerotic processes in obstructive sleep apnea syndrome (OSAS). Sleep Breath. 2010;14(3):261–9.
39. Lattimore JL, Wilcox I, Skilton M, Langenfeld M, Celermajer DS. Treatment of obstructive sleep apnoea leads to improved microvascular endothelial function in the systemic circulation. Thorax. 2006;61(6):491–5.
40. El Solh AA, Akinnusi ME, Baddoura FH, Mankowski CR. Endothelial cell apoptosis in obstructive sleep apnea: a link to endothelial dysfunction. Am J Respir Crit Care Med. 2007;175(11):1186–91.
41. Schulz R, Mahmoudi S, Hattar K, Sibelius U, Olschewski H, Mayer K, Seeger W, Gimminger F. Enhanced release of superoxide from polymorphonuclear neutrophils in obstructive sleep apnea impact of continuous positive airway pressure therapy. Am J Respir Crit Care Med. 2000;162(2 Pt 1):566–70.
42. Yokoe T, Minoguchi K, Matsuo H, Oda N, Minoguchi H, Yoshino G, Hirano T, Adachi M. Elevated levels of C-reactive

protein and interleukin-6 in patients with obstructive sleep apnea syndrome are decreased by nasal continuous positive airway pressure. Circulation. 2003;107(8):1129–34.

43. Schulz R, Schmidt D, Blum A, Lopes-Ribeiro X, Lücke C, Mayer K, Olschewski H, Seeger W, Grimminger F. Decreased plasma levels of nitric oxide derivatives in obstructive sleep apnoea: response to CPAP therapy. Thorax. 2000;55(12):1046–51.
44. Phillips BG, Narkiewicz K, Pesek CA, Haynes WG, Dyken ME, Somers VK. Effects of obstructive sleep apnea on endothelin-1 and blood pressure. J Hypertens. 1999;17(1):61–6.

Part VIII
Dilemmas in Hypertension

Chronic Kidney Disease and BP Goals

39

Debbie L. Cohen and Raymond R. Townsend

Introduction

Patients with chronic kidney disease (CKD) are at particular high risk for cardiovascular (CV) events and the rationale for treatment of hypertension in CKD is to slow ongoing renal injury and delay progression to end-stage renal disease (ESRD). Patients with CKD are more likely to have resistant hypertension and are frequently taking multiple antihypertensive agents therefore achieving the recommended blood pressure (BP) goals in this population is often therapeutically challenging. Patients with CKD are less likely to achieve BP goals and a recent NHANES analysis demonstrated that more patients with CKD have uncontrolled BP compared to non-CKD patients, even when using the higher BP targets suggested by the 2014 Adult Hypertension Management guidelines (BP < 140/90 mmHg) [1, 2]. BP goals in the CKD population are still evolving and there is no definite consensus. The 2014 guidelines [2] were based on evidence from older studies, but these guidelines may change again, targeting lower BP goals based on how data from the recently published SPRINT study is interpreted in the CKD group, representing 28% of the SPRINT cohort [3]. The majority of the current guidelines for BP goals in CKD favor a BP < 140/90 mmHg in CKD without proteinuria; however, most guidelines recommend maintaining a lower BP target for those with more severe proteinuria. This contrasts with JNC 7 [4], which recommended a BP goal of <130/80 mmHg in all patients with CKD. The recommended BP guidelines in CKD from the various guideline committees are shown in Table 39.1 and the rationale for these guidelines will be detailed below [5].

D.L. Cohen (✉) · R.R. Townsend
Renal Division, Perelman School of Medicine at The University of Pennsylvania, 1 Founders Building, 3400 SPpuce Street, Philadelphia, 19104, PA, USA
e-mail: debbie.cohen@uphs.upenn.edu

R.R. Townsend
e-mail: townsend@upenn.edu

J. Rangaswami et al. (eds.), *Cardio-Nephrology*,
DOI 10.1007/978-3-319-56042-7_39

Rationale for BP Guidelines in CKD

The 2014 Evidence-Based Guideline for the Management of High Blood Pressure in Adults (JNC 8) 2014 [1, 2] recommended a BP goal of <140/90 mmHg in CKD, regardless of level of proteinuria and presence of diabetes. They also recommended that in patients with CKD regardless of race or diabetes, initial (or add-on) treatment should include an ACEI or ARB to improve kidney outcomes. The rationale for raising the BP goal in the 2014 evidence-based guidelines was based on data obtained from three randomized, controlled trials: Modification of Diet in Renal Disease (MDRD) Study; African American Study of Kidney Disease and Hypertension (AASK) trial and the Ramipril Efficacy in Nephropathy-2 (REIN-2) trial [12–14] and subsequent meta-analyses based on the same three trials [15–18].

The MDRD study included 585 patients with a GFR of 25–55 mL/min/1.73 m^2 and 255 patients with a GFR of 13–24 mL/min/1.73 m^2. The study was a 2 × 2 factorial design and patients were randomly assigned to an intensive BP target (a mean arterial pressure (MAP) of 92 mmHg corresponding to about 125/75 mmHg) or a standard BP target (MAP of 107 mmHg or approximately 140/90 mmHg) and to 1 of 2 types of diet. The use of all antihypertensives was allowed but angiotensin converting enzyme inhibitors (ACE) ± diuretic were encouraged as first-line agents and calcium channel blockers (CCB) ± diuretics were encouraged as second line agents. Eighty-five percent of patients were white and 97% of patients had nondiabetic CKD. Diabetics requiring insulin were excluded. Achieved BP was 126/77 mmHg in the intensive BP group versus 133/80 mmHg in the standard BP group. A posttrial follow-up of 6.2 years did not show benefit of any specific BP target or antihypertensive regimen. Importantly, the death outcome was not different between the two groups, and patients who reached ESRD were excluded from the analysis. The MDRD findings were largely based on slope of change of GFR (usually halving of GFR or the development of ESRD are the typical renal outcomes), and the original

Table 39.1 BP targets and treatment recommendations in CKD

Guideline source	CKD without proteinuria[a] (mmHg)	CKD with proteinuria (mmHg)	Recommended agents
USA JNC8 [2]	<140/<90	<140/<90	ACEI or ARB
KDIGO [6]	<140/<90	<130/<80	ACEI or ARB
NICE [7]	<140/<90	<130/<80	ACEI or ARB[b]
CHEP [8]	<140/<90	<140/<90	ACEI; ARB if ACEI intolerant
ESC/ESH [9]	<140	<130	ACEI or ARB
ASH/ISH [10]	<140/<90	<140/<90[c]	ARB or ACEI
ISHIB [11]	<130/<80	<130/<80	Diuretic or CCB

[a]Proteinuria definitions vary; the authors recommend using either +1 (by dipstick); more than 500 mg protein per 24 h; or more than 200 mg albumin per 24 h (or the equivalent of these values in a spot urine determination that employs a protein-to-creatinine or albumin-to-creatinine ratio)
[b]The NICE recommendations are to use ACEI or ARB when proteinuria is present; otherwise the guidance is to follow general recommendations for BP control when proteinuria is absent
[c]ASH/ISH guidelines acknowledge that some authorities still recommend <130/<80 mmHg for CKD with proteinuria
Reprinted with permission from Townsend et al. [5]

report did not support a benefit of more aggressive BP reduction for either halving of GFR or ESRD. A follow-up of the MDRD cohort was published in 2005, 12 years after the study finished, and concluded that those randomized to the intensive BP goal had less development of kidney outcomes compared with those in the standard BP target (62 vs. 70% requiring either dialysis initiation or transplantation), however, no BP data was available on the cohort after they completed the trial phase nor is information available indicating specifics of drug therapy in the interval [19].

The AASK trial enrolled 1094 nondiabetic black patients with hypertensive nephrosclerosis. The study had a 3 × 2 factorial design with patients being randomly assigned to an intensive (MAP < 92 mmHg) or standard (MAP 102–107 mmHg) BP target and 1 of 3 initial therapies (ramipril, metoprolol, or amlodipine). The trial allowed sequential addition of furosemide, doxazosin, clonidine, hydralazine, and minoxidil to achieve randomized BP target. The mean BP achieved was 128/78 mmHg in the intensive versus 141/85 mmHg in the standard BP groups. At a mean follow-up of 4 years, the average rate of change (as a slope) in GFR was not different between the BP groups. In the posttrial follow-up for AASK at 8–12 years, patients were treated to a BP goal of less than 130/80 mmHg and used either an ACE or an angiotensin receptor blocker (ARB) if ACE-intolerant. Target BP achieved was 131/78 versus 134/78 mmHg in the intensive versus standard BP groups. Use of ACE and ARB was similar in the both groups. There was no difference between groups in the progression of kidney disease (doubling of serum creatinine, diagnosis of ESRD, or death) in the main cohort.

REIN-2 Trial specifically enrolled 338 patients with proteinuria >1000 mg/day for 3 months. Patients with proteinuria between 1000 and 3000 mg/day were included if GFR was <45 mL/min/1.73 m^2 and patients with proteinuria >3000 mg/day were included if GFR was <70 mL/min/1.73 m^2. Type 1 diabetics were excluded. Patients were assigned to an intensive BP target of <130/80 mmHg or a standard BP target of DBP < 90 mmHg. All patients were treated with ramipril (ACE) 5 mg daily during the trial. Felodipine (dihydropyridine CCB) in the dose of 5–10 mg daily was used as add-on treatment in the intensive BP target. Antihypertensive agents other than ACE, ARB, and dihydropyridine CCB were allowed in both groups. BP achieved was 130/80 versus 134/82 mmHg in the intensive versus standard BP targets. After a median time of 19 months, no significant differences were noted in the percentage of patients who progressed to ESRD (23 vs. 20%, slightly though not significantly higher incidence in the intensive BP target group), the decline in GFR or the effects on proteinuria between the groups.

The MDRD, AASK and REIN-2 all failed to show a benefit from lower BP goals (<140/90 vs. 125–130/75–80 mmHg) in reduction of CV events, slowing progression of CKD to ESRD, and reducing mortality. The AASK trial did prospectively include proteinuria as an end point but lower BP targets did not show any benefit on slowing progression of CKD [13]. The MDRD trial; however, did show a benefit in a post hoc analysis of lower BP goals in the setting of proteinuria (more than 1 g/24 h) on the slope of glomerular filtration rate (GFR) loss [17]. There was, however, an unequal use of ACE inhibitor treatment in the different treatment groups. A systematic review and meta-analysis of the 2272 participants of these three trials comparing lower versus higher BP targets in adults with CKD also did not show any conclusive evidence favoring a lower BP target of 125/75–130/80 versus 140/90 mmHg after a mean follow-up of 2–4 years. There was however a benefit for CKD patients with proteinuria of 300–1000 mg/day [16].

BP Goals in Diabetes

The Action to Control Cardiovascular Risk in Diabetes (ACCORD) trial which randomized type 2 diabetics to a SBP goal of <140 versus <120 mmHg also failed to demonstrate CV protection from a lower BP target, but the rate of stroke was decreased [20]. Renal outcomes were not separately addressed in the ACCORD Trial and serum creatinine levels and estimated GFR were not improved with lower BP goals. Based on the data from MDRD, AASK and REIN, which failed to show a decrease in CV risk, mortality, and progression of CKD or to ESRD, the 2014 Evidence-Based Guideline for the Management of High Blood Pressure in Adults (JNC 8) 2014 [1] committee recommended a BP goal of <140/90 mmHg in all patients with CKD regardless of proteinuria. Although there was some data showing benefit of a lower BP in patients with proteinuria of 300–1000 mg/day, they did not recommend a lower BP goal for CKD patients with macroalbuminuria.

Current BP Guidelines in CKD

The 2012 KDIGO Clinical Practice Guideline for Management of Blood Pressure in CKD [6] was the first guideline to recommend a higher BP goal for patients with CKD. This guideline recommended a BP goal of $\leq$140/90 mmHg in CKD patients without albuminuria. They however recommended a goal BP $\leq$130/80 mmHg in CKD patients with albuminuria $\geq$30 mg/24 h. KDIGO also recommended treatment with RAAS blockade in all CKD patients with an albumin excretion rate of $\geq$30 mg/24 h.

Other guideline groups also raised the BP goals for patients with CKD including the American Diabetes Association (BP target < 140/80 mmHg) [19], Canadian Hypertension Education Program (BP target < 140/90 mmHg for CKD) [8], and European Society of Cardiology/European Society of Hypertension (SBP target < 140 mmHg for CKD) [9]. The National Institute for Health and Clinical Excellence (NICE) guideline advised initiating treatment in those with CKD at BP $\geq$ 140/90 mmHg and treating to a target of 120–139/<90 mmHg [7, 21]. The NICE guidelines also recommended drug treatment for BP $\geq$ 130/80 mmHg for albumin-to-creatinine ratio (ACR) of $\geq$70 mg/mmol and a target of 120–129/<80 mmHg).

Observational Studies in CKD

There are two recent retrospective observational studies from a national CKD database of mostly male US veterans assessing all-cause mortality in veterans with CKD. The first study compared mortality in CKD patients with a treated SBP of <120 mmHg to patients with the currently recommended SBP of <140 mmHg [22]. This study included 77,765 individuals with GFR < 60 mL/min/1.73 m^2 and uncontrolled hypertension (received $\geq$1 BP medication with evidence of a decrease in SBP). Of this cohort, 5760 patients had a treated SBP of <120 mmHg at follow-up and 72,005 patients had a treated SBP of 120–139 mmHg at follow-up. During a median follow-up of 6.0 years, 19,517 patients died (2380 deaths in SBP < 120 mmHg group (death rate of 80.9/1000 patient-years) and 17,137 deaths in SBP of 120–139 mmHg group (death rate, 41.8/1000 patient-years; $p < 0.001$). The mortality hazard ratio associated with follow-up SBP less than 120 versus 120–139 mmHg was 1.70 (95% CI 1.63–1.78). These results suggest that lower SBP levels were associated with higher all-cause mortality in patients with CKD.

The second study assessed the association of BP with death in patients with CKD [23]. They included 651,749 US Veterans with CKD and examined all possible combinations of SBP and DBP from lowest (BP = 80/40 mmHg) to highest (BP = 210/120 mmHg), in 10 mmHg increments. The study demonstrated that patients with SBP of 130–159 mmHg combined with DBP of 70–89 mmHg had the lowest adjusted mortality rates, and those in whom both SBP and DBP were concomitantly very high or very low had the highest mortality rates. Patients with moderately elevated SBP combined with DBP no <70 mmHg had consistently lower mortality rates than patients with DBP < 70 mmHg. Results were consistent in subgroups of patients with normal and elevated ACRs. Overall, the optimal BP in CKD patients in this study appeared to be 130–159/70–89 mmHg. Both these studies are retrospective observational analyses, and are at risk for confounding, but appear to indicate that a SBP <120 mmHg at least observationally is associated with an increased risk of mortality.

The Systolic BP Intervention Trial

The Systolic BP Intervention Trial (SPRINT) may finally answer the ongoing debate about what SBP goal clinicians should be targeting in certain patients with CKD [3, 24].

SPRINT is a large NIH-sponsored, multicenter, randomized, controlled intervention trial that enrolled 9361 subjects with a SBP of at least 130 mmHg. The primary goal of SPRINT was to test whether reducing SBP to a lower goal (SBP < 120 mmHg) than currently recommended (SBP < 140 mmHg) would reduce the occurrence of CV disease events defined as CV death, nonfatal heart attack, nonfatal stroke, acute coronary syndrome without heart attack, and hospitalized heart failure. Subjects enrolled were 50 years or older with SBP of 130 mmHg or higher and at least one of the following: a history of cardiovascular disease, stage 3/4 chronic kidney disease (estimated glomerular filtration rate 20–59 mL/min/1.73 m^2), an intermediate to high risk for CVD other than stroke or age $\geq$ 75 years. A subject was defined as having CVD if they had a prior myocardial infarction, percutaneous coronary intervention, coronary artery bypass grafting, carotid endarterectomy or carotid stenting, peripheral arterial disease with revascularization, acute coronary syndrome, abdominal aortic aneurysm $\geq$ 5 cm with or without repair, a coronary calcium score > 400 or left ventricular hypertrophy. A subject was defined as intermediate or high risk for CVD based on the following: Framingham Risk Score for 10-year CVD risk of 15% based on laboratory work done within the past 12 months for lipids. The primary outcome was a composite of CV events. SPRINT was terminated early after 3.26 years on a recommendation from the data safety monitoring board. The results of the SPRINT study showed a 25% reduction in the primary combined CV outcome and a 27% reduction in mortality in the group randomized to a SBP < 120 mmHg [3, 24]. This obviously has important implications for BP guidelines in this population with CKD. The baseline mean systolic and diastolic blood pressures were 139.7 and 78.1 mmHg. At 1 year, the mean SBP was 121.4 mmHg in the intensive treatment group and 136.2 mmHg in the standard-treatment group. The SPRINT study included 28% of subjects with CKD and 28% of subjects were older than 75 years, 36% were women, and 20% had prior cardiovascular disease. The sample was diverse and included 29.9% Black, 10.5% Hispanic, and 57.7% White subjects. Importantly, SPRINT *excluded* many patients with hypertension and CKD including those with a history of prior stroke, diabetes, polycystic kidney disease, any secondary cause for hypertension, GFR < 20 cc/min, >1 g of proteinuria per 24 h, glomerulonephritis treated with immunosuppressive therapy, symptomatic heart failure within last 6 months or left ventricular ejection fraction <35%, organ transplant recipients, cardiovascular event, procedure, or hospitalization for unstable angina within the last 3 months and patients <50 years of age. Although the SPRINT study will provide important information on managing systolic BP in older nondiabetic subjects with substantial CVD risk, it is important to remember that these results cannot be generalized to the other populations and to all patients with CKD.

Among participants who had CKD at baseline, a prespecified secondary analysis in SPRINT was the number of patients who developed a decrease of GFR of >50%, or end-stage renal disease (ESRD; requiring dialysis or transplantation). There were no significant differences in the intensive versus standard BP group with regards to the composite outcome of a decrease in the eGFR of 50% or more or the development of ESRD. The number of ESRD events was small in both groups (14 and 15 in the intensive group vs. the standard BP group respectively) perhaps due to early termination of the trial and a lower-than-expected decline in the eGFR. Among participants who did not have CKD at baseline, a decrease in the eGFR of $\geq$30% to a eGFR of <60 mL/min/1.73 m^2 occurred more frequently in the intensive treatment group than in the standard-treatment group (1.21 vs. 0.35%/year). This is not unexpected given the need for more intensive antihypertensive therapy in this group. With the currently available data, there is no evidence of substantial permanent kidney injury associated with the lower systolic BP goal; however, the possibility of a long-term adverse renal outcome cannot be excluded. Further more detailed subgroup analysis of CKD patients in the SPRINT study is still being performed and will incorporate longer follow-up and will likely add data to the debate of the "ideal" BP goal in CKD. A comparison of the various studies regarding intensive versus standard BP goals and CKD outcomes are summarized in Table 39.2.

BP Goals in Polycystic Kidney Disease

The HALT-PKD trial has provided some additional data on BP goals in patients with autosomal dominant polycystic kidney disease (APCKD) [25]. This study enrolled patients with hypertension and APCKD with preserved renal function in a double-blind, placebo-controlled trial, and randomly assigned 558 patients with an estimated GFR > 60 mL/min/1.73 m^2 to either a standard BP target (120/70–130/80 mmHg) or an intensive BP target (95/60–110/75 mmHg) and to either combination of ACE and ARB (lisinopril and telmisartan) or ACE plus placebo (lisinopril plus placebo). The primary outcome was the annual percentage change in the total kidney volume. The annual percentage increase in total kidney volume was significantly lower in the intensive BP group than in the standard BP group (5.6 vs. 6.6%, $p = 0.006$), without significant differences between the ACE/ARB and ACE/placebo group. The rate of change in estimated GFR was similar in the two medication groups, with a negative slope difference in the short term in the low-blood-pressure group as compared with the

Table 39.2 Comparison of studies in CKD comparing intensive versus standard BP targets

	MDRD [12]	AASK [13]	REIN-2 [14]	SPRINT [3]
Subject #	840	1094	338	2646
Cause of CKD	Nondiabetic CKD	Hypertensive nephrosclerosis	CKD excluded type 1 DM	Nondiabetic CKD
Stage CKD	3–4	3	3–4	3–4
Proteinuria inclusion	300–1000 mg/day	<300 mg/day	1000–5000 mg/day	<1000 mg/day
BP inclusion	MAP ≤ 125	DBP ≥ 90	Not specified	SBP > 130 mmHg
Baseline proteinuria	Intensive BP target: 390 mg/day Standard BP target: 310 mg/day	Intensive BP target: 0.08 g/g (0.03–0.36 g/g) Standard BP target: 0.08 g/g (0.03–0.37 g/g)	Intensive BP target: 2800 mg/day Standard BP target: 2900 mg/day	Intensive BP target: 44.1 mg/g creatinine Standard BP target: 41.1 mg/g creatinine
Target BP (mmHg)	Intensive BP target: MAP ≤ 92 (125/75) Standard BP target: MAP ≤ 107 (140/90)	Intensive BP target: MAP ≤ 92 Standard BP target: MAP ≤ 102–107	Intensive BP target: <130/80 Standard BP target: DBP <90	Intensive BP target: SBP < 120 Standard BP target: SBP 140
Achieved BP target (mmHg)	Intensive BP target: 126/77 Standard BP target: 133/80	Intensive BP target: 130/78 Standard BP target: 141/86	Intensive BP target: 130/80 Standard BP target: 134/82	Intensive BP target: SBP < 121.5 Standard BP target: SBP 134.6
Primary outcome	Rate of change in GFR	Rate of change in GFR and composite of $\geq 50\%$ (or ≥ 25 mL/min/1.73 m^2) reduction in GFR, ESRD or death	ESRD	$\geq 50\%$ change in GFR, ESRD, transplantation and incident albuminuria

CKD outcomes	MDRD trial [12]	MDRD observational follow-up [17]	AASK trial [13]	AASK observational follow-up [18]	REIN-2 trial [14]	SPRINT [3]
$\geq 50\%$ (or ≥ 25 mL/min/1.73 m^2) reduction in GFR, ESRD or death	Not stated	Not stated	Risk reduction (RR) 2% (95% CI −22 to 21%) $p = 0.85$	HR 0.91 (CI 0.77–1.08) $p = 0.27$	Not stated	HR 0.89 (CI 0.42–1.87) $p = 0.76$
Kidney failure or death	Study A: RR, not stated $p > 0.05$ Study B: RR, 0.85 (CI 0.6–1.22) $p = 0.33$	HR 0.77 (CI 0.65–0.91) $p = 0.002$	RR 12% (CI −13 to 30%) $p = 0.31$	HR 0.85 (CI 0.71–1.02) $p = 0.08$	Not stated	Not stated
50% decrease in GFR or kidney failure	Not stated	Not stated	RR 2% (CI −31 to 20%) $p = 0.87$	HR 0.95 (CI 0.78–1.15) $p = 0.59$	Not stated	HR 0.87 (CI 0.36–2.07) $p = 0.75$
Kidney failure or ESRD	HR 0.76 (CI 0.52–1.1) $p = 0.15$	HR 0.68 (CI 0.57–0.82) $p < 0.001$	RR 6% (CI −29 to 31%) $p = 0.72$	Not stated	23 versus 20% $p = 0.99$	HR 0.57 (CI. 0.19–1.54) $p = 0.27$
Incident albuminuria						HR 0.72 (CI. 0.48–1.07) $p = 0.11$

(continued)

Table 39.2 (continued)

CKD outcomes	MDRD trial [12]	MDRD observational follow-up [17]	AASK trial [13]	AASK observational follow-up [18]	REIN-2 trial [14]	SPRINT [3]
Rate of annual GFR decline, mL/min/1.73 m^2	Study A: 1.6 (CI −0.8 to 3.9) $p = 0.18$ Study B: 0.5 (CI 0.4–1.4) $p = 0.28$	Not stated	0.26 (CI −0.21 to 0.64) $p = 0.25$	Not stated	0.22 versus 0.24 $p = 0.62$	Not stated

MDRD modification of diet in renal disease, *AASK* African American Study of Kidney Disease, *REIN-2* Ramipril efficacy in nephropathy-2, *SPRINT* systolic blood pressure intervention trial, *CKD* chronic kidney disease, *DM* diabetes mellitus, *MAP* mean arterial pressure, *GFR* glomerular filtration rate, *CI* confidence interval, *RR* risk reduction; *HR* hazard ratio

standard-blood-pressure group ($p < 0.001$) and a marginally positive slope difference in the long term ($p = 0.05$). The left ventricular mass index decreased more in the intensive BP versus standard BP group (−1.17 vs. −0.57 g/m^2/year, $p < 0.001$); urinary albumin excretion was reduced by 3.77% with the intensive BP group and increased by 2.43% with the standard BP group ($p < 0.001$). Dizziness and light-headedness were more common in the intensive BP versus standard BP group (80.7 vs. 69.4%, $p = 0.002$). This study showed that a more intensive BP goal of ≤ 110/75 mmHg slowed the increase in total kidney volume, reduced LV mass index, and reduced urinary albumin excretion. Intensive BP control did not affect the change in eGFR. Use of single versus dual RAAS blockade did not affect outcomes.

Summary of BP Goals

In summary, there is no consensus on the ideal BP goal in CKD but most of the current BP guidelines committees currently recommend a BP goal of <140/90 mmHg for most CKD patients and some guidelines recommend a lower BP goal of <130/80 mmHg in CKD patients with proteinuria. Newer studies are now shedding light on this debate with high quality prospective data indicating that a lower BP goal may be indicated in certain populations with CKD. An even lower BP goal of ≤ 110/75 mmHg might be indicated in autosomal dominant PCKD patients with preserved renal function. These studies however still do not apply to a large proportion of CKD patients with diabetic nephropathy. We suggest that a BP range of 120–130 mmHg as recommended by the NICE guidelines is probably a "safe" BP goal to aim for in the interim in most patients with CKD. All the concerns are likely to be incorporated into the next set of guidelines which are likely to be revised in 2017.

References

1. Sakhuja A, Textor SC, Taler SJ. Uncontrolled hypertension by the 2014 evidence-based guideline: results from NHANES 2011–2012. J Hypertens. 2015;33(3):644–51 (discussion 52).
2. James PA, Oparil S, Carter BL, Cushman WC, Dennison-Himmelfarb C, Handler J, et al. 2014 evidence-based guideline for the management of high blood pressure in adults: report from the panel members appointed to the Eighth Joint National Committee (JNC 8). JAMA. 2014;311(5):507–20.
3. SPRINT Research Group, Wright JT Jr, Williamson JD, Whelton PK, Snyder JK, Sink KM, et al. A randomized trial of intensive versus standard blood-pressure control. N Engl J Med. 2015 Nov 26;373(22):2103–16
4. Chobanian AV, Bakris GL, Black HR, Cushman WC, Green LA, Izzo JL Jr, et al. The seventh report of the joint national committee on prevention, detection, evaluation, and treatment of high blood pressure: the JNC 7 report. JAMA. 2003;289(19):2560–72.
5. Townsend RR, Taler SJ. Management of hypertension in chronic kidney disease. Nat Rev Nephrol. 2015;11(9):555–63
6. Wheeler DC, Becker GJ. Summary of KDIGO guideline. What do we really know about management of blood pressure in patients with chronic kidney disease? Kidney Int. 2013;83(3):377–83.
7. Hypertension: The clinical management of primary hypertension in adults: update of clinical guidelines 18 and 34. London; 2011.
8. Hackam DG, Quinn RR, Ravani P, Rabi DM, Dasgupta K, Daskalopoulou SS, et al. The 2013 Canadian Hypertension Education Program recommendations for blood pressure measurement, diagnosis, assessment of risk, prevention, and treatment of hypertension. Can J Cardiol. 2013;29(5):528–42.
9. Mancia G, Fagard R, Narkiewicz K, Redon J, Zanchetti A, Bohm M, et al. 2013 ESH/ESC Guidelines for the management of arterial hypertension: the Task Force for the management of arterial hypertension of the European Society of Hypertension (ESH) and of the European Society of Cardiology (ESC). J Hypertens. 2013;31(7):1281–357.
10. Weber MA, Schiffrin EL, White WB, Mann S, Lindholm LH, Kenerson JG, et al. Clinical practice guidelines for the management of hypertension in the community a statement by the American Society of Hypertension and the International Society of Hypertension. J Hypertens. 2014;32(1):3–15.
11. Flack JM, Sica DA, Bakris G, Brown AL, Ferdinand KC, Grimm RH Jr, et al. Management of high blood pressure in Blacks: an update of the International Society on Hypertension in Blacks consensus statement. Hypertension. 2010;56(5):780–800.

12. Klahr S, Levey AS, Beck GJ, Caggiula AW, Hunsicker L, Kusek JW, et al. The effects of dietary protein restriction and blood-pressure control on the progression of chronic renal disease. Modification of Diet in Renal Disease Study Group. N Engl J Med. 1994;330(13):877–84.
13. Wright JT Jr, Bakris G, Greene T, Agodoa LY, Appel LJ, Charleston J, et al. Effect of blood pressure lowering and antihypertensive drug class on progression of hypertensive kidney disease: results from the AASK trial. JAMA. 2002;288(19):2421–31.
14. Ruggenenti P, Perna A, Loriga G, Ganeva M, Ene-Iordache B, Turturro M, et al. Blood-pressure control for renoprotection in patients with non-diabetic chronic renal disease (REIN-2): multicentre, randomised controlled trial. Lancet. 2005;365(9463):939–46.
15. Jafar TH, Stark PC, Schmid CH, Landa M, Maschio G, de Jong PE, et al. Progression of chronic kidney disease: the role of blood pressure control, proteinuria, and angiotensin-converting enzyme inhibition: a patient-level meta-analysis. Ann Intern Med. 2003;139(4):244–52.
16. Upadhyay A, Earley A, Haynes SM, Uhlig K. Systematic review: blood pressure target in chronic kidney disease and proteinuria as an effect modifier. Ann Intern Med. 2011;154(8):541–8.
17. Peterson JC, Adler S, Burkart JM, Greene T, Hebert LA, Hunsicker LG, et al. Blood pressure control, proteinuria, and the progression of renal disease. The Modification of Diet in Renal Disease Study. Ann Intern Med. 1995;123(10):754–62.
18. Appel LJ, Wright JT Jr, Greene T, Agodoa LY, Astor BC, Bakris GL, et al. Intensive blood-pressure control in hypertensive chronic kidney disease. N Engl J Med. 2010;363(10):918–29.
19. American Diabetes A. Standards of medical care in diabetes—2013. Diabetes Care. 2013;36(Suppl 1):S11–66.
20. Group AS, Cushman WC, Evans GW, Byington RP, Goff DC Jr, Grimm RH Jr, et al. Effects of intensive blood-pressure control in type 2 diabetes mellitus. N Engl J Med. 2010;362(17):1575–85.
21. Carville S, Wonderling D, Stevens P. Guideline Development G. Early identification and management of chronic kidney disease in adults: summary of updated NICE guidance. BMJ. 2014;349: g4507.
22. Kovesdy CP, Lu JL, Molnar MZ, Ma JZ, Canada RB, Streja E, et al. Observational modeling of strict vs. conventional blood pressure control in patients with chronic kidney disease. JAMA Intern Med. 2014;174(9):1442–9.
23. Kovesdy CP, Bleyer AJ, Molnar MZ, Ma JZ, Sim JJ, Cushman WC, et al. Blood pressure and mortality in U.S. veterans with chronic kidney disease: a cohort study. Ann Intern Med. 2013;159 (4):233–42.
24 Ambrosius WT, Sink KM, Foy CG, Berlowitz DR, Cheung AK, Cushman WC, et al. The design and rationale of a multicenter clinical trial comparing two strategies for control of systolic blood pressure: the Systolic Blood Pressure Intervention Trial (SPRINT). Clin Trials. 2014;11(5):532–46.
25 Schrier RW, Abebe KZ, Perrone RD, Torres VE, Braun WE, Steinman TI, et al. Blood pressure in early autosomal dominant polycystic kidney disease. N Engl J Med. 2014;371(24):2255–66.

Renal Artery Stenosis: Diagnosis and Management

40

Harold M. Szerlip and Bhupinder Singh

Introduction

Renal artery stenosis (RAS), narrowing of renal arteries, can be unilateral or bilateral. This narrowing may reduce blood supply to the affected kidney and lead to renovascular hypertension. It needs to be emphasized however, that the presence of renal artery stenosis is not synonymous with renovascular hypertension. RAS is commonly atherosclerotic in origin, and its incidence increases with age. There are three main causes of renal artery stenosis: atherosclerotic disease, fibromuscular dysplasia, and Takayasu's arteritis [1]. Other rare causes of RAS include post-radiation, trauma, neurofibromatosis, vascular bands, complications from renal denervation therapy and congenital vascular abnormalities. We have also encountered a case of cryofibrinogenemia presenting with bilateral RAS caused by fibrin deposition in the renal arteries. Diagnosis and management of clinically significant RAS can be difficult to establish. It is therefore important to understand the epidemiology, risk factors and clinical sequelae associated with the condition.

Etiology

Atherosclerotic Renal Artery Disease

By far the most common cause of renal artery stenosis is atherosclerotic renal artery disease (ARAD), which is responsible for up to 90% of the cases of renovascular disease. Stenosis in atherosclerotic disease occurs most commonly in the proximal renal artery. As with all atherosclerotic diseases the prevalence increases with aging [2]. In addition, the prevalence reported varies depending on the population studied, the percent luminal narrowing considered significant, the reliability of the diagnostic tools used to identify the stenosis and the prevailing community standard regarding the importance of making the diagnosis as far as treatment is concerned.

In 4429, patients referred for evaluation of secondary hypertension the finding of ARAD increased from 1.3% in patients 30–39 years old to 6.5% in patients' age greater than 70 [2]. In 295 patients studied post-mortem with an average age of 61 the overall prevalence of a greater than 50% narrowing of the renal artery was 22%; whereas in those patients over 70 32% had greater than 50% stenosis [3]. In patients with underlying coronary artery disease or peripheral vascular disease the incidence of renal artery stenosis is between 30 and 50% [4–6]. In patients undergoing coronary angiography 38.8% were noted to have greater than a 50% stenosis of one or both renal arteries with 40% of these patients having greater than a 70% narrowing [7]. Similarly, 16.6% of patients undergoing angiography following an acute myocardial infarction and thus with established atherosclerotic disease, had significant renal artery stenosis as defined by greater than 50% narrowing [8]. In another high-risk population, patients initiating chronic hemodialysis, 41% of the patients had a greater than 50% stenosis [9]. Renal artery stenosis appears to be less common in African-Americans [10, 11], although when factored for other co-morbidities race no longer appears to be significant [12].

Review of Medicare data showed that the hazard ratio for the diagnosis of ARAD increased 4.71-fold between 1992 and 2004 [13]. Between 1996 and 2000 the number of renal artery interventions increased 62% [14]. The reason for this increase is unclear, but may have been related to improvements in imaging or the increase in the ease of performing percutaneous interventions. Thus the prevalence of renal artery stenosis varies significantly depending on the

H.M. Szerlip (✉)
Department of Nephrology, Baylor University Medical Center, 3600 Gaston Ave, Barnett Tower, Suite 904, 75246 Dallas, TX, USA
e-mail: Harold.szerlip@baylorhealth.edu

B. Singh
Cardio Renal Society of America, 3219 East Camelback Road, Suite 517, 85018 Phoenix, AZ, USA
e-mail: 100GFR@gmail.com

J. Rangaswami et al. (eds.), *Cardio-Nephrology*,
DOI 10.1007/978-3-319-56042-7_40

population studied. Again it needs to be emphasized that even severe renal artery stenosis of greater than 70–80% does not necessarily equal renovascular hypertension. In fact, significant renal artery stenosis can be found in normotensive patients [3, 7].

Fibromuscular Dysplasia

Fibromuscular dysplasia (FMD) is a non-inflammatory, non-atherosclerotic vascular disease. It most frequently affects the medial portion of the renal and/or carotid arteries. Involvement of the renal arteries occurs in approximately 60–75% of cases. As opposed to atherosclerotic disease, classic medial FMD characteristically occurs in the distal two-third of the renal artery. The cause of FMD is unknown. It is estimated that FMD is responsible for 10% of all cases of renal artery stenosis suggesting a prevalence of 0.4%. However, because many patients are asymptomatic, the prevalence of FMD is even greater. In 3181 potential renal donors 4.4% were noted to have FMD [15]. Classic FMD affecting medial aspect of the artery showing the characteristic "string-of-beads" angiographic appearance occurs 4 times more commonly in women. FMD usually is diagnosed in women between the ages of 20–60 although it has been reported in the both the very young and very elderly. There appears to be a genetic component to this disorder, since it occurs frequently in first degree relatives. An association between smoking and FMD had also been described. The presence of hypertension in woman younger than 40 years, should raise the possibility of FMD.

Takayasu's Arteritis

Takayasu's arteritis is a systemic inflammatory disease involving large arteries that can lead to stenosis, occlusion or aneurysmal dilation. The etiology remains uncertain. Takayasu's arteritis occurs with a worldwide estimate of 2.6 cases per million [16, 17]. The disease is far more common in persons of Asian descent and occurs primarily in woman younger than 40. Disease affecting the renal arteries is defined as Type 3 or 4. In Japan Takayasu's arteritis is the second leading cause of renal artery stenosis [18]. A diagnosis of Takayasu's is made based upon angiographic findings which meet the Ishikawa criteria, or those established by the American College of Rheumatology [19]. Treatment depends upon the extent of the disease, and may include use of corticosteroids and cytotoxic therapy to control inflammation. Anti-IL-6 receptor antibody Tocilizumab has shown promise as a potential treatment of large vessel vasculitis including Takayasu's arteritis.

Consequences of Renal Artery Stenosis

The most common side effects from renal artery stenosis are hypertension and progressive renal failure. A decrease in renal perfusion activates the renin–angiotensin–aldosterone system (RAAS). Although the pathophysiologic mechanism that results in hypertension is somewhat different between the Goldblatt one-clip and two-clip models, for all practical purposes a decrease in renal blood flow increases renal sodium retention and vascocontriction [20, 21]. The presence of significant renal artery stenosis (>70%) does not necessarily cause hypertension and similarly the finding of renal artery stenosis in a hypertensive individual does not always indicate causality. In fact, both autopsy and angiographic studies demonstrate the existence of significant stenosis in the absence of hypertension [3, 7]. Unfortunately, the only definitive way to establish a diagnosis of renovascular hypertension is to show a decrease in blood pressure after relief of the blockage.

A critical decrease in renal perfusion results in activation of numerous cytokines and inflammatory mediators associated with renal injury [22, 23]. These inflammatory and pro-fibrotic cytokines as well as reactive oxygen species leads to rarefication of the renal microvascular structures, glomerular sclerosis, and interstitial fibrosis with tubular atrophy. Ongoing renal ischemia results in progressive kidney disease. Interestingly, even when renal perfusion is restored these inflammatory mediators and markers of renal injury may remain elevated [24].

The presence of critical renal artery stenosis is associated with increased cardiovascular morbidity and mortality even when factored for other comorbid conditions [8, 25, 26]. However, it is unclear if these data are confounded by the extent of overall atherosclerosis, the presence of chronic kidney disease and poorly controlled hypertension. The fact that randomized trials evaluating the use of stents in ARVD do not show improvement in cardiovascular outcomes whereas individuals treated for FMD appear to have an excellent prognosis, supports the role of confounders.

Another entity that appears to occur more frequently in patients with renal artery stenosis is recurrent episodes of flash pulmonary edema [27–29]. This was initially described by Pickering in 11 patients in 1988 [28]. Patients typically present with acute onset pulmonary edema that can be recurrent. BP is invariably markedly elevated and cardiac function is preserved. Pickering syndrome occurs more frequently with bilateral renal artery stenosis than with unilateral involvement [27–30]. This increased incidence is likely related to the sodium and water retention that occurs more frequently with bilateral disease, as opposed to the pressure natriuresis that ensues in unilateral disease. Relief of the obstruction frequently prevents reoccurrence [28–30].

Randomized Trials

The diagnostic challenge for the clinician is to understand who needs to be evaluated for renal artery disease and what diagnostic tools provide the most useful information. Although no randomized trial comparing medical therapy to endovascular repair has shown a clinical benefit for stenting [31–34], all these trials have been faulted [35, 36]. The STAR trial conducted in the Netherlands and France recruited 140 patients with impaired renal function, stable blood pressure, and ostial renal artery stenosis greater than 50% [31]. Patients were randomized to medical therapy with anti-hypertensive agents, atorvastatin and aspirin or medical therapy plus stenting. 25% of the subjects randomized to the stent arm did not receive the therapy. At the conclusion of the study there was no significant difference between the groups in regards to decline in renal function, change in blood pressure or cardiovascular events. Furthermore, two patients in the stent group died of complications from the procedure. This negative study was obviously under-powered and included patients who were not at high risk. Therefore, no definitive conclusion can be made from the results.

The ASTRAL trial was a much larger study with 806 patients enrolled [33]. After initial screening subjects were enrolled if they had "substantial" atherosclerotic stenosis and if the "patient's doctor was uncertain that the patient would definitely have a worthwhile clinical benefit from revascularization." 59% of the subjects had greater than 70% stenosis and 60% had a serum creatinine greater than 1.7 mg/dl. Subjects were randomized to stenting plus medical therapy or medical therapy alone and followed for up to 5 years. At the conclusion of the study there were no differences in renal outcomes, blood pressure control or cardiovascular events. Unfortunately 40% of the enrollees had a stenosis of less than 50% and 25% had normal renal function [36]. Only 79% of the patients randomized to revascularization had a successful procedure. As with the STAR trial the major criticism of ASTRAL is that patients enrolled were not at high risk for outcomes. For any trial to produce reliable data it is important that there be clinical equipoise; meaning there is true uncertainty concerning benefit of the therapeutic maneuver. Because in the ASTRAL trial clinicians could exclude a patient based on whether or not they felt stenting would be beneficial a selection bias was introduced that tainted the results.

The Cardiovascular Outcomes in Renal Atherosclerotic Lesions (CORAL) study was designed to address the methodologic shortcomings raised in the prior studies [32]. To be enrolled in the study subjects had to have a BP greater than 155 mmHg on two or more medications, have stenosis of between 80 and less than 100% of the artery or if between 60 and 80% there needed to be a systolic pressure gradient of at least 20 mmHg. Because of slow recruitment, the BP criteria was dropped as long the patient had an eGFR less than 60 ml/min/1.73 m^2. In addition, significant stenosis could be identified by modalities other than angiography. Subjects were excluded from participation if they had chronic kidney from a cause other than ischemic nephropathy, a creatinine higher than 2 mg/dl or a kidney smaller than 7 cm. 947 subjects were randomized in a 1:1 fashion to medical therapy or medical therapy and revascularization. Medical therapy included the angiotensin receptor blocker, candesartan (with or without hydrochlorothiazide) and combination amlodipine atorvastatin. Goal BP was less than 140/90 in patients without other comorbid conditions and less than 130/80 in those subjects with diabetes or chronic kidney disease. Subjects were followed for a median period of 43 months. As with the other trials there was no significant difference between groups in regards to cardiovascular or renal outcomes. In the patients who had undergone stenting there was a 2.3 mmHg decrease in systolic blood pressure ($p = 0.3$). Although a well-conducted study, because of lack of clinical equipoise the subjects were not high risk. The average stenosis verified by the core laboratory was only 67% [37]. In an unplanned post hoc analysis the investigators examined outcome data from within three subgroups: (1) patients with higher degree of stenosis, (2) patients with higher trans-lesional pressure gradients and (3) patients with higher baseline blood pressure to assess if revascularization was beneficial [38]. In comparisons using either quartiles or predefined thresholds no difference was noted between the two arms. As would be expected this analysis was also considered flawed, because each group was analyzed independently instead of looking specifically at patients who were in the upper range in all three parameters [37].

When interpreting the randomized trials two confounders standout: (1) the studies included many subjects who were not high risk and (2) many patients with atherosclerotic renal vascular disease have essential hypertension and/or underlying renal damage. It would not be expected that revascularization would improve blood pressure or reverse renal disease in these individuals.

Kalra et al. [13] using Medicare data between 1992 and 2004 showed that patients with atherosclerotic renovascular disease who did not undergo revascularization had an adjusted mortality hazard ratio between 1.55 and 2.28. In distinction those patients who had revascularization procedures had an adjusted mortality hazard ratio between 0.65 and 0.88. Although these data do not prove that revascularization is beneficial, they suggest that there may be a population in whom revascularization is favorable to medical therapy.

Pooled data from five prospective, industry sponsored, United States Food and Drug Administration investigational device exemption studies were analyzed for efficacy in reducing blood pressure by Weinberg and colleagues [39]. Subjects were recruited for these trials if they had blood pressures greater than 140/90 on 3 anti-hypertensive medications. At 9 months, systolic BP had dropped from 164 to 146 mmHg ($p < 0.0001$) and diastolic BP from 79 to 76 mmHg ($p < 0.0001$). Baseline systolic BP greater than 150 mmHg was associated with a positive response with revascularization.

Ritchie et al. [40] in an analysis of data from the United Kingdom showed that patients who presented with flash pulmonary edema who underwent revascularization had a reduced risk of death (HR 0.4) versus those who were treated medically (HR 2.2). In patients with rapidly declining renal function or refractory hypertension revascularization did not show a benefit, although if both these conditions were present revascularization was associated with a reduce risk of death (HR 0.2). Again these data need to be interpreted with caution until a randomized trial of high risk patients is conducted.

Diagnosis of Clinically Significant Renal Artery Stenosis

Because renal artery disease in a majority of patients can be successfully treated medically with control of blood pressure and cholesterol lowering agents, it is unnecessary to evaluate most patients for the presence of renal artery stenosis. It is clear from the randomized studies that routine stenting of atherosclerotic renal artery stenosis is not warranted. However, even the most diehard therapeutic nihilists do not believe that there is never an indication for revascularization. There are individuals who do benefit. Practice guidelines from the American College of Cardiology (ACC) [41] and the Society for Cardiac Angiography and Interventions (SCAI) [42] still recommend revascularization in specific patients. The ACC guidelines that were published in 2006 recommend diagnostic evaluation in patients with: (1) Resistant or malignant hypertension, (2) New or worsening azotemia after initiation of an ACE inhibitor or angiotensin blocker, (3) renal asymmetry of greater than 1.5 cm and (4) unexplained sudden onset of pulmonary edema. The SCAI guidelines add little further guidance.

In a meta-analysis of 11 studies no clinical predictors were found that could identify patients who would have improved renal function after revascularization [43]. This is understandable because it is unlikely that ischemic damage can be reversed. In the same study high baseline diastolic pressure was the best predictor of a post-procedure decrease in diastolic pressure; whereas an increased pulse pressure (a marker of arterial stiffness) was a negative predictor of a drop in systolic blood pressure [43].

In high-risk patients (Table 40.1) diagnostic evaluation is aimed at identifying renal artery lesion that limit renal perfusion and produce ischemia. These are the lesions in which a revascularization procedure is most likely to improve clinical outcomes. Most commonly used diagnostic strategies are aimed at initially assessing anatomically significant stenosis (>70–80%) and not the presence of renal ischemia. There are three tests that can be used to screen for the presence of renal artery stenosis: Duplex renal ultrasonography (DUS), computed tomographic angiography (CTA), and magnetic resonance angiography (MRA). Published assessments of these methodologies suffer from publication bias and small size of the study population. The appropriate diagnostic strategy should be based on center expertise, patient habitus and risks of adverse events due to contrast.

Duplex ultrasonography is noninvasive and less costly than other screening tests. The results, however, are extremely operator dependent. Measuring peak systolic velocity has the best performance characteristics [44]. Published investigations report sensitivity between 75–99% and specificity of 90–99% [44–46]. The utility of DUS is limited in the presence of excess bowel gas and in obese subjects. CTA and MRA appear slightly better at diagnosing significant stenosis than DUS, especially involving the branch renal arteries [46–48]. Both these contrast enhanced methods, however, have the potential for adverse effects in patients with significant underlying renal dysfunction. Newer magnetic resonance techniques using time-spatial labeling inversion pulse avoids the need for gadolinium and appears to provide similar results to CTA [49, 50].

The gold standard for the diagnosis of renal artery stenosis is invasive renal arteriography. However, even this "gold standard" does not always accurately predict the severity of the blockage. The calculation of the percent

Table 40.1 Predictors of individuals at high risk for critical renal artery stenosis

Predictors
Flash pulmonary edema
Resistant hypertension
Asymmetry in renal size
Diastolic renal artery bruit
Progressive renal failure
Hypertension in young women

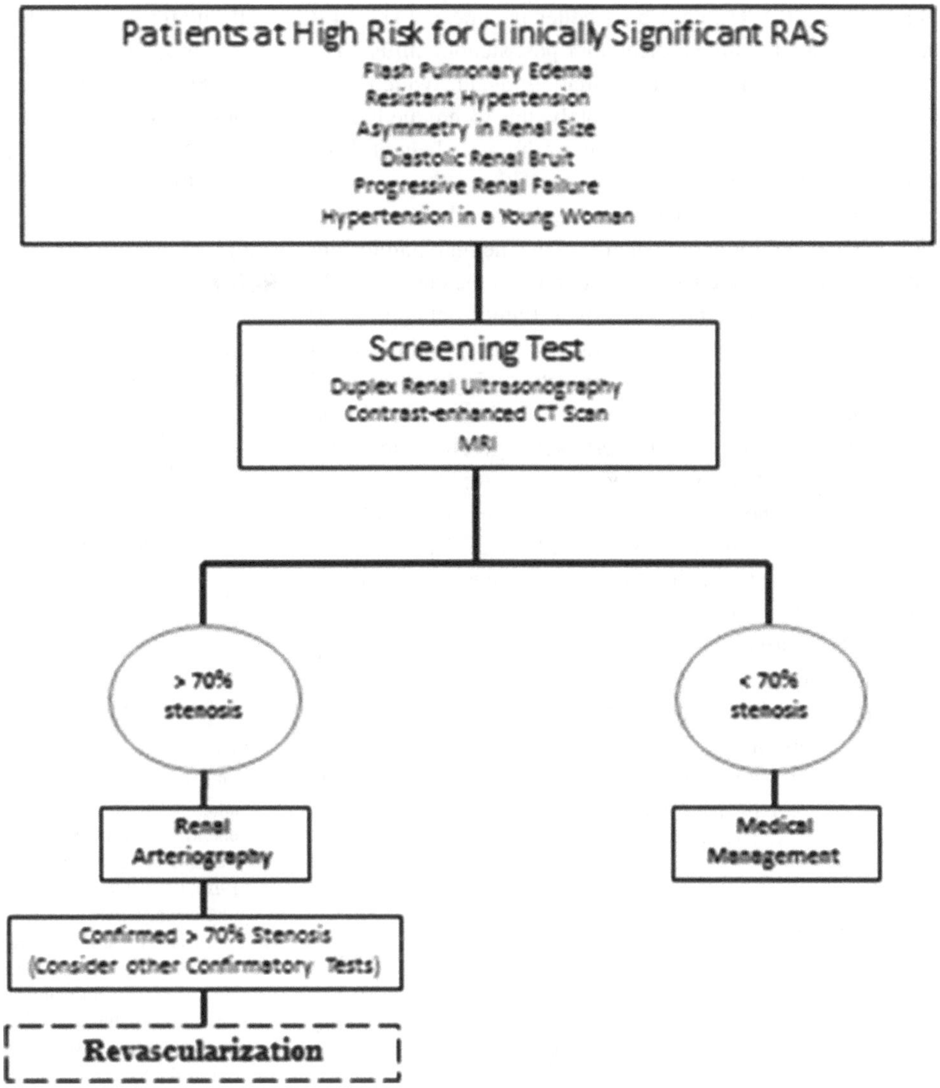

Fig. 40.1 Proposed algorithm for evaluation and management of suspected renal artery stenosis

stenosis based on the two-dimensional image may vary depending on the projection in which the image was obtained and interpretation of the degree of obstruction by the observers. Furthermore, what degree of renal artery stenosis produces renal ischemia is unclear [51]. Because of their function as filtering units, the kidneys receive far more blood than is necessary for metabolic demands. In addition delivery of oxygenated blood beyond an obstruction is dependent on cardiac output and blood pressure [52]. Measurement of tissue oxygenation using blood oxygen level-dependent (BOLD) MRI demonstrates that despite significant decreases in renal perfusion, post-stenosis renal cortical and medullary oxygenation is maintained [53].

The Holy Grail in the evaluation of patients with renal artery disease is to be able to predict which patient will respond to revascularization. Several different methodologies have been developed to better assess renal ischemia. One method to determine if the stenosis is significant enough to limit renal perfusion is to measure the trans-stenotic pressure gradient. In 15 patients with renal artery stenosis, after successful stenting, graded degrees of obstruction were obtained using a balloon catheter and renal vein renin was measured [54]. Increases in renin occurred when the pressure distal to the graded obstruction was less than 90% of aortic pressure and became maximal at 50%. Thus measurement of pressure gradient may provide useful information. However, as already noted the translesional gradient may vary depending on cardiac output, blood pressure and renal vascular resistance. Furthermore, post hoc analysis of the CORAL trial did not show a benefit of stenting over medical therapy based on peak systolic pressure gradient [38]. In a small prospective study, the translesional gradient was unable to predict a beneficial response to stenting in either blood pressure or renal function [55, 56].

In order to avoid the pitfalls associated with the use of a pressure gradient it has been suggested that renal fractional flow reserve (FFR) might be a better parameter [51]. FFR measures the pressure gradient after post-stenotic infusion of an endothelium independent dilating agent, which thus maximizes blood flow. Unfortunately, this technique has not been shown to be able to predict who will benefit from revascularization [55, 56].

Another recently reported methodology that may provides better information regarding the hemodynamic significance of a stenotic lesion is the renal frame count (RFC). This is the number cineangiographic frames obtained at 30 frames/s for radiocontrast to flow from the proximal renal artery to the smallest cortical branches. Naghi et al. [57] found that a RFC > 30 was associated with improved blood pressure control after renal artery stenting. This interesting observation needs to be verified in future studies.

Newer technologies that have future potential are dynamic contrast enhanced MRI and BOLD MRI. Dynamic contrast enhanced MRI has the ability to measure numerous parameters including renal blood flow, single kidney glomerular filtration rate, and extraction fraction [58]. Whether such measurements will be useful for choosing those patients who will benefit from renal artery stenting has yet to be determined. BOLD-MRI can show areas of renal ischemia [59]. Future studies need to examine whether this technology can be useful in identifying patients who will benefit from revascularization.

Conclusions

The incidence of atherosclerotic renal artery stenosis increases with age and affects approximately 7% of the population over the age of 65 and is found far more frequently in individuals with other evidence of atherosclerotic disease. Because of the failure of several large randomized trials to show a benefit of renal revascularization compared to medical therapy, the initial enthusiasm associated with percutaneous interventions have waned. These studies have conclusively demonstrated that the majority of patients with renal artery stenosis can be managed with medical therapy alone. Yet there are clearly patients who will benefit from revascularization. Severely compromised renal perfusion activates an extensive hormonal network that increases blood pressure. Renal ischemia results in loss of microvascular structures, tubular dropout, loss of glomeruli and fibrosis with a decline in renal function. The challenge is to identify those patients who will benefit from revascularization. Although new imaging technologies are being studied, none have yet to be validated as useful to predict successful outcomes from renal stenting. Until we have better diagnostic tools only those patients who are considered high risk should be evaluated (see Fig. 40.1). Initially these patients should be screened noninvasively. If noninvasive techniques confirm the presence of stenosis, the next step is renal angiography. Lesions > 70–80% should be corrected. This protocol will obviously miss patients who might benefit as well as intervene on patients who will not benefit, but overall should provide the best evaluation and management for all.

References

1. Peng M, Jiang XJ, Dong H, et al. Etiology of renal artery stenosis in 2047 patients: a single-center retrospective analysis during a 15-year period in China. J Hum Hypertens. 2016;30:124–8.
2. Anderson GH Jr, Blakeman N, Streeten DH. The effect of age on prevalence of secondary forms of hypertension in 4429 consecutively referred patients. J Hypertens. 1994;12:609–15.
3. Holley KE, Hunt JC, Brown AL Jr, Kincaid OW, Sheps SG. Renal artery stenosis. A clinical-pathologic study in normotensive and hypertensive patients. Am J Med. 1964;37:14–22.
4. Buller CE, Nogareda JG, Ramanathan K, et al. The profile of cardiac patients with renal artery stenosis. J Am Coll Cardiol. 2004;43:1606–13.
5. Harding MB, Smith LR, Himmelstein SI, et al. Renal artery stenosis: prevalence and associated risk factors in patients undergoing routine cardiac catheterization. J Am Soc Nephrol. 1992;2:1608–16.
6. Olin JW, Melia M, Young JR, Graor RA, Risius B. Prevalence of atherosclerotic renal artery stenosis in patients with atherosclerosis elsewhere. Am J Med. 1990;88:46N–51N.
7. Zandparsa A, Habashizadeh M, Moradi Farsani E, Jabbari M, Rezaei R. Relationship between renal artery stenosis and severity of coronary artery disease in patients with coronary atherosclerotic disease. Int Cardiovasc Res J. 2012;6:84–7.
8. Burlacu A, Siriopol D, Voroneanu L, et al. Atherosclerotic renal artery stenosis prevalence and correlations in acute myocardial infarction patients undergoing primary percutaneous coronary interventions: data from nonrandomized single-center study (REN-ACS)—a single center, prospective, observational study. J Am Heart Assoc. 2015;4:e002379.
9. van Ampting JM, Penne EL, Beek FJ, Koomans HA, Boer WH, Beutler JJ. Prevalence of atherosclerotic renal artery stenosis in patients starting dialysis. Nephrol Dial Transplant. 2003;18:1147–51.
10. Detection, evaluation, and treatment of renovascular hypertension. Final report. Working group on renovascular hypertension. Arch Intern Med 1987;147:820–9.
11. Alhaddad IA, Blum S, Heller EN, et al. Renal artery stenosis in minority patients undergoing diagnostic cardiac catheterization: prevalence and risk factors. J Cardiovasc Pharmacol Ther. 2001;6:147–53.
12. Jazrawi A, Darda S, Burke P, et al. Is race a risk factor for the development of renal artery stenosis? Cardiol Res Pract. 2009;2009:817987.
13. Kalra PA, Guo H, Gilbertson DT, et al. Atherosclerotic renovascular disease in the United States. Kidney Int. 2010;77:37–43.
14. Murphy TP, Soares G, Kim M. Increase in utilization of percutaneous renal artery interventions by medicare beneficiaries, 1996–2000. AJR Am J Roentgenol. 2004;183:561–8.
15. Plouin PF, Perdu J, La Batide-Alanore A, Boutouyrie P, Gimenez-Roqueplo AP, Jeunemaitre X. Fibromuscular dysplasia. Orphanet J Rare Dis. 2007;2:28.
16. Alibaz-Oner F, Direskeneli H. Update on Takayasu's arteritis. Presse Med. 2015;44:e259–65.

17. Hall S, Barr W, Lie JT, Stanson AW, Kazmier FJ, Hunder GG. Takayasu arteritis. A study of 32 North American patients. Medicine (Baltimore). 1985;64:89–99.
18. Peng M, Jiang XJ, Dong H, et al. Etiology of renal artery stenosis in 2047 patients: a single-center retrospective analysis during a 15-year period in China. J Hum Hypertens. 2016;30:124–8.
19. Arend WP, Michel BA, Bloch DA, et al. The American College of Rheumatology 1990 criteria for the classification of Takayasu arteritis. Arthritis Rheum. 1990;33:1129–34.
20. Goldblatt H, Lynch J, Hanzal RF, Summerville WW. Studies on experimental hypertension: I. The production of persistent elevation of systolic blood pressure by means of renal ischemia. J Exp Med. 1934;59:347–79.
21. Martinez-Maldonado M. Pathophysiology of renovascular hypertension. Hypertension. 1991;17:707–19.
22. Eirin A, Gloviczki ML, Tang H, et al. Inflammatory and injury signals released from the post-stenotic human kidney. Eur Heart J. 2013;34:540–548a.
23. Eirin A, Gloviczki ML, Tang H, et al. Chronic renovascular hypertension is associated with elevated levels of neutrophil gelatinase-associated lipocalin. Nephrol Dial Transplant. 2012;27:4153–61.
24. Saad A, Herrmann SM, Crane J, et al. Stent revascularization restores cortical blood flow and reverses tissue hypoxia in atherosclerotic renal artery stenosis but fails to reverse inflammatory pathways or glomerular filtration rate. Circ Cardiovasc Interv. 2013;6:428–35.
25. Mui KW, Sleeswijk M, van den Hout H, van Baal J, Navis G, Woittiez AJ. Incidental renal artery stenosis is an independent predictor of mortality in patients with peripheral vascular disease. J Am Soc Nephrol. 2006;17:2069–74.
26. Shafique S, Peixoto AJ. Renal artery stenosis and cardiovascular risk. J Clin Hypertens (Greenwich). 2007;9:201–8.
27. Messerli FH, Bangalore S, Makani H, et al. Flash pulmonary oedema and bilateral renal artery stenosis: the Pickering syndrome. Eur Heart J. 2011;32:2231–5.
28. Pickering TG, Herman L, Devereux RB, et al. Recurrent pulmonary oedema in hypertension due to bilateral renal artery stenosis: treatment by angioplasty or surgical revascularisation. Lancet. 1988;2:551–2.
29. Pelta A, Andersen UB, Just S, Baekgaard N. Flash pulmonary edema in patients with renal artery stenosis—the Pickering syndrome. Blood Press. 2011;20:15–9.
30. Messina LM, Zelenock GB, Yao KA, Stanley JC. Renal revascularization for recurrent pulmonary edema in patients with poorly controlled hypertension and renal insufficiency: a distinct subgroup of patients with arteriosclerotic renal artery occlusive disease. J Vasc Surg. 1992;15:73–80 (discussion-2).
31. Bax L, Woittiez AJ, Kouwenberg HJ, et al. Stent placement in patients with atherosclerotic renal artery stenosis and impaired renal function: a randomized trial. Ann Intern Med. 2009;150(840–8):W150–1.
32. Cooper CJ, Murphy TP, Cutlip DE, et al. Stenting and medical therapy for atherosclerotic renal-artery stenosis. N Engl J Med. 2014;370:13–22.
33. Investigators A, Wheatley K, Ives N, et al. Revascularization versus medical therapy for renal-artery stenosis. N Engl J Med. 2009;361:1953–62.
34. Jenks S, Yeoh SE, Conway BR. Balloon angioplasty, with and without stenting, versus medical therapy for hypertensive patients with renal artery stenosis. Cochrane Database Syst Rev. 2014;12: CD002944.
35. Herrmann SM, Saad A, Textor SC. Management of atherosclerotic renovascular disease after Cardiovascular Outcomes in Renal Atherosclerotic Lesions (CORAL). Nephrol Dial Transplant. 2015;30:366–75.
36. Mohan IV, Bourke V. The management of renal artery stenosis: an alternative interpretation of ASTRAL and CORAL. Eur J Vasc Endovasc Surg. 2015;49:465–73.
37. White CJ. The "chicken little" of renal stent trials: the CORAL trial in perspective. JACC Cardiovasc Interv. 2014;7:111–3.
38. Murphy TP, Cooper CJ, Matsumoto AH, et al. Renal artery stent outcomes: effect of baseline blood pressure, stenosis severity, and translesion pressure gradient. J Am Coll Cardiol. 2015;66: 2487–94.
39. Weinberg I, Keyes MJ, Giri J, et al. Blood pressure response to renal artery stenting in 901 patients from five prospective multicenter FDA-approved trials. Catheter Cardiovasc Interv. 2014;83:603–9.
40. Ritchie J, Green D, Chrysochou C, Chalmers N, Foley RN, Kalra PA. High-risk clinical presentations in atherosclerotic renovascular disease: prognosis and response to renal artery revascularization. Am J Kidney Dis. 2014;63:186–97.
41. Hirsch AT, Haskal ZJ, Hertzer NR, et al. ACC/AHA 2005 guidelines for the management of patients with peripheral arterial disease (lower extremity, renal, mesenteric, and abdominal aortic): executive summary a collaborative report from the American Association for Vascular Surgery/Society for Vascular Surgery, Society for Cardiovascular Angiography and Interventions, Society for Vascular Medicine and Biology, Society of Interventional Radiology, and the ACC/AHA Task Force on Practice Guidelines (Writing Committee to Develop Guidelines for the Management of Patients With Peripheral Arterial Disease) endorsed by the American Association of Cardiovascular and Pulmonary Rehabilitation; National Heart, Lung, and Blood Institute; Society for Vascular Nursing; TransAtlantic Inter-Society Consensus; and Vascular Disease Foundation. J Am Coll Cardiol. 2006;47: 1239–312.
42. Parikh SA, Shishehbor MH, Gray BH, White CJ, Jaff MR. SCAI expert consensus statement for renal artery stenting appropriate use. Catheter Cardiovasc Interv. 2014;84:1163–71.
43. Ronden RA, Houben AJ, Kessels AG, Stehouwer CD, de Leeuw PW, Kroon AA. Predictors of clinical outcome after stent placement in atherosclerotic renal artery stenosis: a systematic review and meta-analysis of prospective studies. J Hypertens. 2010;28:2370–7.
44. Williams GJ, Macaskill P, Chan SF, et al. Comparative accuracy of renal duplex sonographic parameters in the diagnosis of renal artery stenosis: paired and unpaired analysis. AJR Am J Roentgenol. 2007;188:798–811.
45. Olin JW, Piedmonte MR, Young JR, DeAnna S, Grubb M, Childs MB. The utility of duplex ultrasound scanning of the renal arteries for diagnosing significant renal artery stenosis. Ann Intern Med. 1995;122:833–8.
46. Rountas C, Vlychou M, Vassiou K, et al. Imaging modalities for renal artery stenosis in suspected renovascular hypertension: prospective intraindividual comparison of color Doppler US, CT angiography, GD-enhanced MR angiography, and digital substraction angiography. Ren Fail. 2007;29:295–302.
47. Eklof H, Ahlstrom H, Magnusson A, et al. A prospective comparison of duplex ultrasonography, captopril renography, MRA, and CTA in assessing renal artery stenosis. Acta Radiol. 2006;47:764–74.
48. Eriksson P, Mohammed AA, De Geer J, et al. Non-invasive investigations of potential renal artery stenosis in renal insufficiency. Nephrol Dial Transplant. 2010;25:3607–14.
49. Albert TS, Akahane M, Parienty I, et al. An international multicenter comparison of time-SLIP unenhanced MR angiography and contrast-enhanced CT angiography for assessing renal artery stenosis: the renal artery contrast-free trial. AJR Am J Roentgenol. 2015;204:182–8.

50. Angeretti MG, Lumia D, Cani A, et al. Non-enhanced MR angiography of renal arteries: comparison with contrast-enhanced MR angiography. Acta Radiol. 2013;54:749–56.
51. Subramanian R, White CJ, Rosenfield K, et al. Renal fractional flow reserve: a hemodynamic evaluation of moderate renal artery stenoses. Catheter Cardiovasc Interv. 2005;64:480–6.
52. Textor SC, Lerman LO. Paradigm shifts in atherosclerotic renovascular disease: where are we now? J Am Soc Nephrol. 2015;26:2074–80.
53. Gloviczki ML, Glockner JF, Lerman LO, et al. Preserved oxygenation despite reduced blood flow in poststenotic kidneys in human atherosclerotic renal artery stenosis. Hypertension. 2010;55:961–6.
54. De Bruyne B, Manoharan G, Pijls NH, et al. Assessment of renal artery stenosis severity by pressure gradient measurements. J Am Coll Cardiol. 2006;48:1851–5.
55. Kadziela J, Januszewicz A, Prejbisz A, et al. Prognostic value of renal fractional flow reserve in blood pressure response after renal artery stenting (PREFER study). Cardiol J. 2013;20:418–22.
56. Kadziela J, Prejbisz A, Michalowska I, et al. Relationship between hemodynamic parameters of renal artery stenosis and the changes of kidney function after renal artery stenting in patients with hypertension and preserved renal function. Blood Press. 2015;24:30–4.
57. Naghi J, Palakodeti S, Ang L, Reeves R, Patel M, Mahmud E. Renal frame count: a measure of renal flow that predicts success of renal artery stenting in hypertensive patients. Catheter Cardiovasc Interv. 2015;86:304–9.
58. Lim SW, Chrysochou C, Buckley DL, Kalra PA, Sourbron SP. Prediction and assessment of responses to renal artery revascularization with dynamic contrast-enhanced magnetic resonance imaging: a pilot study. Am J Physiol Renal Physiol. 2013;305:F672–8.
59. Gloviczki ML, Saad A, Textor SC. Blood oxygen level-dependent (BOLD) MRI analysis in atherosclerotic renal artery stenosis. Curr Opin Nephrol Hypertens. 2013;22:519–24.

Renal Denervation: Current Opinions and Practice

41

Markus P. Schlaich

The Role of Renal Sympathetic Nerves in Cardiovascular Control

The renal sympathetic nerves consist of efferent sympathetic fibers and afferent sensory fibers. The renal efferent nerves supply all relevant structures including the renal vasculature, the tubules, and the juxtaglomerular apparatus [1]. Accordingly, excitation of the renal efferent sympathetic nerves results in (i) urinary sodium and water retention via enhanced tubular sodium reabsorption, (ii) reduction in renal blood flow and glomerular filtration rate (GFR) through neurally mediated vasoconstriction, and (iii) release of renin by stimulation of β[beta]1-adrenoceptors on the juxtaglomerular apparatus with concomitant engagement of the renin–angiotensin–aldosterone system [2–4].

The renal afferent sensory nerves are predominantly located in the renal pelvic wall [5, 6]. In contrast to renal efferent nerves, afferent nerves project to the ipsilateral dorsal root ganglia at the level of T6-L2 with the majority of the nerve cell bodies residing at the level of T9-L1. Through integrative processes in the paraventricular nuclei, renal afferent nerve stimulation results in alterations of baroreceptor sensitivity, vagal function, and central dopaminergic tone, and an increase in systemic sympathetic nervous activity [7, 8] (Fig. 41.1). Increased renal afferent activity is also known to decrease renal efferent activity through the powerful negative feedback control of reno-renal reflexes via mechano-receptor-mediated pathways [6, 9]. Furthermore, through an elegantly demonstrated feedback loop, increased renal efferent activity increases renal afferent activity [10].

M.P. Schlaich (✉)
Dobney Hypertension Centre, School of Medicine and Pharmacology – Royal Hospital Unit, University of Western Australia, Level 3, MRF Building, 50 Rear Murray Street, Perth, WA 6000, Australia
e-mail: markus.schlaich@uwa.edu.au

J. Rangaswami et al. (eds.), *Cardio-Nephrology*,
DOI 10.1007/978-3-319-56042-7_41

Rationale of Targeting Renal Sympathetic Nerves in Chronic Kidney Disease

Elevated sympathetic nervous system activity has been demonstrated to play a key role in hypertension as well as in various cardiovascular conditions and chronic kidney disease [11]. Stimulation of renal afferent nerves caused by various mechanisms including ischemia and uremic toxins increases systemic sympathetic outflow via central integrative pathways in the hypothalamus. Sustained sympathetic overactivity per se and the associated rise in blood pressure are relevant factors contributing to further deterioration of renal function [12]. The kidneys are, therefore, not only effector organs of sympathetic outflow, but also an important modulator of sympathetic nervous system activity [13].

Targeting renal sympathetic nerves in hypertension and other cardio-renal conditions appears as a logical therapeutic option to block the vicious cycle between renal sympathetic nervous hyperactivity and deterioration of kidney function. In fact, attempts were undertaken to modulate renal sympatho-excitation to relieve symptoms of patients with renal failure since the early 1930s [14]. Despite the demonstration of a survival benefit, surgical denervation, most commonly splanchnicectomy, was plagued by a number of complications relating primarily to its nonspecific nature. Meanwhile, studies in many experimental animal models of hypertension have convincingly demonstrated the blood pressure lowering and renoprotective effects of sympathetic inhibition achieved by renal denervation.

Introduction of Catheter-Based Renal Denervation in Human Resistant Hypertension

Surgical sectioning of sympathetic nerves by thoracic and lumbar sympathectomy and splanchnicectomy has been applied successfully to reduce blood pressure and improve

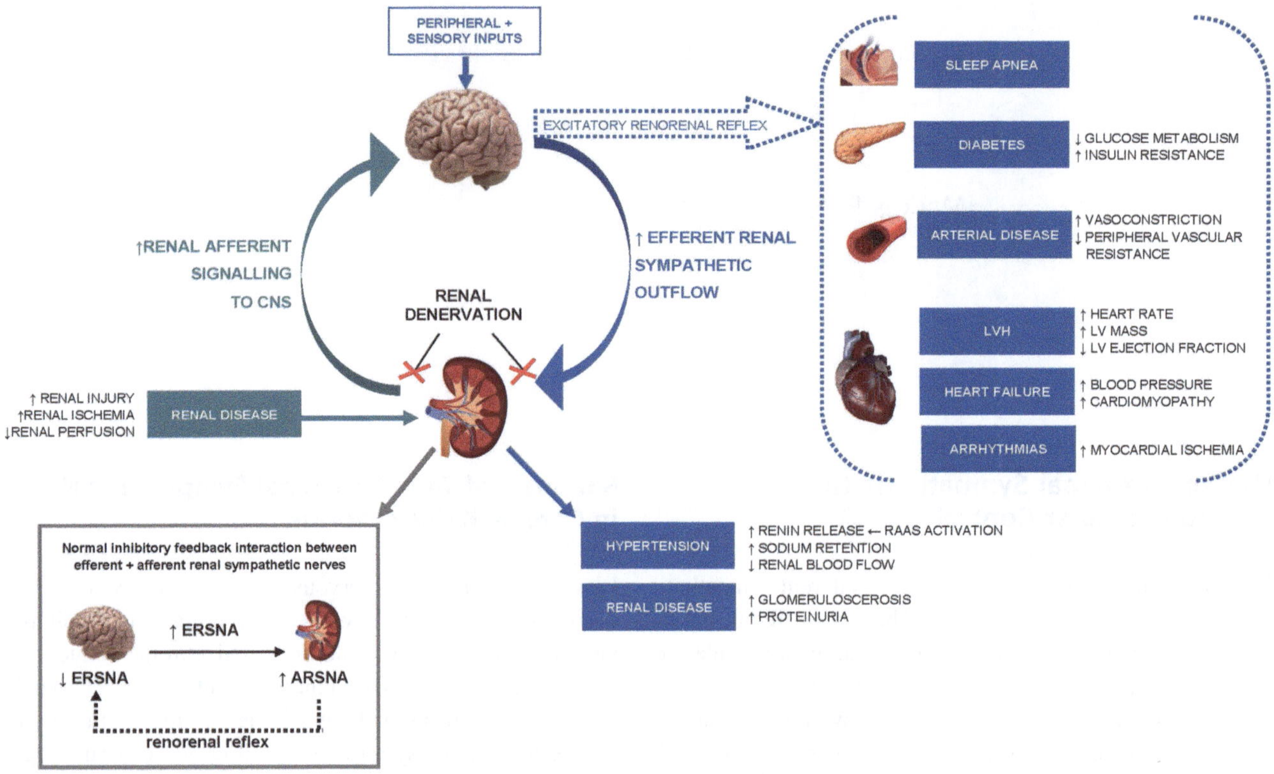

Fig. 41.1 Schematic illustration of the role of increased renal efferent sympathetic outflow and increased renal afferent sensory signaling in the pathophysiology of hypertension and other cardiovascular, renal, and metabolic disease states. *ERSNA* Efferent Renal Sympathetic Nerve Activity, *ARSNA* Afferent Renal Sympathetic Nerve Activity, *RAAS* Renin–Angiotensin–Aldosterone System, *LVH* Left Ventricular Hypertrophy, *LV* Left Ventricular, *CNS* Central Nervous System

the long-term outcome of patients with hypertension [15, 16]. Studies in animals have also demonstrated the significant benefit of reduction in sympathetic nervous activity [17], improvement in natriuresis [18], and improvement in left ventricular function [19]. The introduction of catheter-based radiofrequency ablation of renal sympathetic nerves to clinical medicine has been considered as a promising new avenue to device-based therapies for hypertension. Renal sympathetic efferent and afferent nerves located in the adventitia of the renal arteries are the target of this procedure [5].

The Symplicity HTN Studies

The Symplicity HTN trial program was initiated to assess the safety and utility of a catheter-based approach to achieve renal denervation. The initial proof-of-concept study, Symplicity HTN-1 [20], demonstrated the safety and efficacy of catheter-based renal denervation in 45 patients with resistant hypertension. While only minor procedure-related complications were reported [21], the reduction in office systolic and diastolic blood pressure was substantial (−14/−10, −21/−10, −22/−11, −24/−11 and −27/−17 mmHg at 1, 3, 6, 9 and 12 months follow-up respectively from an average BP of 177/101 mmHg at baseline [20]. A sustained long-term effect of renal denervation on blood pressure (−32/−14 mmHg) was recently described in the 36 months follow-up report [22]. While the office blood pressure fall from baseline did not differ between groups dichotomized by eGFR (>60 and 45–60 ml/min/1.73 m^2), the safety of the procedure could also be confirmed for stage 3b CKD. The release of norepinephrine from the renal sympathetic nerves was measured in ten patients using isotope dilution renal norepinephrine spillover methodology [20]. At 30 days after the procedure, the renal norepinephrine spillover was decreased by 47%, suggesting a substantial albeit incomplete reduction of renal efferent sympathetic nerve traffic [20].

Results from the subsequent Symplicity HTN-2 study, a randomized, controlled clinical trial were reported in 2010 and 2012 [23, 24]. Patients with resistant hypertension were randomized to either undergo RDN with continued pharmacological treatment (n = 52) or to continue their established conventional pharmacological treatment alone (n = 54). In line with the results of Symplicity HTN-1, renal denervation reduced office blood pressure by −32 ± 23/12 ± 11 mmHg at 6 month follow-up [23], with sustained effects reported at 12-month follow-up (−28 ± 25/10 ± 11 mmHg) [24].

In contrast, no significant change was observed in the control group (1 ± 21/0 ± 10 in office blood pressure, and 2 ± 13/7 ± 11 mmHg in home blood pressure) [23]. Mean eGFR was unchanged in both groups at 6 month (0.2 ± 11 ml/min/1.73 m^2 in renal denervation group, and 0.9 ± 12 ml/min/1.73 m^2 in control group) [23].

The results of the latest, largest, and most rigorously designed clinical trial of catheter-based renal denervation, Symplicity HTN-3, have been reported recently [25]. This study was a randomized, blinded, sham-controlled trial. Patients in the control group underwent a renal angiogram and a sham procedure. Stable medication regimens were to be implemented and had to be unchanged for at least 2 weeks prior to enrollment. 24-h ambulatory blood pressure monitoring was performed to confirm an average 24-h systolic blood pressure ≥135 mmHg to exclude white-coat hypertension. Safety and efficacy endpoints were assessed at 6-month follow-up. During the 6-month follow-up period, the regimen of antihypertensive medication was supposed to be kept stable with medication changes allowed only if deemed clinically necessary. Among 535 uncontrolled hypertensive patients, 364 patients were blindly allocated to treatment group and underwent renal denervation across 88 centers in the United States. At 6 months after the procedure, a significant drop in office systolic blood pressure from baseline had occurred in the treatment group, however, this was not statistically significant when compared to the BP fall observed in the sham procedure group (−14.1 ± 23.9 vs. −11.7 ± 25.9 mmHg, $p = 0.26$).

In comparison to Symplicity HTN-1 and HTN-2, the reduction in office blood pressure in the treatment group was less pronounced (−14.1 ± 23.9/−6.6 ± 11.9 in HTN-3 vs. −22/−11 mmHg in HTN-1 20 and −32 ± 23/ −12 ± 11 mmHg in HTN-2) [23]. Furthermore, there was a large BP effect in the sham control group with the drop in office systolic blood pressure being more pronounced than in the non-blinded control group of Symplicity HTN-2; (−11.7 ± 25.3 vs. 1 ± 21 mmHg in HTN-2) [23]. Although the pretreatment blood pressure was similar, the greater range of standard deviation in the treatment group of HTN-3 indicates a wider variation in response. Interestingly, a prespecified subgroup analysis revealed that while no difference in BP changes between RDN and sham control were evident in patients with an African-American background, there was a significant difference in non-African Americans, perhaps indicating that racial background may influence the response to the procedure. Of note, patients of African-American descent have previously been shown to respond less favorably to treatment with angiotensin-converting enzyme (ACE) inhibitors and beta-blockers [26].

Concerns have also been raised in regards to the operator experience in this US trial. The renal denervation procedures carried out as part of the Symplicity HTN-3 trial were performed by a total of 111 operators throughout the United States. Among them, 31% (34 operators) had only performed 1 procedure, and 85 operators had done less than 5 procedures [25]. Although no significant difference was observed in outcomes between operators who performed <5 procedures and others, this may not eliminate the possible influence of the operators' learning curve on relatively marginal reduction of blood pressure in the treatment group. From this point of view, ineffective renal denervation might have contributed to the neutral outcome of this study. Furthermore, the absence of tests to assess the degree of renal denervation makes it difficult to investigate this matter further.

The results from Symplicity HTN-3 raised some important issues that need to be resolved in future renal denervation studies. The procedure of catheter-based renal denervation is substantially different from traditional experimental denervation in animals, in which total renal denervation is accomplished by visually stripping and by painting phenol or xylocaine around the adventitia of the renal artery [18, 27, 28]. In contrast to animal experiments, a reliable test to confirm that renal denervation has been achieved is currently limited to invasive renal norepinephrine spillover methodology which is not suitable for wider clinical application [20, 29, 30].

While evidence for the utility of renal denervation from experimental animal studies is strong, the data from currently available randomized clinical trials is less conclusive and warrants further investigation with a specific focus on improvement of procedural aspects, identification of most suitable patient cohorts, and long-term outcomes.

More recently, several prospective, randomized controlled trials have reported either a modest or no effect of RDN on BP reduction in patients with resistant hypertension, each with their own limitations [31–34]. Two of the studies showed RDN to be at least equally effective [31, 32] to intensive pharmacotherapy in lowering BP in patients with true resistant hypertension, highlighting the ability of RDN to lower BP at least to the extent of additional pharmacologic treatment. The DENERV-HTN [31] study compared RDN in combination with standardized, stepped-care antihypertensive treatment (SSAHT) and observed a modest, albeit significant reduction in 6-month daytime SBP (adjusted mean difference of −5.9 mmHg (95% CI −11.3, −0.5; $p = 0.03$) compared to SSAHT alone [31]. Another study [32] applying a sham-controlled study design not dissimilar to that used in Symplicity HTN-3 found that in the per-protocol analysis, those who underwent RDN experienced a significantly more pronounced reduction in mean 24-h and daytime systolic BP at 6-months follow-up compared to patients treated with a sham procedure (−8.3 ± 8.9 vs. −3.5 ± 9.5 mmHg; $p = 0.04$).

Renal Denervation and Chronic Kidney Disease

The results from the aforementioned studies are of major interest for exploration of the therapeutic utility of renal denervation in the context of CKD. In fact, impaired kidney function is a common feature of patients presenting with resistant hypertension. Furthermore, fluid retention is a relevant pathophysiologic component of resistant hypertension and is promoted by increased sympathetic nerve activity, as is increased renin release. Renal denervation, therefore, appears as a sensible treatment approach in CKD patients with concomitant hypertension. While at this stage no randomized controlled clinical studies are available in this specific cohort, subgroup analyses from larger clinical trials and smaller mechanistic studies have started to explore this further.

While patients in the Symplicity HTN-2 trial had a mean eGFR of 77 ml/min/1.73 m^2 and patients with chronic kidney disease and eGFR <45 ml/min/1.73 m^2 were excluded [23], this study is important in the current context since it demonstrated that renal function assessed by serum creatinine, eGFR, and cystatin C concentrations were unchanged at 6 months, suggesting that the procedure itself and the associated haemodynamic changes have no adverse effects on the kidneys. Furthermore, longer term follow-up data of Symplicity HTN-1, in which again no patients with CKD and eGFR < 45 ml/min/1.73 m^2 were included, reported that during the first year of follow-up, eGFR remained stable [21]. In patients without newly added spironolactone or other diuretic therapy, eGFR changed by −7.8 mL/min/1.73 m^2, for an annualized change of −3.9 mL/min/1.73 m^2. In no case did serum creatinine double. Although it was a non-randomized study, the decline in renal function observed in this 24-month follow-up suggested that there might be an intrinsic beneficial effect of the procedure on the kidney to maintain renal function, which is greater than that achieved via BP reduction alone. In line with this notion is a recent report assessing the influence of renal denervation on renal haemodynamics, renal function, and urinary albumin excretion [35]. In this study, 88 patients with resistant hypertension and normal renal function underwent bilateral renal denervation. Systolic, diastolic, and pulse pressure were reduced by 22.7/26.6, 7.7/9.7, and 15.1/17.5 mmHg at 3 and 6 months follow-up, respectively. Furthermore, renal resistive index decreased from 0.691 ± 0.01 at baseline to 0.674 ± 0.01 and 0.670 ± 0.01 ($p < 0.05$) at 3 and 6 months follow-up, respectively; the proportion of patients with normal urinary albumin excretion increased by 5 and 12%; whereas proportion of patients with micro-albuminuria and macro-albuminuria decreased by 10 and 23%, at 3 and 6 month follow-up without effects on glomerular filtration rate within 6 months.

Whether this approach is safe and effective in patients with an estimated glomerular filtration rate below 45 ml/min/1.73 m^2 remains to be determined in appropriately designed clinical trials. However, preliminary evidence is available from small proof of concept studies. Hering et al. [36] reported the effects of catheter-based renal denervation in patients with resistant hypertension and moderate to severe CKD. An average of 5.0 ± 0.7 ablation treatments per artery were delivered without complications in any of the treated patients. Angiographic evaluation directly after renal denervation did not reveal any compromise of treated arteries. Importantly, eGFR remained stable in this patient cohort with 5 patients being followed up to 12 months. A significant drop in office blood pressure (−34/−14, −25/−11, −32/−15, and −33/−19 mmHg at 1, 3, 6, and 12 months after renal denervation, respectively) was observed without deterioration in renal function and renal blood flow. In contrast to office BP readings, mean 24-h BP and mean day BP were not significantly reduced after the procedure, possibly related to the limited number of valid ABPM available and substantial intra-individual variability. However, radiofrequency ablation treatment had a considerable impact on nocturnal blood pressure control. In addition, significant reduction in the rate of blood pressure rise, blood pressure power surge, and night-day blood pressure ratios were observed. Renal denervation also diminished mean and maximum night-time blood pressure and restored a physiologic dipping pattern in 9 out of 10 patients. The potential clinical relevance of these observations needs to be delineated in future studies.

Kiuchi et al. [37] reported similar beneficial effects of catheter-based renal denervation in 24 patients with CKD and refractory hypertension. Using an irrigated cardiac ablation catheter, a significant improvement in eGFR (from 64.4 ± 23.9 at baseline to 85.4 ± 34.9 ml/min/1.73 m^2 at 6 months follow-up after denervation) was observed. The reduction in office blood pressure (from 186 ± 19/108 ± 13 at baseline to 135 ± 13/88 ± 7 mmHg at 6 months after denervation) was substantial. A reduction in albuminuria was also reported after catheter-based renal denervation in patients with resistant hypertension [38].

Sympathetic nervous overactivity is pronounced not only in ESKD, but also in early stages of renal disease [39, 40]. Urinary albumin excretion, which is a reliable marker of early stage of CKD, correlated positively with elevated plasma norepinephrine levels in a cross-sectional study of 495 subjects from the general population [41]. Catheter-based renal denervation has been associated with a reduction of albuminuria [38].

Whether these beneficial effects may help to slow the progression of CKD is unknown, however, Ott et al. recently provided preliminary evidence from a small uncontrolled study to this effect. A total of 27 patients with CKD stage

3–4 underwent renal denervation for uncontrolled blood pressure [42] and renal function was evaluated for up to 3 years prior and 1 year after renal denervation. The change in estimated glomerular filtration rate (eGFR) was calculated by individual regression slopes for each patient before and after renal denervation. Mean baseline BP was 156 ± 12/82 ± 13 mmHg, despite treatment with 6.2 ± 1.1 antihypertensive drugs. One year after renal denervation, office BP was reduced by 20 ± 20 ($p < 0.001$)/8 ± 14 mmHg ($p = 0.005$) and average 24-h ambulatory BP by 9 ± 14 ($p = 0.009$)/4 ± 7 mmHg ($p = 0.019$). Before renal denervation, eGFR declined by −4.8 ± 3.8 ml/min per 1.73 m per year, and after renal denervation eGFR improved by +1.5 ± 10 ml/min per 1.73 m at 12 months ($p = 0.009$). These results indicate that in patients with CKD stages 3 and 4 renal denervation does not only decrease BP but appears to slow or even halt the decline of renal function.

A possible mechanism for the potential benefit of renal denervation on renal function may be a prominent vasodilatation in pre-glomerular arterioles due to inhibition of renal sympathetic nerve activity [43]. Lohmeier et al. [43] could demonstrate that renal denervation increased GFR without a change in fractional sodium reabsorption in dogs with obesity induced hypertension indicating that renal denervation alters glomerular filtration through the dilation of the renal afferent arteriole.

Another possible mechanism might be related to renalase, a protein reported to be secreted by the kidney and relevant for catecholamine metabolism [44, 45]. Renalase metabolizes circulating catecholamines, and renalase deficiency may therefore play a role in catecholamine excess. Plasma levels of renalase have been reported to be markedly suppressed in patients with renal failure and renalase activation induced by catecholamines appears attenuated in renal failure [46].

Interestingly, Jiang et al. [47] reported that plasma renalase content and renalase expression in the kidneys were higher in SHR after renal denervation than those in sham operated and other control groups, suggesting that renal denervation-induced blood pressure reductions could also be mediated in part by normalized or increased renalase levels.

Renal Denervation and End-Stage Kidney Disease

While substantial evidence supports the benefits of experimental renal denervation in animal models of ESKD [12], little is known about the effects of renal denervation in patients with ESKD. The initial proof-of-concept pilot study of catheter-based renal denervation in ESKD patients on dialysis (average time on dialysis was 3.6 ± 2.6 years) was tested in 12 patients with uncontrolled blood pressure [48]. All patients were on dialysis due to ESKD of various primary renal diseases including nephrosclerosis ($n = 4$), glomerulopathies ($n = 5$), IgA nephropathy ($n = 1$), nephrolithiasis ($n = 1$) and bilateral atrophic kidneys of unknown origin ($n = 1$). Catheter-based renal denervation was only feasible in nine patients whereas the remaining three patients were unable to undergo the procedure due to atrophic renal arteries.

The office systolic blood pressure decreased from 166 ± 16.0 to 148 ± 11, 150 ± 14, and 138 ± 17 mmHg at 3, 6 and 12-month follow-up, respectively, in patients who had undergone renal denervation ($n = 9$), whereas in the remaining 3 whose renal artery anatomy was not suitable, blood pressure remained unchanged (176 ± 7 vs. 172 ± 6 mmHg) at 3 month follow-up. 24-h ambulatory blood pressure measurements (ABPM) revealed a significant reduction in systolic blood pressure at 3 months ($n = 5$). Sympathetic nervous activity was significantly reduced after bilateral renal denervation in two patients in whom microneurography and noardenaline spillover measurements were obtained. The average number of antihypertensive medications following renal denervation was reduced from 4.2 ± 1.9 ($n = 9$) at baseline to 4.0 ± 1.9 ($n = 9$), 3.7 ± 2.3 ($n = 7$), and 2.2 ± 1.0 ($n = 5$) at 3, 6, and 12 months follow-up, respectively.

Several case reports have been published confirming possible benefit of catheter-based renal denervation in ESKD. One report describes a patient on hemodialysis treatment who received a kidney transplant around 4 months after his bilateral renal denervation procedure [48]. In the 3 months after RDN blood pressure was substantially reduced (from 156/95 to 133/81 mmHg) probably as a result of the demonstrated reduction in renal and total body NE spillover. Consistently, a significant reduction of MSNA was observed and was sustained for 33 months after renal denervation, despite both native kidneys still being in situ, but functionally denervated. Another case report of an ESKD patient with nephrosclerosis due to malignant hypertension demonstrated improved blood pressure control (average office blood pressure from 180 ± 15/105 ± 11 to 155 ± 14/90 ± 10 mmHg), reduced plasma renin (13.12–11.06 ng/mL/h) and angiotensin-converting enzyme activity (22.62–14.94 IU/L) at 1 month follow-up [49]. Although these reports have to be interpreted with caution, renal denervation may provide benefits for patients with ESKD. Larger and properly designed clinical trials are now warranted to determine the potential role of this therapeutic approach in ESKD.

Renal Denervation in Heart Failure and Cardiac Arrhythmias

Among the various conditions characterized by sympathetic activation, heart failure plays a crucial role in cardiovascular outcomes and is very common in patients with CKD and ESKD [50, 51]. Remarkably, sympathetic hyperactivity is known to occur in the early stage of asymptomatic heart failure with both preserved and reduced ejection fraction [52]. Given the role of renal denervation in sympathetic hyperactive conditions, renal denervation may possibly improve the outcomes of patients with heart failure. Surgical renal denervation was shown to improve the LV function of heart failure induced by myocardial infarction in Wistar rats [19]. Surgical renal denervation also restored natriuresis in response to atrial natriuretic peptide (ANP) in experimental ischemic heart failure dogs [53].

Several studies in resistant hypertensive patients have demonstrated that renal denervation reduces LV hypertrophy [54] and LV mass index [55]. The recurrence of atrial fibrillation (AF) has also been suggested to be reduced in hypertensive patients with chronic AF [56, 57].

Interestingly, a recent study demonstrated beneficial effects of RDN on atrial electrophysiologic and structural aspects [58]. Renal denervation performed in 14 patients with resistant hypertension not only reduced mean 24-h BP from 152/84 to 141/80 mmHg at 6-month follow-up ($p < 0.01$), but was also associated with increased global conduction velocity (0.98 ± 0.13–1.2 ± 0.16 m/s at 6 months, $p < 0.01$), shortened conduction time (32 ± 5–27 ± 6 ms, $p < 0.01$), and reduced complex fractionated activity (37 ± 14–$19 \pm 12\%$, $p = 0.02$). The changes in conduction velocity correlated positively with changes in 24-h mean systolic BP (R[2] = 0.55, $p = 0.01$) and there was a significant reduction in left ventricular mass (139 ± 37–120 ± 29 g, $p < 0.01$) and diffuse ventricular fibrosis (T1 partition coefficient 0.39 ± 0.07–0.31 ± 0.09, $p = 0.01$) on cardiac magnetic resonance imaging, This study indicates that BP reduction after renal denervation is associated with improvements in regional and global atrial conduction and reductions in ventricular mass and fibrosis. It remains to be determined whether the changes in electrical and structural remodeling are solely due to BP lowering or are due in part to intrinsic effects of renal denervation.

Only a few studies are available that investigated the potential utility of RDN in HF patients.

A first-in-man clinical study of renal denervation in systolic heart failure, the REACH-Pilot Study, was designed to evaluate the safety of catheter-based renal denervation in heart failure patients with reduced ejection fraction [59]. No acute hemodynamic changes occurred that would have interfered with completion of the procedure. In addition, no procedure-related complications were documented. At 6-month follow-up, both symptoms and the 6-min walk test (by 27.1 ± 9.7 m) were improved in all patients. Although there was a nonsignificant trend of reduction in both systolic and diastolic blood pressure at 6 month (-7.1 ± 6.9 and -0.6 ± 4.0 mmHg, respectively), no hypotensive episodes were reported.

Ukena et al. [60] reported that electrical storm was reduced after bilateral renal denervation in two patients with chronic heart failure. Both patients suffered from treatment-resistant tachy-arrhythmias and required a cardioverter defibrillator (ICD) implantation. The etiology of heart failure was non-ischemic. Subsequent to renal denervation, both patients had an event-free period up to 6 months. Interestingly, blood pressure was not decreased with renal denervation in either patient.

In line with evidence from animal studies, natriuretic effects of renal denervation might have contributed to the improvement of functional as well as electrophysiological alterations of the failing myocardium in the above clinical studies of heart failure. However, given the malicious role of sympathetic overactivity, reduced sympathetic nervous activity through renal denervation may well have beneficial effects and deserves further investigation in larger and appropriately designed studies.

Conclusion

As summarized in Fig. 41.1, communication between the kidney and brain involves multiple factors. The etiology of hypertension tends to be multifactorial especially when accompanied by CKD. Several lines of research suggest that renal denervation may exert beneficial effects in the context of CKD. These beneficial effects relate primarily to improved BP control, but may also extend to preservation of renal function and reduction of albuminuria. Several comorbidities that commonly exist in patients with CKD such as heart failure and arrhythmias may also be affected beneficially and strengthen the potential therapeutic utility in CKD. While the experimental evidence to support such notions is convincing, the clinical data available is preliminary and stems mainly from uncontrolled clinical trials and small mechanistic studies and have to be interpreted with the appropriate caution. In light of the results of Symplicity HTN-3 and the questions raised by this study, it will be crucial to perform properly designed randomized controlled studies applying catheter-based renal denervation in an environment with sufficient experience to better understand the potential clinical benefits of renal denervation in CKD.

Conflict of interest MS is supported by a Senior Research Fellowship from the National Health and Medical Research Council (NHMRC) of Australia. This research was funded in part by the grants from the National Health and Research Council of Australia (NHMRC) and the Victorian Government's Operational Infrastructure Support Program. MS is an investigator in studies sponsored by Medtronic and has received honoraria and lecture fees.

References

1. Bertog SC, Sobotka PA, Sievert H. Renal denervation for hypertension. JACC Cardiovasc Interv. 2012;5:249–58.
2. Bell-Reuss E, Trevino D, Gottschalk C. Effect of renal sympathetic nerve stimulation on proximal water and sodium reabsorption. J Clin Invest. 1976;57:1104.
3. Francisco LL, Sawin LL, DiBona GF. Renal sympathetic nerve activity and the exaggerated natriuresis of the spontaneous hypertensive rat. Hypertension. 1981;3:134–8.
4. Kirchheim H, Ehmke H, Persson P. Sympathetic modulation of renal hemodynamics, renin release and sodium excretion. Klin Wochenschr. 1989;67:858–64.
5. Dibona GF, Kopp UC. Neural control of renal function. Physiol Rev. 1997;77:75–197.
6. Kopp UC, Cicha MZ, Smith LA, Mulder J, Hökfelt T. Renal sympathetic nerve activity modulates afferent renal nerve activity by PGE2-dependent activation of α1-and α2-adrenoceptors on renal sensory nerve fibers. Am J Physiol Regul Integr Comp Physiol. 2007;293:R1561–72.
7. Vecchione C, Maffei A, Colella S, Aretini A, Poulet R, Frati G, Gentile MT, Fratta L, Trimarco V, Trimarco B. Leptin effect on endothelial nitric oxide is mediated through Akt–endothelial nitric oxide synthase phosphorylation pathway. Diabetes. 2002;51:168–73.
8. Lembo G, Vecchione C, Fratta L, Marino G, Trimarco V, d'Amati G, Trimarco B. Leptin induces direct vasodilation through distinct endothelial mechanisms. Diabetes. 2000;49:293–7.
9. Kopp UC, Olson LA, DiBona GF. Renorenal reflex responses to mechano-and chemoreceptor stimulation in the dog and rat. Am J Physiol Renal Physiol. 1984;246:F67–77.
10. Kopp UC, Smith LA, DiBona GF. Facilitatory role of efferent renal nerve activity on renal sensory receptors. Am J Physiol Renal Physiol. 1987;253:F767–77.
11. Converse RL Jr, Jacobsen TN, Toto RD, Jost CM, Cosentino F, Fouad-Tarazi F, Victor RG. Sympathetic overactivity in patients with chronic renal failure. N Engl J Med. 1992;327:1912–8.
12. Campese VM, Kogosov E. Renal afferent denervation prevents hypertension in rats with chronic renal failure. Hypertension. 1995;25:878–82.
13. Rao F, Wessel J, Wen G, Zhang L, Rana BK, Kennedy BP, Greenwood TA, Salem RM, Chen Y, Khandrika S, Hamilton BA, Smith DW, Holstein-Rathlou NH, Ziegler MG, Schork NJ, O'Connor DT. Renal albumin excretion: twin studies identify influences of heredity, environment, and adrenergic pathway polymorphism. Hypertension. 2007;49:1015–31.
14. Page IH, Heuer GJ. The effect of renal denervation on patients suffering from nephritis. J Clin Invest. 1935;14:443.
15. Grimson KS, Orgain ES, Anderson B, Broome RA Jr, Longino FH. Results of treatment of patients with hypertension by total thoracic and partial to total lumbar sympathectomy, splanchnicectomy and celiac ganglionectomy. Ann Surg. 1949;129:850.
16. Smithwick RH, Thompson JE. Splanchnicectomy for essential hypertension; results in 1,266 cases. J Am Med Assoc. 1953;152:1501–4.
17. Katholi RE, Winternitz SR, Oparil S. Decrease in peripheral sympathetic nervous system activity following renal denervation or unclipping in the one-kidney one-clip Goldblatt hypertensive rat. J Clin Invest. 1982;69:55–62.
18. Bello-Reuss E, Colindres RE, Pastoriza-Munoz E, Mueller RA, Gottschalk CW. Effects of acute unilateral renal denervation in the rat. J Clin Invest. 1975;56:208–17.
19. Nozawa T, Igawa A, Fujii N, Kato B, Yoshida N, Asanoi H, Inoue H. Effects of long-term renal sympathetic denervation on heart failure after myocardial infarction in rats. Heart Vessels. 2002;16:51–6.
20. Krum H, Schlaich M, Whitbourn R, Sobotka PA, Sadowski J, Bartus K, Kapelak B, Walton A, Sievert H, Thambar S, Abraham WT, Esler M. Catheter-based renal sympathetic denervation for resistant hypertension: a multicentre safety and proof-of-principle cohort study. Lancet. 2009;373:1275–81.
21. Symplicity HTNI. Catheter-based renal sympathetic denervation for resistant hypertension: durability of blood pressure reduction out to 24 months. Hypertension. 2011;57:911–7.
22. Krum H, Schlaich MP, Sobotka PA, Bohm M, Mahfoud F, Rocha-Singh K, Katholi R, Esler MD. Percutaneous renal denervation in patients with treatment-resistant hypertension: final 3-year report of the Symplicity HTN-1 study. Lancet. 2014;383:622–9.
23. Esler MD, Krum H, Sobotka PA, Schlaich MP, Schmieder RE, Bohm M. Renal sympathetic denervation in patients with treatment-resistant hypertension (The Symplicity HTN-2 Trial): a randomised controlled trial. Lancet. 2010;376:1903–9.
24. Esler MD, Krum H, Schlaich M, Schmieder RE, Bohm M, Sobotka PA, Symplicity HTNI. Renal sympathetic denervation for treatment of drug-resistant hypertension: one-year results from the Symplicity HTN-2 randomized, controlled trial. Circulation. 2012;126:2976–82.
25. Bhatt DL, Kandzari DE, O'Neill WW, D'Agostino R, Flack JM, Katzen BT, Leon MB, Liu M, Mauri L, Negoita M, Cohen SA, Oparil S, Rocha-Singh K, Townsend RR and Bakris GL. A controlled trial of renal denervation for resistant hypertension. N Engl J Med. 2014;370(15):1393–401.
26. Materson BJ, Reda DJ, Cushman WC, Massie BM, Freis ED, Kochar MS, Hamburger RJ, Fye C, Lakshman R, Gottdiener J. Single-drug therapy for hypertension in men—A comparison of six antihypertensive agents with Placebo. N Engl J Med. 1993;328:914–21.
27. Blake WD, Jurf AN. Renal sodium reabsorption after acute renal denervation in the rabbit. J Physiol. 1968;196:65–73.
28. Bello-Reuss E, Pastoriza-Munoz E, Colindres RE. Acute unilateral renal denervation in rats with extracellular volume expansion. Am J Physiol. 1977;232:F26–32.
29. Hering D, Lambert EA, Marusic P, Walton AS, Krum H, Lambert GW, Esler MD, Schlaich MP. Substantial reduction in single sympathetic nerve firing after renal denervation in patients with resistant hypertension. Hypertension. 2013;61:457–64.
30. Hering D, Marusic P, Walton AS, Lambert EA, Krum H, Narkiewicz K, Lambert GW, Esler MD, Schlaich MP. Sustained sympathetic and blood pressure reduction 1 year after renal denervation in patients with resistant hypertension. Hypertension. 2014;64:118–24. doi:10.1161/HYPERTENSIONAHA.113.03098.
31. Azizi M, Sapoval M, Gosse P, Monge M, Bobrie G, Delsart P, Midulla M, Mounier-Vehier C, Courand PY, Lantelme P, Denolle T, Dourmap-Collas C, Trillaud H, Pereira H, Plouin PF, Chatellier G. Optimum and stepped care standardised antihypertensive treatment with or without renal denervation for resistant hypertension (DENERHTN): a multicentre, open-label, randomised controlled trial. Lancet. 2015;385(9981):1957–65.
32. Desch S, Okon T, Heinemann D, Kulle K, Rohnert K, Sonnabend M, Petzold M, Muller U, Schuler G, Eitel I,

Thiele H, Lurz P. Randomized sham-controlled trial of renal sympathetic denervation in mild resistant hypertension. Hypertension. 2015;65(6):1202–8.

33. Fadl Elmula FE, Hoffmann P, Larstorp AC, Fossum E, Brekke M, Kjeldsen SE, Gjonnaess E, Hjornholm U, Kjaer VN, Rostrup M, Os I, Stenehjem A, Hoieggen A. Adjusted drug treatment is superior to renal sympathetic denervation in patients with true treatment-resistant hypertension. Hypertension. 2014;63:991–9.
34. Rosa J, Widimsky P, Tousek P, Petrak O, Curila K, Waldauf P, Bednar F, Zelinka T, Holaj R, Strauch B, Somloova Z, Taborsky M, Vaclavik J, Kocianova E, Branny M, Nykl I, Jiravsky O, Widimsky J Jr. Randomized comparison of renal denervation versus intensified pharmacotherapy including spironolactone in true-resistant hypertension: six-month results from the Prague-15 study. Hypertension. 2015;65(2):407–13.
35. Mahfoud F, Cremers B, Janker J, Link B, Vonend O, Ukena C, Linz D, Schmieder R, Rump LC, Kindermann I, Sobotka PA, Krum H, Scheller B, Schlaich M, Laufs U, Bohm M. Renal hemodynamics and renal function after catheter-based renal sympathetic denervation in patients with resistant hypertension. Hypertension. 2012;60:419–24.
36. Hering D, Mahfoud F, Walton AS, Krum H, Lambert GW, Lambert EA, Sobotka PA, Bohm M, Cremers B, Esler MD, Schlaich MP. Renal denervation in moderate to severe CKD. J Am Soc Nephrol. 2012;23:1250–7.
37. Kiuchi MG, Maia GL, de Queiroz Carreira MA, Kiuchi T, Chen S, Andrea BR, Graciano ML, Lugon JR. Effects of renal denervation with a standard irrigated cardiac ablation catheter on blood pressure and renal function in patients with chronic kidney disease and resistant hypertension. Eur Heart J. 2013;34(28):2114–21.
38. Ott C, Mahfoud F, Schmid A, Ditting T, Veelken R, Ewen S, Ukena C, Uder M, Bohm M, Schmieder RE. Improvement of albuminuria after renal denervation. Int J Cardiol. 2014;173:311–5.
39. Masuo K, Mikami H, Ogihara T, Tuck M. Hormonal mechanisms in blood pressure reduction during hemodialysis in patients with chronic renal failure. Hypertens Res. 1995;18(Suppl 1):S201–3.
40. Masuo K, Katsuya T, Sugimoto K, Kawaguchi H, Rakugi H, Ogihara T, Tuck ML. High plasma norepinephrine levels associated with beta2-adrenoceptor polymorphisms predict future renal damage in nonobese normotensive individuals. Hypertens Res. 2007;30:503–11.
41. Mena-Martin FJ, Martin-Escudero JC, Simal-Blanco F, Carretero-Ares JL, Arzua-Mouronte D, Castrodeza Sanz JJ. Influence of sympathetic activity on blood pressure and vascular damage evaluated by means of urinary albumin excretion. J Clin Hypertens (Greenwich). 2006;8:619–24.
42. Ott C, Mahfoud F, Schmid A, Toennes SW, Ewen S, Ditting T, Veelken R, Ukena C, Uder M, Bohm M, Schmieder RE. Renal denervation preserves renal function in patients with chronic kidney disease and resistant hypertension. J Hypertens. 2015;33:1261–6.
43. Lohmeier TE, Iliescu R, Liu B, Henegar JR, Maric-Bilkan C, Irwin ED. Systemic and renal-specific sympathoinhibition in obesity hypertension. Hypertension. 2012;59:331–8.
44. Schlaich MP, Socratous F, Hennebry S, Eikelis N, Lambert EA, Straznicky N, Esler MD, Lambert GW. Sympathetic activation in chronic renal failure. J Am Soc Nephrol. 2009;20:933–9.
45. Eikelis N, Hennebry SC, Lambert GW, Schlaich MP. Does renalase degrade catecholamines? Kidney Int. 2011;79:1380 author reply 1380–1.
46. Li G, Xu J, Wang P, Velazquez H, Li Y, Wu Y, Desir GV. Catecholamines regulate the activity, secretion, and synthesis of renalase. Circulation. 2008;117:1277–82.
47. Jiang W, Guo Y, Tan L, Tang X, Yang Q, Yang K. Impact of renal denervation on renalase expression in adult rats with spontaneous hypertension. Exp Ther Med. 2012;4:493–6.
48. Schlaich MP, Bart B, Hering D, Walton A, Marusic P, Mahfoud F, Bohm M, Lambert EA, Krum H, Sobotka PA, Schmieder RE, Ika-Sari C, Eikelis N, Straznicky N, Lambert GW, Esler MD. Feasibility of catheter-based renal nerve ablation and effects on sympathetic nerve activity and blood pressure in patients with end-stage renal disease. Int J Cardiol. 2013;168(3):2214–20.
49. Di Daniele N, De Francesco M, Violo L, Spinelli A, Simonetti G. Renal sympathetic nerve ablation for the treatment of difficult-to-control or refractory hypertension in a haemodialysis patient. Nephrol Dial Transplant. 2012;27:1689–90.
50. Cohn JN, Levine TB, Olivari MT, Garberg V, Lura D, Francis GS, Simon AB, Rector T. Plasma norepinephrine as a guide to prognosis in patients with chronic congestive heart failure. N Engl J Med. 1984;311:819–23.
51. Mancia G. Sympathetic activation in congestive heart failure. Eur Heart J. 1990;11:3–11.
52. Rundqvist B, Elam M, Bergmann-Sverrisdottir Y, Eisenhofer G, Friberg P. Increased cardiac adrenergic drive precedes generalized sympathetic activation in human heart failure. Circulation. 1997;95:169–75.
53. Pettersson A, Hedner J, Hedner T. Renal interaction between sympathetic activity and ANP in rats with chronic ischaemic heart failure. Acta Physiol Scand. 1989;135:487–92.
54. Brandt MC, Mahfoud F, Reda S, Schirmer SH, Erdmann E, Bohm M, Hoppe UC. Renal sympathetic denervation reduces left ventricular hypertrophy and improves cardiac function in patients with resistant hypertension. J Am Coll Cardiol. 2012;59:901–9.
55. Mahfoud F, Urban D, Teller D, Linz D, Stawowy P, Hassel J-H, Fries P, Dreysse S, Wellnhofer E, Schneider G. Effect of renal denervation on left ventricular mass and function in patients with resistant hypertension: data from a multi-centre cardiovascular magnetic resonance imaging trial. Eur Heart J. 2014:ehu093.
56. Pokushalov E, Romanov A, Corbucci G, Artyomenko S, Baranova V, Turov A, Shirokova N, Karaskov A, Mittal S, Steinberg JS. A randomized comparison of pulmonary vein isolation with versus without concomitant renal artery denervation in patients with refractory symptomatic atrial fibrillation and resistant hypertension. J Am Coll Cardiol. 2012;60:1163–70.
57. Linz D, Mahfoud F, Schotten U, Ukena C, Neuberger H-R, Wirth K, Böhm M. Renal sympathetic denervation suppresses postapneic blood pressure rises and atrial fibrillation in a model for sleep apnea. Hypertension. 2012;60:172–8.
58. McLellan AJ, Schlaich MP, Taylor AJ, Prabhu S, Hering D, Hammond L, Marusic P, Duval J, Sata Y, Ellims A. Reverse cardiac remodelling following renal denervation-atrial electrophysiologic and structural changes associated with blood pressure lowering. Heart Rhythm. 2015.
59. Davies JE, Manisty CH, Petraco R, Barron AJ, Unsworth B, Mayet J, Hamady M, Hughes AD, Sever PS, Sobotka PA, Francis DP. First-in-man safety evaluation of renal denervation for chronic systolic heart failure: primary outcome from REACH-Pilot study. Int J Cardiol. 2013;162:189–92.
60. Ukena C, Bauer A, Mahfoud F, Schreieck J, Neuberger HR, Eick C, Sobotka PA, Gawaz M, Bohm M. Renal sympathetic denervation for treatment of electrical storm: first-in-man experience. Clin Res Cardiol. 2012;101:63–7.

Index

Page numbers followed by "*f*" indicate figures; those followed by "*t*" indicate tables.

A

AA. *See* Arachidonic acid (AA)
ABI. *See* Ankle brachial index (ABI)
Abnormal calcium and phosphate metabolism, 46, 49*f*
Abnormal phosphate metabolism, 264
ACC. *See* American College of Cardiology (ACC)
ACE. *See* Angiotensin converting enzyme (ACE)
Acetylcholine, 4, 5
Acetylsalicylic acid. *See* Aspirin
ACP. *See* Advance care planning (ACP)
ACR. *See* Albumin-to-creatinine ratio (ACR)
ACS. *See* Acute coronary syndrome (ACS)
Action to Control Cardiovascular Risk in Diabetes (ACCORD) trial, 405
Acute and Chronic Therapeutic Impact of a Vasopressin Antagonist (ACTIV in CHF) trial, 178
Acute cardiorenal syndrome. *See* Type 1 Cardiorenal syndrome (CRS-1)
Acute coronary syndrome (ACS), 237
  catalytic (labile) iron in, 110–115
  CKD patients with, 36
  contrast induced nephropathy (CIN) and, 347
  coronary artery disease (CAD) and, 87
  oral antiplatelet agents for, 302
Acute decompensated heart failure (ADHF), 131, 164
  bioimpedance vectorial analyses (BIVA) in, 171, 172
  fluid removal strategies
    diuretics, 177
    tolvaptan, 178–179
    ultrafiltration, 180
  hospitalizations for, 177
  neutral endopeptidase (NEP) inhibitors, 185–187
  novel inotropes
    istaroxime, 185
    levosimendan, 183–185
    omecamtiv mecarbil (OM), 182–183
  novel therapies for, 177–187
  novel vasodilators
    nesiritide, 180–181
    relaxin, 181–182
    rolofylline, 182
  overview, 177
  ultrafiltration (UF) therapy in, 163–169
Acute heart failure syndromes (AHFS)
  bioimpedance vectorial analyses (BIVA) in, 172–173
Acute kidney injury (AKI), 113, 131, 132*f*, 155
  after cardiac surgery, 355–363
    biomarkers role, 357–358
    incidence/prognosis, 355–366
  pathogenesis, 356–357
  pharmacological renal protection, 361–363
  risk factors, 358–361, 359*t*
  contrast induced nephropathy (CIN) and, 347
  definition of, 356, 357*t*
  incidence of, 196*t*
  post-implant, 195–196
  and type 3 cardiorenal syndrome (CRS-3)
    direct effects on cardiac function, 134–135
    indirect effects on heart function, 135
Acute Kidney Injury Network (AKIN), 356
Acute myocardial infarction (AMI), 81
Acute renocardiac syndrome. *See* Type 3 cardiorenal syndrome (CRS-3)
Acute Study of Clinical Effectiveness of Nesiritide and Decompensated Heart Failure (ASCEND-HF) trial, 180, 181*f*
Acute Treatment with Omecamtiv Mecarbil to Increase Contractility in Acute Heart Failure (ATOMIC-AHF) study, 183
Acute tubular necrosis (ATN), 349
Adenosine diphosphate (ADP), 5, 301, 305
Adenosine triphosphate (ATP), 182, 305
ADHERE study, 205
ADHF. *See* Acute decompensated heart failure (ADHF)
ADMA. *See* Asymmetric dimethylarginine (ADMA)
ADP. *See* Adenosine diphosphate (ADP)
Advance care planning (ACP), 213
AF. *See* Atrial fibrillation (AF)
African American Study of Kidney Disease and Hypertension (AASK) trial, 403, 405, 407*t*
AHA. *See* American Heart Association (AHA)
AHD. *See* Atherosclerotic heart disease (AHD)
AHFS. *See* Acute heart failure syndromes (AHFS)
AHI. *See* Apnea–hypopnea index (AHI)
AKI. *See* Acute kidney injury (AKI)
Albumin, 106
Albumin-to-creatinine ratio (ACR), 358
Albuminuria, 148
  and cardiovascular disease, 7–8
  as central marker, 3–8
  and endothelium, 6
  in kidney disease, 6
Aldosterone, 56, 77, 79*t*, 81, 134
Aldosterone receptor antagonists, 83, 83*t*
  plus ACEi/AIIT1RA, 90
Aldosterone receptor blockers (ARBs), 352
Aliskiren, 82, 83*t*, 84, 87–91

J. Rangaswami et al. (eds.), *Cardio-Nephrology*,
DOI 10.1007/978-3-319-56042-7

Allograft dysfunction, on CVD risk post-KT, 264
Alpha-1 collagen, 137
α1-Microglobulin, 149–150
ALTITUDE investigators, 89
Ambrisentan, 248
American College of Cardiology (ACC), 414
American College of Cardiology/American Heart Association (ACC/AHA) task force, 317, 321, 330
American College of Cardiology Foundation/American Heart Association (ACCF/AHA) guidelines, 147
American College of Rheumatology Treatment, 412
American Heart Association (AHA), 219
American Heart Association/American College of Cardiology Foundation (AHA/ACCF), 248, 252*t*, 253–254, 256
AMI. *See* Acute myocardial infarction (AMI)
Anemia, 211
Anemia treatment in patients with CKD
  future of, 126–127
  KDIGO guidelines, 124*t*
  randomized controlled trails in, 122*t*
  target hemoglobin for, 121–122
Angiogenesis, 120
Angioplasty and Stent for Renal Artery Lesions Trial (ASTRAL), 379, 380, 413
Angiopoietins, 7, 8*f*
Angiotensin 1–7, 77, 79*t*, 81–82
Angiotensin 1–9, 77, 79*t*
Angiotensin converting enzyme (ACE), 185
  ACE2, 77, 78*t*, 82
  inhibitor (ACEI), 29, 45, 55, 82, 83*t*, 84, 86, 89–90, 199, 261, 274, 352, 379, 421
Angiotensin I, 77, 78*t*
Angiotensin II (Ang II), 3, 45, 77, 78*t*, 81, 134, 378
Angiotensin II AT1 receptor blockers (AIIT1RA), 82, 83*t*, 84, 86, 89–90
Angiotensin III (Ang III), 77, 79*t*
Angiotensin IV (Ang IV), 77, 79*t*
Angiotensinogen, 77, 78*t*
Angiotensin receptor antagonists, 55
Angiotensin receptor blockers (ARBs), 29, 45, 81, 186, 262, 274, 379, 404
Ankle brachial index (ABI), 337
ANP. *See* Atrial natriuretic peptide (ANP)
ANS. *See* Autonomic nervous system (ANS)
Anticoagulation
  in atrial fibrillation (AF), 284
  direct oral anticoagulants (DOACs) in AF
    laboratory monitoring and management of bleeding for DOACs, 286–288
    pharmacokinetic/pharmacodynamic characteristics, 286
    pivotal clinical trials, summary of, 284–286
    prescribing information and characteristics, 287*t*
    trials for nonvalvular atrial fibrillation, 285*t*, 289*t*
  pragmatic clinical considerations in CKD patients, 291–292
  in stage 3 CKD patients with AF, 288–290
  in stage 4 CKD patients with AF, 290–291
  in stage 5D CKD patients with AF, 291
Anticoagulation-related nephropathy (ARN), 291
  clinical consequences, 298
  diagnosis and work-up, 297–298, 297*f*
  diagnostic criteria, 295
  epidemiology, 295–296
  historical perspective, 295
  importance of, 295
  main risk factor for, 296
  microscopy pathology associated with, 296*f*
  overview, 295
  pathophysiology and mechanism, 296–297
  prevention, 299
  treatment and monitoring, 298, 298*t*
Antidiuretic hormone (ADH). *See* Arginine vasopressin (AVP)
Anti-hypertensive therapy, 231
Antioxidants, 67
Antiplatelet therapy, 231–232
  on cardiovascular outcomes in patients with CKD, 301–310
    antiplatelet monotherapy, 307
    dual antiplatelet therapy, 307–308
  for coronary artery disease (CAD), 38
  oral antiplatelet agents
    aspirin, 302
    P2Y12 receptor blockers, 303
    thrombin receptor antagonists (TRA), 303–304
  platelet biology, 301–302
  platelet dysfunction, in CKD, 305–307
    altered non-renal drug metabolism, 306–307
    cytochrome P450 (CYP) polymorphisms, 306
    dysfunctional von Willebrand factor (VWF), 307
    endogenous derangements of vascular and hemostatic function, 305–306
    high platelet reactivity, 306
    potential mechanisms for impaired antiplatelet response, 306–307
  platelet function assessment, methods for, 304–305
  platelet function testing in CVD, 309
  post-PCI in CKD, 323–331
  vascular thrombosis, 301–302
Antithrombotic Trialists' (ATT), 302
Aortic stenosis (AS), 11
Aortic valve, 17, 18*f*
Aortic valvular calcification (AVC), 17
Aorto iliac disease
  clinical presentation, 338
  endovascular therapy for, 338
  interventional management, 338–339
  non-interventional management, 338
  surgical techniques for, 338
ADPKD. *See* Autosomal dominant polycystic kidney disease (ADPKD)
Apixaban, 285, 286, 287*t*
Apnea–hypopnea index (AHI), 396
Aquadex FlexFlow System, 180
Aquapheresis versus Intravenous Diuretics Hospitalizations for Heart Failure (AVOID-HF) trial, 166*t*, 168
Arachidonic acid (AA), 302
ARAD. *See* Atherosclerotic renal artery disease (ARAD)
ARBs. *See* Aldosterone receptor blockers (ARBs); Angiotensin receptor blockers (ARBs)
ARCTIC study, 309
Arginine vasopressin (AVP), 178
ARISTOTLE trial, 285, 285*t*, 288, 289*t*, 290
ARN. *See* Anticoagulation-related nephropathy (ARN)
Arrhythmia, vitamin D therapy in, 105
Arterial calcification, vitamin D and, 103
Arterial Revascularization Therapies Study (ARTS) trial, 39
Arteriosclerosis, 35–36
Arteriovenous fistulae (AVF), 243, 246–247
ARVD. *See* Atherosclerotic renovascular disease (ARVD)
AS. *See* Aortic stenosis (AS)
ASCVD. *See* Atherosclerotic cardiovascular disease (ASCVD)
Aspirin, 38, 231, 302, 339, 340
Assessment of Dual Antiplatelet Therapy with Drug-Eluting Stents (ADAPT-DES), 308

Assessment of Lescol in Renal Transplantation study (ALERT), 260, 263, 369, 371*t*, 374
Assessment of Survival and Cardiovascular Events (AURORA), 37, 371, 371*t*
AST-120, 67
ASTRONAUT investigators, 90
Asymmetric dimethylarginine (ADMA), 63, 64
ATEROMO-NIRS study, 237
Atherosclerosis, 35
Atherosclerosis Risk in Communities (ARIC) study, 35
Atherosclerotic cardiovascular disease (ASCVD), 370
Atherosclerotic heart disease (AHD), 81
Atherosclerotic renal artery disease (ARAD), 411–412
Atherosclerotic renovascular disease (ARVD)
  cardiac impact of, 377–382
  cardiac remodeling, 378
  epidemiology of, 377
  flash pulmonary edema (FPE), 378
  overview, 377
  pathophysiology of cardiac disease in, 378
  prognosis of, 377
  randomized controlled studies, 379–380
  recommendations and future directions, 382
  retrospective studies, 380–382
  revascularization, 379–382
  treatment of, 378–379
  unstable angina, 378
ATLAS study, 266
ATN. *See* Acute tubular necrosis (ATN)
ATP. *See* Adenosine triphosphate (ATP)
Atrial fibrillation (AF), 105, 137, 424
  anticoagulation, 284
    in advanced CKD, 288–291
    in stage 3 CKD patients with AF, 288–290
    in stage 4 CKD patients with AF, 290–291
    in stage 5D CKD patients with AF, 291
  direct oral anticoagulants (DOACs)
    laboratory monitoring and management of bleeding for DOACs, 286–288
    pharmacokinetic/pharmacodynamic characteristics, 286
    pivotal clinical trials, summary of, 284–286
    prescribing information and characteristics, 287*t*
    trials for nonvalvular atrial fibrillation, 285*t*, 289*t*
  prevalence/incidence in CKD, 283
  risks, 283–284
Atrial natriuretic peptide (ANP), 424
Autonomic nervous system (ANS), 139
Autosomal dominant polycystic kidney disease (ADPKD), 85–86, 406
AVC. *See* Aortic valvular calcification (AVC)
AVERROES trial, 285, 285*t*, 286, 289*t*, 290
AVF. *See* Arteriovenous fistulae (AVF)
AVP. *See* Arginine vasopressin (AVP)

B

Bare metal stent (BMS), 39, 238, 319
  vs. coronary artery bypass grafting (CABG), 321–322
  drug-eluting stents *vs.*, 331–332
    in dialysis patients, 332
BARI-2D trial, 318
Belatacept, 266
Berlin Heart INCOR, LVAD device, 191
Bernoulli equation, 243
Beta-blockers, 421
  for CKD-associated cardiomyopathy, 55
  for SCD prevention, 29
β-Glucuronidase, 71
β1-Adrenoceptors, stimulation of, 419
Bioimpedance vectorial analyses (BIVA)
  in acute heart failure, 172–173
  bioelectrical impedance techniques, principles of, 171–172
  in cardiorenal syndrome, 171–175
  in chronic heart failure (CHF), 174–175
  in chronic kidney disease (CKD), 174–175
  graphic representation of hydration state, 172*f*
  overview, 171
Biomarkers
  of acute kidney injury, 357–358
  in cardiorenal syndrome, 145–146, 147*t*
  clinical implications, 151–152
  definition of, 145
  in heart disease, 148*f*
    B-type natriuretic peptide (BNP), 146
    galectin-3, 147
    high-sensitivity cardiac troponin (cTn), 146
    N-terminal pro-B-type natriuretic peptide (NT-proBNP), 146
    soluble suppressor of tumorigenicity 2 (sST2), 146–147
    urinary angiotensinogen, 148
  in renal disease, 148–151, 149*f*
    albuminuria, 148
    α1-microglobulin, 149–150
    H-type fatty acid-binding protein (H-FABP), 151
    insulin-like growth factor-binding protein 7 (IGFBP7), 150
    interleukin-18 (IL-18), 151
    kidney injury molecule-1 (KIM-1), 151
    L-type fatty acid-binding protein (L-FABP), 151
    neutrophil gelatinase-associated lipocalin (NGAL), 150
    tissue inhibitor of metalloproteinase-2 (TIMP-2), 150
    urine sediment, 148–149
  time-dependent release of, 151–152
  use of, 152
BIVA. *See* Bioimpedance vectorial analyses (BIVA)
Blood oxygen level-dependent (BOLD) MRI, in renal artery stenosis, 415, 416
Blood pressure (BP) goals
  chronic kidney disease (CKD) and, 37–38, 403–408
    in diabetes, 405
    guidelines, 403–405
    intensive *vs.* standard BP targets, 407–408*t*
    observational studies, 405
    overview, 403
    in polycystic kidney disease, 406–408
    summary, 408
    Systolic BP Intervention Trial (SPRINT), 405–406
    targets and treatment recommendations, 404*t*
  in kidney transplant candidates, 231
Blood vessels
  inflammation and oxidative stress, 64–65, 65*f*
BMS. *See* Bare metal stent (BMS)
BNP. *See* B-type natriuretic peptide (BNP)
Bosentan, 248
Bowman's space, 296
BP. *See* Blood pressure (BP)
Bradykinin, 4, 5, 91
Bridge to recovery (BTR) pathway, 191
Bridge to transplantation (BTT) pathway, 191
B-type natriuretic peptide (BNP), 104, 135, 146, 173, 180

C

CABG. *See* Coronary artery bypass graft (CABG)
CAC score. *See* Coronary artery calcium (CAC) score

CAD. *See* Coronary artery disease (CAD)
Calcification. *See* Vascular calcification; Valvular calcification
Calcineurin inhibitors (CNI) choice/minimization, in KT, 261–262, 265
Calcitriol, 15
Calcium channel blockers (CCB), 29, 403
Calcium phosphorus product (CaXP), 16, 71
Calcium regulation, 247
cAMP. *See* Cyclic adenosine monophosphate (cAMP)
CAPD. *See* Continuous ambulatory peritoneal dialysis (CAPD)
Captopril, 87
Cardiac arrhythmias
  renal denervation in, 424
  and sudden cardiac death, 136–137
Cardiac biomarkers, 222–223
Cardiac conduction, 30
Cardiac destabilization syndromes, 380
Cardiac disease
  clinical relevance of RAAS inhibition in
    cardiorenal syndromes, 88–89
    coronary angiogram and contrast induced nephropathy, 88
    coronary artery disease and acute coronary syndromes, 87
    reduced left ventricular systolic function or heart failure, 88
    sudden cardiac death, 88
  pathophysiology in atherosclerotic renovascular disease (ARVD), 378
Cardiac fibrosis, 137–138
Cardiac ischemia-reperfusion injury in animals, catalytic (labile) iron in, 110
Cardiac magnetic resonance (CMR) imaging, 222
  in CKD-associated cardiomyopathy, 45, 54
  in vitamin D therapy for HF treatment, 104
Cardiac muscles, erythropoietin effect on, 121
Cardiac pre-operative evaluation, risk factors optimization in KT, 229–232
  lifestyle interventions, 229
    exercise, 229–230
    malabsorptive interventions, 229
    obesity/diet/bariatric interventions, 229
    recommendations, 230
    smoking cessation, 230
  medical interventions
    anti-hypertensive therapy, 231
    antiplatelet therapy, 231–232
    blood pressure control, 231
    dyslipidemia, 230–231
    hypertension, 231
Cardiac remodeling, 378
Cardiac reserve, CKD and, 273
Cardiac surgery associated acute kidney injury (CSA-AKI), 156
  diagnosis of, 357–358
  pharmacological renal protection
    perioperative, 362
    postoperative, 362–363
    preoperative, 361–362
  risk factors for, 359*t*
    blood transfusion, 361
    events associated with cardiac pulmonary bypass (CPB), 360
    intraoperative events, 359–360
    on-pump *vs.* off-pump, 360–361
    preoperative risk factors for AKI, 358–359
    surgical reexploration, 361
Cardiac surgery-associated NGAL (CSA-NGAL) score, 159
Cardiac surveillance, in transplant candidates, 251–256
  coronary artery disease, 251–253
  left ventricular dysfunction, 254–256
  recommendations on, 252*t*
  valvular heart disease, 253–254
Cardiac troponin (cTn), 146
Cardiac troponin T (cTnT), 222
Cardiomyopathy (CM)*See also* CKD-associated cardiomyopathy
  chronic kidney disease (CKD) and cardiac reserve, 273
  and end stage kidney disease (ESKD)
    diagnosing CHF in, 271–272
    epidemiology, 271
    pathophysiology, 272–273, 272*f*
    treatment, 273–274
  kidney transplantation (KT)
    diastolic dysfunction, 274
    left ventricular dysfunction (LVD) and, 275–277
    systolic dysfunction, 274–275
    work-up, 277*f*
  overview, 271
  in potential kidney transplant candidate, 271–278
Cardiopulmonary bypass (CPB), 359
  events associated with, 360
Cardiopulmonary exercise testing (CPET), 105
Cardiopulmonary stress testing (CPX), 273
Cardiorenal connectors, 134
Cardiorenal Rescue Study in Acute Decompensated Heart Failure (CARRESS-HF) trial, 166*t*, 167, 177, 179*f*, 180
Cardiorenal syndrome (CRS)
  background of, 131
  bioimpedance vectorial analyses (BIVA) in, 171–175
  classification of, 132*t*
  clinical relevance of RAAS inhibition in, 88–89
  hemodynamic cross-talk in, 145–152
  palliative care, 211–212
  type 1, 131–133
  type 2, 133–134
  type 3, 134–135
  type 4, 135–138, 136–137*f*
  type 5, 138–140, 138*t*, 139*f*, 140*f*
Cardiotonic steroids, 50
Cardiovascular disease (CVD)*See also* Cardiovascular risk
  albuminuria and, 7–8
  association of catalytic iron with, 113–115, 113–114*f*, 114*t*
  dyslipidemia as risk factor for, 369
  fibroblast growth factor 23 (FGF23) and, 71, 73
  phosphorus level and, 73
  post-kidney transplant modification
    incidence/prevalence, 259
    risk estimation, 260
    risk factors for, 259–260, 260*t*
    strategies to reducing risk, 265–267
    traditional risk factors, 260–264
    transplant specific risk factors, 264–265
  and preeclampsia, 385
  renal transplantation and, 251
  vitamin D therapy in, 103
Cardiovascular Outcomes in Renal Atherosclerotic Lesions (CORAL) study, 379, 413, 415
Cardiovascular risk
  erythropoiesis stimulating agent (ESA) dose, role of, 124–125
  higher Hb level, role of, 123–124
  hypertension, role of, 125
  iron and thrombocytosis, role of, 125–126
  potential mechanism of, 122–126, 124*f*
Cardiovascular Risk Extended Evaluation in Dialysis Patients (CREED) study, 255
Cardiovascular Risk Reduction by Early Anemia Treatment with Epoetin (CREATE) study, 121

Cardiovascular system, non-hematological effects of erythropoietin on, 120*t*
  angiogenesis, 120
  cardiac effects, 120–121
  hypertension, 121
  thrombosis, 121
Carotid artery endarterectomy, 340
Carotid Stenosis Trial (CREST-2), 340
CASCADE study, 255
Catalytic (labile) iron
  in acute coronary syndrome (ACS), 110–115
  association with cardiovascular diseases, 113–115, 113–114*f*, 114*t*
  in cardiac ischemia-reperfusion injury, in animals, 110
  definition of, 109
  in diagnosis and prognosis of ACS, in humans, 110–113, 111–112*f*, 111–112*t*
  in tissue injury, 109–110
Catheter-based renal denervation
  in heart failure patients, 424
  in human resistant hypertension, 419–420
CaXP. *See* Calcium phosphorus product (CaXP)
CCB. *See* Calcium channel blockers (CCB)
CCF. *See* Congestive cardiac failure (CCF)
CCTA. *See* Coronary computed tomographic angiography (CCTA)
CDC. *See* Centers for Disease Control (CDC)
Centers for Disease Control (CDC), 337
Central venous pressure (CVP), 131, 195, 350
Cerebrovascular accident (CVA), 81
CHF. *See* Chronic heart failure (CHF); Congestive heart failure (CHF)
Cholecalciferol (vitamin D_3), 97
Chronic heart failure (CHF)
  atherosclerotic renovascular disease (ARVD) in, 377–382
  bioimpedance vectorial analyses (BIVA) in, 174–175
  renal denervation in, 424
Chronic kidney disease (CKD)
  anemia treatment in patients with, 126–127
  anticoagulation in patients with AF and, 283–292
  antiplatelet therapy on cardiovascular outcomes in patients with, 301–310
  bioimpedance vectorial analyses (BIVA) in, 174–175
  and blood pressure (BP) goals. *See* Blood pressure (BP) goals
  and cardiac reserve, 273
  CKD-associated cardiomyopathy. *See* CKD-associated cardiomyopathy
  contrast induced nephropathy (CIN) and, 347, 348
  coronary artery disease (CAD) in. *See* Coronary artery disease (CAD)
  depression in, 211
  dyslipidemia in, 369–374
  inflammation and. *See* Inflammation, in chronic kidney disease (CKD)
  obstructive sleep apnea (OSA) and, 395–398
  pain in, 206
  peripheral arterial disease (PAD) in. *See* Peripheral arterial disease (PAD)
  platelet dysfunction in, 305–307
  and preeclampsia, 385
  reducing cardiovascular mortality in patients with, 71
  renal denervation and, 422–423
  revascularization strategies in. *See* Revascularization
  symptom burden of, 205
  target hemoglobin for anemia of, 121–122
  targeting renal sympathetic nerves in, 419
  valvular calcification in, 11–19
  vascular calcification in, 11–19
  vitamin D in. *See* Vitamin D
Chronic Kidney Disease Epidemiology Collaboration (CKD-EPI) equations, 292
Chronic Oral Study of Myosin Activation to Increase Contractility in Heart failure (COSMIC-HF) study, 183
Chronic Renal Insufficiency Cohort (CRIC) study, 137, 255
Chronic renocardiac syndrome. *See* Type 4 Cardiorenal syndrome (CRS-4)
Chronic thromboembolism pulmonary hypertension (CTEPH), 243, 248
CIN. *See* Contrast induced nephropathy (CIN)
Circulating endothelial cells (CEC), 6
CKD-associated cardiomyopathy
  evolution of, 54–55
  histopathology images of, 46*f*
  imaging modalities, 51*t*
    cardiac magnetic resonance (CMR), 54
    computed tomography, 54
    gadolinium-based contrast agents in CKD, 53–54
    late enhancement imaging, 52–53
    left ventricular mass, 50, 51–52*f*
    myocardial fibrosis, 50, 52
    T1 mapping, 53
  interventions for
    aldosterone, 56
    continuous haemodialysis regimes, 55–56
    hyperuricemia and oxidative stress, 56
    parathyroid hormone (PTH), 56
    phosphate, 56
    vitamin D, 56
  molecular mechanisms, 47*f*
    abnormal calcium and phosphate metabolism, 46, 49*f*
    cardiotonic steroids, 50
    fibroblast growth factor 23 (FGF-23), 46–47
    hyperuricemia, 48
    insulin resistance, 50
    parathyroid hormone, 47–48
    phosphate, 46
    protein bound uremic toxins, 48–50
    renin–angiotensin–aldosterone system (RAAS), 45–46
    vitamin D, 48
  novel targets and treatments
    FGF inhibitors, 56
    indoxyl sulphate, 57
    Klotho, 56–57
  overview, 45
  role of aldosterone in, 48*f*
Clinical Outcomes Utilizing Revascularization and Aggressive Drug Evaluation (COURAGE) trial, 38, 318
Clonidine, 404
Clopidogrel, 303, 329–330
Clopidogrel for High Atherothrombotic Risk and Ischemic Stabilization, Management, and Avoidance (CHARISMA) trial, 308
Clopidogrel for the Reduction of Events during Observation (CREDO) trial, 308, 329
Clopidogrel in Unstable Angina to Prevent Recurrent Events (CURE) trial, 308, 329
CMR imaging. *See* Cardiac magnetic resonance (CMR) imaging
Cochrane Database Systematic Review, 84, 86, 87
Colony forming unit-erythrocyte (CFU-E), 120
Communication, with patients, 212–213
Complement-mediated thrombotic microangiopathy (TMA)/hemolytic uremic syndrome (HUS), 5
Computed tomographic angiography (CTA), for renal artery stenosis, 414
Computed tomography, in CKD-associated cardiomyopathy, 54
Congestive cardiac failure (CCF), 255

Congestive heart failure (CHF)
diagnosing in end stage kidney disease (ESKD), 271–272
in end-stage renal disease (ESRD), 253
epidemiology, 271
and left ventricular hypertrophy (LVH), 135–136
risk of contrast induced nephropathy (CIN), 348
Connective tissue diseases (CTD), 246
Continuous ambulatory peritoneal dialysis (CAPD), 174
Continuous haemodialysis regimes, 55–56
Continuous positive airway pressure (CPAP), 397, 398
Continuous renal replacement therapy (CRRT), 175, 193
Continuous Ultrafiltration for Congestive Heart Failure (CUORE) trial, 166*t*, 167–168
Contrast-induced acute kidney injury (CI-AKI), 157
Contrast induced nephropathy (CIN), 16, 88
clinical features/diagnosis of, 349
clinical significance of, 347
overview of, 347
pathogenesis of, 347–348
preventive strategies
contrast volume, 351, 351*t*
intravenous fluids, 349–350
N-acetylcysteine (NAC), 350–351
pathogenic mechanisms and, 348*f*
remote ischemic preconditioning (RIPC) technique, 351–352
renin–angiotensin–aldosterone system (RAAS) blockade, 352
statins, 351
risk factors of, 348–349
risk scoring model for PCI, 349*f*
Contrast volume, minimization, during angiography, 351, 351*t*
Coronary angiography, 88, 224–225
Coronary artery bypass graft (CABG)
in acute kidney injury (AKI), 355–356
bare metal stents (BMS) *vs*., 321–322
in chronic kidney disease (CKD), 28, 35, 238, 320
drug eluting stents (DES) *vs*., 322–323, 322*f*, 323*f*
optimization, 324–325, 325*t*
percutaneous coronary intervention (PCI) *vs*., 36, 321, 321*t*
percutaneous transluminal coronary angioplasty (PTCA) *vs*., 321
Coronary artery calcium (CAC) score, 221
Coronary artery disease (CAD), 251–253, 252*t*
and acute coronary syndromes, 87
cardiovascular features, between CKD and non CKD patients, 40*t*
in chronic kidney disease (CKD), 6, 35–40
clinical presentation, 36
epidemiology of, 35
medical therapy, 37–40
pathophysiology of, 35–36
problems, reasons for, 317, 318*t*
risk reduction, 36–37
traditional and nontraditional risk factors, 36
treatment options, 317–325 *See also* Revascularization
electron-beam CT (EBCT) for, 16
endothelial dysfunction and, 3, 5
medical therapy
antiplatelet therapy, 38
blood pressure management, 37–38
CABG *vs*. PCI, 39
revascularization in CKD patients, 38–40
stable angina, 38
statins, 37
STEMI and NSTEMI, 38–39
screening strategies, in candidates for kidney transplants, 219–225
cardiac biomarkers, 222–223
cardiac magnetic resonance imaging (CMR), 222
coronary angiography, 224–225
coronary artery calcium (CAC) score, 221
coronary computed tomographic angiography (CCTA), 221–222
dobutamine stress echocardiogram (DSE), 223–224
electrocardiogram (ECG), 220–221
exercise stress test (EST), 223
myocardial perfusion scintigraphy (MPS), 223
physical examination, 220
stress cardiac MRI (dobutamine and adenosine), 224
transthoracic echocardiogram (TTE), 221
single-photon emission computed tomography (SPECT) for, 16
sudden cardiac death (SCD) and, 24
vitamin D in. *See* Vitamin D
Coronary atheroma, revascularisation for, 28–29
Coronary atherosclerotic heart disease, 137
Coronary computed tomographic angiography (CCTA), 221–222
Coronary endothelial dysfunction, 5
Coronary stent type, in CKD
drug-eluting stent
vs. bare metal stents, 331–332
in dialysis patients, 332
in dialysis *vs*. non-dialysis patients, 332–333
CORONARY trial, 361
Correction of Hemoglobin and Outcomes in Renal Insufficiency (CHOIR) study, 121–122
Corticosteroids, 261–262
minimization strategy, in KTR, 266
CPAP. *See* Continuous positive airway pressure (CPAP)
CPB. *See* Cardiopulmonary bypass (CPB)
CPET. *See* Cardiopulmonary exercise testing (CPET)
CPX. *See* Cardiopulmonary stress testing (CPX)
C-reactive protein (CRP), 36, 61, 63, 139
Critical limb ischemia (CLI), 16, 339
CRP. *See* C-reactive protein (CRP)
CRRT. *See* Continuous renal replacement therapy (CRRT)
CRS. *See* Cardiorenal syndrome (CRS)
CTA. *See* Computed tomographic angiography (CTA)
CTD. *See* Connective tissue diseases (CTD)
CTEPH. *See* Chronic thromboembolism pulmonary hypertension (CTEPH)
cTn. *See* Cardiac troponin (cTn)
cTnT. *See* Cardiac troponin T (cTnT)
C-type natriuretic peptide, 3
CVA. *See* Cerebrovascular accident (CVA)
CVD. *See* Cardiovascular disease (CVD)
CVP. *See* Central venous pressure (CVP)
Cyclic adenosine monophosphate (cAMP), 303, 305
Cyclooxygenase 1 (COX-1), 302
CYP450. *See* Cytochrome P450 (CYP)
Cystatin C, 358
Cytochrome P450 (CYP) polymorphisms, 306
Cytokines and markers of inflammation in CKD, 62–63

D

D-1α-Hydroxylase, 71
Dabigatran, 284–285, 286, 287*t*, 288
Daily nocturnal HD (DNHD), 66
DAPT. *See* Dual antiplatelet therapy (DAPT)
Dartmouth Atlas, 213
DCT1. *See* Divalent metal transporter 1
DD. *See* Diastolic dysfunction (DD)
"Dead in bed" syndrome, 24
Decompensated heart failure, ultrafiltration (UF) therapy in, 163–169 *See also* Acute decompensated heart failure (ADHF)
Deferasirox (DFRA), 115
Deferiprone, 110, 115

Deferoxamine (DFO), 110, 112, 115
DENERV-HTN study, 421
DES. *See* Drug eluting stents (DES)
Destination therapy (DT) pathway, 191
Detection of Ischemia in Asymptomatic Diabetics (DIAD) trial, 236
DEU. *See* Deuterium dilution (DEU)
Deuterium dilution (DEU), 175
DFO. *See* Deferoxamine (DFO)
DFRA. *See* Deferasirox (DFRA)
Diabetes*See also* Dyslipidemia
  BP goals in, 405
  post-KT, 262–263
  as risk factor for CIN, 348
  as risk factor for CKD, 80, 85, 236, 239
  as risk factor for SCD, 24–25
Dialysis-induced ischemia, 25
Dialysis Infection and Vitamin D in New England (DIVINE) trial, 102
Dialysis Outcomes and Practice Patterns Study (DOPPS) study, 38, 307
Diastolic dysfunction (DD)
  KT in patients with cardiomyopathy, 274
Die Deutsche Diabetes Dialyse (4-D) trial, 37, 230, 370–371, 371*t*
Dietary and microbiota modification, for inflammation and CKD, 66
Dietary phosphorus intake, 71, 72*f*
DIF. *See* Diffuse interstitial fibrosis (DIF)
Diffuse interstitial fibrosis (DIF), 45
Direct oral anticoagulants (DOACs), 295–296, 298
  in atrial fibrillation
    in CKD stage 3 patients, 288–290
    laboratory monitoring and management of bleeding for DOACs, 286–288
    pharmacokinetic/pharmacodynamic characteristics, 286
    pivotal clinical trials, summary of, 284–286
    prescribing information and characteristics, 287*t*
    in stage 5D CKD patients with AF, 291
    trials for nonvalvular atrial fibrillation, 285*t*, 289*t*
Direct renin inhibitors (DRI), 82, 83*t*
  plus ACEi/AIIT1RA, 89
Diuretic Optimization Strategies Evaluation trial (DOSE-AHF), 177, 178*f*
Diuretics, clinical trials and, 165, 166*t*, 177, 180
Divalent metal transporter 1 (DMT1), 109
DOACs. *See* Direct oral anticoagulants (DOACs)
Dobutamine stress cardiac MRI (DSCMR)
  for coronary artery disease (CAD), 224
Dobutamine stress echocardiogram (DSE)
  for coronary artery disease (CAD), 223–224
  for kidney transplantation, 235–236, 253
Dopamine, 362
Doxazosin, 404
Doxercalciferol, 106
DREAM trial investigators, 85
DRI. *See* Direct renin inhibitors (DRI)
Drug eluting stents (DES), 319
  vs. coronary artery bypass grafting (CABG), 322–323, 322*f*, 323*f*
Drug-eluting stents (DES), 39
"Dry weight," 174
Dual antiplatelet therapy (DAPT), 225, 303
  in CKD patients, 307–308, 319, 329, 330
Dual-energy X-ray absorptiometry (DXA), 175
Duplex renal ultrasonography (DUS), for renal artery stenosis, 414
DUS. *See* Duplex renal ultrasonography (DUS)
DXA. *See* Dual-energy X-ray absorptiometry (DXA)
Dyslipidemia
  in chronic kidney disease (CKD), 369
    AURORA trial, 371, 371*t*
    4D trial, 370–371, 371*t*
    other treatments, 372–373
    SHARP trial, 371–372, 371*t*
    statin therapy, 372, 372*f*, 373*f*
    treatment, 370–372
  in end stage kidney disease (ESKD)
    hemodialysis (HD), 370
    peritoneal dialysis (PD), 370
  KDIGO recommendations, 373
  and kidney transplantation, 370, 374
  overview, 369
  in patients with CKD, 64
    interventions, 230–231
  as risk factor for CVD in KTR, 263–264
Dyspnea, 173, 206, 208, 211
Dystrophin, 139

E

EBCT. *See* Electron-beam CT (EBCT)
ECF. *See* Extracellular compartment (ECF)
ECG. *See* Electrocardiogram (ECG)
ECs. *See* Endothelial cells (ECs)
Edmonton Symptom Assessment Scale, 206, 207–208*f*
EDNO. *See* Endothelium-derived nitric oxide (EDNO)
Edoxaban, 285, 286, 287*t*
EES. *See* Everolimus-eluting stents (EES)
Effective circulation fluid volume (ECFV), 131
Effect of Tolvaptan on Hemodynamic Parameters in Subjects with Heart Failure (ECLIPSE) study, 179
Efficacy of Vasopressin Antagonist in Heart Failure Outcome Study with Tolvaptan (EVEREST) trial, 179
ELAMs. *See* Endothelial–leukocyte adhesion molecules (ELAMs)
Electric impedance (Z), 171
Electrocardiogram (ECG), for coronary artery disease (CAD), 220–221
Electron-beam CT (EBCT), for coronary artery disease (CAD), 16
EMPHASIS-HF study group, 88
Endogenous NO synthase (NOS) inhibitor, 63
Endothelial cells (ECs)
  activation, 4
  antigens, 5
  biology of, 3
  dysfunction, 4
  function/injury, 5
  glomerular, 7
  renal, 5
  surface markers, 6
Endothelial dysfunction
  endothelial activation and, 4–5
  evaluation of, 5–6
  and nitric oxide, 3–8
  pulmonary vascular remodeling, 247
Endothelial function, 3–4
  biological spectrum, 4*f*
Endothelial–leukocyte adhesion molecules (ELAMs), 5
Endothelial nitric oxide synthase (eNOS), 6, 81
Endothelial progenitor cells (EPCs), 5, 6, 66, 120
Endothelin-1, 7, 8*f*
Endothelin (ET), 3, 247, 248
Endothelium
  albuminuria and, 6
  complex nature of, 3
  functional changes, 5
  functions of, 3
  nitric oxide and, 6
  structural changes, 5
Endothelium-derived nitric oxide (EDNO), 3

End stage kidney disease (ESKD)
  and cardiomyopathy
    diagnosing CHF, 271–272
    epidemiology, 271
    pathophysiology, 272–273, 272*f*
    treatment, 273–274
  dyslipidemia in, 369–374
  on hemodialysis (HD), 243
  hyperphosphotemia, presence of, 15
  incidence and prevalence of CAD, 251
  PH in patients with, 243
  renal denervation and, 423
  sympathetic nervous overactivity and, 422
  valvular calcification in, 11–19
  vascular calcification in, 11–19
ENGAGE AF-TIMI trial, 285, 285*t*, 289*t*, 290
ENGAGE AF trial, 296
eNOS. *See* Endothelial nitric oxide synthase (eNOS)
EPCs. *See* Endothelial progenitor cells (EPCs)
Epicardial coronary atherosclerosis in CKD patients, 36
Epigenetics
  inflammation and oxidative stress, 65*f*, 66
Epinephrine, 301
Eplerenone Post-Acute Myocardial Infarction Heart Failure Efficacy and Survival Study (EPHESUS), 89
Epoprostenol, 248
Ergosterol, 97
Erythropoiesis stimulating agent (ESA), 121
Erythropoietin (EPO)
  anemia treatment in patients with CKD
    future of, 126–127
    KDIGO guidelines, 124*t*
    randomized controlled trails in, 122*t*
    target hemoglobin for, 121–122
  cardiovascular risk
    erythropoiesis stimulating agent (ESA) dose, role of, 124–125
    higher Hb level, role of, 123–124
    hypertension, role of, 125
    iron and thrombocytosis, role of, 125–126
    potential mechanism of, 122–126, 124*f*
  non-hematological effects on cardiovascular system, 120*t*
    angiogenesis, 120
    cardiac effects, 120–121
    hypertension, 121
    thrombosis, 121
  overview, 119
  physiology, 119–122
  receptor, 119–120
  regulation of production, 120
  site of production, 119
  structure of, 119
ESA. *See* Erythropoiesis stimulating agent (ESA)
E-selectin, 3, 5
ESKD. *See* End stage kidney disease (ESKD)
EST. *See* Exercise stress test (EST)
ET. *See* Endothelin (ET)
European Renal Best Practice (ERBP), 83, 87, 106
  guidelines, 252*t*, 253
Euvolemia, 173
Evaluation of Cinacalet Hydrochloride Therapy to Lower Cardiovascular Events (EVOVLE) study, 56
Everolimus-eluting stents (EES), 323
EVOLVE trial, 73
Exercise stress test (EST), 223
Exercise training, for renal transplantation, 229–230
Extracellular compartment (ECF), 171
Extra cranial carotid artery disease
  clinical presentation, 340
  interventional management, 340
  non interventional management, 340

F

FAME-2 trial, 236, 318
Fat-free mass (FFM), 175
Femoral *vs.* radial artery, in CKD, 333
Fenoldopam, 362
Fentanyl, 206
Fetuin-A, 15
FFM. *See* Fat-free mass (FFM)
FFR. *See* Fractional flow reserve (FFR)
FGF inhibitors, 56
Fibrinogen, 3
Fibroblast growth factor-23 (FGF-23), 15, 46–47, 49*f*, 98, 101, 136, 264
  and cardio vascular disease (CVD), 71, 73
  effect on phosphorus metabolism, 71–72
Fibroblast growth factor receptor (FGFR)-1, 98
Fibromuscular dysplasia (FMD), 412
Fibrotic cardiac remodeling, in ESKD, 27
Flash pulmonary edema (FPE), 378
Flow-mediated dilation (FMD), 4, 104
Flow-mediated vasodilation, 4
FMD. *See* Fibromuscular dysplasia (FMD); Flow-mediated dilation (FMD)
Folic Acid for Vascular Outcome Reduction in Transplantation (FAVORIT) trial, 261, 264
Fosinopril in Dialysis Trial (FOSIDIAL), 29
4D trial, 230, 370–371, 371*t*
FPE. *See* Flash pulmonary edema (FPE)
Fractional flow reserve (FFR), 236, 415–416
Framingham Heart Study score, 220
FREAK trial, 236
FREEDOM trial, 239, 266, 322
Frequent Hemodialysis Network (FHN) trial group, 55, 256
Frizzled-related protein 4 (FRP-4), 98
Furosemide, 208, 404

G

Gadolinium-based contrast agents in CKD, 53–54
Gadolinium-DTPA (Gd-DTPA) metal, 52
Galectin-3, 137–138, 147
Gas microemboli formation, 247
Gestational hypertension, 385
Global Registry of Acute Coronary Events (GRACE) study, 38
Glomerular capillary endotheliosis, 388
Glomerular endothelial cell injury, 7, 8*f*
Glomerular integrity, markers of, 148
Glutathione (GSH), 63
Glutathione redox status (GSSG/GSH), 63–64
Glycocalyx, 7, 8*f*
GRAVITAS study, 309
GSH. *See* Glutathione (GSH)

H

Haemodialysis, 25–26
HALT-PKD trial, 406
HCPOA. *See* Health Care power of attorney (HCPOA)
HD. *See* Hemodialysis (HD)
HDL. *See* High-density lipoprotein (HDL)

Health Care power of attorney (HCPOA), 213
Health related quality of life (HRQOL), 206
Heart and kidney transplantation (HKT), 199
Heart disease, biomarkers in, 146–148, 148*f*
Heart failure (HF)
  clinical relevance of RAAS inhibition in, 88
  palliation with dual burden of, 205–214
  renal denervation in, 424
  UF therapy in. *See* Ultrafiltration (UF) therapy
  vitamin D therapy for, 104–105
Heart, inflammation and oxidative stress, 65–66, 65*f*
HeartMate II, 191–192, 192*f*
HeartMate III, 191
HeartMate I, LVAD device, 191
Heart Outcomes Prevention Evaluation-2 (HOPE-2), 7, 67
Heart rate variability (HRV), 24, 139
HeartWare, LVAD device, 191
HELLP syndrome, 389
Hematuria, 297, 298
Hemodialysis (HD), 62, 86, 174, 237, 370
  and inflammation, associated with CKD, 66–67
Hemodynamic instability, 348
Hemostasis, 3, 231, 301, 303–305
Hepcidin, 126
HF. *See* Heart failure (HF)
HIF-PH inhibitors, 126
HIFs. *See* Hypoxia-inducible factors (HIFs)
High-density lipoprotein (HDL), 64, 369
High homocysteine (HC) level, 63
High platelet reactivity, 306
High residual platelet reactivity (HRPR), 306
High-sensitivity cardiac troponin, 146
Histamine, 5
HKT. *See* Heart and kidney transplantation (HKT)
Holy Grail, 415
Homocysteine study (HOST), 67
HORIZON-HF study, 185, 186*f*
Hospice care, 213–214
HRPR. *See* High residual platelet reactivity (HRPR)
HRQOL. *See* Health related quality of life (HRQOL)
HRV. *See* Heart rate variability (HRV)
HSS. *See* Hypertonic saline solution (HSS)
HTN. *See* Hypertension (HTN)
H-type fatty acid-binding protein (H-FABP), 151
Hydralazine, 404
Hydromorphone-3 glucuronide (H3G), 206
Hydroxyapatite, 15
Hydroxymethylgluaryl-coenzyme A inhibitors, 67
Hyperglycemia, 348
Hyperkalaemia, 26, 26*f*
Hyperkalemia, 135
  RAAS inhibition and, 91
Hyperlipidemia, 374
Hyperparathyroidism, 274
Hypertension (HTN)
  cardiovascular risk and, 125
  erythropoietin effect on cardiovascular system, 121
  optimization in kidney transplant candidates, 231
  post-KT, 261–262, 262*t*
  systemic arterial, 80, 87
  vitamin D and, 103–104
Hypertonic saline solution (HSS), 173
Hypertriglyceridemia, 369
Hypertrophy of distal nephron, avoidance of, 164
Hyperuricemia, 48, 56
Hypokalemia, 26
Hypomagnesemia, 26–27
Hypovolemia
  patient management with ultrafiltration, 169
  risks with ultrafiltration, 164–165
Hypoxia, 120
Hypoxia-inducible factors (HIFs), 120, 126

I

ICD. *See* Implantable cardioverter-defibrillators (ICD); Internal cardioverter defibrillator (ICD)
ICF. *See* Intracellular fluid compartment (ICF)
ICV. *See* Intracellular fluid volume (ICV)
Idarucizimab, 288
IDL. *See* Intermediate-density lipoprotein (IDL)
IFN-α. *See* Interferon-alpha (IFN-α)
IL-1. *See* Interleukin-1 (IL-1)
IL-6. *See* Interleukin-6 (IL-6)
IL-8. *See* Interleukin-8 (IL-8)
IL-10. *See* Interleukin-10 (IL-10)
IL-18. *See* Interleukin-18 (IL-18)
Iloprost, 248
Imaging modalities, in CKD-associated cardiomyopathy, 50–54
Immunosuppression minimization strategies, in KT, 265, 266*t*
Immunosuppressive agents, as transplant specific risk factor for CVD, 261–262, 265
Implantable cardioverter-defibrillators (ICD), 27–28, 28*f*
Indoxyl sulphate (IS), 48, 57, 63
Inflammation, in chronic kidney disease (CKD)
  cytokines and markers of, 62–63
  deficient 02-scavenging capacity, 63–64
  dyslipidemia, 64
  exaggerated 02-generation, 63
  hemodialysis, 62
  malnutrition, 64
  overview of, 61–62, 62*f*
  and oxidative stress, on CVD, 63, 65*f*
    blood vessels, 64–65
    epigenetics, 66
    heart, 65–66
  peritoneal dialysis (PD), 62
  therapeutic interventions
    antioxidants, 67
    AST-120, 67
    dietary and microbiota modification, 66
    hemodialysis frequency, increasing, 66–67
    homocysteine level, lowering, 67
    other therapies, 67
    physical activity and lifestyle modification, 66
    statins, 67
  uremic toxins, 63
Inflammatory cytokines, 248
Inflammatory modulators, 3
Infrainguinal peripheral arterial disease
  clinical presentation, 339
  interventional management, 340
  non interventional management, 339
Inorganic pyrophosphate, 15
Insulin-like growth factor-binding protein 7 (IGFBP7), 150
Insulin resistance
  molecular mechanisms in CKD, 50
Intention to treat (ITT) analyses, 122
Interagency Registry for Mechanically Assisted Circulatory Support (INTERMACS), 192, 193, 195, 196, 199
Intercellular adhesion molecule-1 (ICAM-1), 3, 5, 134
Interferon-alpha (IFN-α), 134

Interleukin-1 (IL-1), 61, 64, 134, 146, 248
Interleukin-6 (IL-6), 61, 63, 64, 66, 67, 134, 139, 248, 398
Interleukin-8 (IL-8), 398
Interleukin-10 (IL-10), 61, 63, 67
Interleukin-18 (IL-18), 151, 159, 358, 359
Intermediate-density lipoprotein (IDL), 369
Internal cardioverter defibrillator (ICD), 272
International normalized ratio (INR), 295
International Study of Comparative Health Effectiveness with Medical and Invasive Approaches–Chronic Kidney Disease (ISCHEMIA-CKD) trial, 318
Intracardiac echocardiography (ICE) catheter, in endovascular aortic repair, 338–339
Intracellular fluid compartment (ICF), 171
Intracellular fluid volume (ICV), 174
Intradialytic myocardial ischemia, 25
Intravascular ultrasound (IVUS), 237
  of coronary plaque in patients with ESKD, 331
  in endovascular aortic repair, 338–339
  minimization of contrast volume, during angiography, 351
Intravenous fluids, for CIN patients, 349–350
Irbesartan, 91
Iron and Atherosclerosis (FeAST) trial, 114
IS. *See* Indoxyl sulphate (IS)
ISCHEMIA-CKD study, 37
Istaroxime, 185
IVUS. *See* Intravascular ultrasound (IVUS)

J
Jarvik 2000, LVAD device, 191

K
Kcentra®, 288
KDIGO. *See* Kidney Disease Improving Global Outcomes (KDIGO)
KDOQI. *See* Kidney Disease Outcomes Quality Initiative (KDOQI)
Kerley B-lines, 172
KI. *See* Kidney impairment (KI)
Kidney attack
  concept of, 155
  neutrophil gelatinase-associated lipocalin. *See* Neutrophil gelatinase-associated lipocalin (NGAL)
  troponin-like biomarker of, 155–156
Kidney Disease Improving Global Outcomes (KDIGO), 37, 83, 106, 126, 291
Kidney Disease Outcomes Quality Initiative (KDOQI), 106, 126, 146, 230, 254–255, 274
Kidney impairment (KI), 192
Kidney injury molecule-1 (KIM-1), 151
Kidney transplantation (KT)*See also* Post-kidney transplant modification, of cardiovascular risk; Pulmonary hypertension (PTH); Revascularization
  cardiac pre-operative evaluation as opportunity to optimizing risk factors in, 229–232
  cardiac surveillance, 251–256
  dyslipidemia and, 370, 374
  heart and, 199
  in patients with cardiomyopathy
    diastolic dysfunction, 274
    left ventricular dysfunction (LVD) and, 275–277
    systolic dysfunction, 274–275
    work-up, 277*f*
  screening strategies for CAD in candidates for, 219–225
  stage 5T CKD, 86–87
Klotho, 46–47, 49*f*, 56–57, 71–73, 98
KT. *See* Kidney transplantation (KT)

L
Labile iron pool, 109
L-Arginine, 247
Late enhancement imaging, in CKD-associated cardiomyopathy, 52–53
Late gadolinium enhancement (LGE), 222
LCBI. *See* Lipid core burden index (LCBI)
LCZ696 therapy, 186–187
LDL. *See* Low-density lipoprotein (LDL)
Left ventricular assist devices (LVADs)
  impact of baseline renal function on outcome after, 192–193, 194*f*
  impact of continuous blood flow on renal outcome, 193–195
  kidney injury in patients with, 191–201
  management of end-stage HF with, 191
  mechanical circulatory support (MCS), 191
  nephrology assessment for patient undergoing, 200*t*, 201
  overview of, 191–192
  post-implant AKI, 195–196
  renal recovery *vs.* CKD post-LVAD, 196–199, 197*f*
  renal replacement therapy with, 199–201
Left ventricular dysfunction (LVD), 252*t*, 254–256, 271
Left ventricular ejection fraction (LVEF), 54, 81, 86, 88, 177, 246, 276, 276*f*
Left ventricular end diastolic pressure (LVEDP), 350
Left ventricular hypertrophy (LVH), 25, 65, 104, 135, 271, 273, 274, 378
  congestive heart failure and, 135–136
  trials evaluating, 275*t*
Left ventricular mass, in CKD-associated cardiomyopathy, 50, 51–52*f*
Left ventricular mass index (LVMI), 104, 272, 274, 381
  trials evaluating, 275*t*
Levosimendan, 183–185
Levosimendan Infusion versus Dobutamine (LIDO) study, 184, 184*f*
LGE. *See* Late gadolinium enhancement (LGE)
LIFE trial, 7
Light transmission aggregometry (LTA), 304
Lipid core burden index (LCBI), 237
Lipid peroxidation, 110
Lipopolysaccharides, 139
Lisbon Conference, 252*t*, 253
Low-density lipoprotein (LDL), 63
  reduction of, 37
Low-density lipoprotein cholesterol (LDL-C), 369
LTA. *See* Light transmission aggregometry (LTA)
L-type fatty acid-binding protein (L-FABP), 151, 358
LVADs. *See* Left ventricular assist devices (LVADs)
LVD. *See* Left ventricular dysfunction (LVD)
LVEDP. *See* Left ventricular end diastolic pressure (LVEDP)
LVEF. *See* Left ventricular ejection fraction (LVEF)
LVH. *See* Left ventricular hypertrophy (LVH)
LVMI. *See* Left ventricular mass index (LVMI)
Lymphocyte function-associated antigen (LFA)-1, 67
Lysophosphatidylcholine (lysoPC), 64

M
MAC. *See* Membrane attack complex (MAC); Mitral annular calcification (MAC)
MACE. *See* Major adverse cardiovascular events (MACE)
Macitentan, 248
Macrophage-colony stimulating factor (MCSCP), 64
Magnetic resonance angiography (MRA)
  for renal artery stenosis, 414
Magnetic resonance imaging (MRI)

for cardiomyopathy, 271
Mahan's equation, 243
Major adverse cardiovascular events (MACE), 110, 236, 239, 259, 260, 332
Malnutrition-inflammation-atherosclerosis (MIA) syndrome, 64
Malnutrition–inflammation complex syndrome (MICS), 15
Mammalian target of rapamycin (mTOR) inhibitors, 66, 265–266
Mannitol, 362
Marinobufagenin (MBG), 50
Matrix extracellular phosphoglycoprotein (MEPE), 98
Matrix Gla protein (MGP), 15
Matrix metalloproteinases (MMP), 12, 15
MBG. *See* Marinobufagenin (MBG)
MCSCP. *See* Macrophage-colony stimulating factor (MCSCP)
MDCT. *See* Multidetector computed tomography (MDCT)
Mean pulmonary artery pressure (mPAP), 243
MECC. *See* Mini-extracorporeal circulation (MECC)
Mechanical circulatory support (MCS), with LVADs, 191, 197, 198*f*
Megestrol acetate, 67
Membrane attack complex (MAC), 5
MEPE. *See* Matrix extracellular phosphoglycoprotein (MEPE)
Mesangial cells, 7, 8*f*
Metabolic syndrome
  obstructive sleep apnea and, 398, 398*f*
  in renal transplantation, 262
Metaregression analysis, 125
Methadone, 206
Metolazone, 208
MGP. *See* Matrix Gla protein (MGP)
MI. *See* Myocardial infarction (MI)
MIA syndrome. *See* Malnutrition-inflammation-atherosclerosis (MIA) syndrome
Microalbuminuria, 6, 84–85
MICS. *See* Malnutrition–inflammation complex syndrome (MICS)
Mineralocorticoid receptor (MR), 77
Mini-extracorporeal circulation (MECC), 361
Minoxidil, 404
Mitral annular calcification (MAC), 11, 13*f*, 17
Mitral stenosis, 17
Mitral valve, 17, 18*f*
MMP. *See* Matrix metalloproteinases (MMP)
Modification of Diet in Renal Disease (MDRD) study, 36, 291, 403, 405, 407*t*
Monocyte chemoattractant protein-1, 64, 398
Morphine, 206
MPO. *See* Myeloperoxidase (MPO)
MPS. *See* Myocardial perfusion scintigraphy (MPS)
MR. *See* Mineralocorticoid receptor (MR)
MRA. *See* Magnetic resonance angiography (MRA)
MRI. *See* Magnetic resonance imaging (MRI)
mTOR inhibitors. *See* Mammalian target of rapamycin (mTOR) inhibitors
Multidetector computed tomography (MDCT)
  in CKD-associated cardiomyopathy, 54
Multiple myeloma, 348
Myeloperoxidase (MPO), 133
Myocardial fibrosis, 50, 52
Myocardial infarction (MI), 16, 229, 235
Myocardial perfusion scintigraphy (MPS), 223, 235, 251

N

NAC. *See* *N*-acetylcysteine (NAC)
N-acetyl-B-d-glucosaminidase (NAG), 358
N-acetylcysteine (NAC), 350–351
NAD(P)H oxidase (NOX), 48, 64, 65–66, 81
NAG. *See* *N*-acetyl-B-d-glucosaminidase (NAG)
National Cardiovascular Data Registry–Acute Coronary Treatment and Intervention Out-comes Network (NCDR-ACTION), 35
National Center for Complementary and Alternative Medicine, 115
National Health and Nutrition Examination Survey (NHANES), 231, 317, 403
National Heart Lung and Blood Institute, 115
National Hospice and Palliative Care Organization (NHPCO), 213
National Kidney Foundation (NKF), 106, 135, 219
National Kidney Foundation/Kidney Disease Outcomes Quality Initiative (NKF/KDOQI), 251, 252*t*
National Registry of Myocardial Infarction (NRMI), 36
Natriuretic peptides (NP), role of, 173
NAVIGATOR study group, 85
Near-infrared spectroscopy (NIRS), 237
Nephrogenic systemic fibrosis (NSF), 222, 272
NEP inhibitors. *See* Neutral endopeptidase (NEP) inhibitors
Neprilysin, 186
Nesiritide, 180–181, 362
Nesiritide Study Group, 180
Neutral endopeptidase (NEP) inhibitors, 185–187
Neutrophil gelatinase-associated lipocalin (NGAL), 150, 357, 359
  as biologically plausible kidney attack biomarker, 156
  clinical platforms for NGAL measurement in kidney attack, 158
  clinical use of NGAL in kidney attack, 158–159, 159*t*
  for differential diagnosis of kidney attack, 157, 157*t*
  for early prediction of kidney attack, 156–157, 156*t*
  economic implications of NGAL use in kidney attack, 158
  for prediction of adverse outcomes after kidney attack, 157–158
  as set for center stage in kidney attack, 160
  use in clinical trials for kidney attack, 159, 159*f*
New onset diabetes after transplantation (NODAT), 262–263, 263*t*
New York Heart Association (NYHA), 88, 175, 275, 381
NGAL. *See* Neutrophil gelatinase-associated lipocalin (NGAL)
NHPCO. *See* National Hospice and Palliative Care Organization (NHPCO)
NIRS. *See* Near-infrared spectroscopy (NIRS)
Nitric oxide (NO), 3, 6, 248
NKF. *See* National Kidney Foundation (NKF)
NO. *See* Nitric oxide (NO)
NODAT. *See* New onset diabetes after transplantation (NODAT)
Noninvasive Doppler ultrasonography (USG), for HTN post-KT, 261
Non-ST-elevation acute coronary syndromes (NSTE-ACS), 303
Non-steroidal anti-inflammatory drugs (NSAIDs), 206, 298
Non-ST segment–elevation myocardial infarction (NSTEMI), 35, 38–39
Norepinephrine, 5
Normal Hematocrit Cardiovascular Trial (NHCT), 121
Novacor, LVAD device, 191
NOX. *See* NAD(P)H oxidase (NOX)
NP. *See* Natriuretic peptides (NP)
NRAMP2. *See* Divalent metal transporter 1
NRMI. *See* National Registry of Myocardial Infarction (NRMI)
NSAIDs. *See* Non-steroidal anti-inflammatory drugs (NSAIDs)
NSF. *See* Nephrogenic systemic fibrosis (NSF)
NSTEMI. *See* Non-ST segment–elevation myocardial infarction (NSTEMI)
N-terminal pro-B-type natriuretic peptide (NT-proBNP), 135, 146, 175
Nuclear factor-κ[kappa]B (NF-κ[kappa]B), 3, 64
NYHA. *See* New York Heart Association (NYHA)

O

Obesity, prevalence of, 229
Obstructive sleep apnea (OSA)
  in chronic kidney disease (CKD)

pathophysiology, 396–398, 397*f*
prevalence, 395–396
studies, 396*t*
and metabolic syndrome, 398*f*
overview, 395
sequence of events in, 397*f*
systemic inflammation and metabolic syndrome, 398
OCT. *See* Optical coherence tomography (OCT)
Ohm's law, 171
Oliguria, 135
OM. *See* Omecamtiv mecarbil (OM)
Omecamtiv mecarbil (OM), 182–183
Omipatrilat Versus Enalapril Randomized Trial of Utility in Reducing Events (OVERTURE) trial, 185–186
OMT. *See* Optimal medical therapy (OMT)
1α-Hydroxylase, 15, 98–101
1,25-Dihydroxyvitamin D, 46, 98–101
1,25-Dihydroxyvitamin D_3 (calcitriol), 15
ONTARGET investigators, 89, 91
Opioids, 211
Optical coherence tomography (OCT) study, 237, 331
Optimal medical therapy (OMT), in CKD patients, 38
Oral hydration, CIN prevention and, 350
OSA. *See* Obstructive sleep apnea (OSA)
Oxidative stress, 56
in CKD, 63
and inflammation, on CVD, 64, 65*f*
type 1 cardiorenal syndrome, 132–133
Oxidized glutathione (GSSG), 63
Oxidized LDL (ox-LDL), 64
Oxidized LDL receptor LOX-1, 64
Oxycodone, 206

P

P2Y12 receptor blockers, 303
PA. *See* "Phase angle" (PA)
PAD. *See* Peripheral arterial disease (PAD)
PAH. *See* Pulmonary arterial hypertension (PAH)
Pain, 206
Palliative care, heart and kidney failure, 211–212
Palliative Performance Scale version 2 (PPSv2), 209–210*f*, 212
PARADIGM study, 187
PARAMOUNT trial, 186
Parathyroid hormone (PTH), 47–48, 56, 98, 247, 273, 305
Paricalcitol and Endothelial Function in Chronic Kidney Disease (PENNY) study, 104
Paricalcitol Capsule Benefits in Renal Failure-Induced Cardiac Morbidity (PRIMO) trial, 104
PARs. *See* Protease-activated receptors (PARs)
PASP. *See* Pulmonary artery systolic pressure (PASP)
Patient Outcomes in Renal Transplantation (PORT) study, 259, 260
Patiromer, 91
PAWP. *See* Pulmonary artery wedge pressure (PAWP)
PCC. *See* Prothrombin complex concentrate (PCC)
PCI. *See* Percutaneous coronary intervention (PCI)
p-Cresyl sulphate, 48
PCWP. *See* Pulmonary capillary wedge pressure (PCWP)
PD. *See* Peritoneal dialysis (PD)
PDGF. *See* Platelet-derived growth factor (PDGF)
Pentoxifylline, 67
PEPPER study, 244
Percutaneous coronary intervention (PCI), in CKD, 319–320
CIN risk scoring model for, 348, 349*f*
complications
stent thrombosis, 333
vascular access complications, 333
vascular closure devices, 333–334
vs. coronary artery bypass grafting (CABG), 321, 321*t*
coronary artery lesions characteristics, 331
early invasive *vs.* conservative PCI strategy in CKD and NSTEMI, 331
vs. fibrinolytic therapy in CKD and STEMI, 331
noninvasive testing in kidney transplantation, 236
optimization, 324, 324*t*
revascularization in CKD patients, 38
Percutaneous transluminal angioplasty with stenting (PTRAS), 379
Percutaneous transluminal coronary angioplasty (PTCA), 86
vs. coronary artery bypass grafting (CABG), 321
Periodontal disease, 61
Peripheral arterial disease (PAD), 16, 86, 236
in chronic kidney disease (CKD), 337–343
clinical presentation and management, 338–341
disease burden, 337–338
impact, 338
outcomes in CKD population, 341–343, 341–342*f*, 342–343*t*
Peripheral vascular intervention (PVI), 16
Peritoneal dialysis (PD), 62, 200, 274, 370
PFT. *See* Platelet function testing (PFT)
"Phase angle" (PA), 172
Phenotypic heterogeneity, 3
Phosphate, 46, 56
Phosphorus metabolism, FGF23 and, 71–72
Physical activity and lifestyle modification, in CKD patients, 66
Placenta, 386, 386*f*
Placental growth factor (PlGF), 387, 389
Plasminogen activator (t-PA), 3
Plasminogen activator inhibitor (PAI-1), 3
Platelet biology, 301–302
Platelet-derived growth factor (PDGF), 378
PDGF-B, 7, 8*f*
Platelet dysfunction, in CKD
altered non-renal drug metabolism, 306–307
cytochrome P450 (CYP) polymorphisms, 306
dysfunctional von Willebrand factor (VWF), 307
endogenous derangements of vascular and hemostatic function, 305–306
high platelet reactivity, 306
Platelet function testing (PFT), in CVD, 301, 304, 309
Platelet Inhibition and Patient Outcomes (PLATO) trial, 308, 330
Platelet–platelet aggregation, 301–302
Platelet rich plasma (PRP), 304
PlGF. *See* Placental growth factor (PlGF)
POC testing. *See* Point-of-care (POC) testing
Podocytes, 7, 8*f*
Point-of-care (POC) testing, 304
Polyunsaturated fatty acids (PUFA), 66
POSEIDON study, 324
Post-kidney transplantation erythrocytosis, 87
Post-kidney transplant modification, of cardiovascular risk
estimation of CVD risk, 260
incidence/prevalence of CVD, 259
overview, 259
risk factors for CVD, 259–260, 260*t*
strategies to reducing CVD risk in KTR
belatacept, 266
calcineurin inhibitors (CNI) choice/minimization, 265
corticosteroid minimization/discontinuation, 266
immunosuppression modification, 265, 266*t*
mammalian target of rapamycin (mTOR) inhibitors, 265–266
pre-emptive and living donor transplantation, 266
traditional risk factors role for CVD

abnormal phosphate metabolism, 264
age, 260–261
diabetes, 262–263
dyslipidemia, 263–264
gender and ethnicity, 261
metabolic syndrome, 262
post-transplantation hypertension, 261–262, 262*t*
tobacco use, 261
transplant specific risk factors for CVD, 264–265
allograft dysfunction, 264
immunosuppressive agents, 265
Post-transplantation hypertension, 261–262, 262*t*
PQRST (presence of pain, quality of pain, radiation, precipitating or relieving factors, and timing), 206
Prasugrel, 303, 330
Preeclampsia
clinical manifestations, 388
definition of, 385
epidemiology of, 385–386
history of, 389*f*
implications for future vascular disease, 388–389
incidence of, 385
overview, 385
pathogenesis of, 386–388
angiogenic factors, 386–388
immune factors, 388
placental factors, 386, 386*f*
risk factors for, 385–386
signs and symptoms of, 388
Pre-emptive and living donor transplantation, 266
Preliminary Study of Relaxin in Acute Heart Failure (Pre-RELAX-AHF) trial, 181
PREVEND study, 7–8
Prevention of Restenosis with Tranilast and its Outcomes (PRESTO) trial, 332
PRIMO trial, 104
Prognostication, 211
PROMETHEUS study, 308
Prostacyclin, 3, 248
Protease-activated receptors (PARs), 304
PROTECT pilot study, 182, 183*f*
Proteinase-activated receptors (PARs), 297
Protein bound "uremic toxins" (PBUTs), 48–50
Protein–energy malnutrition (PEM), 15
Proteinuria, 84–85, 102, 385, 387, 388
Prothrombin complex concentrate (PCC), 288
PRP. *See* Platelet rich plasma (PRP)
P-selectin, 5
Pseudovasculogenesis, 386
PTCA. *See* Percutaneous transluminal coronary angioplasty (PTCA)
PTH. *See* Parathyroid hormone (PTH); Pulmonary hypertension (PTH)
PTRAS. *See* Percutaneous transluminal angioplasty with stenting (PTRAS)
PUFA. *See* Polyunsaturated fatty acids (PUFA)
Pulmonary arterial hypertension (PAH), 243
Pulmonary artery systolic pressure (PASP), 243
Pulmonary artery wedge pressure (PAWP), 243
Pulmonary capillary wedge pressure (PCWP), 179
Pulmonary hypertension (PTH), in potential kidney transplant recipient, 243–249
arteriovenous fistulae, 246–247
classification of, 244*t*
epidemiology
incidence, 244
prevalence, 243–244, 245*t*
prognosis, 244–246
etiology and pathogenesis, 243, 246–248
inflammation, 248
management of, 248
mortality data in patients with, 245–246
overview, 243
pathophysiology of, 246*f*
pulmonary vascular remodeling
endothelial dysfunction, 247
parathyroid hormone and calcium regulation, 247
thromboembolism, 247
Pulmonary vascular resistance (PVR), 243
Pulsatility index, 200
pVHL. *See* von Hippel Lindau protein (pVHL)
PVI. *See* Peripheral vascular intervention (PVI)
PVR. *See* Pulmonary vascular resistance (PVR)
Pyrophosphate, 15

Q

Quality of life (QOL), 126

R

RAAS. *See* Renin–angiotensin–aldosterone system (RAAS)
Ramipril Efficacy in Nephropathy-2 (REIN-2) trial, 403, 405, 407*t*
Randomised Aldactone Evaluation Study (RALES) study, 29, 89
Randomized Evaluation of Intravenous Levosimendan Efficacy (REVIVE-II) trial, 184
RANKL (Receptor Activator for Nuclear Factor kB Ligand), 100
RAS. *See* Renal artery stenosis (RAS)
RBC. *See* Red blood cell (RBC)
REACH-Pilot study, 424
Reactive oxygen species (ROS), 48, 63, 65, 81, 347, 348*f*, 398
and nitric oxide (NO) production, 132
Recombinant human EPO (rHuEPO), 119, 121
Red blood cell (RBC)
production, 119
transfusion risk, 126
Redox cycling, 109
REIN-2 trial, 404
Relaxin, 181–182
Relaxin in Acute Heart Failure (RELAX-AHF) trial, 181
Relief for Acutely Fluid-Overloaded Patients with Decompensated Congestive Heart Failure (Rapid-CHF) trial, 165
RE-LY trial, 285, 285*t*, 288, 289*t*, 290, 296
REMATCH study, 191
Remote ischemic preconditioning (RIPC) technique, 351–352
Renal artery stenosis (RAS)
atherosclerotic renal artery disease (ARAD), 411–412
and atherosclerotic renovascular disease (ARVD), 377, 378
consequences of, 412
diagnosis of clinically significant RAS, 414–416, 414*t*
etiology of, 411–414
evaluation and management of, 415*f*
fibromuscular dysplasia (FMD), 412
overview, 411
randomized trials, 413–414
Takayasu's arteritis, 412
Renal Artery Stenosis in Coronary Artery Disease (RAS-CAD) trial, 379
Renal denervation
catheter-based approach, in human resistant hypertension, 419–420
and chronic kidney disease, 422–423
and end-stage kidney disease, 423
in heart failure and cardiac arrhythmias, 424
renal sympathetic nerves

in cardiovascular control, 419, 420*f*
in chronic kidney disease, 419
Symplicity HTN studies, 420–421
Renal disease, biomarkers in, 148–151, 149*f*
Renal dysfunction, 192
Renal excretion, of water, 171
Renal impairment, 35, 36
Renal morbidity, 298
Renal perfusion, 362
Renal recovery *vs.* CKD post-LVAD, 196–199, 197*f*
Renal replacement therapy (RRT), 195
ESKD patients receiving, 81, 86
with left ventricular assist devices (LVADs), 199–201
Renal revascularization
in patient with heart failure, 380*t*
recommendations for, 381*t*
Renal sympathetic nerves
in cardiovascular control, 419, 420*f*
in chronic kidney disease, 419
Renal tissue oxygenation, 362
Renal transplantation. *See* Kidney transplantation (KT)
Renal tubular epithelium, 132
Renal tubular injury, markers of, 148–149
Renal vein congestion, reduction of, 164
Renin–angiotensin–aldosterone system (RAAS), 45–46, 272, 358, 378, 396, 412
activation, 131, 134
adverse events and safety, 91
in cardiorenal diseases, 82
in cardiovascular risk and disease, 81–82
CIN prevention and, 352
clinical relevance of RAAS inhibition in cardiac disease
cardiorenal syndromes, 88–89
coronary angiogram and contrast induced nephropathy (CIN), 88
coronary artery disease and acute coronary syndromes, 87
reduced left ventricular systolic function or heart failure (HF), 88
sudden cardiac death, 88
clinical relevance of RAAS inhibition in kidney disease
autosomal dominant polycystic kidney disease (ADPKD), 85–86
diabetic kidney disease, 85
insulin sensitivity and diabetic kidney disease, 85
microalbuminuria and proteinuria, 84–85
post-kidney transplantation erythrocytosis, 87
stage 1–5 chronic kidney disease, 83–84
stage 5D CKD renal replacement therapy (RRT) with dialysis, 86
stage 5T CKD kidney transplantation, 86–87
systemic arterial hypertension, 87
combination therapy using classes of RAAS inhibitors, 89–90
elements of, 78–79*t*
and genetics, 90
in health, 77–80, 80*f*
and hyperkalemia, 91
inhibitors, 102, 103
aldosterone receptor antagonists, 83, 83*t*
angiotensin converting enzyme inhibitors (ACEi), 82, 83*t*, 84, 86
angiotensin II AT1 receptor blockers (AIIT1RA), 82, 83*t*, 84, 86
direct renin inhibitors (DRI), 82, 83*t*
in kidney disease, 80–81
and variability by race, 90
Renin–angiotensin system (RAS), 15, 66
blockade, 29
Retinoid X receptor (RXR), 98
Revascularization
atherosclerotic renovascular disease (ARVD), 379–380
in CKD patients, 317–325, 329–334
antiplatelet therapy post-PCI, 323–331
bare metal stents (BMS), 321–322, 331–332
CABG *vs.* PCI, 39
cardiovascular features, between CKD and non CKD patients, 40*t*
challenges, 319
coronary artery bypass grafting (CABG), 320–323, 321*t*, 324–325, 325*t*
coronary artery disease (CAD) in, 317–325
coronary artery lesions characteristics in CKD, 331
coronary stent type, 331–333
drug eluting stents (DES), 322–323, 322*f*, 323*f*, 331–333
dual antiplatelet therapy, 319, 330
early invasive *vs.* conservative PCI strategy, 331
femoral *vs.* radial artery, 333
fibrinolytic therapy *vs.* PCI, 331
medical management, 318, 319*f*
optimization, 324–325
percutaneous coronary intervention (PCI), 319–320, 324, 324*t*, 331, 333–334
percutaneous transluminal coronary angioplasty (PTCA), 321
stable angina, 38
STEMI and NSTEMI, 38–39
treatment options, 317–325
for coronary atheroma, 28–29
evaluation prior to transplantation
invasive testing, 236–237
noninvasive testing, 235
strategies for patients on kidney transplant list, 237–239
RHC. *See* Right heart catheterization (RHC)
Right heart catheterization (RHC), 243
Right ventricular (RV) failure, 199
Riociguat, 248
RIPC technique. *See* Remote ischemic preconditioning (RIPC) technique
Risk, injury, failure, loss of kidney function and end stage kidney disease (RIFLE), 356
Rivaroxaban, 285, 286, 287*t*
ROCKET AF trial, 285, 285*t*, 288, 289*t*, 290, 296
Rolofylline, 182
ROOBY trial, 361
RRT. *See* Renal replacement therapy (RRT)
RV failure. *See* Right ventricular (RV) failure
RXR. *See* Retinoid X receptor (RXR)

S
SADHART CHF trial, 211
SAVR. *See* Surgical aortic valve replacement (SAVR)
SBP. *See* Systolic blood pressure (SBP)
Scavenger receptors, 65
SCD. *See* Sudden cardiac death (SCD)
Scientific Advisory Committee on Nutrition (SACN), 101
Selexipag, 248
Serotonin, 5
Serum creatinine (sCr), 177, 298, 356, 357
Serum phosphate, 73
sESAM. *See* Soluble endothelial cell-selective adhesion molecule (sESAM)
Sevelamer hydrochloride, 67
7-Dehydrocholesterol, 97–98
Sildenafil, 248
Simplified Renal Index (SRI) score, 359
Single nucleotide polymorphisms (SNPs), 90
Single-photon emission computed tomography (SPECT)
for coronary artery disease (CAD), 16
Smoking cessation, 230
post-KT, 261

SNPs. *See* Single nucleotide polymorphisms (SNPs)
SNS activation. *See* Sympathetic nervous system (SNS) activation
Society for Cardiac Angiography and Interventions (SCAI), 414
SOD. *See* Superoxidase dismutase (SOD)
Sodium–phosphorus cotransporter, 71, 72*f*
Sodium–potassium adenosine triphosphate (Na–K ATPase), 185
Sodium zirconium cyclosilicate (ZS-9), 90
Soluble endoglin (sEng), 387
Soluble endothelial cell-selective adhesion molecule (sESAM), 7
Soluble Fms-like tyrosine kinase 1 (sFlt-1), 5, 387
Soluble suppressor of tumorigenicity 2 (sST2), 146–147
"Spare the Nephron" trial, 265
SPECT. *See* Single-photon emission computed tomography (SPECT)
Spironolactone, 30, 83, 84, 90, 91
SPRINT research group, 37, 87
SRI score. *See* Simplified Renal Index (SRI) score
SSAHT. *See* Stepped-care antihypertensive treatment (SSAHT)
SSE. *See* Stroke or systemic embolism (SSE)
Stable angina, 38
Stage 1–5 chronic kidney disease, 83–84
Stage 5D CKD renal replacement therapy (RRT) with dialysis, 86
Stage 5T CKD kidney transplantation, 86–87
STAR trial, 413
Statin therapy
  in CIN prevention, 351
  in CKD, 372, 372*f*, 373*f*
    anti-inflammatory effect, 67
  in coronary artery disease (CAD), 37
  in kidney transplant recipients, 374
ST-elevation myocardial infarction (STEMI), 303
STEMI. *See* ST-elevation myocardial infarction (STEMI)
Stent thrombosis, 333
Stepped-care antihypertensive treatment (SSAHT), 421
Stress cardiac MRI (dobutamine and adenosine)
  for coronary artery disease (CAD), 224
Stroke or systemic embolism (SSE), 285–286
Stroke Prevention in Atrial Fibrillation (SPAF), 288
Stroke risk, among patients with CKD and AF, 283–284
ST segment–elevation myocardial infarction (STEMI), 35, 38–39, 110
Studies of Left Ventricular Dysfunction (SOLVD), 89
Study of Heart and Renal Protection (SHARP) trial, 37, 67, 371–372, 371*t*
Study to Evaluate Challenging Responses to Therapy in Congestive Heart Failure (SECRET of CHF) study, 179
Subjective global assessment (SGA), 174
Sudden cardiac death (SCD)
  associated factors and mechanistic hypotheses
    age, 24, 24*f*
    coronary artery disease (CAD), 24
    diabetes mellitus, 24–25
    dialysis and dialysis modality, 24*f*, 25–26
    hyperkalaemia, 26, 26*f*
    hypokalemia, 26
    hypomagnesemia, 26–27
    left ventricular hypertrophy (LVH), 25
  cardiac arrhythmias and, 136–137
  clinical relevance of RAAS inhibition in, 88
  definition of, 21–22
  in end stage kidney disease (ESKD), 21–31
  event rate in ESKD, 22, 22*f*, 24, 24*f*
  key points, 31*t*
  mechanistic contributions, 25*f*
  overview of, 21
  risk factors, establishing, 21–22, 23*t*
  therapeutic strategies, in ESKD, 31*t*
    beta-blockade, 29
    dialysis prescription, 30
    implantable cardioverter-defibrillators (ICD), 27–28, 28*f*
    other pharmacotherapeutic options, 29–30
    revascularisation for coronary atheroma, 28–29
Superoxidase dismutase (SOD), 63
SUPPORT study, 212
Suppressor of tumorigenicity 2 (ST2), 146–147
Surgical aortic valve replacement (SAVR), 17, 18*f*
Survival and Ventricular Enlargement Trial (SAVE), 89
Survival of Patients with Acute Heart Failure in need of Intravenous Inotropic Support (SURVIVE) trial, 184
Sympathetic nervous system (SNS) activation, 132, 135
  hyperactivity of, 134
Symplicity HTN trial program, 420–421
SYNergy between PCI with TAXus and Cardiac Surgery (SYNTAX) score, 324
SYNTAX trial, 239
Systemic arterial hypertension, 87
Systolic blood pressure (SBP), 181
Systolic BP Intervention Trial (SPRINT), 405–406, 407*t*
Systolic dysfunction
  KT in patients with cardiomyopathy, 274–275

T

T1 mapping, 53, 53*f*
Tadalafil, 248
Takayasu's arteritis, 412
Tamm–Horsfall protein, 195
TARGET-CABG study, 309
Targeting Acute Congestion with Tolvaptan in Congestive Heart Failure Study (TACTICS), 179
Target lesion revascularization (TLR), 238, 332
Target vessel revascularization (TVR), 239
TAVR. *See* Transcatheter aortic valve replacement (TAVR)
TBI. *See* Toe Brachial index (TBI)
TBW. *See* Total body water (TBW)
TEG. *See* Thromboelastography (TEG)
TFPI. *See* Tissue factor pathway inhibitor (TFPI)
TFR. *See* Transferrin receptor (TFR)
Thoratec Paracorporeal Ventricular Assist Device, LVAD, 191
Thrombin, 5, 301, 303
Thrombin receptor antagonist (TRA), 303–304
Thrombin Receptor Antagonist for Clinical Event Reduction (TRA-CER) trial, 304
Thrombin time (TT), 288
Thromboelastography (TEG), for monitoring of antiplatelet therapy, 305
Thromboelastometry, 305
Thromboembolism, 247
Thrombosis, 121
Thrombosis in Myocardial Infarction (TIMI) trial, 111
Thrombotic microangiopathy (TMA), 5
Thromboxane A2 (TXA2), 3, 301, 302, 305
TIA. *See* Transient ischemic attacks (TIA)
Ticagrelor, 303, 330
Ticlopidine, 303
Tissue factor pathway inhibitor (TFPI), 3
Tissue inhibitor of metalloproteinase-1 (TIMP-1), 137
Tissue inhibitor of metalloproteinase-2 (TIMP-2), 150
Tissue injury, catalytic (labile) iron in, 109–110
TKV. *See* Total kidney volume (TKV)
TLR. *See* Target lesion revascularization (TLR)
TMA. *See* Thrombotic microangiopathy (TMA)
TNF-related weak inducer of apoptosis (TWEAK), 66
Tobacco use, 261

Tocilizumab, 412
Toe Brachial index (TBI), 337
Tolvaptan, 178–179
Total body water (TBW), 171, 174
Total kidney volume (TKV), 86
TR. *See* Tricuspid regurgitation (TR)
TRA. *See* Thrombin receptor antagonist (TRA)
Trans-Atlantic Inter Society consensus (TASC) group, 338, 340
  classification of aorto-iliac and femoral popliteal lesions, 339*t*
Transcatheter aortic valve replacement (TAVR), 17, 18*f*
Transferrin receptor (TFR), 109
Transferrin saturation (TSAT), 125
Transforming growth factor-β (TGF-β), 134, 137, 378, 387
Transient ischemic attacks (TIA), 340
Transplantation, kidney. *See* Kidney transplantation (KT)
Transplant renal artery stenosis (TRAS), 261
Transthoracic echocardiogram (TTE)
  for coronary artery disease (CAD), 221
TRAS. *See* Transplant renal artery stenosis (TRAS)
Trepostinil, 248
Trial to Assess Chelation Therapy (TACT), 115
Trial to Reduce Cardiovascular Events with Aranesp Therapy (TREAT), 122
Tricuspid regurgitation (TR), 243
TRIGGER-PCI study, 309
TRITON-TIMI 38 trial, 330
TSAT. *See* Transferrin saturation (TSAT)
TT. *See* Thrombin time (TT)
TTE. *See* Transthoracic echocardiogram (TTE)
Tumor necrosis factor-alpha (TNF-α), 61, 63, 64, 66, 67, 134, 139, 248, 398
25-Hydroxyvitamin D (calcidiol), 97, 101, 104, 105, 106
25-Hydroxyvitamin D-24 hydroxylase, 71
TXA2. *See* Thromboxane A2 (TXA2)
Type 1 cardiorenal syndrome (CRS-1), 131–133, 132*f*, 133*f*
Type 2 cardiorenal syndrome (CRS-2), 133–134
Type 3 cardiorenal syndrome (CRS-3)
  direct/indirect effects of AKI on cardiac function, 134–135
  electrophysiological effects, 135
  pathophysiology of, 134–135
Type 4 cardiorenal syndrome (CRS-4), 136–137*f*
  cardiac arrhythmias and sudden cardiac death, 136–137
  congestive heart failure and left ventricular hypertrophy, 135–136
  coronary atherosclerotic heart disease, 137
  pathophysiology of, 135
  uremia and cardiac fibrosis, 137–138
Type 5 cardiorenal syndrome (CRS-5), 138–140, 138*t*, 139*f*, 140*f*

U
UC. *See* Uremic cardiomyopathy (UC)
Ultrafiltration (UF) therapy
  for acute decompensated heart failure (ADHF), 180
  AVOID-HF trial, 166*t*, 168
  CARRESS-HF trial, 166*t*, 167
  clinical trials and diuretics, 165, 166*t*
  composition of removed fluid, 163
  CUORE trial, 166*t*, 167–168
  in decompensated heart failure, 163–169
  diuretic holiday, 163–164
  hypertrophy of distal nephron, avoidance of, 164
  hypovolemia, avoidance of, 169
  and loop diuretics, 163–165
  mechanical UF, 163
  outcomes for future clinical trials, 169
  overview of, 163, 164*f*
  patient management, 169
  patient selection, 168
  plasma refilling rate (PRR) during, 164, 164*f*
  RAPID-CHF trial, 165
  rehospitalization rates, reduction in, 165, 167*f*
  renal vein congestion, reduction of, 164
  risks of hypovolemia with, 164–165
  UNLOAD trial, 165–167, 166*t*
Ultrafiltration versus Intravenous Diuretics for Patients Hospitalized for Acute Decompensated Heart Failure (UNLOAD) trial, 165–167, 166*t*, 180
United Kingdom Heart and Renal Protection (UK-HARP) trial, 307
United network for organ sharing (UNOS), 199, 274
United States Department of Health and Human Services, 22
United States Renal Data System (USRDS), 22, 36, 80, 213, 235, 259, 271, 283, 321
Unstable angina, 378
UO. *See* Urine output (UO)
Uremia, 273
  and cardiac fibrosis, 137–138
Uremic cardiomyopathy (UC), 45
Uremic dyslipidemia, 369
Uremic toxins, 63
Urinary angiotensinogen, 148
Urine output (UO), 356
Urine sediment, 148–149

V
VADs. *See* Ventricular assist devices (VADs)
Valsartan Heart Failure Trial (Val-HeFT), 89
Valsartan in Acute Myocardial Infarction Trial (VALIANT) trial, 35
Valvular calcification
  clinical impact of, 17
  medical strategies to prevention of calcification, 16
  overview, 11–12
  pathogenesis of, 12
    alteration in inhibitory regulation, 15
    chronic inflammation, 15–16
    in chronic kidney disease (CKD), 12, 14*f*
    disturbance in mineral metabolism, 15
    increase in matrix metalloproteinases (MMP), 15
    mechanical stress, 16
  pathophysiology of, 14*f*
Valvular heart disease (VHD), 252*t*, 253–254
Valvular stenosis, 17
Vascular access complications, 333
Vascular adhesion molecule-1 (VCAM-1), 3, 5
Vascular calcification
  clinical impact of, 16
  medical strategies to prevention of calcification, 16
  overview, 11
  pathogenesis of, 12
    alteration in inhibitory regulation, 15
    chronic inflammation, 15–16
    in chronic kidney disease (CKD), 12, 14*f*
    disturbance in mineral metabolism, 15
    increase in matrix metalloproteinases (MMP), 15
    mechanical stress, 16
  pathophysiology of, 14*f*
Vascular cell adhesion molecule-1 (VACM-1), 64
Vascular closure devices, 333–334
Vascular endothelial growth factor (VEGF), 5, 64, 80, 382, 386, 387, 389
Vascular endothelial growth factor-A (VEGF-A), 7, 8*f*
Vascular smooth muscle cells (VSMCs), 12, 73, 103

Vascular thrombosis, 301–302
Vasoconstriction, 3
Vasodilation in the Management of Acute CHF (VMAC) trial, 180
Vasodilator-stimulated phosphoprotein (VASP), 303
VASP. *See* Vasodilator-stimulated phosphoprotein (VASP)
VDBP. *See* Vitamin D binding protein (VDBP)
VDR. *See* Vitamin D receptor (VDR)
VDRAs. *See* Vitamin D receptor activators (VDRAs)
VDREs. *See* Vitamin D response elements (VDREs)
VEGF. *See* Vascular endothelial growth factor (VEGF)
Venous hypertension, 362
Ventricular assist devices (VADs), 212
Vertebral artery disease
  clinical presentation, 340
  interventional management, 341
  non interventional management, 340
Very-low-density lipoprotein (VLDL), 63, 64, 369
Veterans Affairs High-Density Lipoprotein Intervention Trial (VA-HIT), 372–373
VHD. *See* Valvular heart disease (VHD)
VITAL trial, 104
Vitamin D_2, 97
Vitamin D_3, 97
Vitamin D, 48, 56
  and arterial calcification, 103
  in CKD and CAD, 97–107
  deficiency, in CKD, 101–102
  endocrine and autocrine/paracrine hormonal systems, 100*f*
  functions of, 99–101
  and hypertension, 103–104
  ongoing clinical trials, 107*t*
  overview, 97
  production and metabolism of, 97–98
  regulation of immunity by, 102–103
  replacement therapy, 105–106, 105*f*
  synthesis and regulation of, 98–99, 99*f*
  targeting proteinuria with, 102
  therapy
    in arrhythmia prevention, 105
    in cardiovascular disease (CVD), 103
    in heart failure (HF), 104–105
Vitamin D and Omega-3 (VITAL) trial, 102
Vitamin D binding protein (VDBP), 101, 102, 106
Vitamin D receptor (VDR), 98
Vitamin D receptor activators (VDRAs), 98, 105–106, 105*f*
Vitamin D response elements (VDREs), 98
Vitamin K antagonists (VKAs), 284
VKAs. *See* Vitamin K antagonists (VKAs)
VLDL. *See* Very-low-density lipoprotein (VLDL)
von Hippel Lindau protein (pVHL), 120
von Willebrand factor (vWF), 3, 7, 301, 305, 307
Vorapaxar, 304
VSMCs. *See* Vascular smooth muscle cells (VSMCs)
vWF. *See* von Willebrand factor (vWF)

W

Warfarin, 284, 288, 291, 295
"Warfarin-related nephropathy" (WRN), 295
Water homeostasis, 171
WHO. *See* World Health Organization (WHO)
Women's Health Initiative trial, 104
World Health Organization (WHO), 211, 248
Worsening heart failure (HF), 177
Worsening kidney function (WRF), 89
Worsening renal function (WRF), 167
WRF. *See* Worsening renal function (WRF)
WRN. *See* "Warfarin-related nephropathy" (WRN)

X

Xanthine oxidoreductase activity, 81